LOW BACK PAIN

Bernard E. Finneson, M.D., F.A.C.S.

Director, Crozer-Chester Medical Center Low Back Pain Clinic; Emeritus Chief of Neurological Surgery, Crozer-Chester Medical Center; Sacred Heart Hospital, Chester; Taylor Hospital, Ridley Park; Clinical Associate Professor of Surgery (Neurosurgery), Hahnemann Medical College, Philadelphia, Pennsylvania

15 contributors

illustrations by Barbara Finneson

LOW BACK PAIN

Second Edition

J. B. Lippincott Company Philadelphia · Toronto

Library of Congress Cataloging in Publication Data

Finneson, Bernard E
  Low back pain.

  Bibliography.
  Includes index.
  1. Backache. I. Title. [DNLM: 1. Backache.
WE755 F514L]
RD768.F56   1981   617'.56   80-15914
ISBN 0-397-50493-4

The authors and publisher have exerted every effort to ensure that drug selection and dosage set forth in this text are in accord with current recommendations and practice at the time of publication. However, in view of ongoing research, changes in government regulations, and the constant flow of information relating to drug therapy and drug reactions, the reader is urged to check the package insert for each drug for any change in indications and dosage and for added warnings and precautions. This is particularly important when the recommended agent is a new or infrequently employed drug.

To my wife, Barbara,
Medical Artist in Residence,
who elegantly illustrated this book
and whose talent is a source of great personal pride

Contents

Contributing Authors

Howard J. Barnhard, M.D., Professor of Radiology, University of Arkansas for Medical Sciences, Little Rock, Arkansas; Chapter 4, part 2, Roentgenographic Anatomy of the Lumbar Vertebrae

Ben Maurice Brown, M.D., Department of Radiology, Memorial Hospital Medical Center of Long Beach, Long Beach, California; Chapter 4, part 4, Computerized Body Tomography (CBT) and Evaluation of Lumbosacral Spinal Disease

Mark D. Brown, M.D., PH.D., Department of Orthopaedics and Rehabilitation, University of Miami School of Medicine, Miami, Florida; Chapter 11, Lumbar Spine Fusion

Charles V. Burton, M.D., Director, Low Back Clinic, Sister Kenny Institute, Minneapolis, Minnesota; Chapter 8, The Sister Kenny Institute Gravity Lumbar Reduction Therapy Program

Ralph B. Cloward, M.D., Senior Neurosurgeon, Queen's Medical Center; Clinical Associate Professor of Neurosurgery, John A. Burns School of Medicine, University of Hawaii, Honolulu, Hawaii; Visiting Professor (1978), Departments of Neurosurgery and Orthopedics, Rush Medical College, Chicago, Illinois; Chapter 12, The Cloward Technique

Robert H. Condon, M.D., Director, Department of Physical Medicine and Rehabilitation, Crozer-Chester Medical Center; Clinical Associate Professor of Rehabilitation Medicine, Thomas Jefferson University Hospital, Philadelphia, Pennsylvania; Chapter 6, part 2, Use of Modalities in the Treatment of Acute and Chronic Back Pain

Doyne Dodd, Jr., M.D., Associate Clinical Professor of Radiology, University of Arkansas for Medical Sciences, Little Rock, Arkansas; Chapter 4, part 2, Roentgenographic Anatomy of the Lumbar Vertebrae

William V. Glenn, Jr., Department of Radiology, Memorial Hospital Medical Center of Long Beach, Long Beach, California; Chapter 4, part 4, Computerized Body Tomography (CBT) and Evaluation of Lumbosacral Spinal Disease

Lawrence Green, M.D., Clinical Associate Professor of Neurology, Hahnemann Medical College, Philadelphia; Chief, Division of Neurology and Neurodiagnostic Laboratory, Crozer-Chester Medical Center, Chester, Pennsylvania; Chapter 3, part 2, Electrodiagnostic Studies in Low Back Pain

Scott Haldeman, D.C., PH.D., M.D., Department of Neurology, University of California, Irvine, California; Chapter 7, Spinal Manipulation Therapy

Jerold E. Lancourt, M.D., Department of Radiology, Memorial Hospital Medical Center of Long Beach, Long Beach, California; Chapter 4, part 4, Computerized Body Tomography (CBT) and Evaluation of Lumbosacral Spinal Disease

James M. Morris, M.D., Department of Orthopaedic Surgery, School of Medicine, University of California, San Francisco, California; Chapter 2, Biomechanics of the Lumbar Spine

Michael L. Rhodes, PH.D., Department of Radiology, Memorial Hospital Medical Center of Long Beach, Long Beach, California; Chapter 4, part 4, Computerized Body Tomography (CBT) and Evaluation of Lumbosacral Spinal Disease

Lawrence Wallach, M.D., Clinical Assistant Professor of Medicine, Hahnemann Medical College, Philadelphia; Staff Physician, Division of Endocrinology, Crozer-Chester Medical Center, Chester, Pennsylvania; Chapter 16, Vertebral Osteoporosis

Leon L. Wiltse, M.D., Department of Orthopaedic Surgery, Memorial Hospital Medical Center of Long Beach, Long Beach, California; Clinical Professor of Orthopaedic Surgery, University of California, Irvine, California; Chapter 15, Spondylolisthesis and Its Treatment

Preface

This book is an effort to provide a practical and useful guide for evaluation and management of the various forms of low back dysfunction commonly encountered in practice. Although back pain has probably existed from the time the progenitors of man first assumed the erect stance, it is startling to appreciate how meager and rudimentary is our knowledge of the subject.

Low back dysfunction has been my principal medical interest for almost 30 years, appropriating a progressively increasing apportionment of my time. For the past 8 years, I have been involved in this work exclusively. When I first was exposed to the problem of low back pain, it appeared to be a rather simple mechanical derangement. Now, after having concentrated my interest and time in this field of inquiry, I find that indisputable factual knowledge of the subject appears much less certain than when I was a neophyte. In most instances, I suppose a consciousness of fallibility is less damaging than an ill-founded dogmatism in arriving at a clinical decision.

In the decade that has elapsed since I wrote the first edition, a number of diagnostic and therapeutic advances have either been newly introduced or been made generally available. These include water-soluble myelographic media, lumbar venography, computerized tomography, radioisotope scanning, surgery performed with the aid of magnification and improved lighting, and powered instrumentation. But equal in importance to these technical advances is a critical assessment of the long-term natural history of low back dysfunction and the long-term results of various forms of treatment, including surgery.

A number of sections are written by contributing authors who are experts in their fields. I thank them for their work, cooperation, and patience.

Most of the techniques described are widely accepted, and no claim is made for an original method of treatment. However, a number of unique biases that are based on the trials and errors of personal experience have been insinuated into the text. Foremost is my persuasion that the largest group of treatment failures results either from improper evaluation or from an inadequate trial of conservative management.

BERNARD E. FINNESON, M.D.

Acknowledgments

There are many persons for whose help and encouragement in my writing of this book I am deeply grateful.

Doctor James Loucks, President and Medical Administrator of the Crozer-Chester Medical Center, is responsible for an exciting decade of innovation and growth in the formation of a truly unique and outstanding medical facility. I thank him for his encouragement and support in the development of the Low Back Pain Clinic.

Sister Mary Margaret, administrator of the Sacred Heart Hospital, Chester, Pennsylvania, has supported me in my endeavors and I am grateful.

I am privileged to be associated with Thelma Stauffer, R.N., M.S.N., an outstanding nurse leader and teacher. I am happy to record here my debt for her many helpful suggestions and for sharing with me her considerable insight and understanding of the chronic pain patient.

The illustrations were done by my wife, Barbara, a dedicated and skillful professional medical illustrator. I believe they are so fine that any comment by me would be superfluous. To visualize the surgery properly, Barbara would scrub, be gloved and gowned, and become part of the surgical team. Most of my surgery starts at 7:30 a.m., and her willingness to arise at the time necessary to take part in the procedure was truly a labor of love.

Thanks are due to Doctor Sol Balis, a friend of 31 years, and chief of the Crozer-Chester Medical Center's Anesthesia Department, for his help in reviewing the chapter on Analgesic Blocks.

I am happy to record here my debt to Doctor Rudolph Hecksher, an outstanding physician and dear friend who has been a source of constant encouragement in this project.

My colleagues, Doctor Leonard Hirsh, Chief of Neurosurgery at Crozer-Chester Medical Center, and Doctor V. Shankar, Chief of Neurosurgery at Sacred Heart Hospital, have been most generous in their advice and support.

My fellow members of the International Society for the Study of the Lumbar Spine provided an unequaled source of information and expertise by responding tirelessly to my many questions.

I wish to express my appreciation to Mrs. Eileen Burns, Ms. Janet Iovannacci, Mrs. Esther Cylc, and Mrs. Judy Deaver for cheerfully performing the typing and secretarial tasks.

This book could not have been written without the extensive help provided by the following members of the staff of the J. B. Lippincott Company. Rachel Bedard expertly edited the text with patience and diligence beyond compare. To Lisa Biello, my deepest thanks for her outstanding efforts in my behalf. I thank Stuart Freeman for his unflagging support.

LOW BACK PAIN

Anatomy of the Low Back 1

Development of the Low Back

Embryology

A week after fertilization the embryo comes into direct contact with the uterine mucosa and adheres to it (Figs. 1-1 and 1-2). By digesting the uterine tissue it embeds itself in the endometrium.[3]

After the second week the embryo has become completely buried and the endometrial defect has been closed over by the uterine epithelium.

Demarcation of the embryo begins with formation of the flat oval embryonic disc from the thickened layers of the germ disc. The embryonic disc is composed of ectoderm on the dorsal or amniotic cavity side and of entoderm on the ventral or yolk sac side (Fig. 1-3).

The primitive groove occupies the midline in the caudal portion of the embryonic disc. The primitive node, or Hensen's node, is a clump of cells located at the cephalic end of the primitive groove (Fig. 1-4). The center of the primitive node invaginates to form the primitive pit, from which cells migrate between the ectoderm and entoderm. These cells form a special column of cells in the midline which becomes the notochord. A third embryonic layer, the mesoderm, is formed by cells migrating from the primitive groove between the ectoderm and entoderm.

By the third week the column of mesoderm, which lies along both sides of the notochord, becomes organized into regularly arranged somites or primitive segments, which are the precursors of body segmentation for the skeletal, muscular, and nervous systems (Fig. 1-5). At this time, vertebral column formation begins with the initial mesenchymal or membranous anlage of the vertebrae which is eventually followed by chondrification (the cartilaginous phase), and finally by ossification.

The midline cells of the ectoderm (neural plate) sink inward, become grooved, and form the neural tube, the cranial portion of which differentiates several days later to form the brain. The cephalic flexure develops as the neural folds close rostrally at the anterior neuropore and posteriorly at the posterior neuropore. The posterior neuropore, which closes at approximately 26 or 27 days, is at the level of 1 or 2. By 7 weeks, changes in the primitive tail fold lead to the precursors of the coccygeal medullary vestige and the filum terminale.

The primitive segments are separated by direct arterial branches of the aorta (intersegmental arteries), and each vertebral segment or protovertebra consists of a condensed or dark caudal half and a lighter cephalic half (Figs. 1-6 through 1-9).

The cells nearer the intersegmental arteries receive more nutrition than those farther removed and are more rapid in their differ-

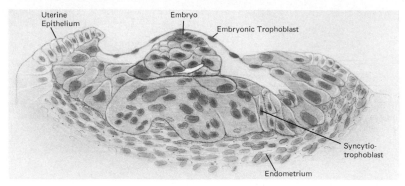

Fig. 1-1. A 1-week-old embryo in process of embedding into the uterine mucosa.

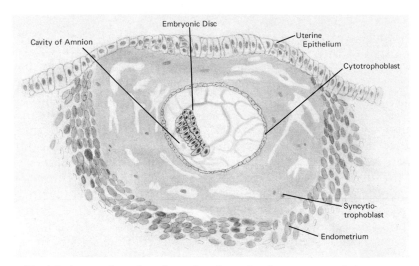

Fig. 1-2. A second-week embryo closed over by the uterine epithelium.

entiation to fuse and form the precursors of the vertebral bodies.

The cranial portion of the condensed caudal mass, being the farthest removed from the nutrition provided by the artery, remains undifferentiated as the precursor of the intervertebral disc. It is significant that the embryologically avascular development of the intervertebral disc is carried through into adult life, with the limited nutritional demands of this tissue fulfilled by diffusion of lymph.

With the rapid addition of cytoplasm to the cells of the vertebral region and fusion of the cephalic and caudal masses to form the vertebral body, the cells of the notochord in this region are obliterated. Some embryologists theorize that there is an actual pressure gradient, with the notochordal cells being extruded or "squeezed" into the intervertebral region where the pressure is less. In any event, the notochordal cells become obliterated within the vertebral body and migrate to the intervertebral region (Fig. 1-10).

After 10 weeks, the cells around the periphery of the intervertebral region begin to differentiate into an elongated fibroblastic type and are arranged along a vertical axis attaching above and below to the vertebral bodies. These cells are formed from the cranial portion of the dark caudal masses and they develop into the annulus fibrosis (Figs. 1-11 and 1-12). Thus, the adult intervertebral disc has a double origin. The central nucleus pulposus is derived from the

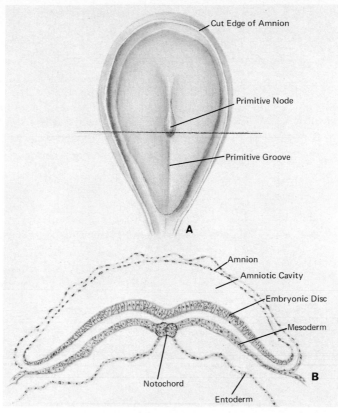

Fig. 1-3. Two views of a 16-day-old presomite human embryo. **(A)** *Embryonic disc with amnion excised.* **(B)** *Cross section of embryo.*

notochord, and the annulus is derived from the fibroblastic extensions of the vertebral bodies.

Ossification of the vertebrae involves both primary and secondary ossification centers. The primary center in the vertebral body encircles the vestigeal mucoid streak. By the 8th week, primary ossification centers form on each side of the vertebral arches. The secondary ossification centers at the tips of the transverse and spinous processes are not seen until the 15th or 16th years and do not fuse until the mid 30s.

Degenerative Effects of Living

The intervertebral disc undergoes progressive changes throughout life, so that its normal biologic state is specifically age-related.[1]

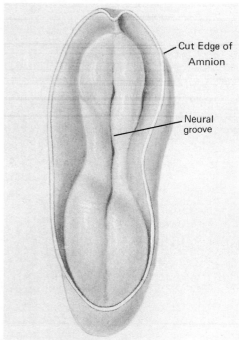

Fig. 1-4. Eighteen-day-old embryo.

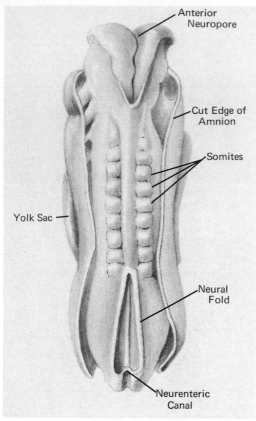
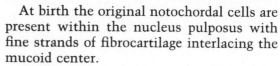

Fig. 1-5. *The somites, or primitive segments, are seen clearly by 3 weeks.*

At birth the original notochordal cells are present within the nucleus pulposus with fine strands of fibrocartilage interlacing the mucoid center.

By the age of 4 years, notochordal cells may be present but are increasingly difficult to find. The fibrous element and cartilage cells are increasingly prominent.

By the age of 12 years, the notochordal cells have been completely replaced by loose fibrocartilage with abundant gelatinous matrix. With the passage of time, the fibrocartilage continues to replace the gelatinous mucoid material of the nucleus pulposus. This process is associated with progressive decrease in resiliency until old age, when the intervertebral disc is composed almost entirely of dense, irregularly arranged fibrocartilage. The water content of the nucleus pulposus decreases progressively with age.[4]

Spinal Curves

The vertebral column is formed by a series of 33 vertebrae: 7 cervical (C1 to C7), 12 thoracic (T1 to T12), 5 lumbar (L1 to L5), 5 sacral (S1 to S5), and 4 coccygeal. The cervical, thoracic, and lumbar vertebrae remain distinct and separate from each other throughout life and may be considered "true" vertebrae. The adult sacral and coc-

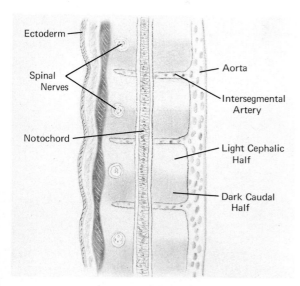

Fig. 1-6. *Diagrammatic representation of the primitive segments and surrounding structures.*

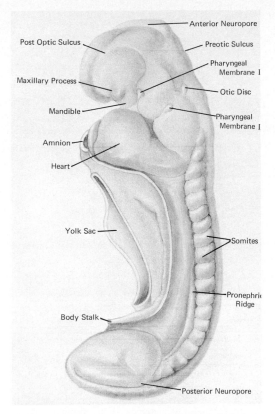

Fig. 1-7. At 3 or 4 weeks, the surface landmarks become recognizable.

Labels: Anterior Neuropore, Post Optic Sulcus, Preotic Sulcus, Maxillary Process, Pharyngeal Membrane I, Otic Disc, Mandible, Pharyngeal Membrane I, Amnion, Heart, Yolk Sac, Somites, Pronephric Ridge, Body Stalk, Posterior Neuropore

cygeal vertebrae are fused or united with each other to form two bones, the sacrum and the coccyx, and can be considered pseudovertebrae. The bodies of the true or movable vertebrae are separated from each other by intervertebral discs, with the exception of C1 and C2.

A lateral view of the vertebral column reveals several curves which are identified by the predominant region in which the curve occurs (Fig. 1-13).

The cervical curve, the least marked of all the curves, is convex anteriorly and extends from C1 to T2.

The thoracic curve extends from T2 to T12 and is concave anteriorly.

The lumbar curve extends from T12 to the lumbosacral articulation and is convex anteriorly.

The pelvic curve begins at the lumbosacral joint and ends at the termination of the coccyx. It is concave anteriorly and is inclined in a somewhat downward direction.

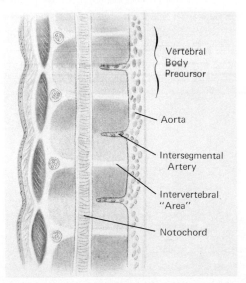

Labels: Vertebral Body Precursor, Aorta, Intersegmental Artery, Intervertebral "Area", Notochord

Fig. 1-8. The cell mass closest to the nutrition afforded by the intersegmental arteries is the precursor of the vertebral bodies.

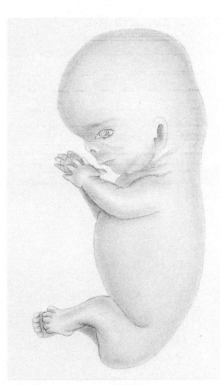

Fig. 1-9. By 8 or 9 weeks, the human embryo is externally well developed.

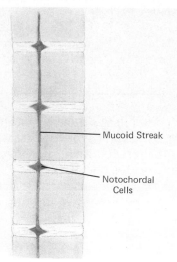

Fig. 1-10. A mucoid streak running through the vertebral body marks the site of the obliterated notochord.

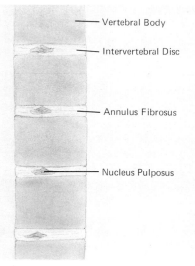

Fig. 1-11. The development of the annulus and the nucleus pulposus.

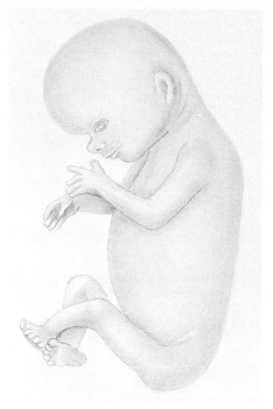

Fig. 1-12. A 12-week fetus.

The early fetal spine, which is completely concave anteriorly, embodies both the thoracic and pelvic curves. These primary curves are shaped by the configuration of the vertebral bodies which are wider posteriorly. The secondary cervical and lumbar curves are formed by the intervertebral discs, which are wider anteriorly.

The thoracic and pelvic curves are termed **primary curves** because they are present during fetal life (Fig. 1-14).

The cervical curve becomes well established at the age of 4 months when the infant is able to hold up its head, the lumbar curve at 12 months when the infant begins to walk. The cervical and lumbar curves are termed **compensatory** or **secondary curves.**

Lumbar Vertebrae

The lumbar vertebrae are heavier and more massive than the other vertebrae, consistent with their primary role of weight bearing. The somewhat kidney-shaped bodies are wider in the transverse than in the antero-posterior diameter. (Fig. 1-15). The five lumbar vertebrae, because of their relatively

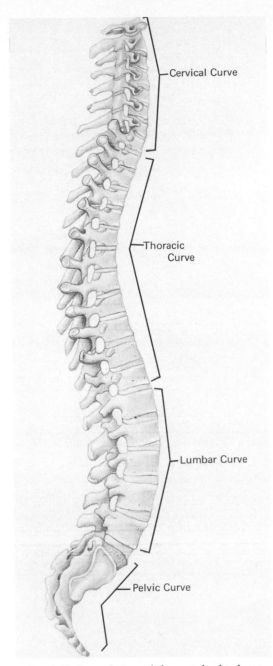

Fig. 1-13. Lateral view of the vertebral column.

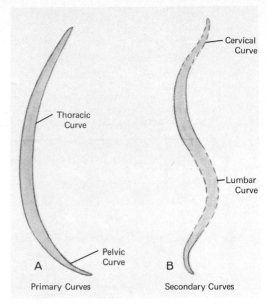

Fig. 1-14. (A) The early fetal supine, which is completely concave anteriorly, embodies both the thoracic and pelvic curves. (B) The secondary cervical and lumbar curves are superimposed.

Vertebral Foramina and the "Lateral Bony Recess"

Changes in configuration of the lumbar vertebral foramina are of considerable clinical and surgical significance. The lumbar vertebral foramina are basically small and triangular in shape, but of prime importance is the progressive pinching of the lateral angles in the L4 and L5 vertebrae.

Prior to exiting from the intervertebral foramina, the nerve root lies snugly within this lateral bony recess (Fig. 1-17).

The L5 and S1 nerve roots lying within this lateral recess are more vulnerable to compression from a protruding intervertebral disc than the higher lumbar roots lying within a rounder vertebral foramen (Fig. 1-18).[2,6]

The minute anatomy of the vertebral foramina exhibits considerable variation, and it is not surprising to find a well-developed lateral bony recess as high as L3 and occasionally even L2.

large size, assume more than their proportionate share of space in the vertebrae spine, representing about 25% of the spine's total length (Fig. 1-16).

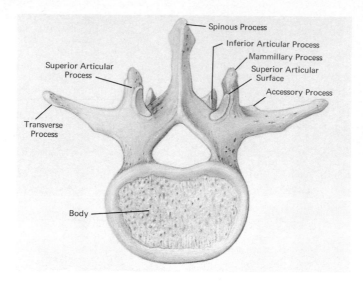

Fig. 1-15. Cephalad view of the fourth lumbar vertebra (L4).

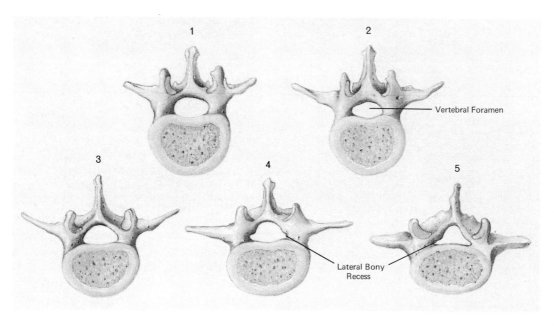

Fig. 1-16. The five lumbar vertebrae. Note the lateral bony recess formed by the last two vertebrae.

Sacrum and Coccyx

The sacrum is a large triangular bone inserted like a wedge between the two hip bones (Fig. 1-19).

The base of the sacrum articulates with L5, producing the rather acute lumbosacral angle formed by the increased anterior width of both the L5 body and the L5–S1 intervertebral disc (Fig. 1-20).

The sacral canal (vertebral canal) encloses the sacral nerves, which pass out of the

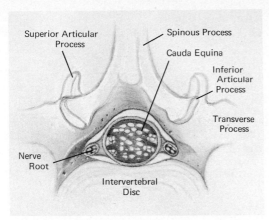

Fig. 1-17. Prior to exiting from the intervertebral foramina, the nerve root lies at the lateral-most portion of the vertebral foramen.

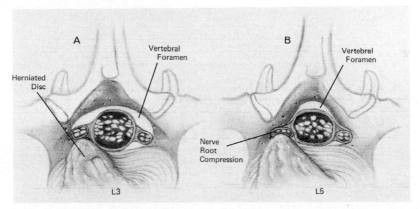

*Fig. 1-18. **(A)** A relatively small intervertebral disc protrusion may not produce significant nerve root compression when the vertebral foramen is oval and may permit elevation of the root. **(B)** When the nerve root lies within a lateral bony recess, even a small disc protrusion may produce severe root compression.*

sacrum through the anterior and posterior sacral foramina.

The coccyx is usually a solid bone formed by the fusion of four rudimentary vertebrae. Occasionally the first coccygeal vertebra exists as a separate segment. The coccygeal cornua project upward and articulate with the sacral cornua to form a foramen through which the first coccygeal nerve passes. No vertebral canal exists within the coccyx itself (Fig. 1-21).

Articulations and Ligaments of the Lumbar Spine

The articulations of the vertebral column consist of two types of joints, the joints between the vertebral bodies (amphiarthrodial) and the joints between the vertebral arches (arthrodial) (Fig. 1-22).

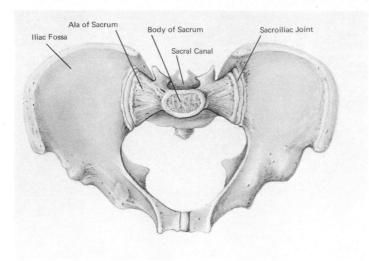

Fig. 1-19. The pelvis viewed from above.

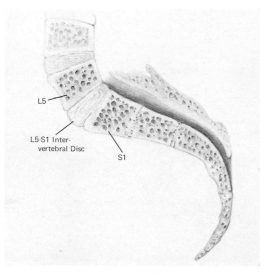

Fig. 1-20. Lumbosacral articulation.

Vertebral Body Articulation

The joint between the vertebral bodies is called an amphiarthrodial joint, a joint in which the contiguous bony surfaces are connected either by discs of fibrocartilage or by an interosseous ligament. This type of joint, of course, permits only very limited movements, but when this slight degree of movement takes place in all of the lumbar ver-

tebrae, the total range of movement is considerable.

There are four ligaments involved in the amphiarthrodial vertebral body articulation:

1. Intervertebral discs
2. Anterior longitudinal ligament
3. Posterior longitudinal ligament
4. Lateral vertebral ligaments

Intervertebral discs contribute approximately one third of the overall length of the lumbar spine, while in the remainder of the vertebral column they contribute just a bit more than one fifth of the overall length (Fig. 1-23).

This striking difference in bone-disc ratio in conjunction with the primary weight-bearing role of the lumbar spine accounts for the unique characteristics of lumbar disc disease (Fig. 1-24). Most lumbar disc lesions are "soft tissue" in nature, resulting from protrusion of the bulky lumbar intervertebral disc and causing nerve root pressure. This is in contrast to cervical nerve root compression syndromes, which are either exclusively bony lesions resulting from hypertrophic osteoarthritic ridging or a combination of bony spurs in association with some soft disc protrusion.

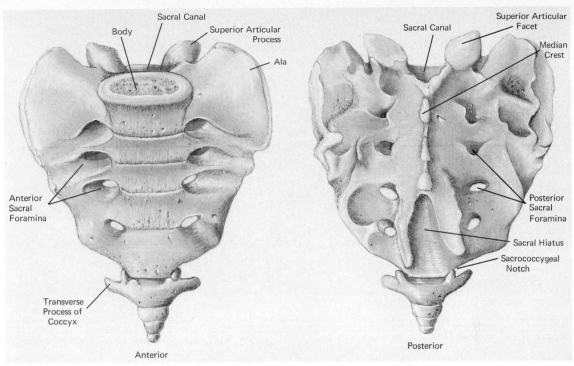

Fig. 1-21. Anterior and posterior views of the sacrum and coccyx.

Structure. The vertebral surface adjacent to the lumbar disc is composed of a thin layer of cortical bone, which is most compact centrally and somewhat more porous at the periphery. A cartilaginous plate composed of hyaline cartilage overlies the cortical bone. This hyaline cartilage ends abruptly in the anterior and lateral regions, when it abuts on the outer raised bony rim of the vertebral body called the **epiphyseal ring.** Posteriorly the cartilaginous plate extends to the margin of the vertebral body. Blended intimately with the cartilaginous plate is a layer of fibrocartilage which gives attachment to the fibers of the annulus fibrosus and nucleus pulposus (Figs. 1-25 and 1-26). The annulus fibrosus forms a dense fibrocartilaginous retaining envelope for the fibrogelatinous nucleus pulposus. It is composed of approximately 12 concentric lamellae with the fibers of one layer running at an angle to those of the preceding layer.

The peripheral fibers of the annulus at the anterior and lateral margins of the vertebral

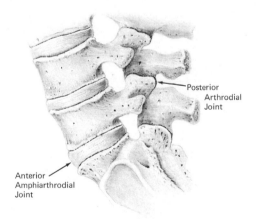

Fig. 1-22. Amphiarthrodial and arthrodial joints.

body become very firmly attached to the outer raised bony rim of the vertebral body (epiphyseal ring).

The anterior fibers of the annulus merge completely to form an intertexture with the anterior longitudinal ligament, creating a powerful and virtually inseparable coupling within the lumbar spine (Fig. 1-27).

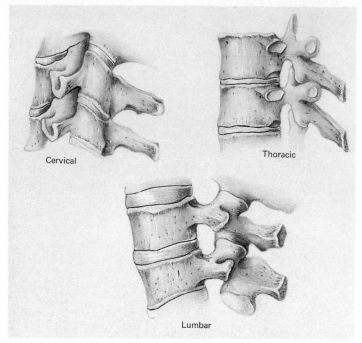

Cervical

Thoracic

Lumbar

Fig. 1-23. Note the striking difference in the bone-to-disc ratio in the cervical, thoracic, and lumbar spines.

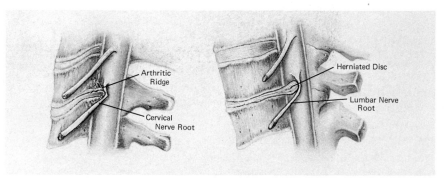

Arthritic Ridge

Cervical Nerve Root

Herniated Disc

Lumbar Nerve Root

Fig. 1-24. The difference in the bone-to-disc ratio between the cervical and the lumbar spines accounts for the different types of root compression lesions found in these two different areas. Most lumbar disc lesions are "soft tissue" in nature, in contrast to the primarily bony lesions seen in the cervical spine.

The posterior juncture is less secure. The annulus fibers are not as dense and firm posteriorly, and the posterior longitudinal ligament is much thinner and less powerful than its anterior counterpart (Fig. 1-28).

The centrally situated nucleus pulposus is composed of a loose network of fibrous tissue within a mucoprotein gel. In its normal state it has a gelatinous consistency and is semitransparent. The degenerated nucleus is denser, more fibrous, and completely opaque.

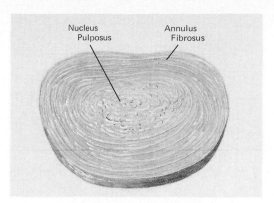

Fig. 1-25. Sectioned lumbar intervetebral disc.

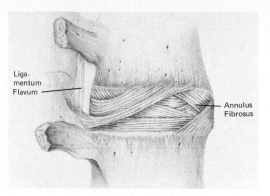

Fig. 1-26. The successive layers of the annulus fibrosus run in alternating oblique directions.

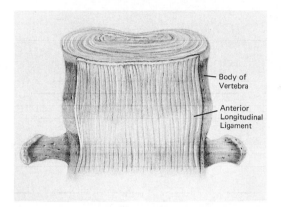

Fig. 1-27. The anterior fibers of the annulus fibrosus, completely merged with the anterior longitudinal ligament fibers.

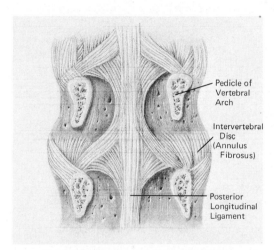

Fig. 1-28. The fibers of the posterior longitudinal ligament are not as broad as the anterior longitudinal ligament. They merge with the annulus fibrosus only in the posteromedial portion of the disc. This leaves the posterolateral portion relatively unsupported.

Anterior longitudinal ligament is a broad, strong band of fibers, extending along the anterior surfaces of the vertebral bodies, from the body of the axis to the upper portion of the anterior sacrum (Fig. 1-29).

It consists of three layers of dense fibers all running in a longitudinal direction. The most superficial fibers are the longest, extending over four or five vertebrae. The middle layer extends between two or three vertebrae. The innermost layer extends from one vertebra to the next, adhering intimately to the intervertebral discs and the outer raised bony rim of the vertebral body (epiphyseal ring) but not to the midportion of the vertebral bodies. The fibers increase in thickness as they pass over the concave anterior surface of the vertebral bodies and fill in the concavities.

Posterior longitudinal ligament lies within the vertebral canal, extending along the posterior surfaces of the vertebral bodies from the axis to the sacrum. This ligament consists of two layers, the superficial layer extending over three or four vertebrae, and a deep layer extending between adjacent vertebrae. The ligament is narrow and thick over the centers of the vertebral bodies where it is only loosely adherent, but at each intervertebral disc it forms a thin lateral extension which is densely adherent to the annulus fibrosis of the intervertebral disc

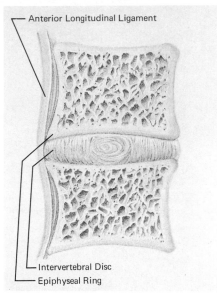

Anterior Longitudinal Ligament

Intervertebral Disc
Epiphyseal Ring

Fig. 1-29. The fibers of the anterior longitudinal ligament increase in thickness as they pass over the concave anterior surface of the vertebral bodies and fill in the concavities.

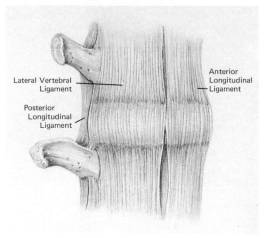

Lateral Vertebral Ligament

Posterior Longitudinal Ligament

Anterior Longitudinal Ligament

Fig. 1-30. The lateral vertebral ligaments consist of short fibers.

and the raised bony rim of the vertebral body.

Lateral vertebral ligaments are situated between the anterior and posterior longitudinal ligaments. They consist of short fibers which adhere firmly to the intervertebral discs and pass over the vertebral body to the adjacent intervertebral disc (Fig. 1-30).

Vertebral Arch Articulation

The joint between the vertebral arches is called an arthrodial joint and permits only a gliding movement.

The articular facets which arise from the vertebral arches form the joint (Fig. 1-31). The superior facet is slightly concave and the inferior facet slightly convex. The lumbar facets lie generally in a sagittal plane, but the lumbosacral facets incline toward the coronal plane.

The gliding nature of the arthrodial joint permits flexion and extension of the lumbar spine. It is widely held that because of the shape and plane of these facets, rotation is not possible. However, the facets are only

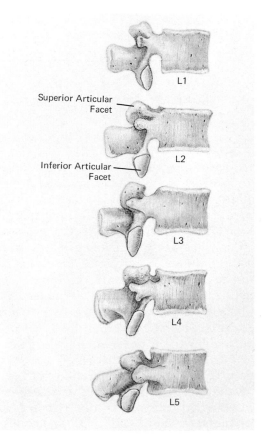

Superior Articular Facet

Inferior Articular Facet

L1

L2

L3

L4

L5

Fig. 1-31. The lumbar superior and inferior articular facets of the lumbar arthrodial joints.

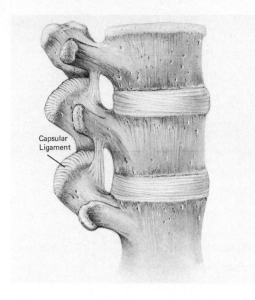

Fig. 1-32. The lumbar articular facets. The capsular ligaments are rather thin and loose, permitting joint mobility.

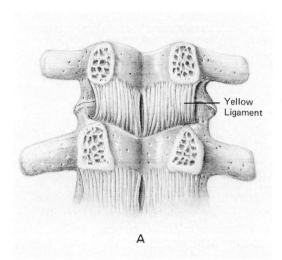

A

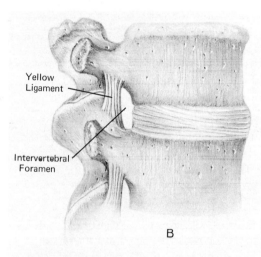

B

Fig. 1-33. (A) The yellow ligaments attach to the anterior surface of the lamina above and extend to the posterior surface and upper margin of the lamina below, producing a "shingle-like" configuration. (B) They form a portion of the foraminal roof.

loosely bound to each other, so that opposing articular facets are not necessarily in close approximation. This limited play allows for slight rotation of the lumbar spine. These joints are enveloped by capsules lined with synovial membranes (Fig. 1-32).

The following ligaments are involved in the vertebral arch articulation:

1. Capsular
2. Yellow
3. Supraspinal
4. Interspinal
5. Intertransverse

Capsular ligaments are composed partly of yellow elastic tissue and partly of white fibrous tissue. They encapsulate the synovial joints between the superior and inferior articular processes of adjacent vertebrae. They are rather thin and loose to permit joint mobility.

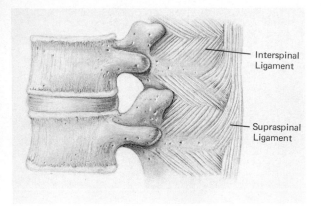

Fig. 1-34. Supraspinal and interspinal ligaments.

Yellow ligaments connecting the laminae of adjacent vertebrae are composed of yellow elastic tissue (Fig. 1-33). The thick, strong fibers are attached to the anterior surface of the lamina above and to the posterior surface and upper margin of the lamina below. They extend laterally to the medial and posterior edge of the intervertebral foramen, forming a portion of the foraminal roof.

Supraspinal ligament is a strong fibrous cord which extends without interruption along the tips of the spinous processes from C7 to the median sacral crest (Fig. 1-34). Between the spinous processes it is continuous with the interspinal ligaments.

Interspinal ligaments are fibers which cross as they pass from the root of one spine to the tip of the next. Although they are thin

and membranous in the cervical and thoracic spine, they are thick and well developed in the lumbar region.

Intertransverse ligaments are flat, membranous bands passing between the apices of the transverse processes (Fig. 1-35). They are relatively weak and unimportant as bonds of union.

Pelvic Articulations and Ligaments

Pelvic-vertebral Articulation

Articulation of the pelvis with the vertebral column occurs at the interspace between L5 and the sacrum (Figs. 1-36 and 1-37). It is similar in almost all respects to those articulations which connect the vertebrae with each other. In addition, the iliolumbar ligament connects the pelvis with the vertebral column on either side.

Sacroiliac Articulation

The sacroiliac articulation is an amphiarthrodial or slightly movable joint. The articular surfaces of the sacrum and ilium are covered with cartilaginous plates in close contact with each other and bound together by fibrous strands. The ligaments of the sacroiliac articulation are the anterior sacroiliac, posterior sacroiliac, and interosseous.

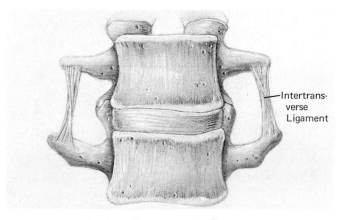

Fig. 1-35. Intertransverse ligament.

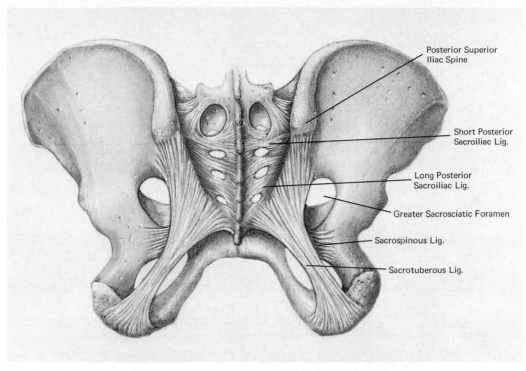

Fig. 1-36. Pelvic joints and ligaments, anterior aspect.

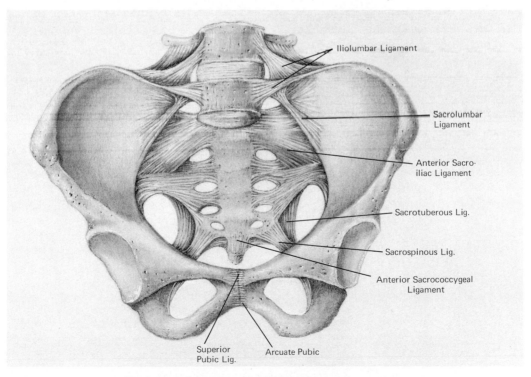

Fig. 1-37. Pelvic joints and ligaments, posterior aspect.

Sacrococcygeal Articulation

The sacrococcygeal articulation is a joint similar to the articulations between vertebral bodies. The ligaments of this symphysis are anterior sacrococcygeal, posterior sacrococcygeal, lateral sacrococcygeal, and interarticular.

Symphysis Pubis

The pubic symphysis is an amphiarthrodial joint formed between the two oval symphyseal surfaces of the pubic bones. The ligaments of this articulation are superior pubic, arcuate pubic, and interpubic fibrocartilaginous lamina.

Blood Supply of the Lumbar Spine

The four lumbar arteries arise in pairs from the posterior aspect of the aorta in front of the bodies of the first four lumbar vertebrae. In front of L5, a fifth pair of arteries may arise from the middle sacral artery. These appear in approximately 50%

of all dissections. This fifth lumbar artery is always smaller than the first four arteries and is frequently unpaired and more often seen on the left side. The right arteries are longer than the left to compensate for the left paramedian position of the aorta. These arteries curve posteriorly around the bodies of the vertebrae to the interspaces between the transverse processes, where a posterior ramus is given off. The posterior ramus, in turn, furnishes the vertebral (spinal) branch which supplies the bodies of the vertebrae and their ligaments.

The spinal rami accompany the spinal nerves through the intervertebral foramina, traverse the dura mater and arachnoid, and divide into radicular branches which supply each nerve root (Fig. 1-38).

Blood Supply of the Intervertebral Disc

The developmental precursor of the disc is that condensed mass most removed from the nutrition provided by the artery. In children and young adults, one can find small vessels within the periphery of the cartilaginous end-plates. These vessels gradually become obliterated so that by the age of 20

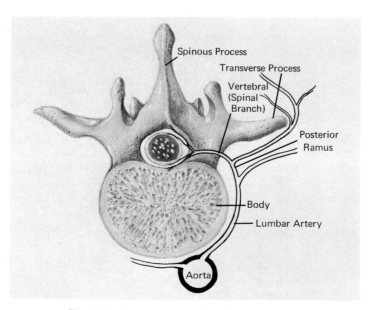

Fig. 1-38. The spinal branch of the lumbar artery.

or 30, the intervertebral disc is found to be completely avascular, in common with most cartilaginous or fibrous tissues subjected to weight-bearing.

The disc's limited nutritional demands are probably fulfilled by the diffusion of lymph through minute perforations from the marrow cavity to the cartilaginous end-plates, which permits a scanty lymph supply to diffuse through the intervertebral disc.

Nerve Supply of the Lumbar Spine

In 1949, as a neurology resident, I assisted in my first neurosurgical procedure, a hemilaminectomy for excision of a herniated lumbar disc. The operation remains keen in my memory. It was performed with the patient under local anesthesia, since, in addition to excising the offending lesion, the surgeon hoped to demonstrate the structures of the lumbar spine which were pain producing. This was to be accomplished by subjecting the various structures and tissues to noxious stimuli prior to anesthetizing them with procaine. He used a hemostat to pinch structures, such as the yellow ligament or the annulus fibrosis, and also exerted pressure upon these tissues.

Other methods for stimulating structures of the lumbar spine can be used, such as injections of minute amounts of hypertonic saline into the various tissues, and a variety of electrical stimuli. These varied noxious stimuli techniques furnish results that are far from conclusive. There are inherent difficulties in working with a partially sedated, intimidated, apprehensive patient undergoing an uncomfortable experience. The patient often is not especially receptive to the imposed demands of clinical research. Of equal importance is the artificial nature of the stimuli, which cannot exactly duplicate the physiological conditions producing pain.

So often it is chronic and persisting pain that tends to erode the physical and emotional defenses of the patient who turns to the physician for help. Because of the many variations in the appreciation of and the reaction to this subjective symptom, many questions remain unanswered.

A number of careful anatomic-histologic studies have been carried out in attempting to trace the nerve supply of the lumbar spine subserving low back pain.[5] It has been demonstrated that nerve strands originate beyond the dorsal root ganglia of the posterior primary division of the root and pass back through the intervertebral foramen, reentering the vertebral canal. This recurrent si-

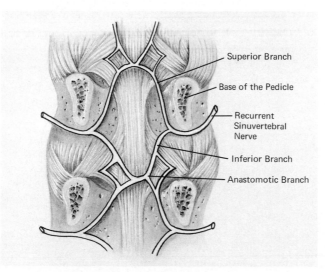

Fig. 1-39. Branches of the recurrent sinuvertebral nerve.

nuvertebral nerve curves around the base of the pedicle and gives off branches which extend to the intervertebral discs above and below (Fig. 1-39). Filaments of this nerve supply the posterior longitudinal ligament, periosteum, epidural blood vessels, and dura mater. The posterior rami of the posterior primary divisions of the spinal nerve roots supply sensory fibers to the skin, muscle, fascia, ligaments, and posterior arthrodial joints.

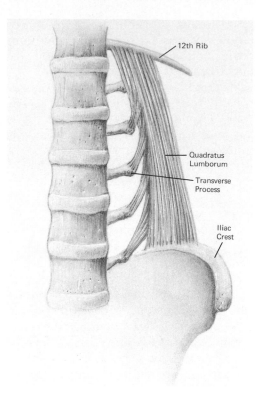

Fig. 1-40. *Quadratus lumborum.*

Low Back Musculature

Determining the exact function of each of the various muscles involved in the low back is difficult. Anatomic studies, the construction of mechanical models, and electrical stimulation of individual muscles are all valuable in investigating this problem. However, the interrelationship of these associated muscles so increases the complexities that we can only approximate the primary function of the individual low back muscles.

Extensors of the Lumbar Spine

Quadratus lumborum derives its name from its irregularly quadrilateral shape, broader at the base than above (Fig. 1-40). It arises from the iliac crest and iliolumbar ligament and inserts into the lower border of the last rib and the transverse process of the first four lumbar vertebrae.

Sacrospinalis muscle, also called the erector spinae, is a long, strong band of muscle running from the sacrum to the occipital portion of the skull and serving as a very powerful extensor of the spine (Fig. 1-41).

It originates from a broad and strong aponeurosis which is attached to the sacrum, iliac crest, the spinous processes of all the lumbar vertebrae, and the last two thoracic vertebrae. The muscle fibers divided in the upper lumbar region into three separate columns. The most lateral slip, the iliocostalis,

is inserted into the angles of the ribs. The intermediate slip, the longissimus, is inserted into the tips of the transverse processes of all the thoracic and cervical vertebrae. The medial slip, the spinalis, is inserted into the spinous processes of the thoracic and cervical vertebrae.

Multifidus muscles extend from the sacrum to the cervical vertebrae but are best developed in the lumbar spine (Fig. 1-42). They consist of numerous small muscular slips or fasciculi which arise from the mammillary process, a small bony prominence on the dorsal margin of each superior articular process; they ascend obliquely toward the midline; and they insert into the spinous process of a vertebrae two to four segments above.

Although categorized as extensors of the lumbar spine, these muscles, acting unilaterally, will abduct and slightly rotate the vertebral column.

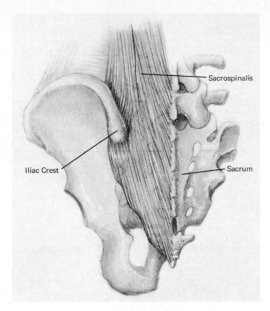

Fig. 1-41. The sacrospinalis muscle.

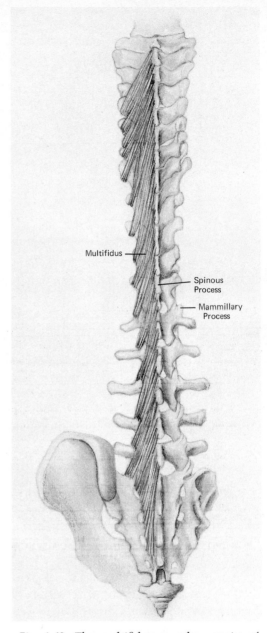

Fig. 1-42. The multifidus muscles consist of numerous small muscular slips which arise from small bony prominences on the articular facet.

Intertransversarii are small muscles between the transverse processes of the vertebrae (Fig. 1-43). In the lumbar region there are three muscle groupings: medial, dorsal lateral, and ventral lateral. They lie between the psoas and sacrospinalis muscles.

The medial intertransverse muscle arises from the accessory process (a minute bony eminence arising at the angle between the superior articular process and the transverse process) of the superior vertebra and is inserted into the mammillary process of the inferior vertebra.

The dorsal lateral slip arises from the accessory process of the superior vertebra and is inserted into the transverse process of the inferior vertebra.

The ventral lateral slip connects the inferior border of one transverse process with the superior border of the next.

Interspinalis muscles consist of short muscular fasciculi that extend from the superior surface of the spinous process below to the inferior surface of the one above (Fig. 1-44). They occur in pairs on either side of the interspinous ligament.

Flexors of the Lumbar Spine

ABDOMINAL MUSCLES

External Oblique. This broad, thin, irregular quadrilateral muscle is the largest and most superficial of the three flat abdominal

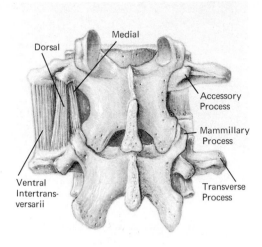

Fig. 1-43. The intertransversarii muscle.

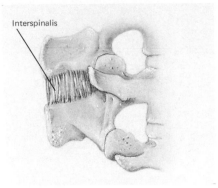

Fig. 1-44. Interspinalis muscle.

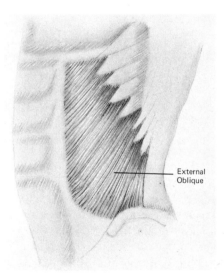

Fig. 1-45. External oblique muscle.

muscles (Fig. 1-45). It originates from eight fleshy digitations from the lower eight ribs and inserts into a broad, strong abdominal aponeurosis that extends over the rectus to the linea alba where the more superficial fibers originating from the last two ribs insert into the anterior wall of the iliac crest.

Internal Oblique. This muscle lies under the external oblique and is smaller and thinner (Fig. 1-46). It originates from the lumbodorsal fascia, the anterior two thirds of the iliac crest, and the lateral half of the inguinal ligament. The fibers, which run perpendicular to the external oblique fibers, pass upward in a vertical direction and insert into the lower three ribs; the remainder extend toward the lateral margin of the rectus muscle and terminate in its sheath.

Transversalis. This muscle is the innermost of the flat abdominal muscles and takes its name from the direction of its fibers (Fig. 1-47). It originates from the lateral third of the inguinal ligament, the anterior three fourths of the iliac crest, the lumbodorsal fascia, and the inner surface of the cartilages of the lower six ribs. The fibers take a nearly transverse course across the abdominal wall, inserting either at the midline in the linea alba or in the lower attachments, curving

behind the spermatic cord, and attaching to the lacunar ligament and pectineal fascia. The chief function of this muscle is to act as a living girdle in supporting the abdominal viscera. It is such support that helps maintain fixation of the lumbar spine.

Rectus Abdominis. This is a long, flat, bandlike muscle which extends along the length of the anterior abdominal wall (Fig. 1-48). It originates as a short, thick tendon which divides into two. The thicker lateral tendon is attached to the crest of the pubis. The muscle inserts into the cartilages of the fifth, sixth, and seventh ribs. The muscle is crossed by three fibrous bands (lineae trans-

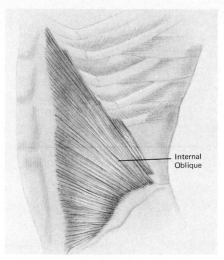

Fig. 1-46. Internal oblique muscle.

versae) passing transversely or obliquely across the muscle.

PSOAS MAJOR

The psoas major is a long, fusiform muscle originating as a series of thick fasciculi attached to the L5 vertebra and the transverse processes of the lumbar vertebrae (Fig. 1-49). The muscle extends downward across the brim of the minor pelvis and ends in a tendon which is inserted into the lesser trochanter of the femur.

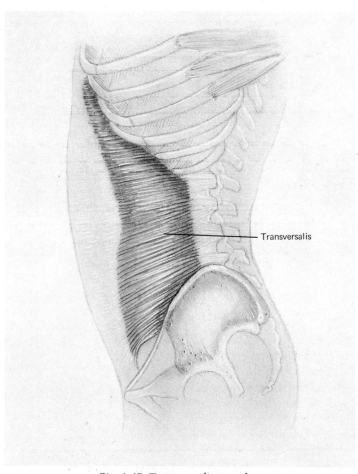

Fig. 1-47. Transversalis muscle.

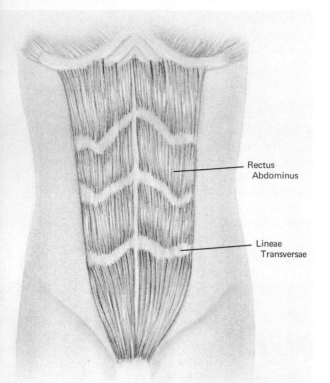

Fig. 1-48. Rectus abdominis muscle.

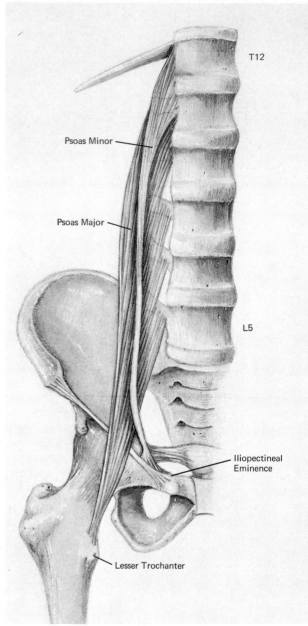

Fig. 1-49. Psoas major and minor.

PSOAS MINOR

The psoas minor is a long, slender muscle lying anterior to the psoas major. It originates from T12 and L1 and the intervening disc. The muscle fibers end in a long flat tendon which inserts into the iliopectineal eminence.

Abductors of the Lumbar Spine

Identifying a muscle as either a flexor or an extensor of the lumbar spine implies bilaterally simultaneous muscle action. Unilateral action will produce abduction or lateral bending of the spine. For example, contraction of the right quadratus lumborum or right psoas major will produce right lumbar abduction (Fig. 1-50).

Abductors of the Lumbar Spine:

Quadratus lumborum
Psoas major and minor
Abdominal muscles
Intertransversarii

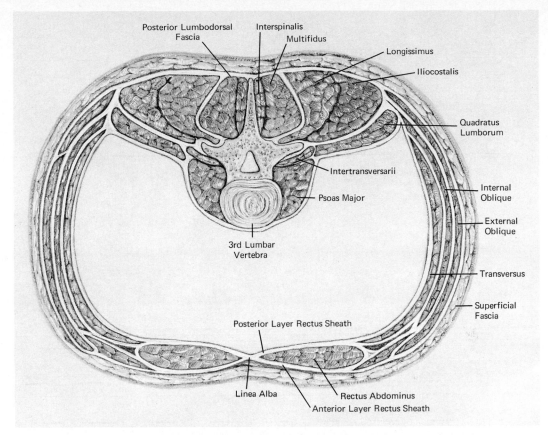

Fig. 1-50. Cross-section of body musculature and fascia through L3, which act as a dynamic girdle to support the abdominal viscera and help maintain fixation of the lumbar spine.

References

1. Comfort A: The Biology of Senescence. New York, Rinehart, 1956
2. Epstein JA, Epstein BS, Rosenthal AD, Carra R, Levine, LS: Sciatica caused by nerve root entrapment in the lateral recess: The superior facet syndrome. J Neurosurg, 36:584, 1972
3. Gray H: Anatomy of the Human Body. ed 27. Philadelphia, Lea & Febiger, 1966
4. Hendry NGC: The hydration of the nucleus pulposus and its relation to intervertebral disc derangement. J Bone Joint Surg, 40B:132, 1958
5. Pederson HE, Blunck CFV, Gardner E: The anatomy of the lumbosacral posterior rami and meningeal branches of spinal nerves (sinu-vertebral nerves). J Bone Joint Surg, 38A:377, 1956
6. Schlesinger PT: Incarceration of the first sacral nerve in a lateral bony recess of the spinal canal as a cause of sciatica: Anatomy—Two case reports. J Bone Joint Surg, 37A:115, 1955

Biomechanics of the Lumbar Spine 2

James M. Morris

Disc degeneration, by far the most common cause of low back pain, is a complex process. It results from biochemical and metabolic changes in the nucleus and annulus, repetitive mechanical stresses, and perhaps from auto-immune reactions. The importance of mechanical factors in the process of disc degeneration has been questioned. If, however, we recognize that the preponderance of disc problems occurs at the base of the lumbar spine (L4–5 and L5–S1), and that the greatest mechanical forces occur at these levels, we must conclude that these mechanical forces have a significant effect on the degenerative process. The spinal column, which serves as a sustaining rod for the maintenance of the upright position of the body, is subjected to many different forces (e.g., compression, tension, shear, bending, and rotation). It is the purpose of this chapter to review the forces imposed upon the lumbar spine and their possible relationship to disc degeneration.

Mechanical Considerations of the Anatomy of the Vertebral Column

The spinal column is a remarkable mechanism and structure. As a mechanism it may be quite flexible, and as a structure it can be rigid and capable of withstanding great force. Consider, for example, the function of the spinal column in a gymnast compared with that in a weightlifter.

The spinal column consists of 24 presacral vertebrae, the sacrum, and the coccyx. The presacral segments increase in size from C1 to L5, whereas the sacral and coccygeal segments decrease in size from S1 caudally. From a simple mechanical standpoint, a typical presacral vertebra may be considered to be composed of four parts: (1) the body, which ordinarily transmits 70% of any imposed load; (2) the laminae and pedicles which, with the body, enclose the spinal canal; (3) the spinous and transverse processes, for attachments of ligaments and muscles which move one segment upon the other; (4) the posterior articular processes or facets, which guide and limit motion between adjacent vertebrae, and which transmit approximately 30% of any imposed load.

The intervertebral disc, which gives the spine its flexibility, is generally considered to consist of three components: the nucleus pulposus, which occupies the central 50% to 60% of the cross-sectional area of the disc; the surrounding, thick annulus fibrosus; and the two cartilaginous end-plates, which separate each disc from the vertebral bodies above and below it. Many authors consider the end-plates to be a portion of the vertebral body rather than of the disc. There is no doubt, however, that the integrity of the nucleus depends on the integrity of the end-plates.

27

Located in the posterior central portion of the disc, the **nucleus pulposus** is an oval gelatinous mass consisting of chondrocyte-like cell bodies. These cell bodies are dispersed within an intercellular matrix that is made up of poorly differentiated collagen fibrils surrounded by a protein polysaccharide complex. The polysaccharide is generally chondroitin sulfate. Because of its polar (−OH) groups, the nucleus has a great capacity to imbibe and bind water. Depending on its age, the nucleus pulposus contains 69% to 88% water by weight.

The **annulus fibrosus** is formed of successive layers of collagenous and fibrocartilaginous tissue that are firmly anchored to the vertebrae above and below. The fibers within each layer are directed obliquely between the vertebrae, and successive layers of fibers are perpendicular to those of the adjacent layer, an orientation which gives the disc its elasticity. The layers of fibrous tissue are normally firmly bound together by an intercellular cementlike substance. The anterior and lateral portions of the annulus are approximately twice as thick as the posterior portion, where the layers are fewer in number and the fibers are oriented in a direction more nearly parallel to those of the adjacent level. There is also less binding substance in the posterior portion. These conditions no doubt contribute to the propensity of the disc to herniate posteriorly. Fibers of the innermost layers in the annulus pass into the nucleus and blend with the intercellular matrix, resulting in a lack of demarcation of the annulus and nucleus.

From an engineering standpoint, the spinal column is unique. It is not a homogeneous structure, but instead is composed of relatively rigid units (vertebrae) interspersed with highly deformable discs and arranged within a complex of guiding and restraining facet joints. This combination of strength and flexibility is a workable compromise that affords maximal protection for the spinal cord and nerves with minimal restriction of mobility. The isolated ligamentous spine devoid of its musculature behaves as a modified elastic rod. Despite the fact that it is a tapered column, its flexibility is quite uniform throughout its length, because flexibility is dependent upon the geometry of the elastic components, the discs. Flexibility varies directly with the height and inversely with the cross-sectional area of the disc. For example, in the thoracic region, the height and cross-section of the disc are smaller than in the lumbar region, but the combination of the two provides the relative uniformity of flexibility. Another interesting feature of the spinal column is that it is not straight in the sagittal plane but rather possesses the typical curves as a result of adaptation to the upright position. This feature allows the column to absorb vertical shocks (e.g., those imposed by running and jumping) more efficiently. If the spine were straight, these shocks would be transmitted along the axis of the spine and would jolt the head.

Viscoelasticity

The disc and, to a lesser extent, the vertebral body demonstrate viscoelastic properties characteristic of biological materials in general. These properties are probably best demonstrated by the load-deflection curve for pure compression (Fig. 2-1). When a compression load is plotted against deflection or deformation of the disc, the curve does not show the steady increase in deflection proportionate to the increasing force that would be indicated by a straight line. Instead it demonstrates stiffening behavior, the stiffness being the slope or rate of increase of load, with deformation measured in units of kilograms per millimeter (kg/mm) or pounds per inch (lb/in). The tangent or slope of the curve increases as the curve bends upward, indicating stiffening of the disc as a result of loading. Most engineering materials have a curve that tends to flatten or "soften" for high loads; thus, the vertebral disc is unique as a compressive unit.

Another important feature of the load-deflection curve is its dependence on the loading rate. The disc becomes stiffer the faster it is loaded. This response is valuable

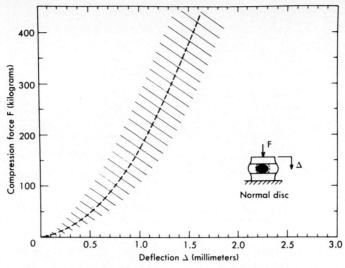

Fig. 2-1. An average force-deflection curve for compression of 24 normal discs. Range of variation is indicated by the shaded area. (Morris M, Markolf KL: Biomechanics of the lumbosacral spine. In American Academy of Orthopaedic Surgeons: Atlas of Orthotics. Biomechanical Principles and Applications, p. 315. Saint Louis, CV Mosby, 1975)

in such instances as high-speed ejection from jet aircraft.

The disc exhibits other phenomena characteristic of viscoelasticity, namely, creep and load relaxation (Fig. 2-2). **Creep** refers to the tendency to compress with time under constant compressive loading. This long-term compressive deformation of the disc is responsible for the change in height of an individual between morning and evening. The creep behavior of the spinal column is probably due to fluid transfer into and out of the disc as a result of the hydrophilic nature of the nucleus. **Load relaxation** refers to the decrease of load over time for a constant deformation.

The contributions to spinal mechanics of the components of the intervertebral disc (i.e., the nucleus and the annulus) have been studied, with interesting results.[7] It has been observed that the first time a disc is compressed in a load-deflection test after a small defect has been made in the annulus, nuclear material is extruded through the opening and the deflection curve is much softer, indicating that the disc is more compressible than normal for a given load. If the load is removed and the disc is loaded a second time

in the same manner, the disc becomes stiffer. By the third loading cycle, normal compressive behavior is restored. However, because of loss of nuclear material, the disc is now slightly diminished in height despite a normal load-deflection curve. Similar findings have been observed when the nucleus pulposus is removed, as would be done in a laminotomy or discectomy.

Of particular interest in the study mentioned above was the behavior of the annulus after removal of the nucleus, the end-plates, and the supporting bone above and below the end-plates (Fig. 2-3). This preparation excluded any possibility of a self-contained generation of pressure within the nucleus. Again, the first time the disc was compressed a very soft curve was revealed, demonstrating that the annulus was compressed into a new configuration. By the third loading cycle, the load-deflection curve approached that of a normal disc. These results indicate that the annulus alone is strong enough to carry the compressive force on the disc in a normal fashion. The role of the nucleus therefore appears to be one of load distribution rather than of direct load carrying. In addition, the imbibition pressure of the nu-

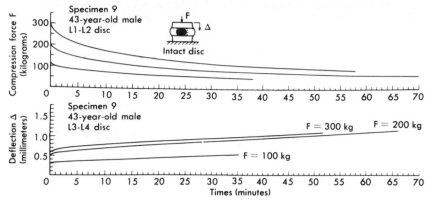

Fig. 2-2. Long-term creep curve for the disc of a 43-year-old man. (Markolf KL, Morris JM: The structural components of the intervertebral disc: A study of their contributions to the ability of the disc to withstand compressive forces. J Bone Joint Surg 56A: 675–687, 1974)

cleus serves to maintain the height of a normal disc and to preserve normal ligament tension and facet alignment. This study helps to explain how most patients, at least initially, do well after discectomy. Note, however, that this is an *in vitro* study, and the effects of rotation and shear stresses have not been determined.

Intrinsic and Extrinsic Stability of the Spine

Intrinsic stability is provided by opposing forces. Those within the nucleus tend to push adjacent vertebrae apart, while those in the binding longitudinal ligaments (the tensile forces) hold them together. Thus, the isolated ligamentous spine has a certain intrinsic stability.

Extrinsic stability of the spine and load reduction are provided by the trunk musculature and will be discussed in some detail later.

Biomechanics of the Intervertebral Disc

The unique construction and composition of the intervertebral disc enables this structure to withstand stresses of various duration and magnitude. Both the annulus and the nucleus absorb forces that occur primarily in a vertical axis, and they redistribute them evenly in all directions. This redistribution is possible because the nucleus pulposus alters its shape freely under pressure, transmitting some forces radially to the annulus and the rest to the entire cartilaginous endplate. The liquid character of the nucleus renders it almost incompressible and is the basis of this shape-altering property.

The importance of the entire phenomenon of fluid exchange as it affects the intervertebral discs has been the subject of considerable investigation since the pioneer papers of Püschel and DePukey. It was originally postulated that fluid exchange was governed by osmotic pressure. The cartilaginous endplates were thought to act as semipermeable membranes, with the nucleus drawing water from the vertebral bodies.[1] It is presently thought that the hydrodynamics of the disc depends upon the nucleus pulposus possessing the properties of a gel, rather than upon osmosis.[4] This gel contains some cartilaginous cells, fibroblasts, collagen framework, and the ground substance, which is mostly mucopolysaccharide protein complexes or proteoglycans with varying amounts of salts and water. A high imbibition pressure is produced by the gel, which can bind almost nine times its volume of water. This water content is not chemically bonded, as demonstrated by the expression of significant

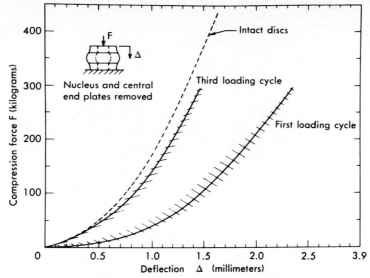

Fig. 2-3. *Average force-deflection curves for discs with the annulus only remaining, repeated loading. Ranges of variation are indicated by the shaded areas. (Markolf KL, Morris JM: The structural components of the intervertebral disc: A study of their contributions to the ability of the disc to withstand compressive forces. J Bone Joint Surg 56A: 675–687, 1974)*

quantities of water from the nucleus by prolonged mechanical pressure. The daily oscillation in body length (the average person is 1% shorter at the end of the day than in the morning) is the most striking example of this phenomenon.

The normal nucleus, occupying about half of the disc surface area, bears most of the vertical load, while the annulus bears the tangential load. When degeneration of the nucleus results in impairment of the gel's imbibition pressure, a marked change occurs in the transmission of forces along the vertical axis of the spine. The degenerated nucleus is less able to redistribute the load radially, causing the annulus to sustain most of the vertical load and little tangential load (Fig. 2-4).

Kinematics

The intervertebral joint complex has six possible degrees of freedom, three in rotation and three in translation (Fig. 2-5). Because of the anatomic configuration of the joint complex, certain motions occur more easily than others. Compression, lateral bending, and anterior or posterior bending and torsion occur most readily, whereas tension and anteroposterior and lateral shear are more restricted in the normal joint. Compression of the disc with low loads has been discussed under viscoelasticity. It should be pointed out that these motions are not pure, but rather, because of the orientation of the facet joints, are coupled. For example, rotation at the intervertebral joint is associated with lateral bending (Fig. 2-6). The possible clinical significance of this is unknown.

Bending (i.e., flexion, extension, and lateral bending) is the second most common motion of the intervertebral joint complex. The mechanics of these motions may be characterized by a curve similar to that of force versus deflection for axial compression. In bending movements the motion observed is rotation (measured in degrees), and the force acting to produce this rotation is called **moment.** A moment is a force applied in such a way as to produce rotation about a fixed point: the value of the moment (in units of newton-meters or in ft-lb) is force times distance of the lever arm. A curve of

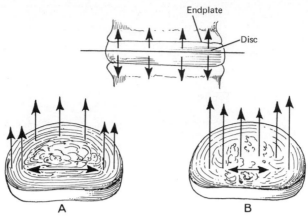

Fig. 2-4. **(A)** *The normal nucleus bears about half the vertical load, while the annulus bears the other half tangentially.* **(B)** *The degenerated nucleus is unable to redistribute much of the load radially, causing the annulus to sustain much of the vertical load.*

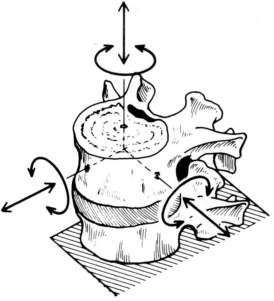

Fig. 2-5. *The intervertebral joint has six degrees of freedom on the three axes of the coordinate system. (After White AA, III, Panjabi MM: Clinical Biomechanics of the Spine, p. 38. Philadelphia, JB Lippincott, 1978.)*

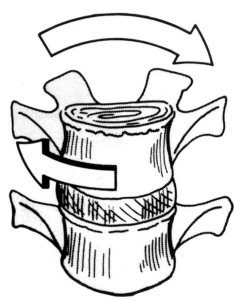

Fig. 2-6. *Representation of a coupling pattern in the lumbar spine. Lateral bending (θz) is coupled with axial rotation (θy). (White, AA, Panjabi MM: Clinical Biomechanics of the Spine, p. 79. Philadelphia, JB Lippincott, 1978. After Krag MH: Three Dimensional Flexibility Measurements of Preloaded Human Vertebral Motion Segments. MD thesis, Yale University School of Medicine, New Haven, 1975)*

a moment-rotation test is similar to that of a force-deflection test (Fig. 2-7). The rotation response of an *in vitro* intervertebral joint demonstrates behavior characteristic of collagenous biological materials. The curves are nonlinear, displaying increasing stiffness, as noted in the force-deflection curves. The importance of the posterior facets for

bending varies with the particular motion. For lateral bending and flexion, the curves vary slightly but are essentially the same. The facets, however, have a definite stiffening influence on extension in both the

Biomechanics of the Intervertebral Disc **33**

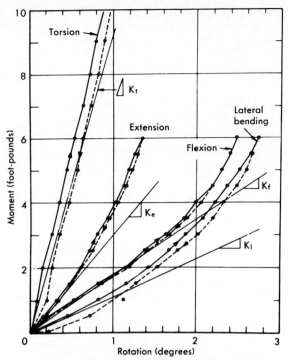

Fig. 2-7. *Moment-rotation curves for a typical disc, the one between T12 and L1, showing the relative initial stiffness for lateral bending (K_1); flexion (K_f); extension (K_e); and torsion (K_t). Solid lines are the loading cycles. Broken lines are the unloading cycles. (1 ft-lb = 0.138 kg-meter.) (Markolf KL: Deformation of the thoracolumbar intervertebral joints in response to external loads: A biomechanical study using autopsy material. J Bone Joint Surg 54A: 511–533, 1972)*

lumbar and thoracic regions (approximately three times that of a joint with the facets removed). This stiffening effect appears to be attributable to facet joint compression and impingement as the joint is extended and resistance to further rotation results.

Torsion, or rotation, of the intervertebral joint about its long axis is a complex motion that is dependent on the structural features of the posterior facets. Torsion in the thoracic and lumbar joints differs significantly because of differences in the facet orientation (Fig. 2-8). In the thoracic spine, the center of rotation lies within the nucleus, and the disc is subjected to rotation forces. In the lumbar spine, the center of axial rotation lies posterior to the disc, and the disc is thus subjected to translational shear-

ing forces. In the case of bending, stiffening characterizes the response to a moment.

The torsional behavior of the thoracic and lumbar discs was investigated before and after removal of posterior facets (Fig. 2-9)[6]. The thoracic joint showed little change in torsional (moment rotation) behavior as a result of facet removal. This was to be expected, because the facet articulating surfaces of the thoracic facets are horizontal in orientation and thus offer little resistance to torsion. The lumbar facets, however, are aligned in the sagittal plane and do resist torsional or rotational motions. Torsional tests by Farfan indicated an average failure torque of 881×10^6 dyne-cm, or 8.99 kg/meter.[2] He estimated that the disc provides 40% to 50% of the torsional stiffness, with the remainder provided by the posterior facet joints. When torsion was applied to the point of failure (Fig. 2-10), it was found that intervertebral joints with degenerated discs were, as expected, weaker than normal specimens.

Axial Rotation of the Spine *in vivo*

Gregersen and Lucas studied axial rotation of the spine *in vivo* while the trunk was rotated from side to side.[3] Steinmann pins were inserted into the spinous processes under local anesthesia, and angular displacement between various vertebral segments was measured by special transducers designed to measure only rotation. Approximately 74 degrees of rotation occurred between T1 and T12, and the average cumulative rotation from the sacrum to T1 was 102 degrees (Fig. 2-11). Very little rotation occurs in the lumbar as compared with the thoracic spine, and again this is a reflection of the orientation of the facet joints. Measurements of rotation obtained during walking indicated the following:

1. The pelvis and the lumbar spine rotate as a functional unit.
2. In the lower thoracic spine, rotation diminishes gradually up to T7.

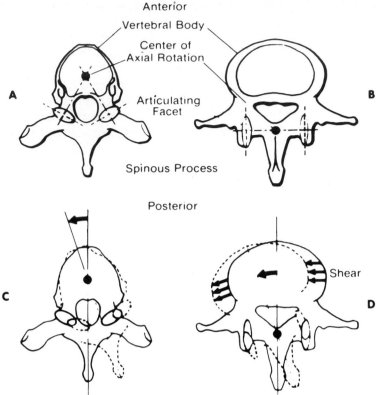

Anterior
Vertebral Body
Center of
Axial Rotation
Articulating
Facet
Spinous Process
Posterior
Shear

*Fig. 2-8. Mechanism of axial rotation (**C** and **D**) in a thoracic (left) and a lumbar (right) vertebra. (Gregersen GG, Lucas DB: An in vivo study of the axial rotation of the human thoracolumbar spine. J Bone Joint Surg 49A: 247–262, 1967)*

3. T7 represents the area of transition from vertebral rotation in the direction of the pelvis to rotation in the opposite direction, that of the shoulder girdle (Fig. 2-12).

4. The amount of rotation in the upper thoracic spine increases gradually from T7 to T1.

Using a specially designed transducer, Lumsden and Morris measured axial rotation at the lumbosacral level *in vivo.*[5] Approximately 6 degrees of rotation occurred at the lumbosacral joint during maximal rotation. With the pelvis fixed, the subject stood or straddled a bicycle seat. Approximately 1.5 degrees of rotation occurred during normal walking. Rotation at the lumbosacral joint was not measurably affected by asymmetrically oriented lumbar facets (tropism). It was always associated with flexion of L5 on the sacrum.

The Ligamentous Spine

The isolated spinal column, devoid of musculature, demonstrates an intrinsic stability and behaves as a modified elastic rod. Although the spinal column is nonuniform in size, bending and compression stiffnesses are nearly constant throughout the dorsolumbar spine.

Torsional stiffness, however, is not uniform. As a result of the orientation of their facets, the lower lumbar joints are far stiffer than the thoracic joints. The upper thoracic vertebrae (T10 and above) articulate with the rib cage in such a manner that resistance to torsional motion is increased. The thoracic vertebrae may be visualized as a rigid unit bound together by the rib cage. Since the lumbar vertebrae possess an inherently high torsional stiffness, they may also be

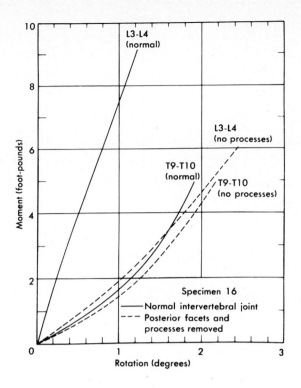

considered as a stiff structural unit. This leaves the discs T10 to T12 as the intermediate elastic elements when sudden torsional movements are applied, such as might occur during a fall or during acceleration. These intermediate discs are likely to absorb a great deal of energy since rotation is greatest at these levels. Thus, the lowest thoracic discs are the most prone to injuries involving torsion.

As mentioned, the ligamentous spine possesses an intrinsic stability. This stability, however, is minimal so far as the entire column is concerned, for although the liga-

Fig. 2-9. Effect of articular processes and posterior elements on moment-rotation behavior of a thoracic and a lumbar intervertebral joint in torsion. (1 ft-lb = 0.138 kg-meter) (Markolf KL: Deformation of the thoracolumbar intervertebral joints in response to external loads: A biomechanical study using autopsy material. J Bone Joint Surg 54A: 511–533, 1972)

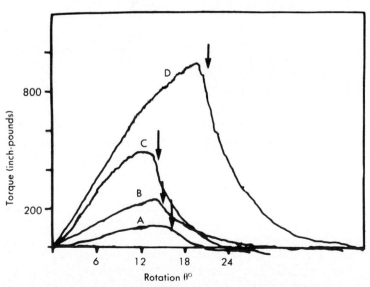

Fig. 2-10. Typical moment-rotation curves for intact intervertebral disc and its components, loaded to failure. (A) Intact joints between articular processes with capsule of contralateral articular process removed. (B) Ruptured isolated disc. (C) Intact (normal) isolated disc. (D) Intact intervertebral joint with a normal discogram. (1 in-lb = 0.0115 kg-meter) (Farfan HF, Cossette JW, Robertson GH, Wells RV, Kraus H: The effects of torsion of the lumbar intervertebral joints: The role of torsion in the production of disc degeneration. J Bone Joint Surg 52A: 468–497, 1970).

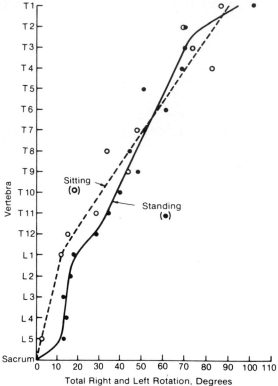

Fig. 2-11. Maximum total axial rotation of thoracolumbar spine in standing and sitting positions, pelvis immobilized. (Gregersen GG, Lucas
DB: An in vivo study of the axial rotation of the
human thoracolumbar spine. J Bone Joint Surg
49A: 247–262, 1967)

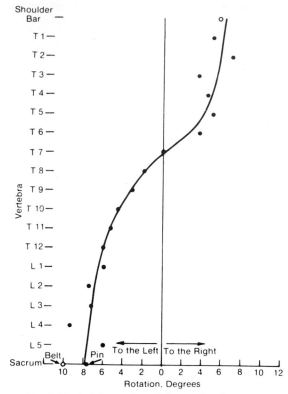

Fig. 2-12. Axial rotation of thoracolumbar spine
during locomotion. Left heel strike to right heel
strike is 4.38 km per hr. Solid circles are values
for readings from pins. Open circles are readings
from the belt. (Gregersen GG, Lucas DB: An in
vivo study of the axial rotation of the human
thoracolumbar spine. J Bone Joint Surg 49A:
247–262, 1967)

mentous spine is capable of standing erect without external support, a compressive force of only 2.04 kg (4.4 lb) applied to the top is enough to buckle the column laterally (Fig. 2-13).

Role of the Trunk in Spine Stability

If the ligamentous spine is able to withstand only very small loads, it is apparent that the extrinsic support provided by the trunk musculature is responsible for the ability of the spinal column to withstand the great loads to which it may be subjected. When an individual bends forward to lift a heavy weight, a large force is generated at the lumbosacral level. This force can be

calculated by means of a free body diagram (Fig. 2-14). The weight lifted and the weight of the trunk, head, and upper extremities act at a distance (lever arm) from the base of the spine (fulcrum).

Lifting occurs by contraction of the erector spinae and gluteus maximus musculature acting through a much shorter lever arm (i.e., from the disc center to the spinous process). For example, if 90.7 kg (200 lb) is lifted, there is theoretically a force of 939.4 kg (over 2000 lb) at the lumbosacral level. However, a number of biomechanical experiments have been carried out to determine the strength of the discs and vertebral bodies, and it has been demonstrated that they cannot tolerate such great forces. By

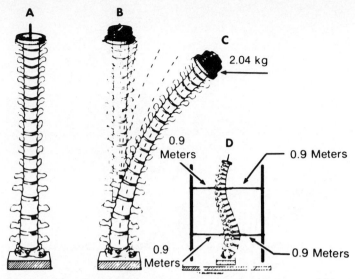

Fig. 2-13. *Adult thoracolumbar ligamentous spine, fixed at the base and free at the top, under vertical loading, and restrained at midthoracic and midlumbar levels in anteroposterior plane. (A) Before loading. (B) During loading. (C) Stability failure occurring under 2.04 kg load. (D) Lateral view showing anteroposterior restrains. (Morris M, Markolf KL: Biomechanics of the lumbosacral spine. In American Academy of Orthopaedic Surgeons: Atlas of Orthotics. Biomechanical Principles and Application, p. 32. Saint Louis, CV Mosby, 1975)*

placing two vertebral bodies and their intervening disc in a materials-testing compression machine or by subjecting them to sudden dynamic forces, considerable information has been obtained. Compression forces have been imposed up to the point of failure of the segment of the spine being studied. This failure is characterized by an audible crack, followed by sanguineous leakage from one of the vertebrae (usually the superior) through the vascular foramen and occasionally along the attachment of the peripheral fibers of the annulus to the vertebral body. The evidence of failure is often difficult to visualize by either gross examination or roentgenography. It may consist of compression of a few spicules of bone, cracks in the end-plate, or collapse of the plate. It has been shown that failure occurs in specimens from young persons at a compressive load of 453.6 to 771.1 kg (1000 to 1700 lb). When specimens from older persons were studied, the critical load was found to be much less, even as little as 136.1 kg (300 lb). However, it is important to note

that when the annulus is intact, its elastic limits cannot be exceeded without vertebral fracture. The end-plate is the component most susceptible to fracture as a result of the forces exerted on the spine and generally is the first to give way (Fig. 2-15). It is most likely to fracture centrally when the disc is normal and when the resistance of the vertebral body is greater than the pressure generated within the nucleus. This type of end-plate failure might explain the origin of Schmorl's nodules in young people. Peripheral plate fractures or fissures across the end-plate occur when various degrees of disc degeneration lead to an abnormal distribution of forces across the disc space.

The vertebral body itself, the next most susceptible part of the segment under study, usually collapses before herniation of the nucleus occurs through the annulus. Even when well-developed defects of the annulus are present, end-plate or vertebral fractures are more likely to occur than disc herniation. (Note that the above values are not *in vivo* measurements.) It has been shown experi-

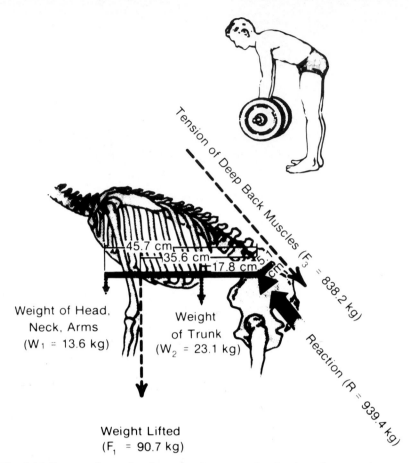

Fig. 2-14. Force on lower lumbar part of spine, with role of trunk omitted. (Morris JM, Lucas DB, Bresler B: Role of the trunk in stability of the spine. J Bone Joint Surg 43A: 327–351, 1961)

mentally in dogs that a single violent impact causes fracture of the vertebra more often than it causes disc herniation. This finding supports the opinion that trauma per se seldom causes disc herniation. Organic as well as inorganic materials generally are able to withstand stresses applied for a short period more readily than stresses exerted over a longer period of time. It has also been demonstrated that an approximately equal number of end-plate fractures occur when a static force of approximately 589.7 kg (1300 lb) is exerted as when dynamic stresses of 1179.3 kg (2600 lb) are applied.[11] This is no doubt related to the viscoelastic properties of the structures involved.

How, then, can the spine support the theoretical loads to which it may be sub-

jected? One explanation is to consider the spine as a segmented elastic column supported by the paraspinal muscles, situated within and attached to the sides of two chambers (the abdominal and thoracic cavities) which are separated by the diaphragm. The abdominal cavity is filled with a combination of solids and liquids, whereas the thoracic cavity is filled largely with fluids and air. The action of the trunk musculature converts these chambers into semirigid walled cylinders of air and semisolids, which are capable of transmitting forces generated in loading the spine, and thereby of relieving the spinal column itself.

The above hypothesis was studied by utilizing small balloon-tip catheters to measure the intrathoracic (esophageal) and intra-ab-

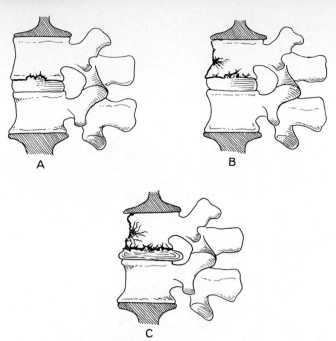

Fig. 2-15. (A) *The cartilaginous end-plates are most susceptible to spinal compression.* (B) *The vertebral body is the second most susceptible unit of the spine.* (C) *The normal nucleus pulposus and annulus fibrosus are least susceptible to pressure.*

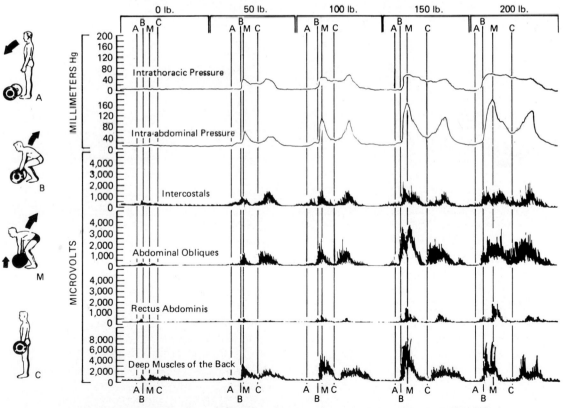

Fig. 2-16. *Dynamic loading of the spine. (Morris JM, Lucas DB, Bresler B: Role of the trunk in stability of the spine. J Bone Joint Surg 43A: 327–351, 1961)*

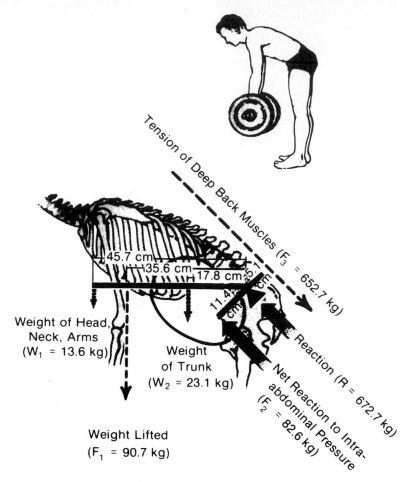

Tension of Deep Back Muscles (F_3 = 652.7 kg)

Reaction (R = 672.7 kg)

Net Reaction to Intra-abdominal Pressure (F_2 = 82.6 kg)

45.7 cm
35.6 cm
17.8 cm
11.4 cm

Weight of Head, Neck, Arms (W_1 = 13.6 kg)

Weight of Trunk (W_2 = 23.1 kg)

Weight Lifted (F_1 = 90.7 kg)

Fig. 2-17. Force on lower lumbar part of spine, with role of trunk included. (Morris JM, Lucas DB, Bresler B: Role of the trunk in stability of the spine. J Bone Joint Surg 43A: 327–351, 1961)

dominal (stomach) pressures.[8] It was possible to show that during the act of lifting, the action of intercostal muscles and muscles of the shoulder girdle rendered the thoracic cage quite rigid. An increase in thoracic pressure resulted, converting the thoracic cage and the spine into a sturdy unit capable of transmitting large forces. The abdominal contents were compressed into a semirigid mass by contraction of the diaphragm and the muscles of the abdominal wall, which made the abdominal cavity a semirigid cylinder. The force of the weights lifted by the arms was thus transmitted to the spinal column by the muscles of the shoulder

girdle, principally by the trapezius, and then to the abdominal cylinder and the pelvis, partly through the spinal column and partly through the rigid rib cage and abdomen. The larger the weight lifted, the greater was the activity of the trunk musculature (Fig. 2-16). When the effects of the increased cavitary pressures were included (using the free body diagram) in the calculations of the forces imposed on the spine during heavy lifting, the load on the lumbosacral disc was decreased by approximately 30% and the load at the thoracolumbar level was reduced by 50%. Thus when 90.7 kg (200 lb) is lifted, only 672.7 kg (1483 lb) of force are actually

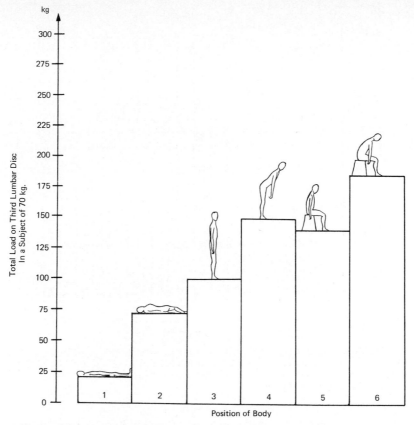

Fig. 2-18. Total load on the L3 disc in different positions in a subject weighing 70 kg. Positions shown are (1) reclining (relaxed, supine), (2) reclining (lateral decubitus), (3) standing upright, (4) standing and 20° forward leaning, (5) sitting upright, arms and back unsupported, (6) sitting and 20° forward leaning.

transmitted along the spine to the lumbosacral level, instead of the theoretical force of approximately 939.4 kg (2071 lb) (Fig. 2-17). It is interesting to note that when a tight corset was worn about the abdomen, an increase in the intra-abdominal and intrathoracic pressures resulted from tightening of the corset. At the same time, during the act of lifting there was a decrease in activity of the thoracic and abdominal muscles, indicating that the effect of the muscle could be replaced by such an external appliance.

In an attempt to confirm the above calculations, intradiscal pressures were measured *in vivo* by Nachemson and Morris.[10] A needle with a pressure-sensitive polyethylene membrane tip was inserted into the disc under study. Intradiscal pressure of 10 to 15 kg/cm² was found in normal discs with subjects in a sitting position. There was approximately 30% less pressure during standing, and 50% less in a reclining position (Fig. 2-18). From the measurements, one can determine that the lower lumbar discs of adults must support total loads of as much as 99.8 to 174.6 kg (220 to 385 lb) when the subjects are seated. For the standing position, total loads of 90.7 to 120.2 kg (200 to 265 lb) were calculated from the pressure values obtained. The intradiscal pressure was significantly elevated when weights were lifted and especially when lifting involved forward flexion of the trunk.

In 1970, Nachemson and Elfström published a study on intravital dynamic

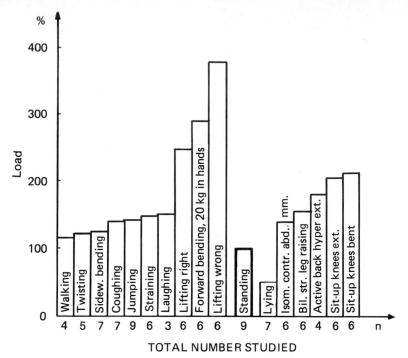

Fig. 2-19. Mean change in load (%) compared with that obtained in the upright standing position. (Nachemson A, Elfström G: Intravital dynamic pressure measurements in lumbar discs: A study of common movements, maneuvers and exercises. Scand J Rehabil Med (Suppl) 1: 32, 1970)

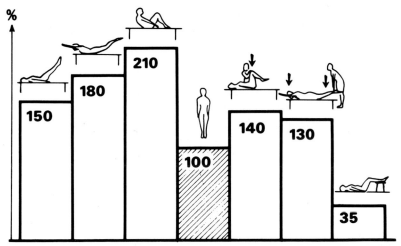

Fig. 2-20. Relative change in pressure (or load) in L3 in various muscle-strengthening exercises in living subjects. (Nachemson AL: The lumbar spine: An orthopaedic challenge. Spine, 1: 59–71, 1976)

pressure measurements in lumbar discs.[9] Using a smaller, more flexible needle with a pressure-sensitive tip, they were able to measure pressures while the subjects were engaged in a number of activities such as bending, sitting, lifting (Fig. 2-19) and performing various back exercises (Fig. 2-20). The figures obtained agree closely with the theoretical calculations of forces on the spine which we have mentioned previously.

References

1. Charnley J: Imbibition of fluid as a cause of herniation of the nucleus pulposus. Lancet 1:124–127, 1952.
2. Farfan HF, Cossette JW, Robertson GH, Wells RV, Kraus H: The effects of torsion on the lumbar intervertebral joints: The role of torsion in the production of disc degeneration. J Bone Joint Surg, 52A: 468–497, 1970
3. Gregersen GG, Lucas DB: An in vivo study of the axial rotation of the human thoracolumbar spine. J Bone Joint Surg, 49A: 247–262, 1967
4. Hendry NGC: The hydration of the nucleus pulposus and its relation to intervertebral disc derangement. J Bone Joint Surg, 40B: 132–144, 1958
5. Lumsden RM II, Morris JM: An in vivo study of axial rotation and immobilization at the lumbosacral joint. J Bone Joint Surg, 50A: 1591–1602, 1968
6. Markolf KL: Deformation of the thoracolumbar intervertebral joints in response to external loads: A biomechanical study using autopsy material. J Bone Joint Surg, 54A: 511–533, 1972
7. Markolf KL, Morris JM: The structural components of the intervertebral disc: A study of their contributions to the ability of the disc to withstand compressive forces. J Bone Joint Surg, 56A: 675–687, 1974
8. Morris JM, Lucas DB, Bresler B: Role of the trunk in stability of the spine. J Bone Joint Surg, 43A: 327–351, 1961
9. Nachemson A, Elfström G: Intravital dynamic pressure measurements in lumbar discs: A study of common movements, maneuvers and exercises. Scand J Rehabil Med (Suppl) 1: 1970
10. Nachemson A, Morris JM: In vivo measurements of intradiscal pressure: Discometry, a method for the determination of pressure in the lower lumbar discs. J Bone Joint Surg, 46A: 1077–1092, 1964
11. Perey O: Fracture of the vertebral endplate in the lumbar spine: An experimental biomechanical investigation. Acta Orthop Scand (Suppl) 25: 1957

PART I

Examination of the Patient

History

When Thomas Carlyle, the Scottish author, wrote in 1845 "histories are as perfect as the historian is wise and is gifted with an eye and a soul," he assuredly did not have low back dysfunction in mind. However, the quotation is quite apt and appropriate when applied to this clinical problem.

Sit Back and Listen

In evaluating a patient with low back pain, a most searching and deliberate history is required to appraise the problem properly. As with any pain syndrome, the examiner should keep in mind the importance of allowing the patient free expression, since pain is a subjective entity and a preoccupied physician may often misinterpret the patient's statements. The examiner should maintain an open mind and not prejudge every patient with back and sciatic pain as having a "disc problem." Although lumbar disc disease is a fairly common cause for back and sciatic pain, many other entities need to be considered.

Low Back Pain

In eliciting a history from a patient who is being seen for low back pain, one commonly finds that the patient is most eager to speak about the most recent episode of pain for which treatment is being sought. The current painful condition may so dominate the history that it obscures previous episodes of similar, but possibly less severe, attacks. For this reason, even when previous episodes of low back pain are denied, it may be advisable to pursue the point a bit further with leading questions, such as whether long auto trips, heavy lifting, or extended periods of stooping had ever previously produced low back dysfunction.

How the symptoms develop is of interest. We may tend to think of the spontaneous onset of low back pain as caused by an entity such as tumor, or expect the onset of a herniated disc to be associated with an injury. Many patients with low back pain can, in hindsight, name some injury to the low back that may have been responsible for the symptoms; it may have been a direct fall, lifting heavy weights, or merely leaning forward to pick up something of negligible weight from the floor.

Attributing too much importance to mode of onset, however, may be misleading. In reviewing a recent series of 14 patients presenting with low back pain as the initial symptom caused by unsuspected metastatic

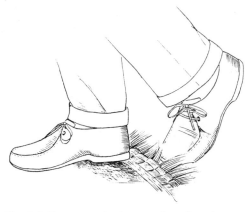

Fig. 3-1. *Frequent tripping on the edge of a rug with the painfully affected limb may indicate a partial foot drop.*

neoplasm, five attributed the onset of their symptoms to trauma. A history of injury or trauma is of interest but must be considered in its proper perspective.

Are the low back symptoms intermittent? Is the patient completely free of any discomfort between episodes of back pain? Is it a pain of gradual onset and unremitting progression? (Certainly, this last history should alert one to the possibility of neoplasm.)

What is the relationship of the pain to mechanical factors? Is the pain eased by bed rest and made worse with physical activities, or is the pain worse at night while lying supine in bed, as is true of many tumors? What type of activity aggravates the pain most? Is standing worse than sitting? Does bending forward or stooping aggravate the pain? It is usually necessary to ask specific and sometimes leading questions to elicit such details. Recently, a medical student noted on the chart that a patient under my care for very severe lumbar disc pain was not adversely affected by heavy lifting or stooping. On reviewing the chart and seeing this unexpected allegation, I went back to the patient's room and asked if such strenuous activities increased his pain. The patient denied such aggravation. However, when I expressed surprise at this answer, he explained that he never did heavy lifting or stooping because of his low back pain.

It is important to find out what relieves the pain. Is it eased when sitting or standing? Is there any specific body position that relieves it? What medications are helpful? Does aspirin help, or is it necessary to take more powerful analgesics? Learning the type of medication required helps the physician assess the intensity of pain.

What previous treatment has been carried out? Was low back manipulation helpful, or did it seem to aggravate the symptoms? Have low back supports or girdles been of help?

Does the patient have a spinal list or scoliosis? Is it always to the same side or does it alternate? Does one leg seem longer than the other?

Sciatica

Sciatica can occur with or without back pain, and the following questions can help in diagnosis. Where is the sciatic radiation? (The distribution of the sciatic radiation may be helpful in diagnosing the level of the lesion.) Is the symptom exclusively one of pain, or is it associated with numbness and tingling? Did back and leg pain occur simultaneously, or did the back pain occur first and the leg pain occur subsequently? Did sciatica occur without a previous history of low back pain?

To determine the aggravating effect of increased intraspinal pressure, the examiner asks if coughing, sneezing, or straining at stool causes either increased pain in the back or sciatic distribution of the pain. One must be cautious in attributing the effects of increased intraspinal pressure to a vigorous cough or sneeze, since it can produce a sudden body movement which might aggravate pain of any sort. For example, a sneeze might aggravate the pain of a fractured limb, which would have nothing to do with increased intraspinal pressure. Straining at stool or a Valsalva maneuver is not likely to cause any sudden body movement. If either of these causes pain, one is more likely to consider increased intraspinal pressure as the aggravating factor.

Motor Impairment

It is sometimes difficult to differentiate weakness from pain. The patient may state: "I'm paralyzed and can't move my legs." Examination may disclose no actual motor dysfunction but such severe muscle spasm and pain that it is almost impossible for the patient to move. Oftentimes, the patient is not aware of any specific weakness, and the examiner must search for subtle clues to decide whether a motor deficit does exist. For example, if a patient has a partial foot drop, an increased unilateral shoe slap may be heard when walking on hard surfaces. Another clue to a partial foot drop is the tendency to trip over small surface elevations such as curbs, rocks, or even the edge of rugs and carpets (Fig. 3-1). The patient has habitually cleared these obstacles in the past without using any special precautions and, not realizing that the extensors are a bit weaker as a result of a partial foot drop, the tip of the shoe will catch against rugs or curbs.

Once aware of this phenomenon, some patients habitually overcorrect by lifting the affected foot a bit higher with each step to avoid tripping, thus producing a characteristic gait abnormality.

Weakness of the quadriceps is often first noted on climbing stairs, when it is necessary to elevate the weight of the body using primarily the quadriceps and gluteus muscles. Oftentimes, the patient will complain, "My leg gives out from under me unexpectedly."

Sensory Impairment

As a rule, sciatic pain is most severe proximally, since it begins in the hip and decreases in intensity as it progresses distally. Although sensory symptoms may follow a similar course, the predominant site of symptoms is usually the reverse of pain (Fig. 3-2). Oftentimes, numbness is primarily appreciated distally, and the patient will be

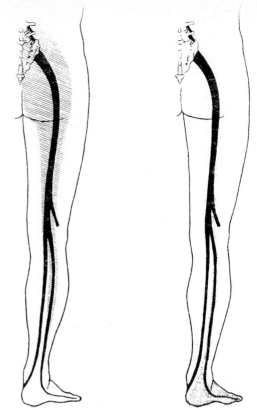

Fig. 3-2. Predominant site reversal of nerve root pain and sensory symptoms. Pain is most severe proximally, and numbness is most severe distally.

aware of what is described as a "pins and needles feeling" in the foot or lower leg.

The subjective distal sensory symptoms are of much greater diagnostic help than those more proximal. It is almost impossible to differentiate clinically the L5 from the S1 roots in the posterior thigh; but when these dermatomes extend down to the foot, they assume a relatively consistent distribution. Sometimes no objective sensory changes can be elicited by examination, and we have only the subjective sensation of numbness to help us localize a lesion.

The number of dermatomes affected is of great importance. Whenever more than one root is involved, either unilaterally, affecting a major portion of one lower extremity, or with bilateral sciatica, the possibility of neoplasm exists.

Sphincter Impairment

Sphincter changes are usually elicited in the history only by direct questions. The patient is not apt to volunteer inadequacy of sphincter mechanisms, particularly if these are not severe, since no relationship between back pain and increased difficulty in voiding may be comprehended. A recent onset of constipation is of interest and may be the initial evidence of sphincter impairment.

True Sciatica Versus Musculoligamentous Pain

It is important to differentiate the pain of true sciatica from hip disease, which is associated with an ill-defined, diffuse, deep, dull, aching discomfort extending into the buttock or posterior thigh, and which is due to ligamentous, periosteal, and joint capsule dysfunction. In the case of hip joint pain, internal and external rotation of the hip is productive of pain. As a rule, the radiating pain of sciatic neuralgia is readily distinguished from the musculoligamentous pain of hip disease. However, nerve root compression may produce a reflex spasm of those muscles innervated by the irritated root, and this occasionally makes differentiation of these two entities a problem.

Medical History

In addition to questions relating specifically to low back dysfunction, additional information must be elicited before the problem can be properly evaluated. The medical history must include a review of previous hospitalizations. Such information may furnish special insight into the patient's personal characteristics and may round out the overall medical picture. For example, was the patient hospitalized for vague gastrointestinal complaints on one occasion and again for vague chest pains, and were the studies performed during both of these hospital stays negative? A history of multiple surgical procedures performed for obscure indications should ring a warning bell in the mind of the examiner. Is litigation anticipated, or is the amount of compensation to be received likely to be an issue? Potential secondary gain may be a factor in prolongation of symptoms.

Physical Examination

Systematic Approach

Examination of the patient with low back pain should take no more than 15 minutes, and yet, if properly done, it can be most comprehensive. An orderly and systematic approach is more than a time-saver. It develops into an aid in proper evaluation. When the examining physician becomes accustomed to a somewhat fixed and specific examining routine, each positive or negative finding falls into a pattern, so that by the end of the examination the physician will find it easy to reach a diagnostic opinion. In contrast, if the examination is done in a haphazard fashion, instead of having a group of patterned findings the physician has a jumble of facts to sort out and try to piece together.

The following 12-point examination is quite comprehensive and can easily be performed in 15 minutes.

1. Inspection. Examination begins when the patient enters the office. Often a great deal can be learned by observing the patient walking the short distance to a chair and sitting down while he or she is not overly self-conscious about being scrutinized. While taking the history, it is good to note external manifestations of pain and any unusual features of stance or carriage.

Exposure of the patient should enable the examiner to visualize the entire spine and both buttocks. Inspect the back for any evidence of midline congenital defect, such as a tuft of hair or a scar indicating a spina bifida occulta. If the patient is having severe discomfort at the time of examination, the lumbar spine may be splinted by severe paraspinal muscle spasm. This produces a flattening of the normal lumbar lordotic curvature which may be associated with slight flexion of both the thoracic and the cervical spines. With a thoracolumbar scoliosis, the hip on the side of the convexity protrudes laterally.

2. Gait. Observe the patient walking back and forth. Even moderately severe back pain usually decreases the mobility of the lumbar spine and produces restriction of normal spinal movement. When lumbar paraspinal muscle spasm is so severe that a "poker spine" or "frozen spine" is present, both lumbar flexion and extension may be completely absent. Even in the presence of severe muscle spasm, a certain degree of lateral flexion and rotation of the spine is usually retained. The patient often walks in a stiff, guarded fashion depending mainly on hip movement and lateral spine flexion rather than using the normal gait involving a more complete range of active spinal movement.

After observing the patient's gait, the physician asks the patient to walk on his toes away from the physician (Fig. 3-3). The examiner observes and compares the height of the heels and notes any tendency for one heel to drop closer to the floor with weight-bearing, indicating some weakness of the gastrocnemius, soleus, and plantaris muscles. Weakness of this muscle group is compatible with S1 nerve root compression.

The patient then walks back toward the physician on the heels permitting the physician to determine whether one foot consistently drops with weight-bearing in comparison to the other foot. This is indicative of weakness of the tibialis anterior, the extensor digitorum longus, and the extensor hallucis longus muscles. Weakness of this muscle group is compatible with L5 nerve root compression.

3. Mobility. When examining the patient for mobility of the lumbar spine, the examiner is seated with the patient standing in front of him (Fig. 3-4). The examiner's

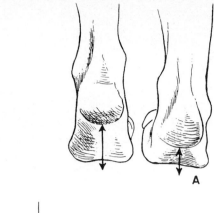

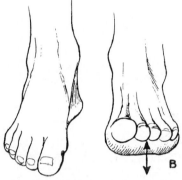

Fig. 3-3. **(A)** The patient "toe walks" away from the examiner for determination of plantar flexion weakness. **(B)** The patient "heel walks" back toward the examiner for determination of foot extensor weakness.

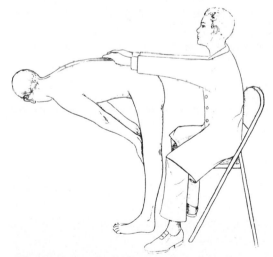

Fig. 3-4. Lumbar mobility can be assessed visually and by palpation.

hand is placed on the patient's lumbar spine, and the patient is asked to bend forward, backward, and to either side. During these

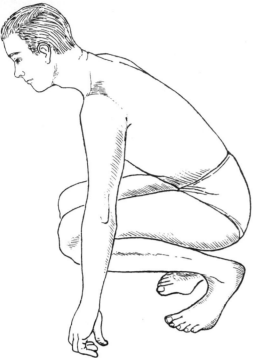

Fig. 3-5. *If hip and knee dysfunction are present, squatting is usually pain producing at the pathologic joint.*

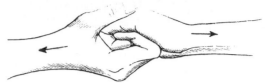

Fig. 3-6. *Opposing hand pull for reinforcement of deep tendon reflexes.*

movements, the examiner determines by palpation whether increased paraspinal muscle spasm develops with any specific movement. The degree of lumbar mobility can be assessed visually and by palpation.

Total spinal mobility is of lesser importance than the specific extent of lumbar spine mobility. Some individuals with a surgically fused lumbar spine can actually bend forward and touch their toes by compensating for the lack of lumbar mobility with hip movement and hypermobility of the remaining vertebrae. For this reason, during flexion, one should observe very carefully any changes in the lumbar spine. Place the thumb and third fingertips over the L2 and L5 spinous processes during flexion. In the presence of good spinal mobility, one will normally see approximately a one-inch spread of these fingertips when the patient demonstrates an adequate reversal of the normal lumbar lordosis. If mobility of the lumbar spine is poor, little or no apparent separation of the fingertips occurs.

Limited flexion may occur when any lumbar spine dysfunction associated with paraspinal muscle spasm, such as lumbar disc protrusions or hypertrophic spurring. Occasionally, flexion can be performed quite freely without limitation or discomfort; but on attempting to resume the erect position, the patient may feel increased discomfort. If, in association with this finding, hyperextension of the spine produces increased pain, the differential diagnosis should include stenotic lumbar spinal canal, midline lumbar disc herniation, or lumbar neoplasm.

Rotation and lateral flexion are not specifically affected by any of the more common lesions causing low back or sciatic pain. Such movements may be limited as a result of extensive paraspinal muscle spasm, which would tend to limit any mobility of the lumbar spine. This is a specific finding in iliac-transverse process pseudoarthrosis.

When a specific movement produces either pain in the back or sciatic radiation, determine as accurately as possible the exact location and nature of the pain so produced.

The range of mobility of the lumbar spine is not usually recorded in degrees but as normal, or slightly, moderately, or markedly limited.

4. Squatting. The patient is asked to squat with complete flexion of the knees and hips (Fig. 3-5). Does this action cause pain in the low back or does it cause pain in hip or knee joints? If dysfunction is present involving the knee or hip, this movement is usually pain producing at the site of the pathology.

5. Reflexes. Reflex examination can be carried out with the patient in a sitting position. If the deep tendon reflexes are difficult to elicit, they can sometimes be

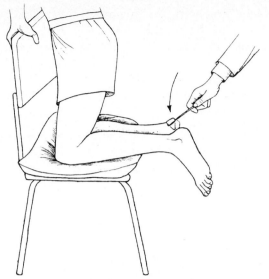

Fig. 3-7. Comparison of Achilles reflexes is best done with patient kneeling on a cushioned chair.

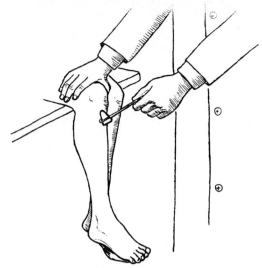

Fig. 3-8. Comparison of patellar reflexes is best done with the legs hanging freely over the edge of an examining table or bed.

brought out by various forms of reinforcement. Most commonly, this consists of an opposing hand pull, but almost any muscular activity can be used which will direct the patient's concentration away from the area to be tested (Fig. 3-6).

If the ankle jerks cannot be elicited or if there is difficulty in doing so, kneeling the patient on a cushioned chair with reinforcement is usually helpful (Fig. 3-7).

A diminished or absent patellar jerk usually implicates the L3 or L4 nerve root, while a diminished or absent ankle jerk implicates the S1 nerve root (Fig. 3-8).

6. Leg Length. Measure leg length from the anterosuperior iliac spine to the medial malleolus. Occasionally, a patient with low back pain derives relief from use of a shoe lift on the short side.

7. Sensation. Test sensation with a wisp of cotton for light touch, and the gently applied sharp end of a pin for pain. If the patient has no subjective appreciation of paresthesia, the examiner is less likely to elicit a dermatomal sensory impairment. Occasionally, even when one of the primary complaints is annoying paresthesia extending into a specific dermatomal distribution,

a most careful examination will not demonstrate any objective change. When mapping out a sensory dermatome, it is useful to go from the zone of numbness toward the area of sensitivity.

Because of the considerable variation in dermatomal patterns, there are no charts of the dermatomes that can be considered absolute (Fig. 3-9). It is generally agreed that the lateral portion of the foot is subserved by the S1 root, and that the dorsum of the foot extending toward the great toe is subserved by the L5 root. Beyond this stage, the dermatomal charts become more disparate.

8. Motor Strength. Loss of lower extremity muscle tone is determined by palpating the quadriceps and calf muscles, with the patient in the erect position, to elicit any significant differences in muscle mass or tone.

Measurement of thigh and calf circumference is carried out with the patient laying supine and the muscles relaxed. The thigh circumference is measured at a specific distance above the upper pole of the patella and compared with similar measurements on the opposite leg. The calf circumference is measured in one leg at the level of estimated

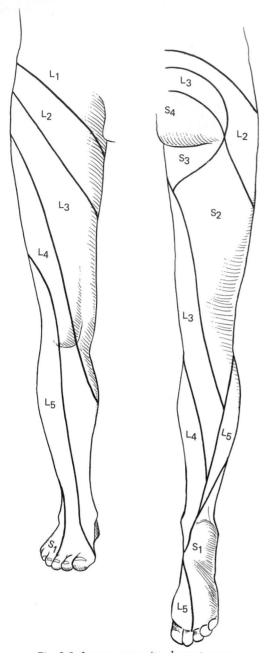

Fig. 3-9. Lower extremity dermatomes.

body, first with the presumed normal thigh and then the suspected one.

Flexion and extension strength of the knee joint can also be tested with the patient in a sitting position with both feet free of the floor (Figs. 3-10 and 3-11). The examiner

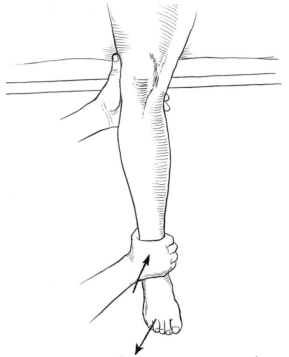

Fig. 3-10. Testing knee joint extensor strength.

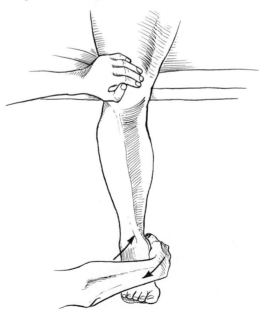

Fig. 3-11. Testing knee joint flexor strength.

greatest circumference. Then, using the same distance from that point to the tibial tuberosity, the opposite calf is measured.

To determine flexion and extension power of the knee joint, the patient grasps the back of a chair or tabletop to maintain balance and attempts squatting and elevating the

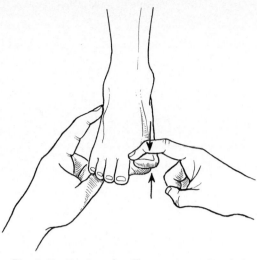

Fig. 3-12. Testing dorsiflexion strength of the great toe.

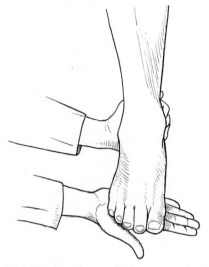

Fig. 3-13. Testing plantar flexion strength of the ankle.

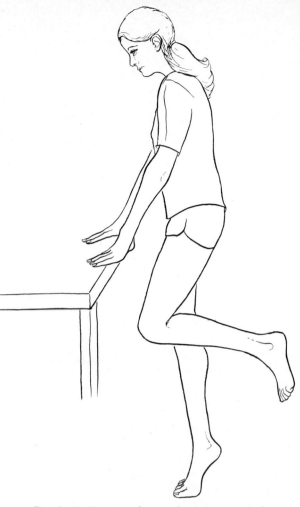

Fig. 3-14. Testing plantar flexion strength by comparing ability to bear weight on toes of each foot.

grasps one ankle at a time and asks the patient to flex and extend the knee joint against resistance.

Test dorsiflexion strength of the great toe and foot (Fig. 3-12). Normally the average patient should be able to dorsiflex the foot despite moderate opposition of the examiner. Weakness of these muscles implicates the L5 and sometimes the L4 nerve roots.

Plantar flexion of the ankle can usually be maintained by the average patient despite moderate resistance (Fig. 3-13). The muscles involved in this movement are primarily subserved by the S1 nerve root (Fig. 3-14).

Larger muscles are usually subserved by more than one nerve root. The quadriceps muscle, which is innervated by the L3, L4, and L5 roots, would be less affected by a single root lesion than the extensor hallucis longus, which is primarily innervated by the L5 root. The gastrocnemius, also a larger muscle, is innervated by the S1 and S2 roots so that although some weakness may be caused by S1 root involvement, it is not as apparent as the extensor hallucis longus. Gluteal muscle weakness may be present

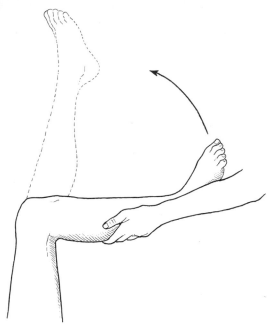

Fig. 3-15. The Lasègue test.

and is usually apparent by comparative inspection and palpation of the buttocks while the patient is in a standing position.

9. Straight Leg Raising. The straight leg raising test is often mistakingly identified as the Lasègue sign (Fig. 3-15). Ernest Charles Lasègue, who wrote a paper in 1864 commenting upon the physical signs of patients with sciatic neuritis, described the following test.[39] With the patient supine he flexed both the knee and hip; after the hip had been flexed to 90 degrees, he slowly extended the knee, producing severe pain in the patient suffering from sciatica. The Lasègue is less valuable than the straight leg raising test, since the movements of two joints are involved, causing increased difficulty in interpretation.

The more valuable straight leg raising test was first described by J. J. Forst, a pupil of Lasègue, 17 years later. This test is done with the patient lying supine. The examiner elevates the straight leg to approximately 90 degrees, which would normally cause no discomfort other than a feeling of tightness behind the knees and in the hamstrings. Straight leg raising performed in the presence

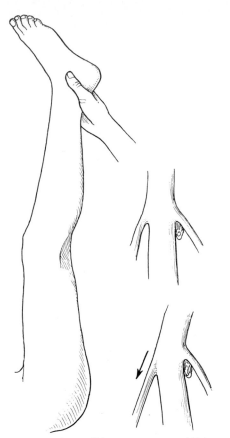

Fig. 3-16. The well-leg-raising test of Fajerstajn.

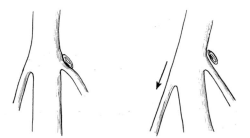

Fig. 3-17. Mechanism of pain relief with straight leg raising of the unaffected leg.

of sciatica caused by nerve root pressure will produce severe pain in the back, in the sciatic distribution of the affected leg, or in both. As a rule, with unilateral root involvement, straight leg raising is diminished on the affected side. In some cases, where the root pressure is extensive as a result of a sizable disc protrusion within the "axilla" between the spinal dura and the exiting root

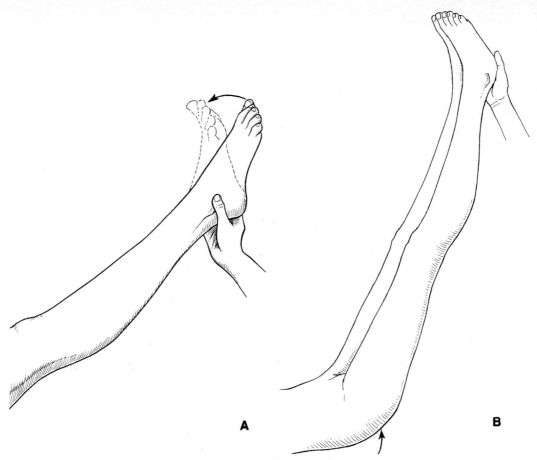

Fig. 3-18. (A) Confirmation of sciatica. (B) Raising both legs together produces an upward tilt of the pelvis and diminishes the desired angulation of straight leg raising.

sleeve, straight leg raising of the unaffected leg may aggravate pain in the involved leg. This phenomenon, which is sometimes identified as the well leg raising test of Fajerstajn (Fig. 3-16), occurs when elevation of the unaffected leg causes a tug on the cauda equina and presses the already compromised root against the protruding disc.[25]

On the other hand, when sciatic pain is caused by a laterally placed disc protrusion, straight leg raising of the unaffected leg may act to relieve root compression and so to reduce sciatic pain (Fig. 3-17).

If the straight leg raising test appears to be positive, sciatica can be confirmed by lowering the raised leg an inch or two until the pain is no longer present and pushing the foot into dorsiflexion. This will produce a recurrence of pain. In carrying out this confirmation test, pain produced by ligamentous or muscle pull is ruled out, since it is presumed that dorsiflexion of the ankle will stretch the sciatic nerve by tightening the posterior tibial branch of this nerve.

When performing the straight leg raising test, each leg should be tested separately, since when both legs are raised together, an upward tilt of the pelvis occurs, diminishing the desired angulation of straight leg raising (Fig. 3-18). The straight leg raising test is recorded in degrees, 90 degrees being considered normal. In addition, one should record the location and intensity of pain produced by this maneuver.

When straight leg raising is painful, the popliteal pressure sign may also be helpful

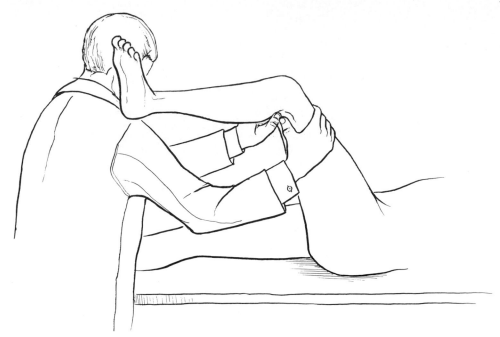

Fig. 3-19. Popliteal pressure sign. Raise straight leg until pain is elicited and then flex the knee sufficiently to ease the pain. Sudden firm pressure over the sciatic nerve in the popliteal fossa will produce sciatica or low back pain in the pressure of nerve root tension.

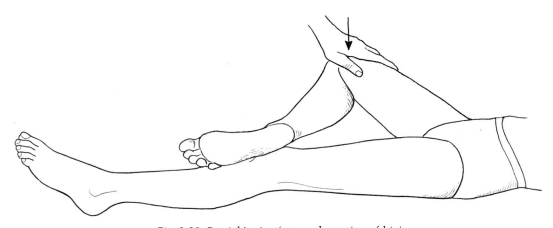

Fig. 3-20. Patrick's sign (external rotation of hip).

in confirming nerve root irritation (Fig. 3-19). This is easily done by maintaining hip angulation at the level where straight leg raising pain was appreciated, and allowing the knee to flex slightly to the point where pain eases. With the elevated heel resting on the examiner's shoulder, place both thumbs in the popliteal fossa and exert a sudden, firm pressure over the sciatic nerve. Produc-

tion of low back or sciatic pain is indicative of nerve root involvement.

10. Hip Rotation. Internal and external rotation of the hip is performed to rule out hip disease (Figs. 3-20 and 3-21). External rotation was originally described by Hugh Talbot Patrick, a Chicago neurologist, and is carried out with the patient supine. The

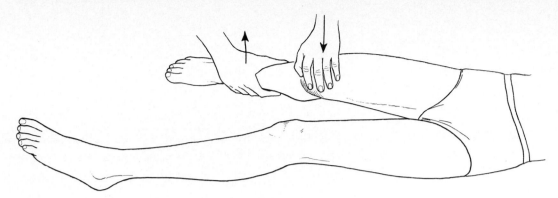

Fig. 3-21. Internal rotation of hip.

thigh and knee are flexed, the external malleolus is placed over the patella of the opposite leg, and the knee is forcibly depressed. If pain is produced by this maneuver, hip disease is indicated. Doctor Patrick originally called this test, the "fabere sign," from the initial letters of movements necessary to elicit it: namely, flexion, abduction, external rotation, and extension.

Internal rotation of the hip produces distraction of the sacroiliac joint and, if painful, may be compatible with sacroiliac dysfunction.

11. Spinal Pressure. With the patient in the prone position, pressure is exerted over the spinous processes of the lumbar spine and sacrum. No tenderness should be elicited over the sacrum, unless neoplasm involving the sacrum or nonorganic disease is present. In the presence of nerve root pressure and irritation, paraspinal pressure on the side of involvement at the affected interspace may cause a twinge of sciatic pain.

12. Arterial Pulses. Every patient who is suspected of having sciatica should have a careful examination of the arterial pulses in the inguinal, popliteal, and dorsalis pedis sites. It is rarely difficult to differentiate vascular occlusive disease from sciatica, but confusion in this regard can occur and may not only be embarrassing to the physician but also be a considerable detriment to the patient.

PART II

Electrodiagnostic Studies in Low Back Pain

LAWRENCE GREEN

Historical Perspective

Electrodiagnostic techniques provide a physiological avenue for evaluation of patients with motor and sensory disorders. These techniques are subdivided generally into methods for measurement of nerve conduction velocity (NCV) and the specific study of muscle known as electromyography (EMG).

The foundations for the study of the electrical activity of nerve and muscle can be traced to the work of Luigi Galvani in the late 18th century. Galvani first demonstrated the natural presence of electricity and the association of electricity with muscular contraction in frog muscle. The first application of *in situ* electrical stimulation of muscles in humans, however, was developed by Duchenne in the 1860s. The development in the middle 19th century of sensitive galvanometers allowed a more accurate demonstration of the small electrical potentials generated by electrically active human tissues (nerve and muscle).

As investigations progressed, the concept of electrical excitation as the initiating factor for muscle contraction was developed and sub-stantiated in the laboratory. It was also demonstrated at this time that electrical stimulation of peripheral nerves resulted in predictable contraction of appropriately innervated muscles.

In the early 1900s, Sherrington developed the concept of the motor unit, joining the motor neuron of the spinal cord via its axon to the nerve terminals in the muscle fibers; and the reflex arc which added a receptor organ, an afferent neuron, and a path in the central nervous system to join with the motor neuron (Fig. 3-22). He also introduced the term **synapse** to describe the contact between the two neurons. In 1929, Adrian and Bronk provided a major technical advance with development of the concentric needle electrode to permit accurate appreciation of electrical potentials within the muscle itself. The previous techniques had recorded only from the surface of the muscle. A report in 1938 by Denny-Brown and Pennypacker cleared much of the confusion about the spontaneous activity of denervated muscle (fibrillations). The appreciation of the characteristics and origins of such spontaneous activity was basic for understanding the EMG changes in denervation.

The study of NCV can be dated to the work

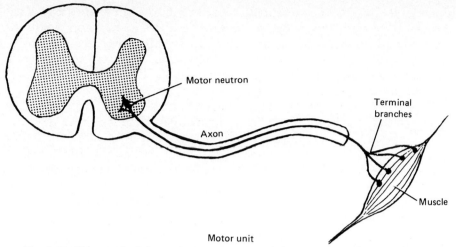

Fig. 3-22. Motor unit. Schematic representation of the motor unit showing the anterior horn cell, the long myelinated axon (peripheral nerve), nerve terminals, and muscle.

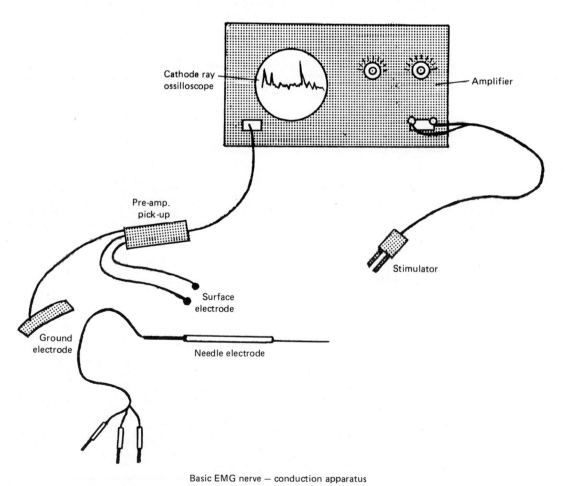

Basic EMG nerve — conduction apparatus

Fig. 3-23. Basic apparatus for electromyelogram-nerve conduction (EMG-NC) study.

of VonHelmholtz in the 1850s, who measured motor nerve conduction with reasonable accuracy in experimental animals and in humans. It was not until the 1930s however, that NCVs in sensory and motor nerves were accurately recorded and published, and it was the middle 1940s when Hodes reported reliable use of motor nerve conduction techniques in assessment of normal and injured peripheral nerves. In 1956, Simpson further defined methods for localization of nerve conduction delay using motor nerve conduction studies in patients with carpal tunnel syndrome.

Work by Buchthal, Kugelberg, Lambert, Desmedt, and many others developed methods for differentiation of nerve disorders from those of primary muscle origin. Techniques for repetitive stimulation of peripheral nerve in diagnosis of disorders of neuromuscular transmission were demonstrated in the 1960s, and further development of methods for studying individual muscle fiber characteristics utilizing special electrodes and improved methods of data storage and display has evolved (Fig. 3-23).

More recent technical advances have provided improved display of electrical data through use of computer storage banks, averaging techniques, computer analysis of EMG characteristics, and somatosensory cerebral-evoked potentials.

This rapid development of electrophysiological technique has moved neurodiagnostic methods from the research laboratory into the routine clinical laboratory where they assist in evaluation of patients with common clinical nerve and muscle disorders.

Basic Anatomy and Pathophysiology

The anatomical basis of EMG and nerve conduction involves the study of the motor unit. As stated above, this consists of the anterior horn motor neuron, its myelinated axon, terminal branches, myoneurojunction, and end organ muscle fibers. EMG is the study of the muscle fibers themselves by means of fine needle electrodes which are used to sample multiple areas of the specific muscle fibers in question. Knowledge of the muscular anatomy, patterns of segmental innervation, and understanding of muscle kinesiology are essential for performance and interpretation of this technique. Motor nerve injuries at all levels (cell body to distal axon) are reflected in the end organ (muscle), although sufficient time for axonal degeneration is required before positive changes can be detected. This usually requires 10 to 14 days from the initial insult. Consequently, timing of the study in relationship to the time of onset of symptoms is crucial.

Electromyography

The EMG study itself begins with the insertion of the recording needle electrode. At this point the electromyographer searches for signs of spontaneous muscle activity. These signs of nerve injury appear in the form of fibrillation potentials and positive sharp waves (denervation potentials). The next step in the study involves voluntary contraction of the muscles with visual analysis of the shape and dimensions of the elicited motor unit potentials (Fig. 3-24). Normal potentials display two to four phases of excursion above and below an arbitrary base line. Abnormal potentials exceed four phases and are called polyphasic units. With increase in the number of phases in these

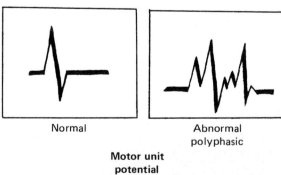

Normal   Abnormal polyphasic

Motor unit potential

Individual units

Fig. 3-24. Individual motor units. Schematic example of cathode ray ossilloscope display of normal and abnormal (polyphasic) motor units.

so-called neuropathic units, there is also an increase in duration of the potential. This characteristic provides differentiation from the short-duration polyphasic potentials seen in the myopathies.

Maximum voluntary contraction is then encouraged to study the recruitment of additional motor units. Maximum effort should produce a high-voltage, high-frequency display known as the interference pattern (Fig. 3-25). In neuropathic disease the loss of small distal fibers, sprouting of new fibers from remaining nerve slips, and reinnervation of the abandoned muscle fibers results in a decrease in the number of motor units and an increase in the size of the surviving units. This explains the long-duration polyphasic individual motor units. The decreased number of units is presented on the EMG screen in the form of gaps or a reduction in the completeness of the interference pattern. The display of neuropathic changes in muscles which anatomically conform to a single peripheral nerve or spinal segment has obvious diagnostic value. Furthermore, the demonstration of neuropathic changes diffusely or in only distal muscles without a segmental pattern indicated polyneuropathy rather than single nerve or root injury.

Nerve Conduction Studies

The direct electrical stimulation of peripheral motor nerves allows for measurement of motor NCV over the course of accessible nerves (Fig. 3-26). A sufficiently long superficial course of the nerve to be studied is necessary, as well as a readily defined distal innervated muscle which can be used as the motor end point. The direct electrical stimulation of the peripheral nerve produces a predictable electrical response in the pickup muscle. Stimulation distally and proximally along the course of this nerve allows for calculation of the motor conduction velocity in the intermediate segment. Peripheral nerves whose anatomical characteristics lend themselves to this method

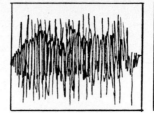 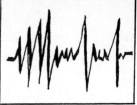

| Full normal interference pattern | Incomplete interference pattern |

Maximum contraction

Fig. 3-25. Interference Pattern. Schematic cathode ray ossilloscope display of normal and abnormal (incomplete) response to maximal muscle contraction.

include the peroneal and tibial nerves in the lower extremities and the median and ulnar nerves in the arms. The sciatic, femoral, and radial nerves may also be studied but with more difficulty and less reproducible results.

Demyelinative nerve injury produces the most significant slowing of NCV. Pure axonal disorders without significant loss of myelin may result in normal NCVs. (EMG, however, will demonstrate features of neuropathic change.) There is considerable variation in the range of normal nerve conduction values from laboratory to laboratory, and the velocities in the upper extremities tend to be faster than those in the legs. Generally, motor conduction velocity less than 41 to 44 meters per second (approximately 20% reduction from normal) should be considered abnormal, assuming room temperature operation. Cold produces a predictable slowing of NCV. In peripheral nerve disorders, conduction velocity is usually affected early and significantly. This is especially true with distal lesions as in compression of the peroneal nerve at the fibular head. Conversely, proximal neuropathic disorders such as radiculopathy and anterior horn cell disease produce distal myelin changes only very late, if at all, and so motor NCVs are usually normal.

Sensory conduction studies are performed by stimulating distal pure sensory fibers and recording the potential passing proximally

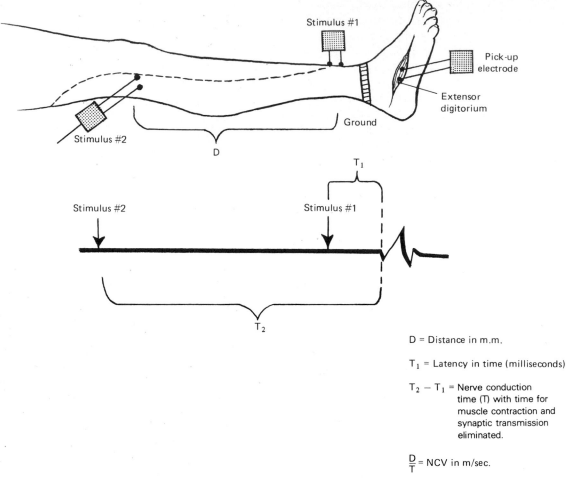

D = Distance in m.m.

T_1 = Latency in time (milliseconds)

$T_2 - T_1$ = Nerve conduction time (T) with time for muscle contraction and synaptic transmission eliminated.

$\dfrac{D}{T}$ = NCV in m/sec.

Fig. 3-26. Technique for motor nerve conduction velocity (NCV), in the peroneal nerve.

(orthodromic) (Fig. 3-27). Antidromic potentials may also be studied, but these are less specific since motor fibers are also included. Sensory-evoked potentials are typically studied in the upper extremities by stimulating the digital nerves and recording over the ulnar and median nerves at superficial sites. In the legs, the sural nerve can be studied but with more difficulty and less reliability. New techniques for measurement of sensory-evoked potentials elicited in the digital nerves of the toes require computer averaging and are just becoming clinically applicable. Sensory conduction is more sensitive than motor velocity for detection of early demyelination of peripheral nerve, providing careful technique is observed. Sensory-

evoked potentials may be abnormal in proximal nerve lesions, if the dorsal root ganglion is involved and secondary demyelinative changes have occurred. This may develop more readily than in motor neuron disease owing to the small safety factor for display of the sensory-evoked potential as compared to the gross motor unit potential.

Late Responses

Late responses include "F" wave and "H" reflex (Fig. 3-28). The F wave appears to be a "backfiring" of anterior horn cells, elicited by distal stimulation of a motor nerve. When these inconstant responses can be evoked

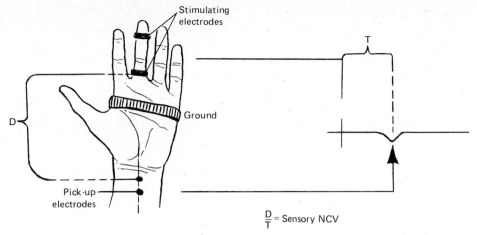

Fig. 3-27. *Technique for sensory-evoked potential and measurement of sensory CV, in the median nerve.*

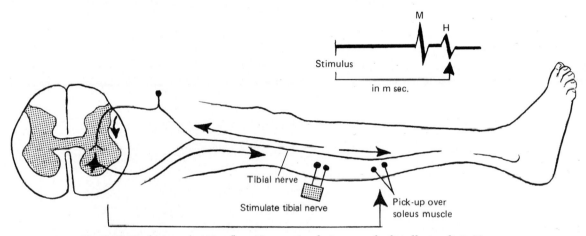

Fig. 3-28. *Technique for H reflex. Nerve stimulation travels distally to elicit M-wave and proximally across monosynaptic pathway and returns to soleus muscle to evoke later H-wave.*

they can offer a means of measurement of proximal NCV. These responses are more readily and reliably induced in the upper extremities than in the lower extremities. The H reflex is the electrophysiological representation of the monosynaptic reflex. This is most reliably elicited in the lower extremities by stimulation of the tibial nerve and can be used to assess a component comparable to the ankle jerk for comparison of symmetry and presence or absence of response.

Neurological Examination

It should be stressed that electrodiagnostic techniques can be utilized only in conjunction with careful clinical neurological examination. This should be the first step in the performance of the EMG-NC study. A careful history must be taken. Observation of muscle bulk, trophic changes, and local limb characteristics must be noted. Careful examination of the deep tendon reflexes and examination for pathological reflexes are obvious components. Careful specific muscle testing must be performed for development of the clinical conclusion and direction for the sites of EMG examination. The sensory examination is of course essential and gives important clues for the differentiation of peripheral nerve from root or plexis lesions.

Limitations of EMG

The limitations of electrodiagnostic techniques include the following:

1. Limited information regarding the etiology of the abnormality
2. Persistence of neuropathic changes after clinical improvement
3. The necessity for a skilled and experienced examiner to perform the study

The persistence of neuropathic changes makes dating of the time of onset of the disorder unreliable. The necessary delay of 7 to 14 days before the appearance of neuropathic changes adds another problem which must be considered in evaluation of the results of EMG. Nerve conduction studies, on the other hand, usually show impaired conduction early in the course of nerve injury (3 to 5 days). Improvement in velocity, although delayed compared to the clinical response, usually accompanies recovery. Finally, it should be appeciated that EMG cannot be relied upon for definite localization of the exact level of root compression, as demonstrated by studies comparing results of EMG, myelography, and surgical exploration.

It must be understood also that these techniques may be unpleasant and painful. It is important that the patient cooperate fully with the electromyographer to obtain a complete and accurate result. Patients with severe pain, low pain threshold, excessive

Table 3-1. TYPICAL EMG-NC FINDINGS IN COMMON NERVE MUSCLE PROBLEMS

	Nerve Conduction	EMG	F Wave H Reflex
Peripheral Neuropathy	*Abnormal:* Slow velocity if demyelinative	*Abnormal:* Long duration polyphasic units; May be fibrillations and positive waves; Incomplete interference pattern	Often abnormal
Entrapment Neuropathy	*Abnormal:* Slow velocity; May be unobtainable	Abnormal only after 14 to 21 days	Abnormal if applicable
Proximal Neuropathy (Radiculopathy)	Usually normal	*Abnormal:* Long duration polyphasic units; May be fibrillations and positive waves; Incomplete interference pattern	May be abnormal
Anterior Horn Cell Disorders	Usually normal	*Abnormal:* Fasciculations, fibrillations, and positive waves; Very large polyphasic units; Incomplete interference pattern	May be abnormal
Upper Motor Neuron Disorders	Normal	*Normal:* Interference pattern may be incomplete	May be abnormal
Muscle Disorders	Normal	*Abnormal:* Short duration, high frequency, polyphasic units; Complete low amplitude interference pattern; Occasional fibrillations	Normal

anxiety, or conflicting emotional symptoms may not be able to participate fully in the examination and the result will be an incomplete or inconclusive study. Instruction and preparation of the patient by the referring physician will often improve the likelihood of a successful evaluation (Table 3-1).

An understanding of the capabilities and limitations of electrodiagnostic techniques will permit intelligent interpretation of the results. Ideally all electrodiagnostic techniques should be employed in an individual study for maximal yield of information. The demonstration of neuropathic EMG findings in a clear segmental pattern should suggest proximal root localization. Further finding of denervation potentials in paraspinous EMG would point to involvement of posterior primary radicals as additional evidence of a proximal neuropathic process. Normal motor conduction velocities would further indicate a proximal rather than distal site of the disorder. Conversely, fibrillations and polyphasic motor unit potentials on needle EMG with slow NCVs would indicate peripheral neuropathy, especially if diffuse and nonsegmental in location. Sensory and late responses should be appreciated to reinforce or support one or the other localization. A normal EMG and nerve conduction would exclude significant neuropathic disorder at any level, but need not rule out ligamentous muscular or osseous cause of pain.

In using these methods for assessment of patients with lumbar disc protrusion syndrome, certain generalizations are valid. A normal EMG excludes radiculopathy and so should direct the physician's attention to musculoskeletal causes of lower extremity pain such as hip disease. When the EMG is abnormal, precise interspace localization can never be as definite as demonstrated by contrast radiological methods, owing to anatomic variation in muscle innervation and nerve root interspace. Patients with sciatic syndromes primarily related to peripheral neuropathy of vascular, metabolic, or post-traumatic etiology will demonstrate specific abnormalities on nerve conduction study and allow differentiation from nerve root involvement caused by disc disease.

PART I

Introduction

Careful study of plain lumbosacral spine x-ray films is routinely carried out by almost all physicians in clinical evaluation of the patient with low back pain and sciatica. Certain conditions, such as fractures, dislocations, infections, tumors, and certain metabolic diseases, are clearly seen on x-ray film and will enable the clinician to demonstrate roentgenographically the specific cause of back pain. These entities account for a small portion of the backache patients encountered in a general hospital population. In the vast majority of patients, the specific cause of low back symptomatology is not clearly demonstrated by roentgenograms.

Retrograde Reasoning

The physician is trained to document symptomatology with objective evidence relating to the etiology of the symptoms. A patient manifesting symptoms of low back symptomatology with anatomical variations of the lumbar spine demonstrated by x-ray film induces the physician to rely upon a form of retrograde reasoning in which he seizes upon this anatomical variant and des-

ignates it as the cause of the patient's problems. Opportunities to compare spine films of patients with and without back pain are limited, because persons without low back dysfunction rarely have roentgenograms of the spine. One of the first papers to bring this to our attention was written by Dr. C. A. Splitoff.[55] Since that time, a number of other investigators have demonstrated a discrepancy between factual knowledge and the physician's inclination to attribute low back symptoms to a number of anatomical variations which have been demonstrated roentgenographically.[22,32,33]

Common Roentgenographic Abnormalities

A review of some of the common roentgenographic abnormalities noted on lumbar spine x-ray film and a discussion of their clinical significance follow (Fig. 4-1).

Transitional Vertebrae

By transitional vertebrae we mean either a sacralized lumbar vertebra or a lumbarized sacral vertebra. This anatomical variant oc-

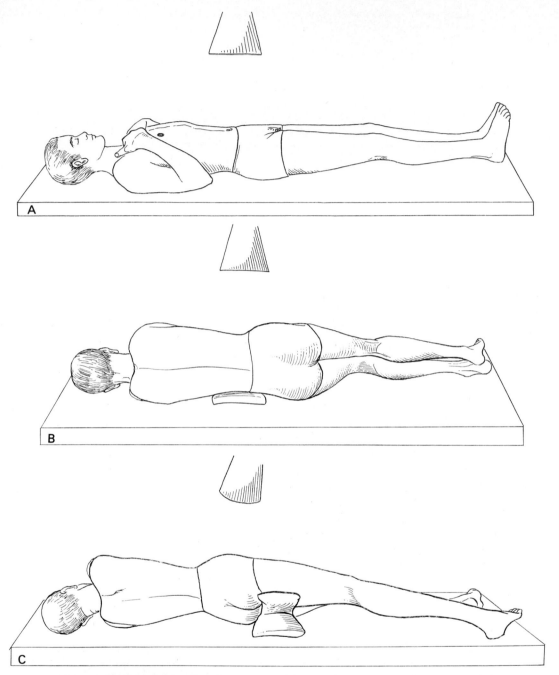

Fig. 4-1. **(A)** AP roentgenographic position. **(B)** Lateral roentgenographic position. **(C)** Left posterior oblique roentgenographic position.

curs in 5% to 7% of the population as a whole.[17] Some physicians give considerable importance to this roentgenographic finding and believe it is associated with an increased incidence of low back dysfunction. One in-

dustrial physician actually considers this finding sufficient grounds to prevent an employee applicant from carrying out heavy duties. However, there are no statistics to demonstrate a significantly increased incidence of low back dysfunction with transitional vertebrae; from my own experience, I feel that there is no direct relationship.

Spina Bifida

With the posterior elements either partially or completely absent, one might anticipate some loss of stability, which would normally be furnished by the muscle and tendinous attachments to these missing posterior elements. Available statistics, however, do not indicate an increased incidence of back pain. This finding is compatible with my personal experience.

Increased Lumbar Lordosis

The patient with chronic lumbosacral strain traditionally has been noted to have an increased lumbar lordosis. This finding is also present in patients with a protuberant abdomen due either to pregnancy or to obesity. What statistics we do have in the population as a whole are equivocal but may indicate that this is more than an incidental finding and that these conditions could conceivably be related to an increased incidence of low back pain.

Scoliosis

When a physician sees a patient with low back pain, and the x-ray films show a scoliosis in the lumbodorsal area, he cannot help considering a direct relationship between what is seen on the films and the presenting symptoms. However, a significant discrepancy in this line of reasoning is demonstrated by the fact that scoliosis clinics in which predominantly young patients are seen have a remarkable infrequency of low back complaints in their patients. There is no question that the intervertebral disc at the apex of the scoliosis has an increased tendency toward degeneration, since it is at the site of greatest stress. Despite this fact, statistics are not clear regarding the incidence of back pain in long-range studies of scoliotic patients.

The severity of the scoliosis probably is significant as the patient ages. A lumbar scoliosis greater than 80 degrees may be associated with an increased incidence of low back pain.

Intervertebral Disc Narrowing

Narrowing at the L5 to S1 interspace is a relatively common finding in patients over the age of 50. There is certainly a very direct relationship between such narrowing and age. Degenerative changes at the disc interspace are also associated with this finding. Less commonly, one sees roentgenographic evidence of disc degeneration and narrowing at the L4–5 interspace, and this is seen even less frequently above that level. There does seem to be a definite relationship between such findings and an increased tendency toward low back pain. However, one must keep in mind the fact that a large number of patients with these incidental findings do not have low back dysfunction.

Pars Defects

Defects in the pars interarticularis are associated with an increased incidence of low back pain. This condition increases the mechanical stress upon the intervertebral disc and may be followed by disc degeneration, producing increased stress upon the annulus fibrosis and a greater tendency toward low back dysfunction.

Asymmetrical Lumbosacral Facets

The condition of asymmetrical lumbosacral facets has been called tropism, which derives from the Greek word tropē, meaning turning. When one of the lumbosacral facets is in a more coronal plane than the other, an abnormal rotary motion acts on the annulus in addition to the normal flexion and extension movements. The torque stress on the annulus is increased and is probably associated with an earlier breakdown, since rotational stresses are not as well tolerated by the lumbar discs as are flexion and extension.

Osteoarthritis

Hypertrophic osteoarthritis of the lumbar spine is associated with an increased incidence of low back pain.[10] However, it must be emphasized that many people with osteoarthritis do not have a great deal of pain. Spine x-ray films of the vast majority of elderly patients in rest homes or nursing homes will reveal rather advanced hypertrophic osteoarthritic changes, yet most of these patients do not have low back pain.

Spondylolisthesis

The condition of spondylolisthesis is definitely associated with an increased incidence of low back pain. An individual with spondylolisthesis may be symptom free until a specific body action or relatively mild trauma will trigger a severe low back syndrome. These incapacitating symptoms may be rather persistent and may seem disproportionate to the relatively innocuous trauma that initiated the illness.

PART II

Roentgenographic Anatomy of the Lumbar Vertebrae

HOWARD J. BARNHARD
DOYNE DODD, JR.

Roentgenographic anatomy of the vertebral column is difficult to learn because the complex parts overlap and appear quite different in various conventional views. Indeed, it is probably safe to assume that many observers either have significant misconceptions about the anatomy of this region or look at only a limited portion of a vertebra in each view because of their uncertainty about the anatomy.

The objective of this study was to facilitate the learning process by presenting vertebral anatomy in a step-by-step fashion. Serendipitously, new information was gained about the contribution of different structures to the images seen in various conventional views.

This article will demonstrate the contribution that each part of the lumbar vertebra makes to the roentgenographic image as seen in the anteroposterior view, the lateral view, the left anterior oblique view, and the right anterior oblique view.

Technique

The lumbar vertebrae were chosen for study because they are representative of the majority of vertebrae and do not have specialized features. Also, the lumbar vertebrae are sturdy and are easily dissected.

The three vertebrae illustrated in this article are L2, L3, and L4 from a woman. They were placed in as exact an anatomic position as possible and were joined with a fast-setting resin. Single vertebrae were also studied; they are not shown because of the limitations of space. The vertebrae were held in position by an apparatus that permitted rotation of the subject with stops every 45 degrees.

Parts were meticulously removed from the L3 using a high-speed electric tool that had assorted attachments for cutting and abrading. Following the removal of each part, roentgenographs and photographs were made in the anteroposterior, the lateral, the left anterior oblique, and the right anterior oblique position. The x-ray tube, which had a 1-mm focal spot, was 6 feet from the subject, and the subject was 2 inches from the film. The best contrast and detail were obtained with 90 kvp, 5 ma, and a 6-second exposure. Kodak Industrex M Film was used to make direct roentgenographic exposures.

Discussion

The roentgenograms made at each step of the study are reproduced as Figures 4-2 to 4-13. They are not, however, presented in the order in which they were made. Instead, the chronologic order has been reversed. Roentgenographs of the two intact vertebrae with the dissected vertebral body between

(Text continues on p. 84.)

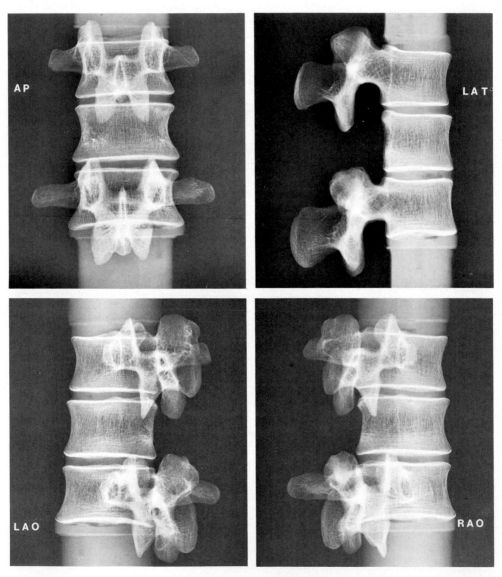

Fig. 4-2. Dissected lumbar vertebra. L2, L3, and L4 from a woman. All appendages have been removed from L3; L2 and L4 are intact. (Barnhard HJ, Dodd D Jr: Radiographic anatomy of the lumbar vertebrae. Med Radiogr Photgr 49(1): 7–20, 1973.)

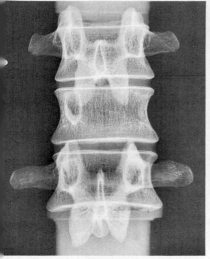
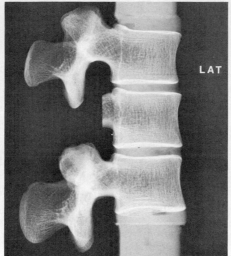
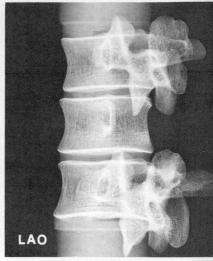
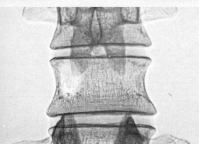
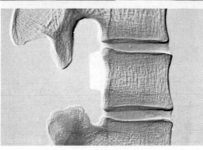
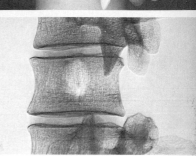
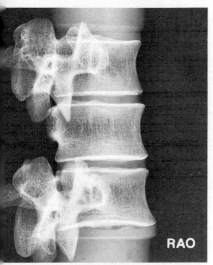

Fig. 4-3. Right pedicle. **(AP)** *The oval cortex of the pedicle is seen well, because the pedicle is tangentially oriented.* **(LAT)** *The pedicle appears relatively short.* **(LAO)** *The image of the pedicle projects through the middle of the vertebral body. The subtracted roentgenograph shows that the pedicle contributes more to the roentgenographic image than just the well-defined oval density seen in the AP view.* **(RAO)** *The image of the pedicle falls just to the right lateral margin of the vertebral body. (Barnhard HJ, Dodd D Jr: Radiographic anatomy of the lumbar vertebrae. Med Radiogr Photogr 49(1): 7–20, 1973.)*

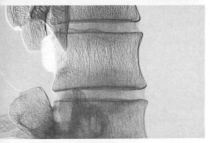

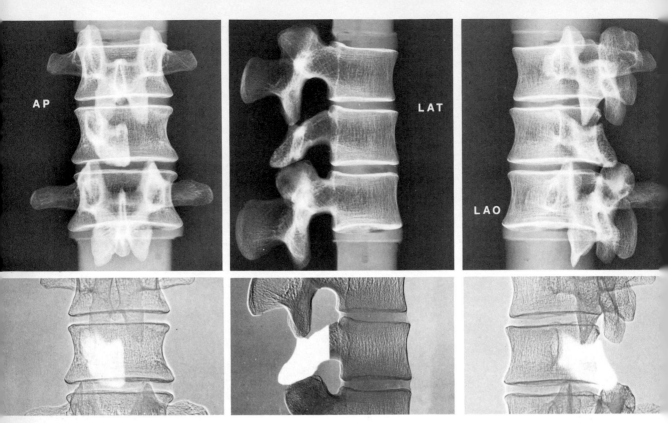

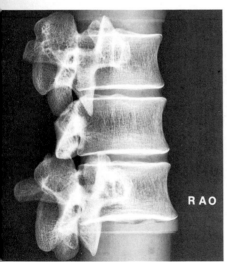

Fig. 4-4. Right lamina. **(AP)** The lamina extends medially, obliquely, and inferiorly from the right pedicle. **(LAT)** The lamina is seen in foreshortened perspective. **(LAO)** The lamina is seen best in this view. Note that the lamina does not quite abut the sharply demarcated margin of the right pedicle, a finding that substantiates the statement in Fig. 4-3 that the right pedicle contributes more to the roentgenographic image than just the oval density seen in the AP view. **(RAO)** The lamina is markedly foreshortened, and its gentle sigmoid configuration is not apparent. (Barnhard HJ, Dodd D Jr: Radiographic anatomy of the lumbar vertebrae. Med Radiogr Photgr 49(1): 7–20, 1973.)

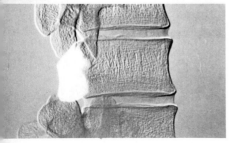

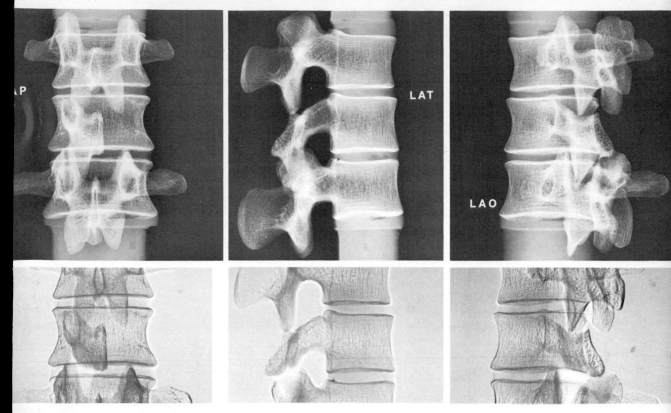

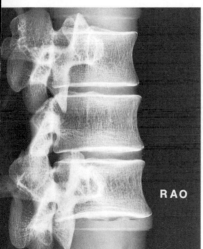

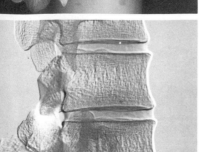

Fig. 4-5. Right inferior articular process. **(AP)** The process drops from the lamina in a perpendicular fashion, and its lateral margin begins near the midportion of the lamina. The medial margin of the process extends to the midportion of the neural arch. **(LAT)** Note the extent of posterior separation of the process from the body of the vertebra and the contribution that the process makes to the bony ring surrounding the intervertebral foramen. **(LAO)** The articulating facet of the process appears smooth and triangular. **(RAO)** Considerable overlap normally makes this area difficult to appreciate. (Barnhard HJ, Dodd D Jr: Radiographic anatomy of the lumbar vertebrae. Med Radiogr Photogr 49(1): 7–20, 1973.)

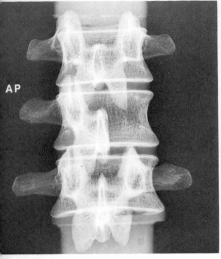

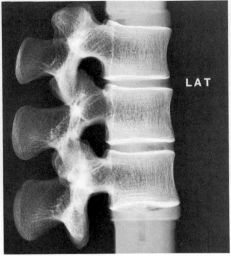

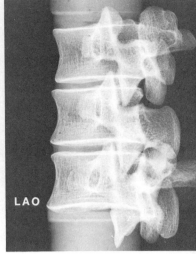

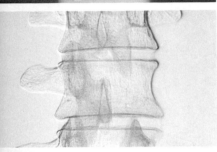

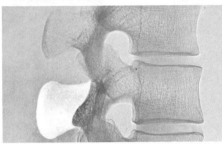

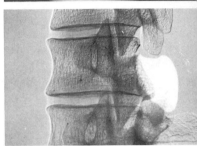

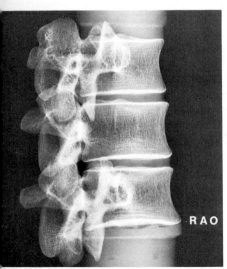

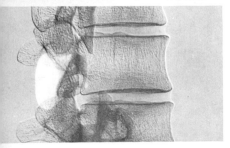

*Fig. 4-8. Spinous process. **(AP)** The process looks like a vertical teardrop in the middle of the vertebral body. Its lower margin extends inferiorly beyond the body, but not so much as the inferior articular process does. **(LAT)** The spinous process is seen best in this view because there are no overlying structures. **(LAO)** The image of the process is not superimposed on the vertebral body, but it is foreshortened. Again, note that the transverse process extends beyond it. **(RAO)** The image of the process extends beyond the vertebral body. The degree of foreshortening is about the same as in the LAO view. (Barnhard HJ, Dodd D Jr: Radiographic anatomy of the lumbar vertebrae. Med Radiogr Photogr 49(1):7–20, 1973)*

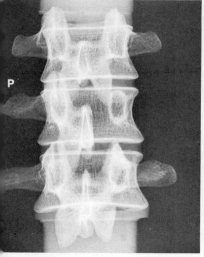

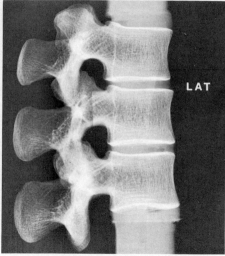

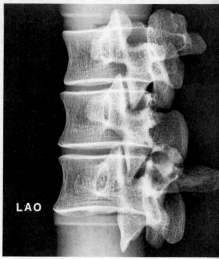

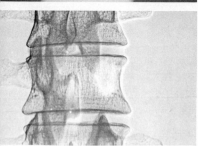

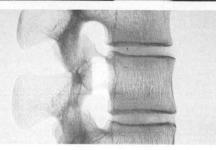

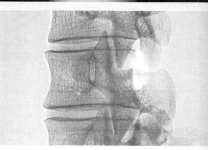

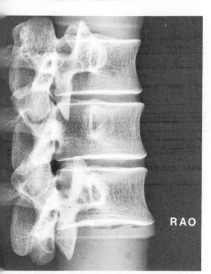

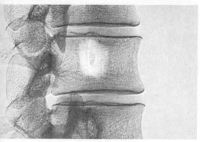

Fig. 4-9. Left pedicle. **(AP)** *The addition of the left pedicle provides symmetry with the right pedicle.* **(LAT)** *The left pedicle is almost exactly superimposed on the right pedicle.* **(LAO)** *The left pedicle extends from the vertebral body. It is partially obscured by the right lamina and the spinous process as well as by a portion of the inferior articular process of the vertebra above.* **(RAO)** *The left pedicle is seen through the middle of the vertebral body. (Barnhard HJ, Dodd D Jr: Radiographic anatomy of the lumbar vertebrae. Med Radiogr Photogr 49(1):7–20,1973)*

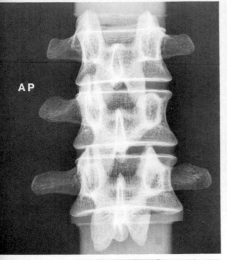
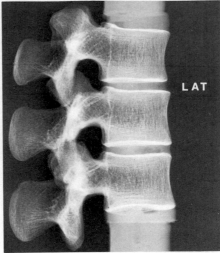
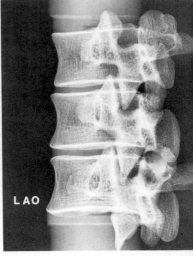
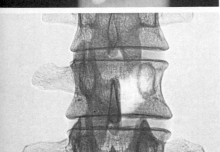
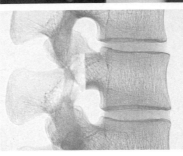
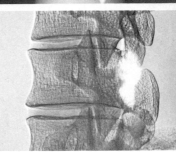
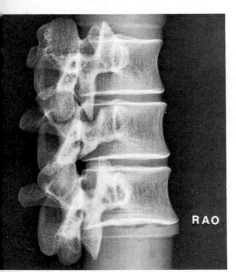
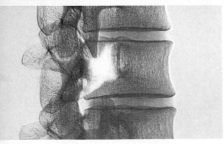

*Fig. 4-10. Left lamina. **(AP)** The left lamina presents a mirror image of the right lamina, joining the pedicle laterally and the teardrop of the spinous process medially. **(LAT)** The left lamina is superimposed on the right lamina. **(LAO)** The left lamina is quite obscured in this view by many overlying structures. **(RAO)** The left lamina is seen well through the vertebral body without interference from other overlying structures. The subtracted radiograph shows that the lamina does not quite reach the sharply delineated oval of the pedicle; this suggests that the pedicle-laminar junction is a continuum and its dissection is necessarily somewhat arbitrary. (Barnhard HJ, Dodd D Jr: Radiographic anatomy of the lumbar vertebrae. Med Radiogr Photogr 49(1):7–20,1973)*

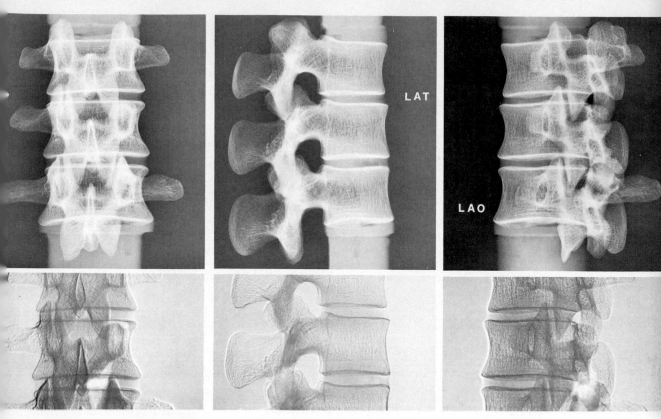

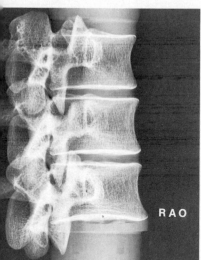

Fig. 4-11. Left inferior articular process. **(AP)** The process is readily seen extending inferiorly from the left lamina. **(LAT)** The process is superimposed on the opposite inferior articular process and is difficult to see even in subtracted radiographs. **(LAO)** The right inferior articular process is seen well, but the left extends slightly away from the vertebral body and is lost amidst the other structures. **(RAO)** The left inferior articular process is seen well here even though it overlaps the interspace. (Barnhard HJ, Dodd D Jr: Radiographic anatomy of the lumbar vertebrae. Med Radiogr Photogr 49(1):7–20,1973)

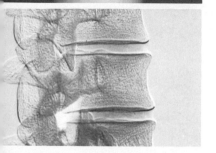

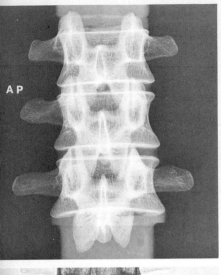
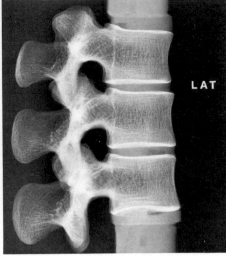
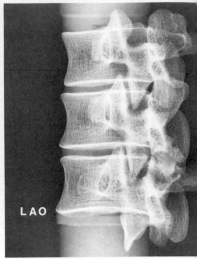

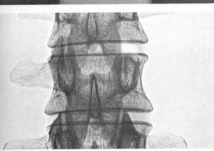
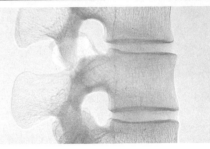
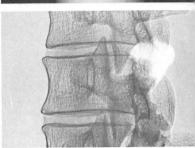

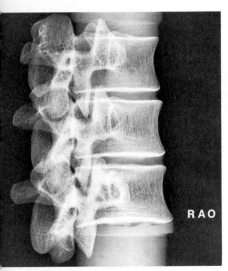

Fig. 4-12. Left superior articular process. *(AP)* The process is superior to the left pedicle, and its flat articulating facet faces medially. The facet is so short that in the subtracted radiograph one sees only a white area at the level of the interspace. *(LAT)* The left superior articular process appears fan-shaped and much larger than the process it abuts. *(LAO)* The process is almost round and stands out well amidst the overlying structures. *(RAO)* The process forms the "ear" of the Scotty dog. The "neck" of the dog is the pars interarticularis, where the defect of spondylolysis occurs. The flat articulating portion of the process is seen well in this view. (Barnhard HJ, Dodd D Jr: Radiographic anatomy of the lumbar vertebrae. Med Radiogr Photogr 49(1):7–20,1973)

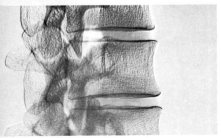

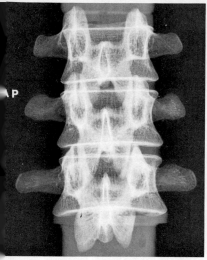

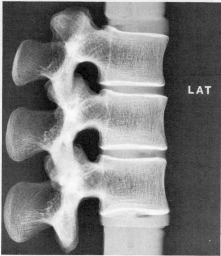

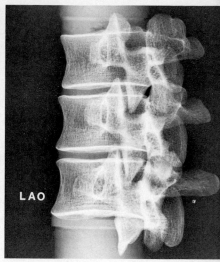

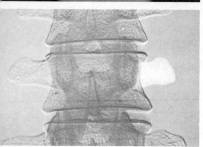

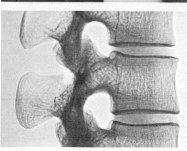

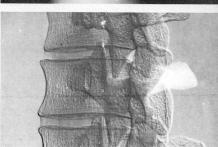

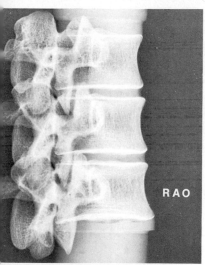

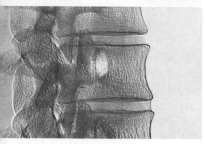

Fig. 4-13. Left transverse process. With the addition of this process, the vertebra is complete. (AP) The transverse processes are frequently somewhat asymmetric. (LAT) The left transverse process is almost indistinguishable because it is seen on end and is overlapped by other structures. Its contribution is evident only in the subtracted radiograph in which its tip is seen as a small white oval at the anterosuperior border of the spinous process. (LAO) The process is seen well as it extends beyond the other structures. (RAO) Again, note the significant contribution of this process to the anterior part of the eye of the "Scotty dog" from which it extends to form the nose of the dog. (Barnhard HJ, Dodd D Jr: Radiographic anatomy of the lumbar vertebrae. Med Radiogr Photogr 49(1):7–20,1973)

them (the roentgenographs made after all the parts had been removed from the middle vertebrae) are shown first (Fig. 4-2); roentgenographs of the three complete vertebrae (the roentgenographs made before any parts had been removed from the middle vertebra) are shown last (Fig. 4-13).

This building-block method of presentation aids comprehension of this complex region. It creates the illusion of adding structures in a sequential fashion and illustrates the contribution of each structure in steps of increasing complexity.

As a further aid to an understanding of the contribution each part makes to the roentgenographic image, Figures 4-3 to 4-13 also contain subtracted roentgenographs. These subtracted roentgenographs were possible because positioning of the subject was carefully controlled. A few of the subtracted roentgenographs have extraneous areas of whiteness caused by slight variations in the position of the vertebrae in the holding device, but this is a rare occurrence that causes little distraction.

Figures 4-2 to 4-13 contain roentgenographs made in four different projections: anteroposterior, lateral, left anterior oblique, and right anterior oblique. In each figure, the anteroposterior roentgenograph (labeled AP) is reproduced at the upper left; the lateral (**LAT**) at the upper right; the left anterior oblique (**LAO**) at the lower left; and the right anterior oblique (**RAO**) at the lower right. Each subtracted roentgenograph in Figures 4-3 to 4-13 appears directly beneath the conventional roentgenogram to which it corresponds.

The four parts of each figure are referred to in the captions as **AP**, **LAT**, **LAO**, and **RAO**, and each caption begins with key words that serve as a title for the figure. These key words quickly show what part has been added and, it is hoped, will be of help to the reader who later wishes to refer to the roentgenograms made at a particular step of the study or to review the contribution a specific part makes to the overall image.

This section first appeared as an article under the title of "Radiographic Anatomy of the Lumbar Vertebrae," in *Medical Radiography and Photography*, Volume 29, Number 1, 7–20, 1973.

Acknowledgment: The authors wish to express their appreciation for technical assistance to Jeannette Baskin, R.T., and Jack Rush, R.T., Department of Radiology, and Calvin Jackson, Division of Instrumentation, all of the University of Arkansas for Medical Sciences, Little Rock, Arkansas.

PART III

Roentgenographic Contrast Studies

Myelogram

History

In the early 1900's, when greater attention was directed to the surgery of spinal lesions, the limitations of plain roentgenography of the spine became increasingly clear. In 1919, Dr. Walter Dandy described the use of air injected into the lumbar subarachnoid space to delineate the cerebral ventricles, pointing out its use as a contrast agent in the spinal canal.[15] Within two years, Binge in Germany, and Jacobaeus and Wideroe in Norway, unaware of Dandy's work, independently carried out air myelography to demonstrate tumors of the spinal cord.[6,34,58] However, air myelography never became universally popular, because the contrast was not great and the air shadow was often indistinct.

The introduction of lipiodol myelography by Sicard and Forestier in 1922 gave such satisfactory visualization of the spinal canal that air was largely neglected as a spinal contrast medium.[52] Adversely, however, this compound of iodine and poppy-seed oil produced meningeal irritation when allowed to remain in the subarachnoid space and be-cause of its high viscosity, removal of this substance was difficult and often painful.

In 1944, Pantopaque, a medium containing iodine in organic combination, was introduced by the University of Rochester group.[56] Because of its lower viscosity, it outlined the finer structures of the spinal canal, such as the root sleeves, and was more easily removed by gentle aspiration. This material received widespread and general acceptance in America. In Europe, especially in the Scandinavian countries, Pantopaque myelography never gained universal acceptance and water soluble contrast agents were preferred.

Water-soluble Contrast Agents

Water-soluble contrast media offer two immediate advantages over iophendylate meglumine (Pantopaque). First, because of their low viscosity, they will readily flow into and delineate nerve root sheaths, demonstrating disc protrusions or other sources of nerve root compression that may lie lateral to the central subarachnoid dye column. Since they are miscible with cerebrospinal fluid (CSF), they are readily absorbed into the CSF circulation, so aspiration from the subarachnoid space at the completion of myelography is not required.[10]

Second, animal experimentation reveals that all contrast materials injected intrathecally produce some degree of inflammatory reaction leading to adhesive arachnoiditis.[18] The reaction in animal experiments that occurs with Pantopaque is more severe than that which occurs with the water-soluble media. Human correlation is somewhat uncertain, primarily because the vast majority of humans who undergo myelography and eventually are diagnosed as having adhesive arachnoiditis also undergo some variety of lumbar spine surgery. Debate over the relative roles of surgery versus myelography in the causation of adhesive arachnoiditis continues.

The first water-soluble contrast agent, methiodal sodium (Abrodil), was introduced in Sweden in 1931 by Arnell and Lidstrom.[3] This agent was painful and was also associated with a high incidence of segmental convulsive myoclonus; it was necessary to combine the material with a spinal anesthetic before it could be tolerated by the patient. Because of this epileptogenic effect, it was not used to demonstrate lesions above the lumbar level. Even with this limitation, permanent lesions of the cauda equina and medullary cone were reported. During my all-too-short sojourns in Sweden, Norway, and Denmark, I had the opportunity to observe the execution of a number of Abrodil myelograms. I recall the difficulties encountered by the radiologist in attempting to tilt the table head up with the patient under spinal anesthesia. I have an even livelier memory of the radiologist's concern for and apprehension about a patient who developed convulsive seizures several hours after the myelogram had been completed. It is a mystery to me why this particular contrast material remained the myelographic agent of choice in Scandinavia until 1964, but since Abrodil is no longer in active use, this will probably be one of the many questions I will take with me to my grave.

In 1963, meglumine iothalamate (Conray)

was introduced as "a new intravascular radiopaque medium with unusual pharmacotoxic inertness," and a year later Campbell and associates used this material for water-soluble myelography.[36] Because this was not as painful as Abrodil, a spinal anesthetic agent was not necessary. Although this new material was somewhat less epileptogenic than Abrodil, severe muscle spasms and paresthesia remained a significant complication.

Because it was felt that much of the epileptogenic irritability of Conray was due to the hyperosmolarity of the agent, a dimer of Conray was produced by linking two molecules of meglumine iothalamate with an adepic acid bridge, forming meglumine iocarmate (Dimer-X).[7] This dimer had half the ionic strength of its predecessor and was less epileptogenic.[25,26] However, it was withdrawn from general usage in the United States in July, 1977, after several postmyelogram deaths resulted from a combination of seizures and hypotension.[2,7,8]

In 1972, metrizamide (Amipaque) was introduced in Scandinavia as a water-soluble agent for myelography.[43] All of the previous water-soluble agents had been (dissociated) ionized salts of iodinated acids which were hypertonic to both blood and CSF. Metrizamide was developed in an effort to avoid the untoward biological effects of a hypertonic solution. Metrizamide is the first commercially available nonionic agent which is practically isotonic with blood and CSF when used in a solution containing 170 mg iodine per ml. For lumbar myelography, concentrations of 170 to 190 mg iodine per ml in volumes of 10 to 15 cc are recommended. For visualization of the thoracic and cervical areas, higher concentrations are recommended to compensate for dilution of Amipaque with CSF. Amipaque is supplied as a lyophilized powder which is combined with a diluent (a solution of sodium bicarbonate) immediately before intrathecal injection.

The adverse effects of an Amipaque lumbar myelogram are significantly greater than a Pantopaque lumbar myelogram. Headache, nausea, and vomiting are approximately twice as frequent in Amipaque as in Pantopaque myelography. Several adverse central nervous system (CNS) effects that are not usually seen with Pantopaque myelography include hallucinations, confusion, and a 1% incidence of generalized convulsive seizures.[45,46,47]

Arachnoiditis due to Amipaque has been demonstrated in animal experimentation but requires relatively high concentrations and occurs less frequently than Pantopaque reactions (Table 4-1).

CHOICE OF CONTRAST AGENT

The ideal contrast agent should be miscible with CSF, both to delineate accurately the structures within the spinal subarachnoid space including the nerve roots, and to be resorbable so that withdrawal after its use is unnecessary. It should not have acute or chronic toxicity either locally or generally. This ideal agent has not yet been developed.

Since the recent approval of Amipaque for general use, the myelographer now has the opportunity to choose either Pantopaque or Amipaque. With this new freedom, he or she incurs an increased degree of responsibility for any complications caused by the selected contrast agent, if the mishap could not have occurred had the alternative agent been employed. If a patient develops adhesive arachnoiditis 10 or 20 years after a Pantopaque myelogram, the myelographer might be held responsible for not using Amipaque, which is presumed to have a decreased incidence of inflammatory reaction. Conversely, if the patient who had an Amipaque myelogram suffers a convulsive seizure which leads to his death, the myelographer may be criticized for not using Pantopaque. These medical, ethical, and legal questions are as yet unanswered.

The problem of which agent to use remains unsettled. The immediate advantages of Amipaque over Pantopaque are the improved root sleeve visualization plus the resorbable quality of the agent which makes withdrawal unnecessary. Local tissue reaction producing adhesive arachnoiditis in humans remains uncertain, but since animal experimentation strongly favors Amipaque in this regard, Amipaque may have long-term advantages.

The incidence of Amipaque-induced convulsive seizures, which is variously reported as 1% or 2%, remains a source of uneasiness and concern. These episodes usually occur several hours after the study has been completed, with the patient "safely" back in his room. The list of potential complications

Table 4-1. COMPARISON OF PANTOPAQUE AND AMIPAQUE

	Pantopaque	Amipaque
X-ray technique	Speed not a factor; if initial films inadequate may repeat the study	Progressive absorption requires rapid roentgenographic technique; if initial films not satisfactory may be too dilute to repeat study
CNS symptoms	None	Hallucinations Confusion 1%–2% seizures
Required withdrawal of contrast after completion of study	Yes	No
Root sleeve delineation	Not completely satisfactory	Good
Adhesive arachnoiditis	Possibly increased incidence in humans	Possibly decreased incidence in humans

from convulsive seizures, including death, is formidable.

The translucent contrast of Amipaque is significantly different from the more opaque image provided by the denser Pantopaque. This difference may present some initial difficulties in interpretation to those who are making a switch to Amipaque.

At this time, Amipaque is gradually replacing Pantopaque for lumbar myelography with Pantopaque still being favored for visualization above the low thoracic level. Several newer contrast agents are in various stages of investigation, and some of these may soon be released for clinical use. Questions and differences of opinion regarding the relative merits of various contrast agents for myelography can be anticipated over the next several years.

Patient Apprehension

Most patients with a prolonged history of low back dysfunction have heard the term myelogram. Some of them view the test with fear and apprehension because of the horror stories they have been told, which are usually pure fantasy. Occasionally, someone does suffer an unfortunate experience, but with few exceptions this study can be performed in a relatively painless fashion.

A few years ago, there remained a number of specialists who advocated proceeding with lumbar spine surgery after a careful clinical evaluation of the presenting signs and symptoms. Myelography was reserved for situations in which the clinical picture was not clear or when neoplasm was suspected.

I am not aware of any significant body of clinicians who now hold such a position. The fallibility of the neurological examination, the increased awareness of the irreversible consequences of lumbar spine surgery, the potential legal implications of carrying out a surgical procedure with less than complete documentation of a specific lesion, all have combined to create a clinical environment in which at least one type of roentgenographic contrast study is generally considered essential prior to a surgical decision.

Possible Complications of Myelography

The incidence of complications resulting from myelography is relatively rare and the likelihood of long-term serious after-effects is extremely low:

1. Pain during the performance of the myelogram, which usually relates to nerve root irritation either from direct trauma of the lumbar puncture (LP) needle when Pantopaque is used or, more frequently, from removal of the radiocontrast material when the root is aspirated against the needle bevel.

2. Postmyelogram radiculitis resulting from nerve root trauma, which may be the cause of persistent pain for a variable period of time.

3. Postspinal headache, which may produce considerable discomfort and be quite disabling to some patients.

4. Meningeal irritation, in reaction to introduction of a foreign material into the subarachnoid space. Infrequently, this may take the form of an aseptic meningitis with nuchal rigidity, severe headache, and increased white cells in the CSF.

5. Rarely, bacterial meningitis, which may result from faulty technique.

6. The irritative effects of the Pantopaque, which may produce adhesive arachnoiditis years after the myelogram has been performed. This complication is more likely to occur if a traumatic lumbar puncture produces subarachnoid bleeding, and if inadequate withdrawal of Pantopaque results in a blood-Pantopaque mixture which remains in the subarachnoid space. When complete removal of this material is not achieved, serial roentgenograms taken at yearly intervals will usually demonstrate gradual diminution in the quantity of visible radiopaque material. The rate of absorption of this material is estimated to be approximately 1 cc per year. The absorption rate varies. Some patients have very little absorption over a

period of many years, while others may absorb it more rapidly.

7. Pantopaque retained in the subarachnoid space which, when the patient lies with the head lower than the lumbar spine, may flow into the basilar cisterns and cerebral ventricles and produce a basilar adhesive arachnoiditis. This, in turn, may lead to obstructive hydrocephalus with all the potential complications of this condition.

8. Faulty lumbar puncture technique used in performing the myelogram, which may deposit Pantopaque outside the subarachnoid space making removal much more difficult and, at times, impossible. This may create a localized tissue reaction at the site of the deposited Pantopaque.

9. When using Pantopaque, a 10% to 15% error, due to inability to visualize laterally placed discs, where they may impinge against the root within the lateral recess. This false negative interpretation may cause the surgeon to withhold indicated surgery.

10. Pantopaque or Amipaque sensitivity.[13,15] Spinal fluid examination 1 or 2 days following myelography will usually demonstrate from 10 to 20 white blood cells per cubic centimeter, associated with a moderate increase in the spinal fluid protein. Symptoms resulting from these spinal fluid changes are not commonly apparent, but occasionally a patient will develop nuchal rigidity, headache, low-grade temperature elevation, and malaise. Spinal fluid culture will reveal no organisms, and the clinical course is self-limiting, responding to bed rest and analgesics within a week or two.

Several reports of more severe and even fatal reactions attributed to a unique hypersensitivity to Pantopaque have appeared in the literature. As a result of the increased sensitivity to this radiopaque material, a widespread aseptic leptomeningitis may occur, involving not only the spine but also the brain, particularly the posterior fossa. This may produce an obstructive hydrocephalus with some cases terminating in death.

The rarity of these tragedies makes it impossible to establish reasonable criteria to prevent similar future complications. Intradermal Pantopaque skin tests have been used but have proven to be unreliable. I will occasionally, and always with some hesitation, perform a Pantopaque myelogram on a patient who has experienced an allergic reaction during an intravenous pyelogram. There seems to be no direct relationship between the sensitivity to intravenous injection of an iodine containing intravascular radiopaque medium and the subarachnoid instillation and subsequent removal of a nonmiscible substance like Pantopaque. Despite my good fortune in avoiding complications up to this point, I carry out this procedure with some reluctance and believe that a decision to perform it can only be made on a case-to-case basis. Though premedication may not be necessary or effective, I do use systematic steroids and antihistamines prior to the procedure.

11. A low grade acute and chronic neurotoxicity with Amipaque. This pharmacological property may give rise to neurological side-effects which are significantly higher than the anticipated symptoms following a Pantopaque myelogram. The following list of symptoms is in order of frequency:

Symptom	Percent
Headache	37
Nausea	27
Vomiting	16
Neck and shoulder pain	15
Back pain	14
Leg pain	9
Mental confusion and hallucinations	2
Dizziness	1
Seizures	1
Hypotension	1
Fever	1
Tinnitus	1

12. The so-called false positive interpretation. Patients who were free of low back and sciatic symptoms but who had subarachnoid instillation of Pantopaque for assessment of cervical or cerebral symptoms

were found to have a 20% to 30% incidence of lumbar myelographic abnormalities. It can be assumed that the lower viscosity Amipaque, which is more sensitive and presents improved opacification of the nerve root sleeves, will reveal many abnormalities which are not symptom producing. Interpretation of abnormal myelographic findings must be done cautiously and only in conjunction with the clinical picture. Using a clinically unsupported myelographic defect as the prime indication for surgery is injudicious and may lead to a disappointing result.

Reviewing the rather formidable list of objections to myelography, one should rightly pause before considering the use of this test. The physician must be cognizant of every objection to the use of myelography, because it is not totally innocuous and carries with it a number of potential risks to the patient.

The alternative to myelography is, however, even more formidable (namely, exploratory surgery of the spine). The potential complications of exploring an extra interspace needlessly, removing one protruding disc when two are present, operating for lumbar disc disease when the symptoms are produced by a stenotic lumbar spinal canal, or not being aware of the presence of neoplasm are all so serious that they far outweigh the recognizably serious, but rare, complications of myelography. Exploring a "negative" interspace and retracting a root medially ever so gently to determine whether a disc is, indeed, protruded, is far more likely to produce persisting symptoms than is myelography.

Indications for Myelography

1. Clinical evidence of a protruding lumbar disc in patients who fail to respond to conservative treatment and who, on the basis of this failure, are being considered for surgery.

2. Significant motor weakness resulting from nerve root compression.

3. A long-standing history of low back pain which has not responded to conservative management.

4. Diagnostic possibility of a neoplasm.

Preparation of Patient

Prior to Pantopaque myelography, no premedication is ordinarily given, unless the patient is suffering from severe pain and is receiving large amounts of medication for pain during bed rest. If this is the case, a dose of the same medication is adminstered prior to being sent for x-ray film. Meals are not routinely withheld. Pantopaque is used for patients with low seizure thresholds or a history of epilepsy.

To avoid the risk of seizures with Amipaque myelography, sodium phenobarbital (60 mg) is used as a sleeping pill the night before and given at 6-hr intervals the day of the myelogram. If the patient has been on drugs which might lower the seizure threshold, such as the phenothiazine derivatives, these are discontinued at least 24 hours before myelography and are not resumed until 24 hours after the procedure.

Allergy to Local Anesthesia

Question the patient about previous dental surgery carried out under local anesthesia and ask whether any untoward reaction resulted from this or other local anesthetic blocks. If a hypersensitivity or allergic history is elicited, use no local anesthetic. In the absence of local anesthesia, one can usually pinch the skin overlying the proposed puncture site and then very quickly introduce the point of the LP needle employing vocal anesthesia in the form of reassurance. Once the needle is beneath the skin, there is usually no significant discomfort.

Myelogram Technique

A number of changes in myelographic technique have evolved in the past several years. Because a smaller-gauge needle is

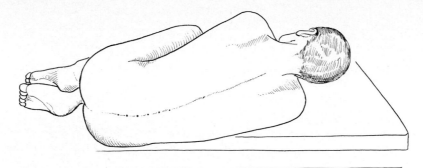

Fig. 4-14. *Accurate midline placement of the lumbar puncture needle is best done with the patient in the prone position. The distortion of spinal alignment with the patient in the lateral decubitus position creates increased difficulty in midline needle placement.*

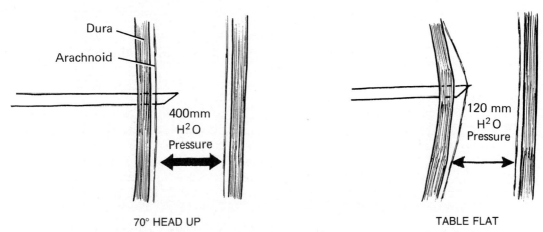

Dura

Arachnoid

400mm H^2O Pressure

70° HEAD UP

120 mm H^2O Pressure

TABLE FLAT

Fig. 4-15. *Meningeal distension of the caudal sac, produced by increased subarachnoid pressure when the x-ray film table is angled 70 degrees head up, allows the lumbar puncture needle to penetrate the dura and arachnoid cleanly, with less tenting of these membranes, decreasing the possibility of epidural or subdural Pantopaque injection.*

associated with a decreased incidence of post-spinal headaches, we now use a 20-gauge lumbar puncture (LP) needle instead of the 18-gauge originally preferred. However, the thinner, more flexible needle may curve as it is being advanced so that a midline insertion may deflect laterally, causing painful impingement upon a nerve root and possibly creating a false (needle) defect in the contrast column. Avoidance of undesirable lateral deflection is easily managed by roentgenographic guidance during needle placement (Figs. 4-14 and 4-15).

The patient is placed in a prone position on the table. A triangular sponge is placed under the abdomen to reduce the lumbar lordosis (Fig. 4-16). The skin is appropriately cleansed, shaving being reserved only for those with unusually luxuriant hair growth. The blunt needle that was used to aspirate the contrast medium into the syringe is placed on the skin as a convenient x-ray marker. This is positioned over the desired interspace and precisely at the lower margin of the space between the tips of the spinous processes. All modifications of marker and needle position are, of course, done with the x-ray inactive, checking each new position with the myelographer's hands completely out of the field, avoiding direct x-ray exposure. After the desired interspace has been roentgenographically localized, a lidocaine

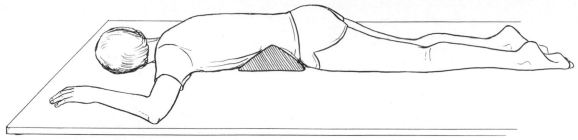

Fig. 4-16. Patient in prone position with triangular sponge under the abdomen to reduce the lumbar lordosis.

skin wheal is made at that exact point, leaving the 25-gauge hypodermic needle in place as a site marker. The 20-gauge disposable LP needle is introduced through the wheal until it is estimated that the tip of the needle has been advanced to a depth beyond three quarters of the length of the spinous processes. At this time, the table, which was flat, is angled "head up" approximately 60 or 70 degrees. This partially standing, weight-bearing body position will increase the lumbar lordosis and alter the angulation of the LP needle so that it is directed slightly more cranially. The advantages of elevating the table (Fig. 4-17) are:

1. In the head up position, the dura and arachnoid are distended, owing to hydrostatic pressure produced by the upright spinal subarachnoid canal. When penetrating this distended dura with a spinal needle, the myelographer is more likely to be altered to the puncture by a dural "ping."

2. As a result of increased compression of the arachnoid against the dura, the needle is less likely to press the arachnoid out into a tent-shape and create a subdural injection (see Fig. 4-15).

3. Increased spinal fluid pressure in the head up position produces a free flow of spinal fluid, with proper placement of the needle tip. When the spinal fluid flow is noted to be less copious and to escape drop by drop, there may be partial obstruction at the needle bevel, which can often be cleared by replacing the stylet and rotating the needle or advancing it a millimeter.

The prime disadvantage to elevating the head of the table is the possibility that the patient will become apprehensive and syncopal. Because of this possibility, it is necessary to have either a nurse or an x-ray technician attentive to the patient, providing reassurance and, if necessary, promptly lowering the table.

As long as the tip of the needle retains the desired midline position, advance the needle slowly, checking its position fluoroscopically with each move. The typical feeling of dural resistance may not be as clearly discernable with the thinner needle, so the stylet should be removed with each advancement to be sure the dura has not yet been reached. Once the dural penetration has occurred, as signaled by CSF flow, advance the needle an additional millimeter to position the bevel well within the subarachnoid space.

Once the LP needle is in satisfactory position, attach a length of plastic tubing for collection of the CSF specimen and for injection of contrast medium. The syringe should never be connected directly to the LP needle either for injection or for aspiration. A flexible connection between the needle and the syringe is advisable to avoid the possibility of altering the position of a well-placed needle, either because of an unanticipated patient's movement or because of a sticky syringe requiring increased pressure.

When Pantopaque is used, it is necessary to withdraw the medium (at completion of the myelogram) with gentle syringe aspiration, since the mere siphoning action of a

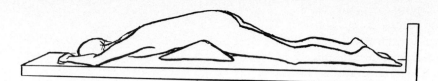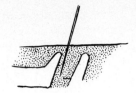

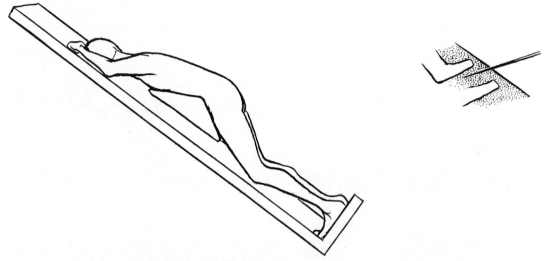

Fig. 4-17. Lumbar puncture (LP) needle is partially inserted with x-ray film table flat; head-up elevation of the table increases the lumbar lordosis and alters angulation of the LP needle, causing it to be directed more cranially.

length of plastic tube is ineffective with the 20-gauge needle. However, a well-placed, 20-gauge, needle provides excellent mechanics for Pantopaque removal and creates much less discomfort than an 18-gauge needle, which has a larger bevel and a greater capacity to irritate a nerve root. Since adoption of the thinner needle, we have not found it necessary to use any of the 18- or 17-gauge needles specifically designed for myelograms.

Needle Placement

DISPOSABLE NEEDLE

A disposable LP needle is used to insure against burs or blunting by previous use. A dull or burred needle may impinge the dura, pushing it forward and reducing the AP diameter of the subarachnoid space to a width sometimes less than the length of the bevel; or after perforating the dura, it may tent the arachnoid away from the dura, creating a false subdural space.

The site at which the lumbar puncture is performed is determined by the level of the suspected lesion. As a rule, the L3–4 interspace is the preferred needle placement site since both the L4–5 and L5–S1 interspaces comprise 90% of all lumbar disc lesions.

The interlaminar space becomes smaller as we go higher, so the lumbar puncture becomes a bit more difficult above the L3–4 level. Pantopaque is more difficult to remove when needle placement is above the L3–4 level, since the column begins to break up at the L2–3 level. When there is clinical evidence that the lesion is in the middle or upper lumbar levels, the injection site can electively be the L4–5 or L5–S1 interspaces.

The patient with a stenotic lumbar spinal canal syndrome and widespread hypertrophic osteoarthritic degenerative changes involving the lumbar spine often presents a technical problem. Because the dural sac and its contents are usually constricted at multiple levels, it may be difficult to obtain a satisfactory needle placement at the L3–4 level. Also, if the needle is inserted at the level of a stricture, interpretation is indecisive since it is not clear if the defect is caused by the needle or was present prior to the lumbar puncture. The spinal canal at the L5–S1 level is usually more capacious than the rest of the lumbar spine. Unless there are specific neurological signs implicating this level, needle insertion at L5–S1 is usually best in the patient with stenotic lumbar spinal canal syndrome, even if the hypertrophic bony changes on the plain x-ray films are severe at the lumbosacral junction.

Occasionally, it is necessary to introduce the dye from above, in which case two methods are suitable.

1. Cisternal Tap. A cisternal tap can be done with the patient in the sitting position (Fig. 4-18). Pantopaque introduced through this needle will drop to the lumbar region. After the contrast medium has been injected, the needle is withdrawn. At the termination of the myelogram, the Pantopaque can be removed by means of a lumbar puncture. If small amounts are used, some physicians make no effort to remove this substance and allow it to remain in the subarachnoid space.

Technique of cisternal puncture. The spinous process of C2 can usually be palpated by having the patient flex gently and extend the neck. The C1 spinous process can be palpated only in extremely thin individuals. A small area is shaved and cleansed with alcohol. With the patient in the sitting position, the head is held firmly in a slightly

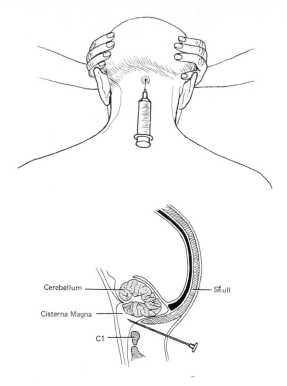

Fig. 4-18. Cisternal puncture.

flexed position by an assistant. Using 1% Xylocaine, a skin wheal is placed exactly in the midline, ½ in above the C2 process. The syringe is removed, and the hypodermic needle is left in place to mark the site. An 18-gauge spinal needle is introduced through the skin wheal and aimed toward the supraorbital ridge. The needle is advanced slowly and carefully until the characteristic snap or ping indicates penetration of the posterior atlanto-occipital ligament. At the time of ligamentous penetration, the immediately adjacent dura may also be penetrated or it may be necessary carefully to advance the needle further until a second ping is appreciated, signaling dural penetration.

It should be noted that the CSF pressure at the level of the cisterna magna may be zero in the erect position, so occasionally CSF will flow sluggishly from the needle. For this reason it is advisable to remove the stylet at regular intervals and aspirate gently, using a 1 or 2 cc syringe. Occasionally, I am

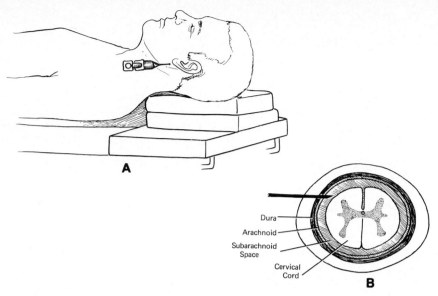

Fig. 4-19. **(A)** *Site of Xylocaine wheal for high cervical lateral puncture.* **(B)** *Diagrammatic cross section of high cervical lateral puncture.*

surprised at aspirating spinal fluid without having appreciated penetration of either the atlanto-occipital ligament or the dura. Depending upon the thickness of the neck and angulation of the spinal needle, the cisterna magna may vary from 3 to 6 cm beneath the skin.

2. High Cervical Lateral Puncture. The lumbar puncture needle can also be introduced laterally between C1 and C2, employing a technique originally devised for percutaneous cordotomy.

Technique of high cervical lateral puncture. With the patient lying supine on the biplane roentgenograph table, a 25-gauge hypodermic needle is inserted 1 cm below and behind the tip of the mastoid process, and 1% Xylocaine is used to infiltrate the skin and subcutaneous tissue (Fig. 4-19). An 18-gauge, short-beveled LP needle is introduced through the anesthetized skin and slowly advanced medially as 1% Xylocaine is infiltrated along the needle pathway. After some experience, the surgeon is able to appreciate the various layers penetrated; but it is wise to check the position of the needle at various levels of penetration by AP and lateral films of the high cervical spine using Polaroid film. Penetration of the dura is signaled by the typical sensation of resistance and then perforation of a parchmentlike membrane. Once the dura is penetrated, CSF will flow freely from the needle when the stylet is withdrawn. AP and lateral films are obtained to check the position of the needle. Optimal placement of the needle tip is approximately 10 mm behind the posterior border of the body of C2, and 10 to 12 mm from the midline.

After satisfactory needle position has been established, a short plastic connector tube is attached to the needle and allowed to fill with CSF. The head of the table is then elevated approximately 35 degrees; and under TV-image intensification, Pantopaque is injected into the subarachnoid space.

This method has the advantage of allowing the injection to be carried out with the patient lying supine. In this position the Pantopaque can be injected under fluoroscopic guidance until a sufficient quantity has been introduced to establish an adequate contrast column. As with cisternal tap, the spinal needle is removed after injection of the Pantopaque; if contrast material recov-

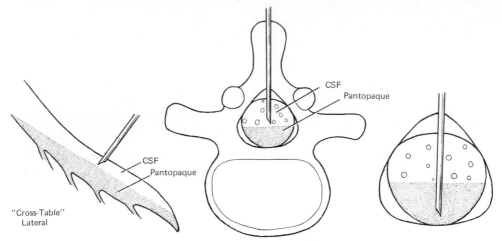

Fig. 4-20. Lateral film. The needle can be depressed for Pantopaque removal, if the needle is in good midline position.

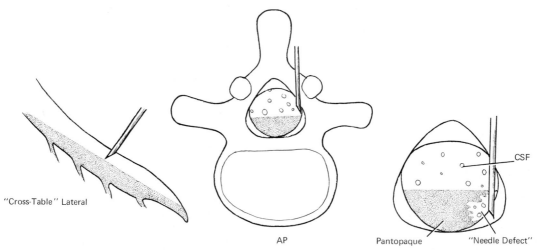

Fig. 4-21. Needle laterally placed at the edge of the subarachnoid space.

ery is carried out, it must be done by means of a standard lumbar puncture at the termination of the myelogram. The disadvantage of this technique is the possibility of injury to the high cervical cord. This procedure is best performed by a physician familiar with the technique of high cervical percutaneous cordotomy.

Pantopaque Removal

After the spinal segment to be surveyed has been fluoroscopically visualized and documented with spot-films, including oblique views and the cross-table lateral, it is helpful to examine the lateral film to visualize the tip of the needle in relationship to the floor of the canal. When the lateral film reveals the needle tip to be a distance from the floor of the subarachnoid space, it can be depressed, if the needle is in good midline position (Fig. 4-20).

If the tip of the needle is laterally placed at the edge of the subarachnoid space, it is a mistake to depress the tip to the level of the floor of the canal as visualized on the cross-table lateral film, since this will result in a needle defect (Fig. 4-21).

In such instances, allow the needle to remain undisturbed and place the patient in an oblique position so that the Pantopaque is pooled beneath the needle bevel (Fig. 4-22).

Using a long plastic connector tube, slowly and gently aspirate as the dye is pooled under the needle tip fluoroscopically. Rapid aspiration will produce a convection current and may cause a root to float up against and be aspirated into the needle bevel, producing pain (Fig. 4-23).

It is important to use a syringe that will not stick, since an irregular, jerky withdrawal may aspirate a root against the needle bevel. After the tubing has been filled, it should no longer be necessary to aspirate, since the siphon effect of the tubing is usually sufficient for removal of the remaining Pantopaque when using an #18-gauge spinal needle. Aspiration of CSF is likely to float up a root against the needle bevel causing pain. This can be avoided by maintaining the dye pool beneath the needle at all times during the removal. The normal, bouyant mobility of the cauda equina roots floating in CSF is dampened by the oily Pantopaque.

Special Myelography Needle

To facilitate Pantopaque withdrawal, the Cuatico myelography needle was designed for myelography (Fig. 4-24).[2]*

The needle set consists of an 18- or 17-gauge needle with the usual solid, sharp-pointed stylet conforming to the bevel of the needle which fits snugly into the needle shaft. This portion of the set is used to perform a lumbar puncture and injection of Pantopaque in the usual fashion.

At the completion of the myelogram, removal of the contrast material is attempted in the ordinary manner. If difficulty is encountered, because of either nerve root or arachnoid adherence at the bevel, then a

---

*Cuatico myelography needle (Becton-Dickinson Company).

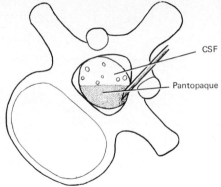

Fig. 4-22. Pantopaque is pooled beneath the needle bevel.

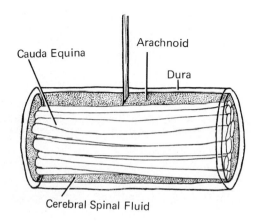

Fig. 4-23. Convection current causes a root to float up against and be aspirated into the needle bevel, producing pain.

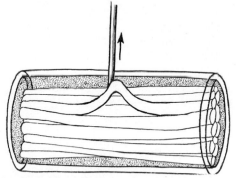

hollow blunt-end aspiration cannula, which fits into the inner bore of the needle, is used. This aspiration cannula is 19-gauge, with multiple openings spaced within the first 5 mm of the distal end. By using this cannula, whatever is adherent to the bevel is pushed

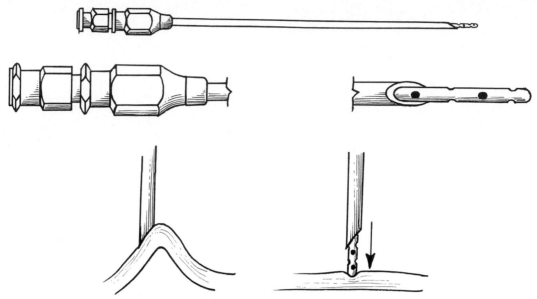

Fig. 4-24. The Cuatico myelography needle.

aside. Gentle aspiration using a plastic venatube removes the Pantopaque easily through the holes at the tip of the cannula.

I have used the Cuatico needle in approximately 100 myelograms and found it particularly helpful in patients with stenotic lumbar spinal canals or adhesive arachnoiditis. The latter causes the nerve roots to be closely adherent, making even gentle aspiration with an 18-gauge LP needle either difficult or painful. However, since switching to the thinner 20-gauge needle, introduced under radiographic guidance, I have not found it necessary to resort to a special needle.

Technical Problems

If in the performance of the lumbar puncture a traumatic tap causes bleeding, discontinue the procedure and wait a week before rescheduling the myelogram. A mixture of blood and Pantopaque is thought to increase the likelihood of adhesive arachnoiditis.

If a lumbar puncture is performed but the CSF flow does not seem satisfactory, attempt a second lumbar puncture at the interspace above or below the original needle. However,

do not remove the first needle, since this may cause a spinal fluid extravasation between the arachnoid and the dura, creating a false space, so that the second puncture would be technically unsuccessful.

If Pantopaque is inadvertently deposited in the subdural space, do not move the needle at all but very gently attempt to aspirate as much Pantopaque as possible. Occasionally, a surprising amount, if not all, the Pantopaque, can be removed in this fashion. However, in an attempt to remove more Pantopaque, do not rotate the needle or manipulate it in any way, since a second lumbar puncture may be performed above or below the original needle site. If a satisfactory flow of spinal fluid is obtained with the second lumbar puncture, inject 6 cc of Pantopaque and proceed with the examination. This procedure may not be as technically satisfactory as desired, but oftentimes a lesion can be identified clearly and the situation retrieved. Allow both needles to remain undisturbed until the study has been completed, after which the subarachnoid dye should be removed initially through the second needle. Following this, rotate or manipulate the original needle in the subdural space to remove the dye that could not be removed on the initial attempt. Both needles are to be removed only after no further dye can be withdrawn.

If, during the aspiration of Pantopaque at the end of the myelogram procedure, severe pain occurs with each aspiration, replace the stylet and turn the needle. If this does not successfully relieve the pain with subsequent aspiration, allow the needle to remain in place and insert a second needle above or below the original needle. Once identification of a lesion has been made or the presence of a lesion ruled out, the needle can be placed into any interspace; and in fact, the myelogram should be helpful, since you now know the configuration of the subarachnoid space. For this reason, dropping a second needle into a subarachnoid space filled with Pantopaque should be easy, since it can be visualized completely.

Postmyelogram Depo-Medrol

During the late 1960s and early 1970s, when the contrast material had been removed and the myelogram completed, a number of physicians routinely injected 40 to 80 mg Depo-Medrol (methylprednisolone acetate) via the LP needle before removing it. This subarachnoid steroid injection seemed to reduce the incidence of post-spinal headaches and postmyelogram discomfort. In some instances, it provided a significant remission of sciatic symptoms. In the past several years, however, we have been much more aware of possible adhesive arachnoiditis as a long-term consequence of intrathecal instillation of medication. In light of our present concerns, the disadvantages of this practice appear to outweigh the advantages.

Postmyelogram Tattoo

At the termination of the myelogram, if a lesion has been demonstrated which may require surgical management, I routinely mark the site with a cutaneous tattoo. This is done by placing a drop of india ink approximately an inch lateral to the involved interspace on the symptomatic side. Several superficial cutaneous punctures through this drop will serve to produce a discernible black dot on the skin which is permanent. This cutaneous mark is most helpful in determining the proper site for the skin incision, particularly when performing lumbar disc surgery with either an operating microscope or an operating telescope, and when desiring a small incision. The tattoo also serves as a presurgical check in proper lateralization, helping to avoid the possibility of exploring the right interspace on the wrong side.

Myelogram Tracing

When the myelogram is abnormal, it may be useful to have a graphic representation of the myelographic defect in the patient's office records. It serves as a helpful reminder of the lesion during follow-up visits. Occasionally, when a patient requires a second myelogram years later, the original films may be lost or destroyed by the radiology department to save storage space, making it impossible to compare the new and old films.

A practical and simple method of dealing with this problem was kindly demonstrated to me by Dr. William B. Scoville of Hartford, Connecticut. He routinely traces the myelographic defect on a sheet of tracing paper which he includes in the patient's office chart (Fig. 4-25). I now follow this practice and find it profitable.

Discogram

Basic Principles

Discography involves introducing a needle under roentgenographic guidance into the nucleus of the intervertebral disc and injecting 2 cc of a water-soluble contrast material such as Diodrast, Hypaque or Conray. The roentgenologic configurations assumed by this injected material are studied to eval-

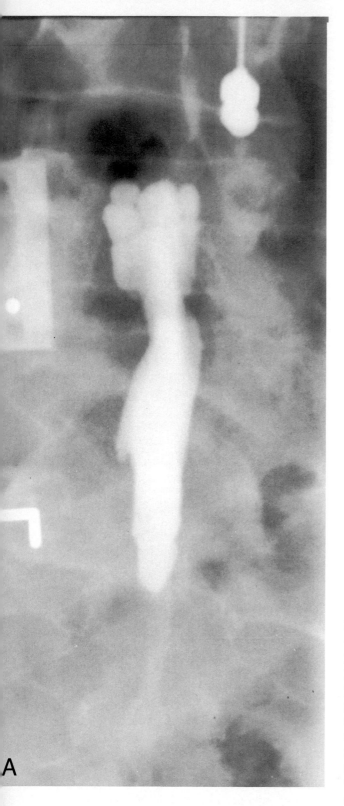

A

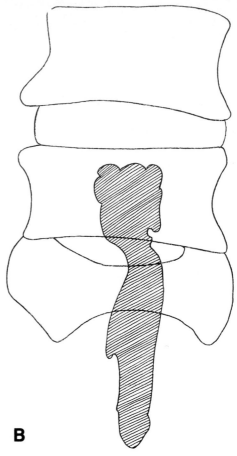

B

*Fig. 4-25. **(A)** Myelogram. **(B)** Tracing of myelographic defect.*

uate the pathology of the disc. In addition to the roentgenologic patterns, radicular symptoms produced by the injection are considered of diagnostic importance. The injection is normally followed by some low back discomfort, but if the injection is carried out into a pathologic disc which is the cause of radicular symptomatology, the injection will precipitate not only low back pain but also sciatic radiation. The pain produced by injection will reduplicate the patient's radicular complaints. A third diagnostic criterion is the injection pressure necessary to instill 1 cc of contrast material into the nucleus and the amount of the material accepted by the disc. A normal disc will accept up to 1 cc of dye with a fairly strong terminal pressure while injecting the last fraction of this dye. A degenerated disc will accept as much as 4 cc of dye, and a ruptured disc will accept 6 cc or more dye without severe pressure.

History of Discography

The discography concept of evaluating the physical state of the intervertebral disc was initially developed by Schmorl as part of his elaborate and painstaking autopsy studies of the human spine. His technique involved postmortem injection of red lead into the intervertebral discs, followed by radiography of the spine, in order to differentiate normal from pathologic intervertebral discs.

Years later, Knut Lindblom, working in the famous Karolinska Institute of Stockholm, became involved in the physiologic aspects of disc disease and pursued this interest for many years. Working on cadaver material, he carried out anatomical studies on discs by injecting them anteriorly with red lead. This paint filled the central cavities of the nucleus pulposus. If the disc was herniated, the dye would pass through the rupture of the annulus fibrosis, spreading concentrically under the outermost layer of the annulus, or in some cases going outside the annulus, and spreading along the nerve roots and epidural tissues.[36] After carrying out these anatomic studies, Lindblom, who had originally intended to continue this type of investigation clinically, was discouraged from doing so by reports of disc lesions caused by lumbar punctures. However, his interest in clinical discography was revived in 1941 by Dr. E. Lindgren who read a paper before the Swedish Radiologic Society demonstrating x-ray films of a patient whose normal disc he had injected with contrast material. It was later demonstrated by Dr. Karl Hirsch that intentionally performed disc puncture during surgery caused no immediate prolapses through the puncture canal, and on subsequent followup no obvious dysfunction was noted. On the basis of these observations, Lindblom was encouraged to perform diagnostic disc punctures on patients. His original technique utilized the prone position with the needle inserted by means of the usual spinal puncture method, passing through the posterior and anterior dural walls and then into the disc itself. He utilized a two-needle method, penetrating the posterior longitudinal ligament with a larger-gauge outer needle through which a thinner needle was introduced to penetrate the disc itself into the nucleus pulposus. Discography was first presented as a clinical diagnostic study by Lindblom in Sweden in 1948.[36] This method was first done in the United States in 1950 by R. E. Wise and E. C. Weiford of the Cleveland Clinic.[24] They carried out discography on the three lower lumbar discs and reported a normal L3–4 disc and herniated L4–5 and L5–S1 discs, findings which were subsequently confirmed at surgery. Interestingly enough, although the procedure was initially developed in Sweden, its use in that country is on a less than routine basis. In the United States the study received a more enthusiastic reception by a number of specialists and clinics which utilized this diagnostic method with great frequency.

In the late 1960s and early 1970s some clinics employed discography in the place of myelography, in most instances performing this study in the three lowest lumbar interspaces. The water-soluble contrast agents with improved delineation of nerve root sheaths, lumbar venography, and computerized axial tomography of the lumbar spine have all provided increased capability for roentgenographic assessment of the spine. These recent advances have decreased the use of discography.

Technique of Midline Lumbar Discography

PREPARATION OF PATIENT

This procedure is a more painful one than myelography, so the patient is sedated prior to the examination. However, he is not so heavily sedated that he is unable to cooperate during the examination and to report on the

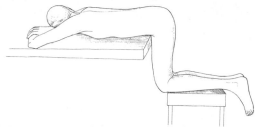

Fig. 4-26. Patient must be flexed over the end of the x-ray film table.

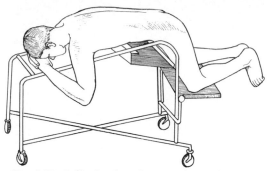

Fig. 4-27. Collis lumbar discography table. (Orthopedic Equipment Company, Bourbon, Indiana)

symptoms attendant to the procedure. Most patients are adequately sedated with 100 mg of Nembutal and 100 mg of Demerol given intramuscularly 1 hour before undergoing lumbar discography.

POSITIONING

The patient is placed in a kneeling-prone position on the table with both hips flexed over the end of the table and knees resting on a padded bench placed at the end of the table (Figs. 4-26 and 4-27). Biplane roentgenographic positioning is important so that an AP and lateral view of the lower lumbar spine can be obtained.

In clinics where discography is performed on a routine basis, a table specifically designed for lumbar discography is commercially available. The knee rest of this table adjusts to the patient's size and comfort and thus facilitates the study.[17]

Positioning the patient prone on the table is likely to provide inadequate reduction of the lumbar lordosis. Even with several pillows or pads under the abdomen, inadequate lumbar flexion may result, making lumbar discography difficult to perform.

INTERSPACE IDENTIFICATION

The skin in the lumbar region is prepared in the usual fashion by shaving the hair and cleansing with antiseptic solution. A 25-gauge hypodermic needle is used to infiltrate the skin and subcutaneous tissues with 1% Xylocaine over what is judged to be the L4–5

interspinous space. The hypodermic needle is allowed to remain in place and roentgenographic verification of the needle placement site is obtained. If the estimated L4–5 interspace is found to be incorrect on x-ray film check, the miscalculation will probably not be greater than one interspace. Since the proposed sites of injection are the L3–4, L4–5, and L5–S1 interspaces, the hypodermic needle will be roentgenographically visualized over one of these sites; and using this marker as a guide, the other two interspaces will similarly be infiltrated with Xylocaine leaving all three hypodermic needles in place. The three hypodermic needles can serve as a subsequent roentgenographic check, if deemed necessary, or as indicators of the exact spot through which the 21-gauge spinal needles are to be introduced.

NEEDLE PLACEMENT

Three 3-inch, 21-gauge spinal needles are inserted through the interspinous ligaments, to provide rigid support for the longer, thinner 26-gauge needles. These, because of their greater flexibility, could not be directed accurately for more than a short distance. Some specialists prefer to advance the heavier, 21-gauge needle only through the interspinous ligaments and use the thinner needle to penetrate the ligamentum flavum, posterior dura, subarachnoid space, and anterior dura, in the belief that penetration of these important structures is best done with the finest needle possible (Fig. 4-28). I prefer to

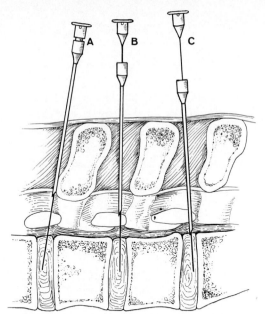

Fig. 4-28. *The penetration depth of the 21-gauge needle is left to the discographer's choice.* **(A)** *Through the interspinous ligament.* **(B)** *Penetrating the posterior dura.* **(C)** *Penetrating the anterior and posterior dura to the posterior longitudinal ligament.*

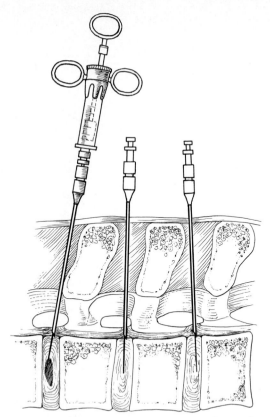

Fig. 4-29. *Injection of contrast material into the nucleus pulposus.*

penetrate all of the above structures down to the posterior longitudinal ligament immediately over the intervertebral disc with the 21-gauge needle, because of the greater control afforded by a more rigid needle. As the needles are slowly advanced, biplane (AP and lateral) roentgenographic guidance is necessary. The needle must be located in the center of the spinal canal to decrease nerve root trauma. The more laterally placed roots of the cauda equina are less apt to slip away from the needle tip, because they are more firmly fixed in their position, exiting laterally from the dural sac. The more medially positioned roots seem to have somewhat more "play," making them less vulnerable to needle impingement.

AP and lateral films are obtained to confirm the correct position of the 21-gauge needles, either set immediately over or directed toward the interspaces, depending on the preference of the physician. When satisfied with needle position, the 5-inch, 26-gauge spinal needles are passed through the

21-gauge needles into the intervertebral discs. As the needle penetrates the annulus fibrosus, slightly increased resistance is appreciated. If a firmer resistance is encountered, the tip of the needle is impinging upon either bone or the subchondral space and must be repositioned. Before injection of contrast material, another AP and lateral film is obtained. A properly placed needle tip is near the midline and does not impinge upon the vertebral body or the cartilaginous plate.

INJECTION OF CONTRAST MATERIAL

A 5 cc "3-ring finger guard" syringe with a Luer-Lok tip is used to inject the 50% Hypaque or water-soluble contrast material of preference into the intervertebral disc to the point of resistance (Fig. 4-29). The normal

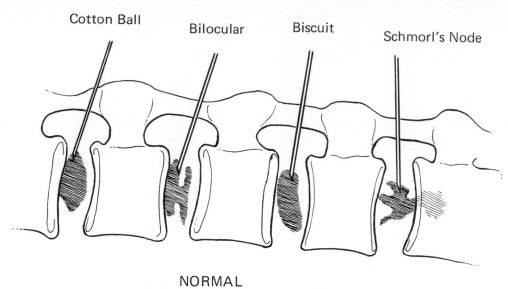

NORMAL

Fig. 4-30. Some normal discogram configurations. The Schmorl's node was included in the "normals" since it is not usually symptom productive.

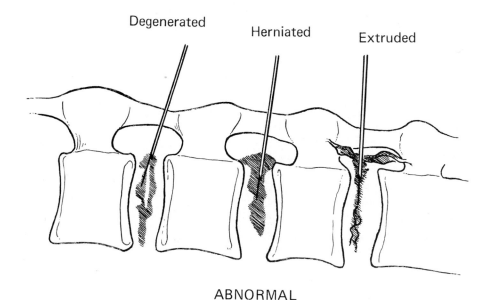

ABNORMAL

Fig. 4-31. Some abnormal discogram configurations.

disc will accept approximately 1 cc of solution with some difficulty (Fig. 4-30). In the absence of resistance, 3 cc of contrast material is injected.

As a rule, the least suspected disc, which is usually the L3–4 disc, is injected with dye first. The disc most suspected is deferred until last, so if the L4–5 disc is clinically symptomatic, the next disc to be injected following the L3–4 disc is the L5–S1 disc.

Immediately following each disc injection, a lateral x-ray film is taken; and after injection of all three discs, a lateral and AP film is obtained. Films taken 15 or 20 minutes after the last injection reveal absorption of most of the contrast material.

Interpretation of Discogram

The distribution and severity of pain produced by the injection is noted, along with the volume of dye accepted by the disc and the pressure required for injection.

The patient with a normal disc may experience some moderate discomfort during the injection unless excessive pressure is used, which may cause extravasation of solution anteriorly extending under the anterior longitudinal ligament or along the course of the needle tract. Such excessively applied pressure may bring about severe back pain.

The x-ray film appearance of the injected material is by far the most important single factor in discogram interpretation. In a normal discogram, the injection pain response is disregarded. It is only in the presence of an abnormal discogram that pain response is interpreted as being of clinical significance (Fig. 4-31). Then, if some reduplication of the patient's symptoms is produced by the injection, with radiation into the clinically affected leg, the pain response is considered positive.

Lateral Approach

The advantage of performing a lumbar discogram by means of the lateral approach is that the spinal canal is not entered and the dura remains intact (Fig. 4-32). This method is specifically adaptable to the use of Chymopapain for chemolysis of the nucleus pulposus. When using this chemolytic agent, great care must be taken to avoid introducing any of the material into the subarachnoid space, so a technique that completely skirts the spinal canal is required. The Federal Drug Administration has banned the clinical employment of Chymopapain in the U.S. but our Canadian neighbors are active in its use.

A posterolateral extradural approach, which was first described by Erlacher in 1952, has been largely replaced by the lateral approach.[6]

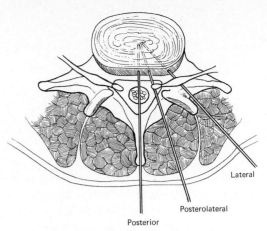

Fig. 4-32. The posterior, posterolateral, and lateral approaches for intradiscal injection.

TECHNIQUE

The patient is positioned right side up on the filming table, and 6-inch, 18-guage spinal needles are directed from a point 8 cm lateral to the spinous process of the disc to be injected, with the needle maintained at an angle of 45 degrees toward the disc (Fig. 4-33). Injection of the L5–S1 disc requires a 35 degree caudal angulation. Sometimes it is impossible to inject the L5–S1 disc using the lateral approach, and in such a case the posterior approach is required.

Advantages and Disadvantages of Discography

The advantages of discography are:

1. It is the only roentgenographic contrast study that examines the discs themselves.
2. Pain response associated with an abnormal discogram can be correlated with the clinical picture.
3. It avoids immediate or delayed reactions to contrast material injected into the subarachnoid space.

The disadvantages of discography are:

1. It is invariably associated with some degree of pain.

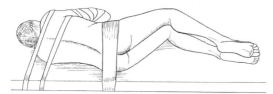

Fig. 4-33. *Position for lateral approach for intradiscal injection.*

2. Possible nerve root trauma may result.

3. The possibility exists that long-term, untoward effects of injecting a needle into a normal disc may accelerate the normal degenerative changes of age and stress.

4. There is the possibility of infection following injection into an interspace.

Postmortem Discography

Dr. Jack L. Gresham and Dr. Roy Miller carried out postmortem discography on 63 fresh autopsy specimens of patients from 14 to 80 years old with relatively asymptomatic "normal" backs.[23] These were divided into four age groups with the following results:

Group I: 14-34 years of age—90% normal and 10% degenerated discs.

Group II: 35-45 years of age—25% normal discograms, majority at the L3–4 level.

Group III: 46-59 years of age—25% normal discograms, majority of normal discs at the L3–4 level and none normal at the L5–S1 level.

Group IV: Over 60 years of age—5% normal discograms, none at L5–S1 level, one at L4–5 level, and two at L3–4 level out of 60 specimens.

The authors conclude that discography has its greatest clinical significance in the younger patient, with less weight given to this study if the patient is beyond the age of 35 years.

Role of Discography

Hazards and discomfort aside, the role assumed by any diagnostic test must be determined primarily by its clinical value in providing direction for proper management of the patient. This test, which is the only roentgenographic contrast study that actually examines the integrity of the disc, has provided us with important information on the degenerative effects of age upon the lower lumbar discs. The majority of symptom-free patients over the age of 35 reveal roentgenographic evidence of lumbar disc degeneration when subjected to this study.

As clinicians, we are principally concerned with the relationship between test findings and symptom-producing lesions. The discrepancy between roentgenographically demonstrated discogram lesions and clinical findings is controvertible. For this reason, universal acceptance of this study as a routine diagnostic measure is not general and widespread; most clinicians reserve its use to unusual diagnostic problems. In those countries where the use of Chymopapain is permitted, discography is routinely performed prior to the intradiscal injection of this chemolytic agent.

Lumbar Epidural Venography

For more than 20 years opacification of the lumbar epidural veins was recognized as a reliable radiological method for assessing lumbar disc disease. At the outset, intraosseous injection of the contrast material was the method of choice.[45,46,47] Because the intraosseous technique was awkward, with satisfactory venous opacification sometimes perversely inadequate, and since it was associated with a significant degree of patient discomfort, it never achieved general acceptance.

In the early and mid1970s a number of reports described opacification of the lumbar epidural venous plexus using the transfemoral approach with selective catheterization and injection of contrast material into the ascending lumbar or internal iliac veins. In the past decade the era of the "special procedure radiologist" has created an increasing number of specialists who possess a unique competence in the technique and interpretation of angiographic studies in various areas of the body. The availability of these specialists who had previously acquired the basic skills necessary for selective catheterization of the ascending lumbar vein made lumbar epidural venography a relatively standard procedure in every medical center within a surprisingly brief time.

Lumbar venography is made possible by the plexus of valveless veins (often identified as Batson's plexus) extending from the occiput down to the sacrum within the vertebral canal. The valveless nature of this plexus allows blood flow in any direction, depending entirely on internal or external body pressures, pressure gradients produced by body positions, or artificially created flow forces such as pressure injection techniques.

Although the anatomy of the epidural veins varies greatly from one individual to another, in a specific individual the right and left sides are remarkably symmetrical. Because the anterior internal vertebral veins bear a constant and intimate relationship to the vertebral bodies and hence to the intervertebral discs, any localized asymmetry can be interpreted as possibly being caused by an abnormality.

For a number of years all of the early literature on this subject described a right and left posterior epidural vein equal in size to the anterior epidural veins. Illustrations were created demonstrating this point of anatomy. The descriptions and illustrations were copied from the anatomy texts, all of which described such a venous system surrounding the dura both anteriorly and posteriorly. All lumbar spine surgeons are aware of the presence of veins traversing the anterior portion of the spinal canal. If this anatomical fact should be forgotten, the surgeon is reacquainted with it when he retracts a nerve root medially to explore a disc and runs into some unwelcome bleeding. Despite the fact that posterior epidural veins were never visualized at surgery, neither the anatomy texts nor the early roentgenographic reports on this subject were challenged. It required several years of reviewing epidural venograms to realize that we could not identify the posterior epidural veins because they didn't exist.

Routes of Catheterization

Catheterization of the femoral vein with a 5 or 6 French catheter is performed using the Seldinger technique. Either unilateral or bilateral catheters can be used. The left femoral vein is preferred over the right, since the left ascending lumbar vein is usually more readily located and selectively catheterized (Fig. 4-34). The left vein has a straighter "take off" from the common iliac vein and may be a bit larger than the right ascending lumbar vein. If the ascending lumbar veins are too small to catheterize, or if injection into these veins provides inadequate visualization of the vertebral plexus, injection of the left or right internal iliac (hypogastric) vein or small sacral branches of the internal iliac vein will also opacify the epidural venous plexus.

Contrast Medium

Any intravascular contrast medium can be used. The denser 76% iodide (Renographin 76, Conray 76) will provide better contrast, but the injection is associated with half a minute of severe low back pain. Injection of 60% iodide (Renographin 60, Conray 60) is relatively painless and is sufficiently dense to provide satisfactory filling. It is important for the patient to remain immobile during the procedure in order to obtain satisfactory "subtraction films." If the patient appears tense or unduly apprehensive, the 60% solution may be advisable to avoid undesirable movement.

Injection Technique

The injection is performed at a rate of 5 ml per sec for a total of 30–50 ml. To decrease the reflux into the inferior vena cava, exter-

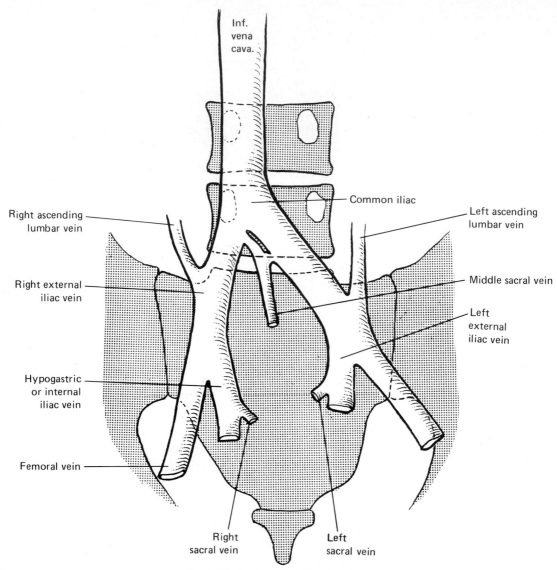

Fig. 4-34. Routes of catheterization.

nal abdominal compression using a binder and "IVP balloons" is invariably helpful. A simultaneous Valsalva maneuver, in which a forcible expiratory effort is made with mouth and nose closed, throughout the duration of the injection, is sometimes of further help in providing improved epidural venous filling, but occasionally it seems to be detrimental.

To a somewhat greater extent than with myelography, the technical aspects of the procedure are related to the interpretation of the films. For example, if there is an unfilled anterior internal vertebral vein, the radiologist must decide if this represents a disc protrusion or is due to a technical problem in which the contrast medium has not been adequately presented to that vein. Ideally, all of the epidural veins proximal and distal to the unfilled vein must be well opacified before they can be interpreted as revealing a lesion. If this prerequisite is not satisfied, further contrast injections are necessary. This type of problem is most apt to

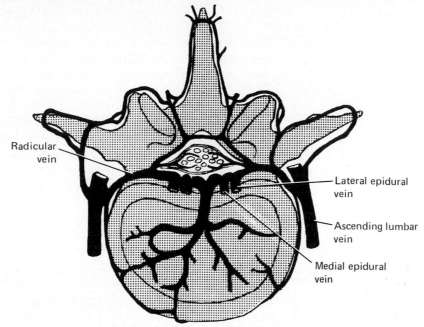

Fig. 4-35. Vertebral venous system.

occur at the L5–S1 level where cross-filling of the anterior internal vertebral veins is not as consistent as at the higher levels. When this occurs, the ipsilateral internal iliac vein should then be selectively catheterized and injected. If the situation remains unresolved and opacification is still unsatisfactory, the contralateral internal iliac vein should be catheterized.

Epidural Veins

The two epidural veins of primary radiological interest are the radicular and the anterior veins (Fig. 4-36 & 4-37). The **radicular veins** pass through the intervertebral foramina to bridge the ascending lumbar vein to the epidural veins. These minute vessels often occur in pairs, and are a source of considerable confusion because of the variations in nomenclature for describing them. The upper and lower veins of each pair are designated as superior and inferior bridging veins, radicular veins, foraminal veins, intervertebral veins, lateral foramen veins, and supra- or infrapedicular veins. To

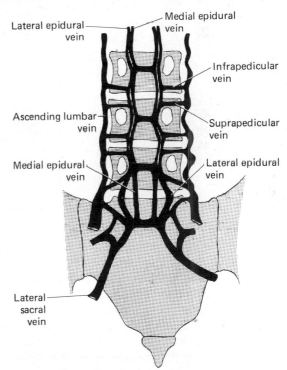

Fig. 4-36. Vertebral venous system.

compound the confusion, the suprapedicular vein is the inferior bridging, radicular vein; while the infrapedicular vein is the superior bridging vein. At this time, the terms supra- and infrapedicular seem to prevail.

The **anterior veins** are most often described as a paired grouping of internal and external (medial and lateral) anterior epidural veins. Occasionally one can demonstrate three parallel veins and, not infrequently, two ribbonlike, broad sheaths of veins, one on each side, covering the anterior portion of the spinal canal. When the anterior epidural veins are paired, they usually retain their parallel position until the L5–S1 level, at which point they diverge. The external anterior epidural veins continue to veer laterally between vertebrae so that with the cross-connection between the right and left sides, they will reproduce the hexagonal pattern present in the higher lumbar segments. The internal anterior epidural veins assume a straight medial course.

Interpretation

All of the anterior epidural and radicular veins are in juxtaposition to the dorsal portion of the vertebral bodies and discs. This close adherence to these structures warrants interpretation of changes in the venous pattern as being compatible with lesions within the spinal canal. The two most important diagnostic signs are:

1. Lateral or, less frequently, medial deviation of an internal anterior epidural vein (Figs. 4-37 & 4-38).
2. Occlusion of the internal anterior epidural vein (either unilateral or bilateral). In some instances thinning, diminished filling, venous dilatation, and evidence of collateral venous circulation may be suspicious or considered as supplementary findings.

The frontal (AP) projection contains most of the diagnostic information. However, when attempting to document spinal stenosis, a lateral view which demonstrates occlusion of the veins at multiple disc levels and venous filling at the level of the vertebral bodies may be helpful.

Previous lumbar disc surgery is almost invariably associated with occlusion of the epidural veins at the level of the original surgery. This could be anticipated, since in the process of excising an intervertebral disc, exposure of the anterior spine can cause direct and indirect trauma to the epidural veins with subsequent obliteration of these vessels. Contrary to my expectations, there are widespread venous occlusive changes following a decompressive laminectomy when no exposure of the anterior spinal canal was performed. I presume that the postoperative perineural and peridural scar tissue extends anteriorly and the fragility of these thin-walled veins will not withstand this encroachment. Because of these postoperative changes in venous flow, interpretation of a lumbar epidural venogram performed on a patient who has previously undergone spine surgery should be provisional.

Indications for Lumbar Epidural Venography

At this time most institutions and clinics are using lumbar epidural venography as a secondary roentgenographic contrast study; the myelogram remains the primary contrast study. The usual order of events occurs with a patient who has a good clinical picture of lumbar disc disease with a nondiagnostic myelogram. This may be a technically adequate myelogram that demonstrates no abnormalities or a technically unsatisfactory myelogram which yields a conjectural diagnostic impression.

When used in this manner, with a technically adequate myelogram, lumbar epidural venography is most helpful in revealing disc herniations at the L5–S1 level. This is the interspace where the myelogram is least reliable and where we see the greatest percentage of false negative interpretations. So in the face of a nondiagnostic myelogram, the clinician should seriously consider venography if the patient has a clinical picture implicating the L5–S1 level.

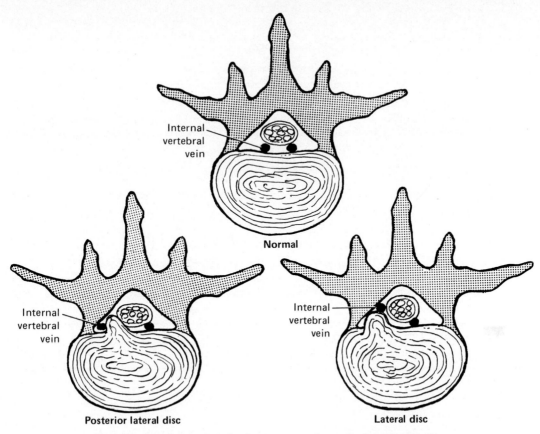

Fig. 4-37. Disc herniation displacing internal vertebral (epidural) vein.

Some institutions use lumbar epidural venography as their primary roentgenographic contrast study. The following reasons are submitted to support their preference:

1. Lumbar epidural venography is approximately equal in diagnostic accuracy to myelography, when performed by experienced specialists who can provide competence in both technical and interpretive aspects of the study.

2. Injecting contrast material through a needle introduced into the vicinity of a suspected spinal lesion may aggravate preexisting symptoms or cause new symptoms by direct or indirect nerve root trauma.

3. Adhesive arachnoiditis may be a long-term complication of the subarachnoid injection of Pantopaque.

4. Central nervous system symptoms (hallucinations, headaches, convulsive seizures) may be possible complications of instilling the miscible, slightly neurotoxic Metrizamide into the freely circulating cerebrospinal fluid.

5. Venography presents a relatively low incidence of complications: an allergic reaction as may occur with an IVP or any intravenous injection of iodinated contrast material, or hemorrhage or extravasation in the soft tissues at the puncture of injection site in the groin or pelvis which is not usually of long-term consequence.

6. Avoidance of postspinal headaches is another reason for choice of venography.

On specific occasions, venography may be performed initially by a physician who would ordinarily employ myelography as the

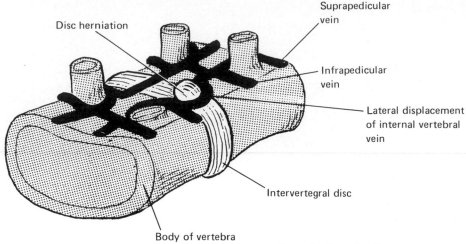

Fig. 4-38. Disc herniation displacing internal vertebral (epidural) vein.

primary x-ray film contrast study. When a contrast study is desired to rule out a lumbar disc protrusion but it seems wise to avoid the hazards of injecting contrast material into the subarachnoid space for medicolegal reasons, a venogram can be considered. It should be recognized, however, that this study is a sensitive indicator of disc disease and may demonstrate abnormalities at asymptomatic levels. In such a situation, what was initially regarded as a solution is merely a bridge to subsequent problems.

Roentgenographic Abnormalities and Symptoms

The specific relationship between x-ray film findings and symptoms remains open to considerable discussion. A normal lumbar spine x-ray film does not rule out a symptom-producing lesion, and a roentgenographic abnormality may not be a cause of symptoms. An awareness of this possible discrepancy is most important when assessing x-ray film contrast studies. These tests are usually performed after an interval of unsuccessful conservative treatment when surgery is being contemplated. When using any x-ray film contrast study as an important determining factor in making a decision regarding surgery, the surgeon must be com-

pletely satisfied that the x-ray film abnormality corroborates the clinical picture.

Until several years ago, most of the myelograms were carried out by the surgeon who would presumably perform the surgery if a disc protrusion was demonstrated. In the past five years, a progressively increasing number of myelograms and virtually all lumbar venograms are being performed by special study radiologists. I raise no issue regarding the technical competence of radiologists and welcome the entry of these worthy individuals into the arena of low back pain. My only caution is the disjunction between interpretation and results. In comparing one type of contrast study to another, considerable importance is attached to the statistical accuracy of each test. These statistics are based on surgical verification of a disc protrusion. Such information is obtained either by contacting the surgeon shortly after he has performed the procedure or by checking the operative note on the chart after the patient has been discharged. Although, data of this sort is of interest, it falls short of the mark.

All lumbar disc surgeons will encounter a vast spectrum of findings in the course of their surgery, ranging from the massively extruded disc compressing the nerve root into a ribbon, to the equivocal nonbulging but possibly somewhat softened annulus.

Most surgical findings range between these extremes; specific interpretations and methods of dealing with these findings vary from surgeon to surgeon. Some surgeons acknowledge a reluctance to document "on the chart" surgical exploration of a normal disc, so once they have made a decision to operate, the finding of an abnormality is almost assured.

We sometimes must remind ourselves that the only basis for all of our endeavors is to relieve patients of their symptoms. A correlation between preoperative roentgenographic findings and long-term surgical results would reach the core of the issue. Such data has yet to be developed.

Diagnostic Ultrasound

Dr. R. W. Porter, an orthopedic surgeon at the Doncaster Royal Infirmary in England, has developed the use of diagnostic ultrasound to measure the oblique sagittal diameter of the lumbar spinal canal (Fig. 4-39). This use of ultrasound is now being assessed by several clinics both in the United States and in Europe. Dr. Porter points out that the available space within the spinal canal is highly significant in the symptomatology of disc disease. He is able to demonstrate a significant difference in the spinal canal measurements of individuals who are asymptomatic and those who present with lumbar disc syndromes. He further demonstrates that of those individuals with lumbar disc syndromes, failure to respond to conservative treatment is related to the size of the spinal canal, with the patients who required surgery having the narrowest canals.

The three methods presently in general use to measure the bony spinal canal each have certain impediments:

1. Special measuring methods employing lateral spine films are not particularly accurate (Fig. 4-40).

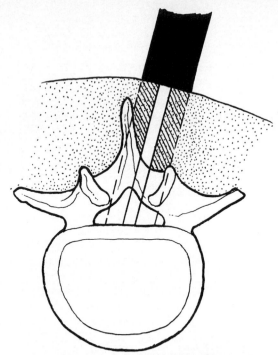

Fig. 4-39. Ultrasound measurement of oblique diameter of spinal canal through the lamina "window."

2. Computerized axial tomography is time-consuming, extremely costly and, at this time, controversial. Because of the expense involved in the use of the CAT scanners, a variety of legislative and legal adversary actions have developed. These usually involve hospitals and physicians who wish to acquire and employ these expensive devices, pitted against a coalition of forces primarily committed to reducing the cost of medical care. The cost-cutting group is usually composed of one or more health insurance plans such as Blue Cross and Blue Shield, a community health planning agency, and a variety of politically oriented individuals. Those opposed to the hospitals and physicians have a somewhat broader base with more favorable access to public opinion forums, so at this time the contention is weighted in their favor.

3. Myelography, which is presently accepted as the best method of demonstrating a compressive encroachment upon the contents of the spinal canal, has two significant

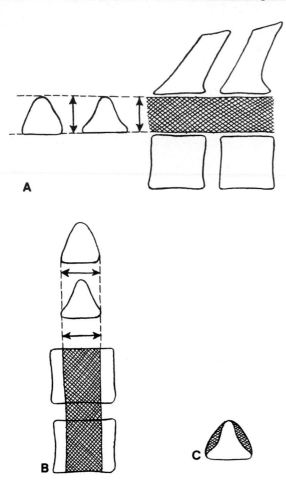

disadvantages. Because it requires a lumbar puncture, the increased risks associated with such an invasive technique preclude its use with those patients who are potential surgical candidates. A second serious limitation of myelography is its inability to demonstrate a large reduction in the cross-sectional area of the spinal canal due to a trefoil configuration (Fig. 4-40).

The use of pulsed echo ultrasound is simple, safe, and in Dr. Porter's hands seems to have a high degree of accuracy. If Dr. Porter's techniques can be reduplicated, they would create a simple, safe, and accurate method to identify, prior to the development of symptoms, those individuals who may be prone to low back dysfunction. For example, ultrasound spinal canal screening could conceivably be done during a youngster's school years. At that early time, vocational counseling is feasible, and those individuals who are potentially more vulnerable to low back dysfunction than the population at large, can be advised to avoid an occupation which may be hazardous to their low back health.

For his innovative use of ultrasound in low back dysfunction, Dr. Porter and his associates received the Volvo Award in Basic Sciences Relevant to Back Pain at the International Association for the Investigation of the Lumbar Spine Meeting in Gotenburg, Sweden, in April of 1979.

Fig. 4-40. Spinal canals of differing capaciousness and configuration may have deceptively similar myelograms.

PART IV

Computerized Body Tomography and Evaluation of Lumbosacral Spinal Disease

WILLIAM V. GLENN, JR.
BEN MAURICE BROWN
MICHAEL L. RHODES
JEROLD E. LANCOURT

New diagnostic tools in clinical medicine gain increasing acceptance as they are noted to provide improved diagnostic accuracy, lower patient risk, and competitive cost. Computerized tomograph (CT) has convincingly demonstrated such benefits over the past decade to a growing segment of the scientific medical community. During the 1970s, the range of CT's applications broadened greatly to include an enormous spectrum of clinical conditions, initially in neurosurgery and neurology, and more recently in orthopedic surgery, general surgery, and internal medicine.

Early developments in CT were focused on the use of CT head scanning which evolved, by the end of 1979, into the dominant roentgenographic technique for diagnosing intracranial lesions. Currently, the CT head scan has largely supplanted two invasive imaging methods (pneumoencephalography and ventriculography), encouraged less widespread and more selective use of a third invasive technique (cerebral an-giography), and greatly increased the accuracy of intracranial lesion detection following initial evaluation by physical examination and plain skull roentgenograms.[5,6,9,53,83,89] There are three major reasons for the preeminence of CT head scanning in modern neurological and neurosurgical diagnosis.

1. CT scanning is noninvasive, so the risk of invasive puncture and catheterization is avoided.
2. CT scanning permits visualization of fine anatomical detail by providing displays of thin slices of various planes.
3. CT scanning permits discrimination of more differing tissue densities than conventional x-ray film techniques, so a greater variety of densities including soft tissue organs and muscle, bone, fat, blood, metal, and iodinated contrast material can be clearly distiguished. It also permits discrimination of soft tissue densities enclosed by dense bone.

The combination of thin tissue slice display and high contrast resolution constitutes a specialized imaging capability unique to CT. This capability was first applied by CT head scanners to the diagnosis of intracranial lesions by generating head slice images which permitted visualization of brain structures inside the skull. Soft tissue abnormalities in the brain, including neoplasm, abscess, and hematoma, thus for the first time became accessible in roentgenographic display without invasive procedures. Subsequent technological advances led to the development of larger and more complex scanners aimed at applying the same specialized CT imaging capabilities to the body. Over the past 5 years, computerized body tomography (CBT) has increasingly demonstrated its usefulness in detecting organic lesions in the chest, abdomen, and pelvis.[2,8,24,25,44,68,72,73,118,133,147,148,157,169] More recently, a variety of orthopedic lesions, especially those located in the lumbosacral verterbral column, have shown an increasing detection rate on CBT. A number of investigations have supported the emergence of CBT as an important and often primary diagnostic method in lumbosacral spinal disease.[1, 4, 15, 18, 23, 27–32, 34–36, 43, 46, 47, 51, 61, 65, 66, 71, 74, 75, 77, 87, 88, 91, 93, 95–99, 102, 104, 106, 108, 111, 112, 119, 121–123, 125, 134–138, 141–144, 146, 152, 153, 159, 160, 163, 165–168, 171]

In fact, the recent development of CBT of the lumbosacral spine (CBT–LS) in selected medical institutions parallels the early history of CT head scanning in several respects. CBT of the spine has permitted supplantation as well as more selective use of invasive imaging procedures, such as lumbar myelography and epidural venography. CBT–LS has greatly increased the detection rate of occult soft tissue lesions adjacent to and inside the bony vertebral column following initial physical examination and plain spine x-ray films. Futhermore, the cost effectiveness and availability of CBT–LS has become increasingly competitive with earlier, less sensitive imaging methods.

Thus, surgeons actively involved in the management of low back pain patients in modern hospital settings can expect to utilize CBT–LS increasingly for a variety of everyday tasks.

1. Surgical candidate selection
2. Surgical procedure planning
3. Postoperative diagnostic evaluation

Surgeons will need to become familiar with the range of normal and abnormal CBT findings in lumbosacral spinal disease, as well as with the application of CBT–LS to the planning and evaluation of surgical intervention. Proper utilization of CBT–LS data will in turn promote a higher success rate in therapeutic interventions, because such interventions will be based upon far more accurate and detailed localization of anatomical abnormalities than was previously possible.

Methods of CBT

Initial studies on the use of CBT in the spine have been based on limited numbers of patients and on the use of transverse images only. Obtaining transverse sections at 1- to 2-cm intervals is adequate for survey purposes, but this approach often does not provide sufficient data for, nor realize CBT's full potential in, the meticulous evaluations required in the diagnosis of spinal disorders.[61,65]

The CBT scanner used at our institution is an EMI 5005 Body Scanner. This second-generation scanner has proven adequate for CBT spine studies, even though more sophisticated, third- and fourth-generation scanners permitting much faster scan time are now available. For CBT exams of the lumbosacral spine utilizing the EMI 5005 scanner, the patient lies supine on the scanner couch for 40 to 50 minutes. Closely-spaced transverse images (8mm thick) are obtained every 3 mm from S1 to midbody L3. Then multiplanar displays (MPD) including sagittal and coronal sections are

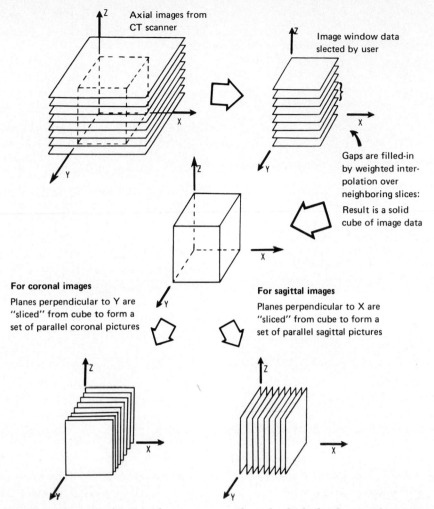

Fig. 4-41. Schematic diagram showing process through which closely spaced transverse axial images are first transformed into a solid cube of image data by interpolation and then redisplayed in alternately coronal and sagittal formats. The original transverse slice thickness is 8 mm. These transverse images are obtained at 3 mm intervals. The resulting coronal and sagittal image thickness is 0.75 mm. (Glenn, WV Jr, Rhodes ML, Altschuler EM, et al: Multiplanar display computerized body tomography applications in the lumbar spine. Spine 4(4): 282–352, 1979)

reconstructed by the computer from the original transverse sections.[61–67,102,103] Lumbar segments L3 to L1 are surveyed with images taken at 1-cm intervals.

The process of transposing horizontal image data into other display orientations is shown schematically in Figure 4-41. The MPD format is the simultaneous presentation of transverse (horizontal), coronal (frontal), and sagittal (lateral) anatomic views.[60–67,103] As shown in Figures 4-41 to 4-44, these different views are perpendicular to each other; each view in the MPD format is represented by one plane from its series of parallel planes (Fig. 4-43). Reference lines indicate the intersection of any two planes. The single pixel common to all three planes can be highlighted as a blinking dot in each corresponding plane, thus providing precise image-to-image registration of small anatomic structures. Simple keyboard interactions and use of various analog diodes are described elsewhere.[61,65]

Careful case analysis requires rapid back-

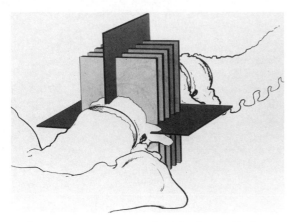

Fig. 4-42. Orientation of Multiplanar display (MPD) views. The transverse image is seen from below, the coronal image from the front, and the sagittal image from the left. (Glenn, WV Jr, Rhodes ML, Altschuler EM, et al: Multiplanar display computerized body tomography applications in the lumbar spine. Spine 4(4): 282–352, 1979)

and-forth display of several adjacent transverse, sagittal, and coronal images. MPD-like implementations which are not responsive may see little clinical use. Large-capacity, on-line disc storage coupled with a point-addressable cathrode ray tube (CRT) is essential. The several hundred image planes comprising a single case study should be quickly accessible for immediate display. Physicians' acceptance and utilization de-

pend to a large extent on agile, flexible software that presents new images very rapidly.

The importance of closely spaced transverse images is illustrated in Figure 4-45 where two images 6 mm apart demonstrate completely different appearances regarding the patency of L5 foramina. Likewise in Figure 4-46, the key finding of a central and left-sided L4 disc bulge is identified in only one or two images. In subtle but crucial CT findings in the head or body, this is the rule rather than the exception. For maximum detail, close spacing is absolutely essential. First, with close spacing diagnostic accuracy is gained simply from having partially redundant transverse images. Second, there is a direct relationship between transverse image spacing and spatial resolution of the coronal and sagittal images.

Through the clinical use of the above basic MPD functions in nearly 2000 cases, several additional refinements have been developed and then grafted into the MPD software package. These include variable thickness coronal and sagittal images, composite CT picture files, a universal oblique plane capability, and various measurement functions.[100]

The composite CT images in Figures 4-47 to 4-49 are derived from the data cube of

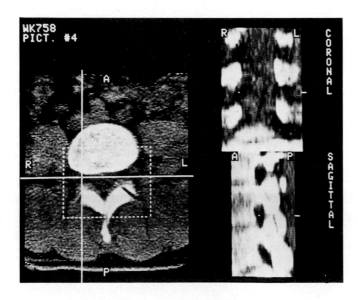

Fig. 4-43. Standard three-way multiplanar views with attention centered on the right L3 spinal nerve canal and foramen. Note the appearance of the lumbar canal and also the axial view of the L3, L4, and L5 pedicles seen in the coronal image. The same image is seen in Fig. 4-44 with reference lines removed and the blinking dot highlighted. The tick mark along the right margin of both the sagittal and the coronal images indicates the craniocaudal position of the current transverse sections. (Glenn, WV Jr, Rhodes ML, Altschuler EM, et al: Multiplanar display computerized body tomography applications in the lumbar spine. Spine 4(4): 282–352, 1979)

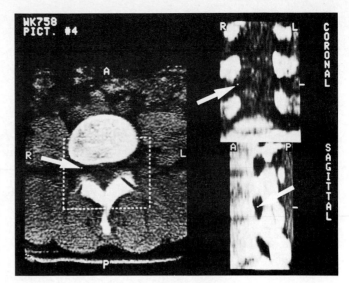

Fig. 4-44. Same as Fig. 4-43, but the reference lines have been removed. The blinking dot **(arrows)** indicates the single pixel common to all three planes. Here the blinking pixel is centered within the right L4 foramen. (Glenn, WV Jr, Rhodes ML, Altschuler EM, et al: Multiplanar display computerized body tomography applications in the lumbar spine. Spine 4(4): 282–352, 1979)

transverse, coronal, and sagittal files shown in Figure 4-41. This feature was created for only one reason: to reduce the time required to analyze a given case. After the current case has been processed into MPD format, the CT technologist can automatically make and photograph each series of composite pictures. Starting with the set of composite pictures on film, the following options become available.

1. Dictate the case from films without an interactive display session when CT images either are completely normal or show only minor abnormalities (time required: 5 min).

2. Briefly review composite pictures of display console for window-width and window-level adjustments, measurements, or labeling (time required: 5–10 min).

3. Review composite images as in (2) but also select a specific area or structure of interest for MPD display, labeling, and so on. This requires linkage of the composite display option with basic MPD options, as shown in Figures 4-49 to 4-50 (time required: 10–15 min).

Fig. 4-45. Two transverse images through the L5 foramina indicate the importance of closely spaced images. **(A)** Complete obliteration of the foramina suggested. **(B)** Six mm higher the image shows both foramina to be open. Neither image alone is sufficient. (Glenn, WV Jr, Rhodes ML, Altschuler EM, et al: Multiplanar display computerized body tomography applications in the lumbar spine. Spine 4(4): 282–352, 1979)

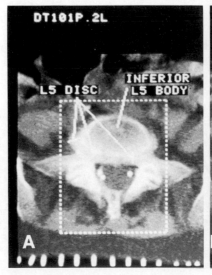

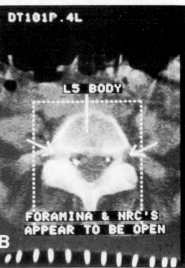

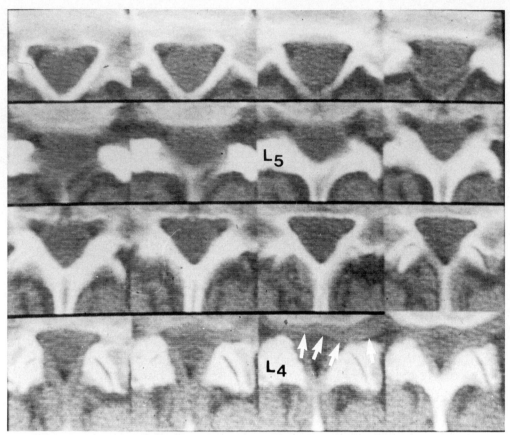

*Fig. 4-46. Spinal canal portions of closely spaced, 8-mm thick transverse images taken every 3 mm. The bulging L4 disc or annulus **(arrows)** is seen on only one or two views. (Glenn, WV Jr, Rhodes ML, Altschuler EM, et al: Multiplanar display computerized body tomography applications in the lumbar spine. Spine 4(4): 282–352, 1979)*

4. Analyze entire case with MPD; this requires careful filming (by the radiologist) of each foramen medially and laterally, 'as well as filming and optional labeling of any other suspected bony or soft tissue abnormality (time required: 30–40 min).

The universal oblique plane capability replaces with software the attributes of a tilting gantry. The software approach shown schematically in Figure 4-51 provides the flexibility of obtaining any desired plane from the original image data cube in Figure 4-41. These programs provide interactive selection of a plane oblique to any of the three conventional transverse, coronal, and sagittal MPD data sets. Though geometric techniques for defining oblique planes are well established, extensive processing time and difficulties with interactive oblique plane specification have limited their clinical implementation. Methodology outlined in references 97, 139, and 140 resolves both obstacles, thus making oblique plane capability a useful option in the MPD software package.

The example in Figure 4-52 shows how the sagittal reference line can be adjusted on a transverse image in order to specify a "tilted" sagittal view. One use for this feature is to provide a true axial view of cervical foramina (Fig. 4-52B) which emerge at 45 and 135 degrees rather than at 0 and 180 degrees as in the lumbar region. For maximal

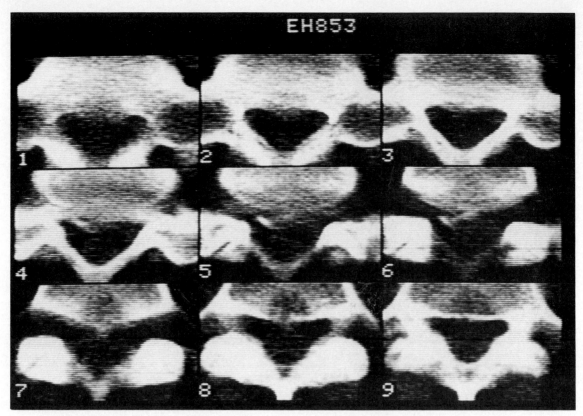

Fig. 4-47. Transverse image, composite image file.

flexibility, the reference line for this type of tilted sagittal oblique plane is specified by adjusting two analog dials. Each dial moves one end of the reference line around the dashed box on the transverse image.

The example shown in Figure 4-53 illustrates tilted axial views of the lumbar canal. The transverse image represents a true axial view of the lumbar canal at an L5–S1 spondylolisthesis. Similar corrected views can be made for each of the disc spaces and should help increase accuracy both in AP canal measurements and in the diagnosis of lumbar disc abnormalities (particularly at L5–S1). As shown in Figure 4-53A and B, the orientation of the new views has been specified by user adjustment of a reference line on the sagittal image only. The example in Figure 4-53C goes one step further. Here the titled axial is specified by reference lines on both the sagittal and coronal images. The

result in Figure 4-53C is truly oblique to each of the transverse, sagittal, and coronal data sets. It is anticipated that the oblique plane capability used in this fashion may be helpful in CT examination of scoliotic spines. This type of software has some very logical and useful extensions in several other areas of the body, including petrous bones, orbits, and retroperitoneum.

Objective measurements can be made on CT images as shown in Figure 4-54 by using a track-ball analog device to position a crosshair. This procedure makes it possible to locate endpoints of a measurement line. After measurements are taken on a series of transverse images, a video plot of the data can be shown as data points alone (Fig. 4-55), straight-line point connection (Fig.4-56), and multiple measurement plots of either the same parameter for several cases (not shown) or several different parameters for

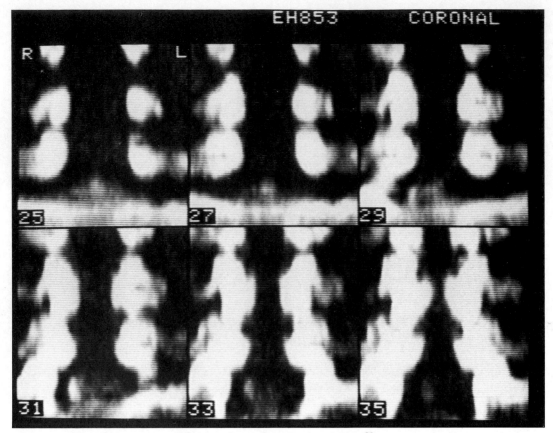

Fig. 4-48. Coronal composite picture file.

the same case (Fig. 4-57). Elsewhere there has been discussion of the three-dimensional graphic presentation of case-to-case measurement comparisons, and the requirement for "rubber-band" compression or expansion of such curves to accommodate the variable number of data points between the same two interspaces in tall versus short people.[100]

CBT Findings in Major Operable Lesions of the Lumbosacral Spine

This section presents a series of cases demonstrating CBT-LS findings in three groups of individuals:

1. Normal anatomy (cadaver specimens)
2. Abnormal anatomy (preoperative patients)
3. Abnormal anatomy (postoperative patients)

Normal Anatomy

While there are significant variations in the configuration of the canal, the spinal column is largely a repetitive series of intra-pedicular and intraforaminal segments. Here we will confine the discussion to a single segment, the right side of the L4 spinal segment. Figure 4-58 is a demonstration of the normal cross-sectional, or axial, anatomy. The first section (Fig. 4-58A and B) shows the bottom of the L3 disc and the top of the L4 cortex. Note the top of the pedicle and the good definition of the apophyseal joint. (The computer reverses the images so that the right is on the reader's left. For ease

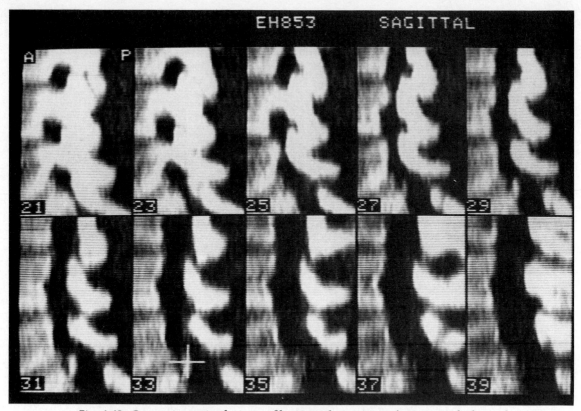

Fig. 4-49. Composite sagittal picture file. Note the position of interactively located cross hair on picture 33. The location of the cross hair within this single sagittal image defines a corresponding transverse and coronal view. The user can immediately switch to MPD format as shown in Fig. 4-50 where the single pixel common to all three planes was defined by the cross hairs shown here.

of comparison, the specimen photographs have been reversed in a similar fashion.)

In the next section (not shown here), the pedicle is slightly thicker. The inferior articular process is now at its distal tip. In the following section (Fig. 4-58C and D), the pedicle and lamina form a continuous osseous ring. This is in the midbody of L4. Looking at the undersurface of this section (Fig. 4-58E and F), note the pedicle fading away to form the smooth lateral wall of the nerve root canal.

Below the pedicle is the foramen (Fig. 4-58G and H). The cuts are slightly oblique on both the CT sections and the specimen, showing the bottom of the pedicle and the nerve root canal on the contralateral side.

One section, or approximately 0.5 cm, lower than this level (not shown here), the

middle of the foramen is still depicted. This demonstrates that the foramen has height as well as other dimensions. The fact that the foramen is open on one view does not establish its normality (see Fig. 4-45). To be normal, it must be open on a number of views sufficient to include its total height.

The superior articular process (SAP) of L5 is more prominent on the next section, in which it will begin to close off the foramen. The L5 pedicle forms the floor of the foramen (Fig. 4-58I and J). Notice the posterior disc margin and the SAP coming together to help close off the foramen. In subsequent sections, the pedicle gets thicker and the L4–5 foramen is completely closed.

So far, only the axial section of the spine has been considered. The axial specimen sections can be reassembled to show the

(Text continues on p. 128.)

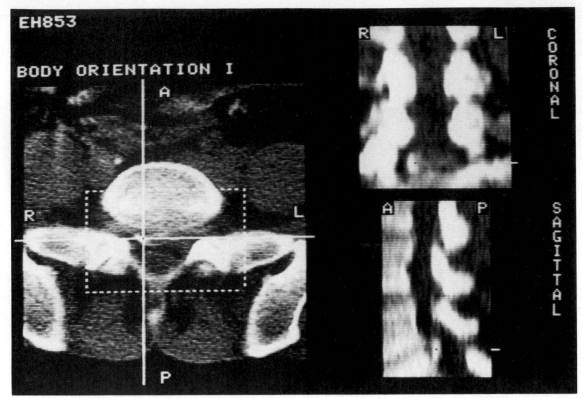

Fig. 4-50. MPD combination defined by cross hair position in Fig. 4-49. The abnormality is a partially calcified, severe, right-sided, L5–S1 disc bulge or rupture.

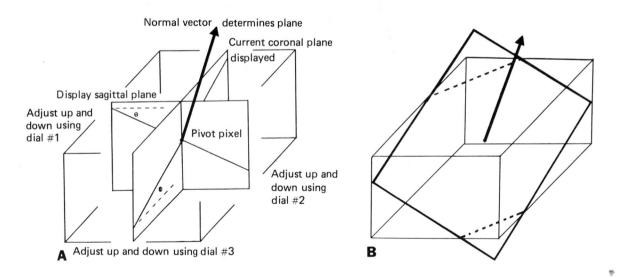

Fig. 4-51. Schematic diagram showing extraction of any desired oblique plane **(B)** *from the solid cube of image data* **(A).** *(Glenn, WV Jr, Rhodes ML, Altschuler EM, et al: Multiplanar display computerized body tomography applications in the lumbar spine. Spine 4(4): 282–352, 1979)*

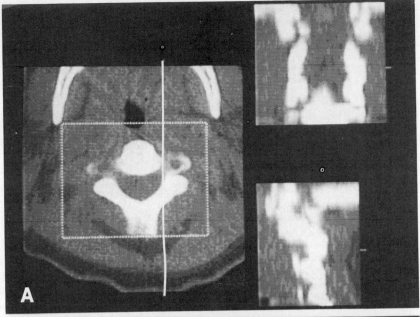

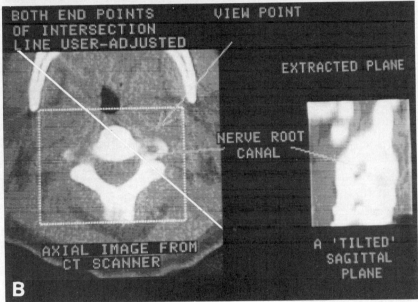

Fig. 4-52. **(A)** *The reconstructed sagittal image does not represent a true axial view of the cervical spinal nerve canals and foramina.* **(B)** *The 45-degree angle or "tilted" sagittal plane does represent a true axial view of the spinal nerve canal and foramina. (Glenn, WV Jr, Rhodes ML, Altschuler EM, et al: Multiplanar display computerized body tomography applications in the lumbar spine. Spine 4(4): 282–352, 1979)*

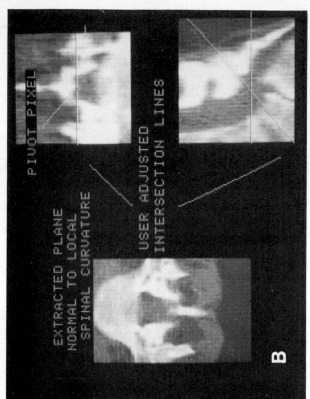

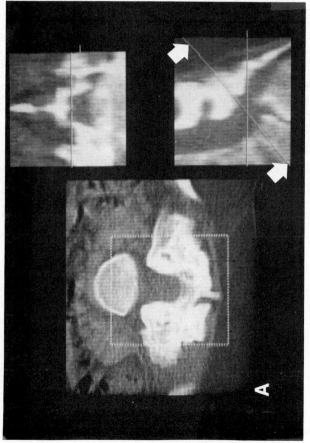

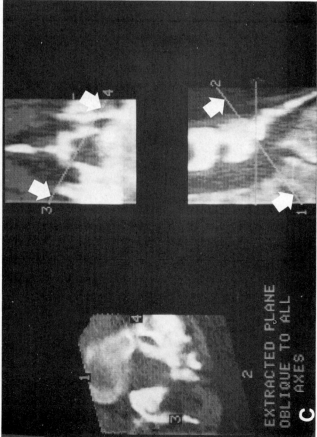

Fig. 4-53. The transverse and sagittal images show a significant L5–S1 spondylolisthesis. The horizontal lines on both coronal and sagittal images represent the craniocaudal position of the transverse section similar to the tick mark described in Fig. 4-43. The appearance of the spinal canal on both the transverse and sagittal views is artificially elongated in the AP dimension owing to the spondylolisthesis. (A) By interactively adjusting an oblique orientation on the sagittal image (arrows) the user can specify a desired true axial "transverse" projection through the canal. (B) The transverse image thus created is shown on the left. The anticipated correction in AP diameter is obvious. (C) A transverse plane which is oblique to both the saggital and coronal axes (arrows). Use of this last imaging technique in cases of severe scoliosis is obviously valuable. (Glenn, WV Jr, Rhodes ML, Altschuler EM, et al: Multiplanar display computerized body tomography applications in the lumbar spine. Spine 4(4): 282–352, 1979)

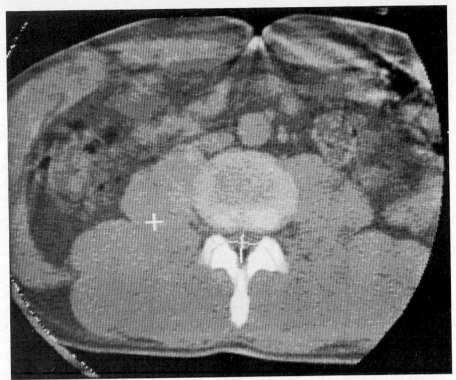

Fig. 4-54. Midsagittal (AP) and transverse canal measurement line. Note the cross-hair, end-point localizer on the left.

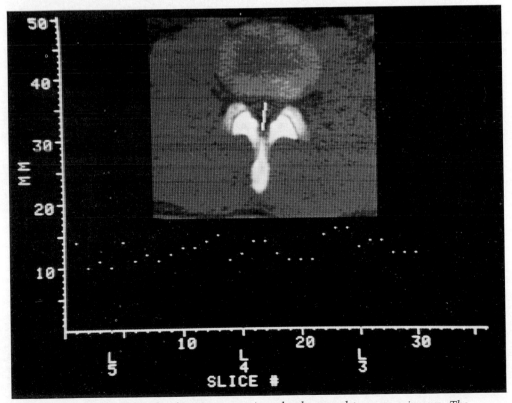

Fig. 4-55. Data point plot for 30 consecutive, closely spaced transverse images. The image inset represents that one data point which is blinking. The blinking data point can be moved left or right with an analog dial; the inset transverse image changes accordingly.

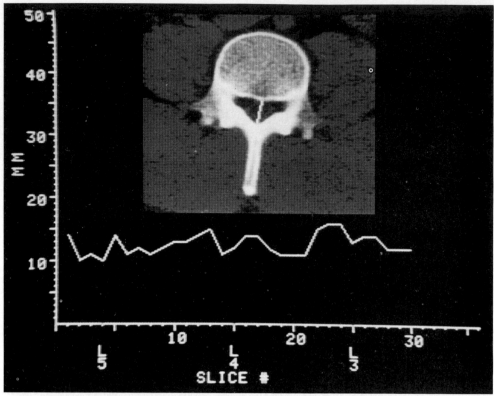

Fig. 4-56. Same graph as in Fig. 4-55 but with straight-line point connection and a different transverse image (inset).

foramen in its sagittal orientation (Fig. 4-59). The computer reasembles the CBT data gathered on the axial sections and constructs images in the sagittal and coronal planes.

Figure 4-60 shows a normal specimen cut sagittally. In part A, the L3, L4, and L5 foramina are open wide. There are no osteophytes in the lateral recesses. The surfaces of the pedicles are smooth. There is adequate room for each nerve root in the foramen. In part B, note that the sagittal image chosen for display is approximately the same distance from the midline as the level of section of the anatomic specimen. The L5 SAP and the L5 foramen have been labeled as reference points. On the coronal reconstruction, note the medial swing of the L5 SAP just above the wide-open L5 foramen. Furthermore, it is possible on a more lateral sagittal scan (Fig. 4-60C) to analyze precisely the

boundaries of the foramen. Note particularly the SAP of L5, the pars of L5, and the SAP of S1. This can be compared point-to-point with the corresponding structures on the anatomic specimen.

It is important to understand the relation of the nerve roots to the superior articular processes. The medial swing of the SAP of L5 is in close proximity to the L5 nerve root at its takeoff. In addition, in the L4 foramen, the superiormost aspect of the L5 SAP is in relative proximity to the L4 nerve root. Should this space be lessened it could easily compromise the nerve root.

To analyze foraminal boundaries, it is helpful to see a close-up view of the L4 foramen of the specimen under consideration (Fig. 4-61). The intervertebral foramen is bounded above and below by the pedicles, anteriorly by the vertebral body and discs,

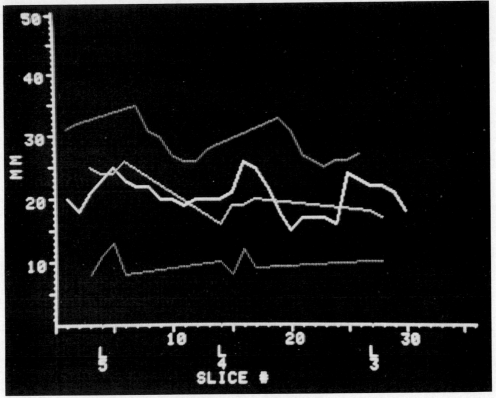

Fig. 4-57. Multiple measurement plot of different parameters from the same patient.

and posteriorly by the pars, flavum, and SAP, (in descending order). Note the wide-open foramen and, particularly, the distance between the tip of the SAP and the pedicle above. Figure 4-61B shows the same specimen after a discectomy has been performed and the spine has been pushed in from both ends, in a very gross sense simulating disc resorption. In particular, note the decreased distance from the SAP to the pedicle above. Note also how the annulus has bulged to decrease further the already compromised foramen. The shape of the intervertebral foramen is determined to a major extent by the height of the intervertebral disc space. In disc resorption, facet subluxation occurs, so the apex of the superior facet of the inferior vertebral body moves upward. This results in deformation of the intervertebral foramen as shown in Figure 4-62.

Abnormal Anatomy

In this section, cases are presented with emphasis on disc disease and bony stenosis of the central canal and foramina. Correlation with myelography, venography, and surgery is provided when available. Other lesions for which CBT has proven extremely beneficial are covered elsewhere, including trauma, spinal dysrhaphia, syringomyelia, cord and nerve root tumors, and infectious processes involving the spinal axis and associated paraspinal soft tissues.[24,32,34,43,46,51,65,72,75,91,95,111,121,122,134–137,141,159,160,168,171]

Figure 4-63 demonstrates a midsagittal appearance of a large L4 disc bulge similar to the unrelated specimen photograph in Figure 4-61B. Other MPD views not shown here confirmed bilateral L4 foraminal encroachment due to lateral extensions of this

(Text continues on p. 133.)

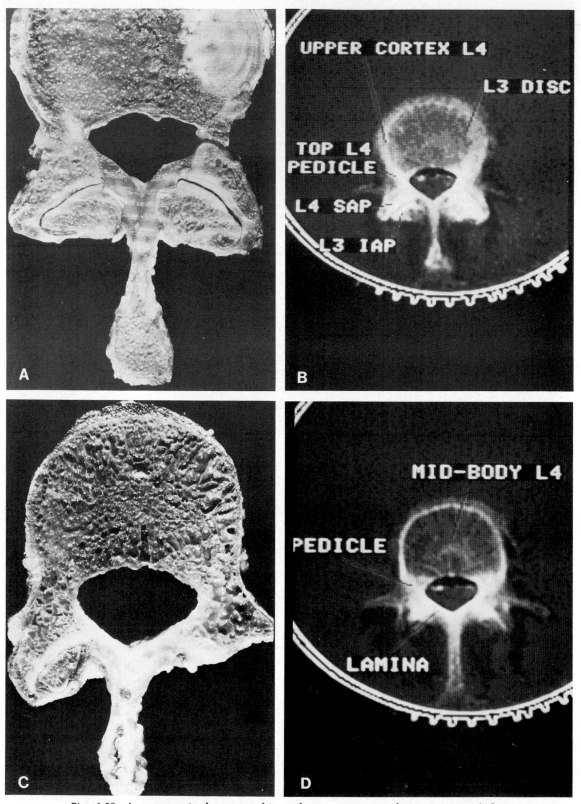

Fig. 4-58. A computerized tomographic and gross anatomic demonstration of the normal axial anatomy of an L4 spinal segment. (A and B) Top of the L4 cortex, bottom of the L3 disc, top of the pedicle, and a good definition of the facet joint are shown. (C and D) The midbody of L4. The pedicle and lamina form a continuous osseous ring. (Caption continues on opposite page)

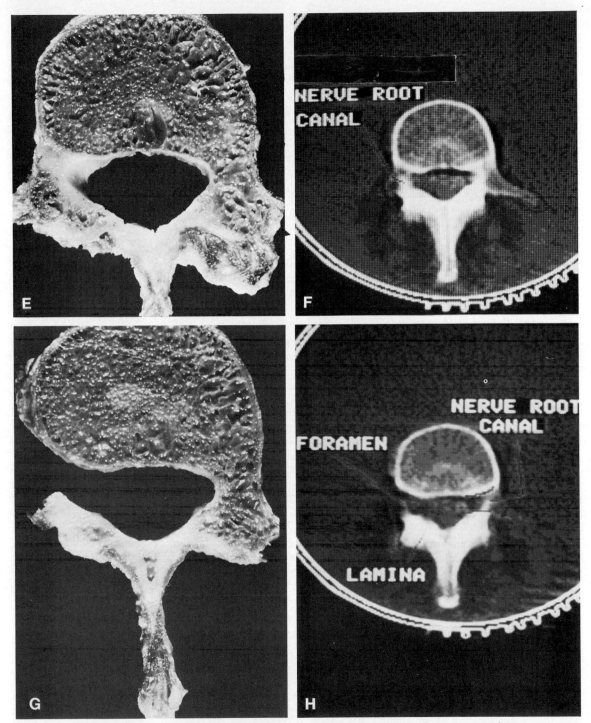

Fig. 4-58. (E and F) (Continued) *Under the surface of the sections shown in C and D. The pedicle is fading away to form the smooth lateral wall of the nerve root canal. (G and H) Below the pedicle, the foramen is entered. The cuts are slightly oblique, showing the bottom of the pedicle and the nerve root canal on the contralateral side. (Caption continues on overleaf page)*

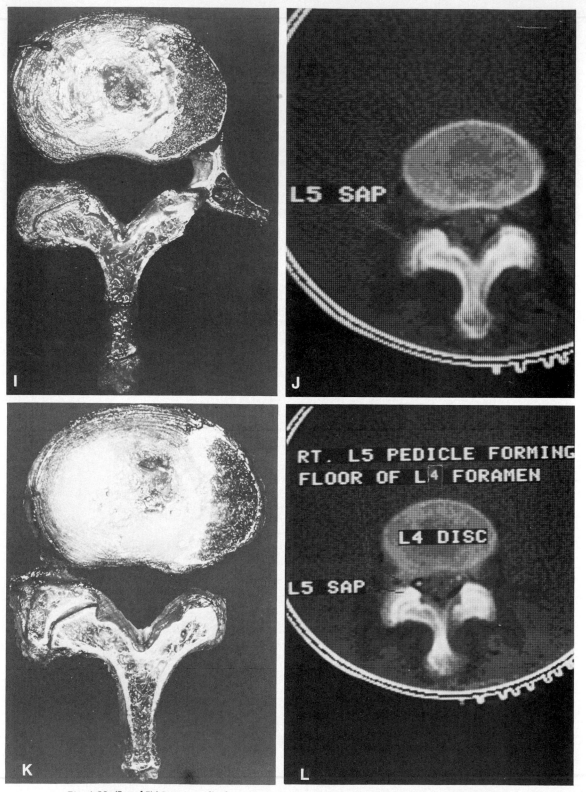

Fig. 4-58. (I and J) (Continued) The L5 superior articular process (SAP) is now prominent. It will begin to play a considerable role in closing the foramen. (K and L) The L5 pedicle forms the floor of the foramen. Notice the posterior disc margin and the SAP coming together to help close the foramen.(Figs. 4-58 through 4-61 ref. 102)

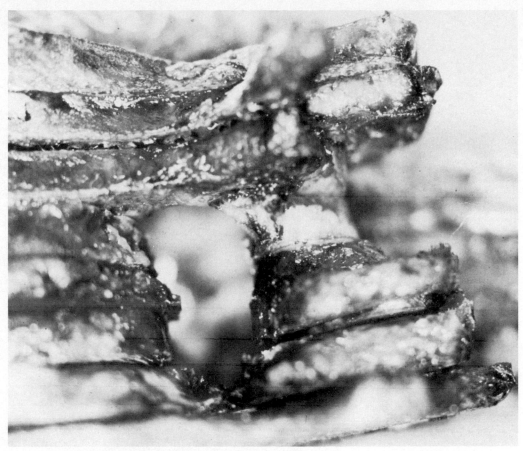

Fig. 4-59. The axial specimen sections of Fig. 4-58 have been reassembled to demonstrate the foramen in its sagittal orientation.

large disc. Because of the history of severe allergic reaction to iodine, this patient's condition precluded standard myelography.

Figure 4-64 is from an 8-year-old boy with L4 disc symptoms following a skateboard accident. The referring physician elected CBT to avoid the general anesthesia required for myelography. Surgery was performed solely on the basis of the CBT examination and plain films, which showed a narrowed L4 disc space. Surgery confirmed the CBT findings of a large bulging L4 disc with lateral extension into both L4 spinal nerve canals and foramina.

Figure 4-65 shows a patient with a large central and right-sided L4 disc with extension into the right L4 spinal nerve canal and foramen. The Metrizamide myelogram and

epidural venogram in Figure 4-66 both confirmed the CBT findings. The epidural venogram was done first, with great difficulty because of the patient's extreme fear of needles; the CBT examination was done next. Following CBT, surgery was advised to alleviate the patient's almost complete incapacitation. Even after the myelogram shown in Figure 4-66, the patient still refused surgery and is currently doing poorly on conservative treatment.

Figures 4-67 to 4-69 show another patient with a large bilateral L4 disc bulge. The midsagittal CBT presentation in Figure 4-68 is particularly striking and corresponds with the lateral myelographic view in Figure 4-69. The fact that the abnormal disc bulge is convincingly seen on only two of the over-

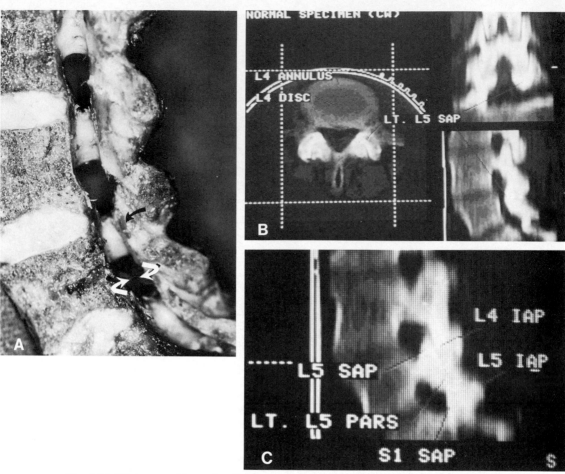

Fig. 4-60. **(A)** *A normal lower lumbar spine cut parasagitally. Note the normal foramina at L3, L4, and L5. The lateral recesses are smooth and are not compromised by osteophytes. Arrows have been placed on the L5 SAP and the L5 foramen to facilitate orientation.* **(B)** *On CT, the axial image is at the level of the L5 SAP. The sagittal image is at approximately the same distance from the midline as the anatomic section in A. On the coronal image, note the medial swing of the SAP, just above the open L5 foramen.* **(C)** *A more lateral sagittal image permits precise analysis of the boundaries of the foramen as labeled.*

lapped images at 3-mm intervals (see Fig. 4-67) reiterates the necessity for close transverse spacing.

Figures 4-70 and 4-71 represent a case in which CBT examination indicated a right L4 disc abnormality only, which corresponded to the clinical picture. The myelogram, however, suggested a more central L4 abnormality, and the epidural venogram was interpreted as abnormal on the right at L5 (Fig. 4-71). Surgery confirmed the unilateral nature of the problem at L4 as seen by CBT.

Figures 4-72 to 4-74 show a case with left L3 symptoms in which the CBT examination was done to resolve a discrepancy between the Metrizamide myelogram and the epidural venogram. On the myelogram only one view, the left lateral decubitus (Fig. 4-74), showed an extradural defect on the left at L3. The epidural venogram in Figure 4-74 was interpreted as showing a possible abnormality on the opposite side, one level lower at L4. The key CBT finding shown in Figures 4-72 and 4-73 is a soft tissue density

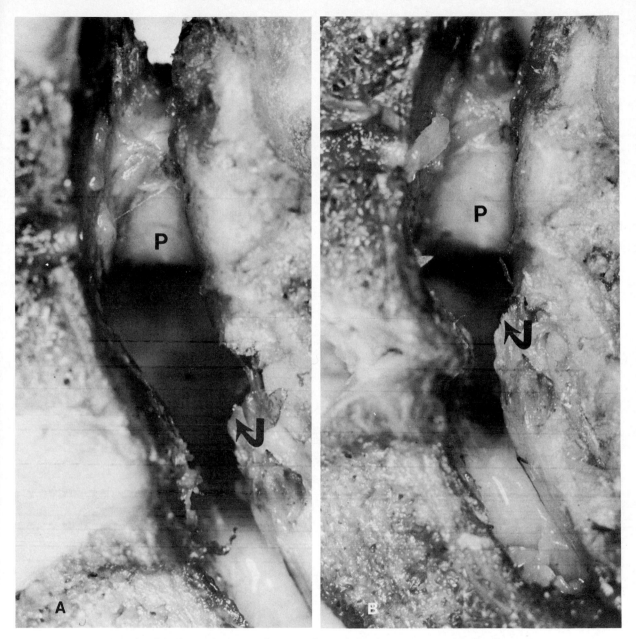

Fig. 4-61. *(A) The L4 foramen of a normal specimen. Note in particular the distance between the tip of the L5 SAP (arrow) and the pedicle above (P). (B) In the same specimen, a discectomy has been performed, simulating disc resorption. Note decreased distance from SAP to pedicle above. The foramen is markedly compromised.*

obscuring the left anterior epidural fat. This abnormality was present with certainty on only two of the transverse images obtained at 3-mm intervals. The coronal appearance in Figure 4-73 was particularly helpful and led to a CBT interpretation of a swollen left L3 nerve root, laterally extruded disc material, or both. The epidural venogram was reevaluated with three CBT findings in mind. The consensus was a possible lateral

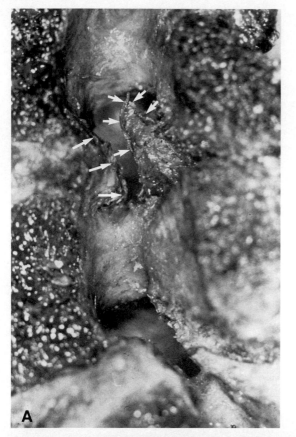

abnormality on the left at L3, in keeping with the clinical symptoms, the lateral decubitus view of the myelogram, and the CBT examination. Surgery confirmed the CBT results: a swollen left L3 nerve root and a laterally extruded disc fragment.

Figure 4-75 represents a patient with symptoms at L5–S1 who had had two previous myelograms. An iophendylate study several months prior to admission showed an extradural defect on the right at L4–5, while a Metrizamide myelogram at the time of admission was completely normal. The CBT examination was interpreted as showing a calcified density in the left anterior portion of the L5–S1 canal, probably a calcified disc fragment. In addition, other CBT images not shown here indicated a mild L4 central disc bulge. At surgery, both the L4 and L5 levels were opened; mild disc protrusion at L4 plus a left-sided calcified disc fragment at L5 confirmed the CBT findings.

Figures 4-76 and 4-77 show a trauma case in which bone from a superior end-plate compression fracture of L2 has been extruded into the upper lumbar canal, almost com-

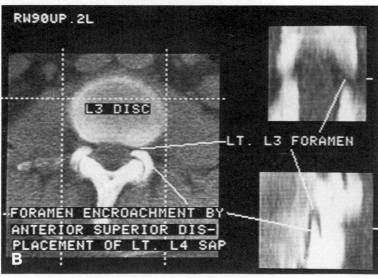

RW90UP.2L

L3 DISC

LT. L3 FORAMEN

FORAMEN ENCROACHMENT BY ANTERIOR SUPERIOR DIS- PLACEMENT OF LT. L4 SAP

Fig. 4-62. MPD views showing encroachment of the left L3 SAP into the left L2 spinal nerve canal and foramen. (All remaining figs. except 4-76 and 4-77 ref. 65.)

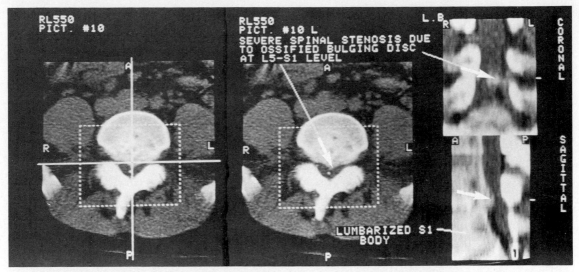

Fig. 4-63. MPD views showing large disc or annulus bulge at L4 **(arrows)**. Midsagittal view is most dramatic and corresponds well to unrelated specimen photograph in Fig. 4-61B showing similar gross finding at L5. Transverse image indicates bilateral extension into L4 spinal nerve canals and foramina.

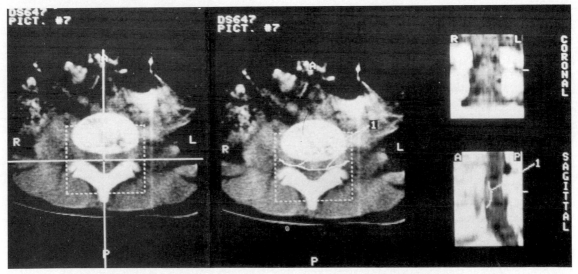

Fig. 4-64. MPD views showing a large L4 disc or annulus bulge with lateral extension into both nerve root canals and foramina. Transverse and midsagittal soft-tissue bulge is highlighted. Sagittal images (not shown) through either the left or the right L4 foramen showed abnormal soft tissue (disc and annulus) when compared with the normal appearance of L3 or L5 foramina on the same side. (Hounsfield GN: Computerized transverse axial scanning [tomography]. Part 1: Description of System. Br J Radiol 46:1016–1022, 1973)

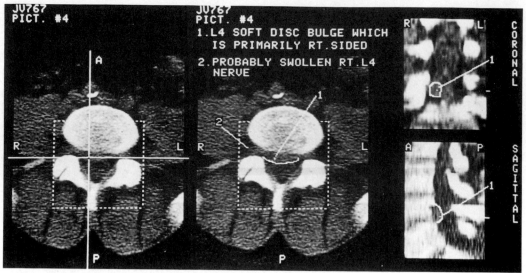

Fig. 4-65. *MPD views showing large central and larger right-sided L4 disc or annulus bulge. The soft tissue density in the right L4 spinal nerve canal and foramen was thought to represent a swollen right L4 nerve, a laterally extruded disc fragment, or both. (Hounsfield GN: Computerized transverse axial scanning [tomography]. Part I: Description of system. Br J Radiol 46:1016⅓1022, 1973; Ambrose J: Computerized transverse scanning [tomography]. Part 2: Clinical applications. Br J Radiol 46:1023–1047, 1973)*

pletely occluding the canal at and just below the disc space of L1–L2. There was a significant second finding in this case, which would have been completely missed without the benefit of the sagittal images. On the sagittal view of Figure 4-77 note the soft tissue density corresponding to the L2–L3 disc space, one level below the traumatic bone fragments. This soft tissue was felt to represent a moderately severe traumatic disc bulge warranting surgery at two levels rather than one.

Figures 4-78 and 4-79 are two cases of bilateral L5 pars defects. There was no evidence of spondylolisthesis in either case. Both examples show the typical bony ridge immediately anterior to the cleft in the pars interarticularis. In the reconstructed sagittal view, this bony ridge acts as a vertical bar dividing the spinal nerve canal and foramen into anterior and posterior compartments, with the nerve occupying the anterior compartment. In many cases of pars defect, the anterior compartment becomes compromised further laterally.

The patient in Figure 4-80 shows moderate degenerative changes consisting of sclerotic bulbous articular processes, posterior laminar thickening, lateral recess stenosis, and apophyseal joint osteophytes. The central canal is mildly compromised. These findings are typical of degenerative disease with or without spondylolisthesis. This particular patient has a grade I L4–5 spondylolisthesis, shown in Figure 4-81. In Figure 4-82, the left L4 spinal nerve canal is partly encroached by an osteophytic ridge on the posterior margin of the vertebral body anteriorly, and by an osteophyte on the left L4 inferior articular process posteriorly. In this situation, the L4 nerve root may be normal, but the L5 nerve root could easily be trapped between the left L4 inferior articular process and the upper posterior margin of the L5 body. Another example is shown in Figure 4-83. Figures 4-84 and 4-85 illustrate moderate circumferential bony encroachment in the medial portion of the spinal nerve canal, with severe lateral encroachment. This stresses the importance of visualizing a se-

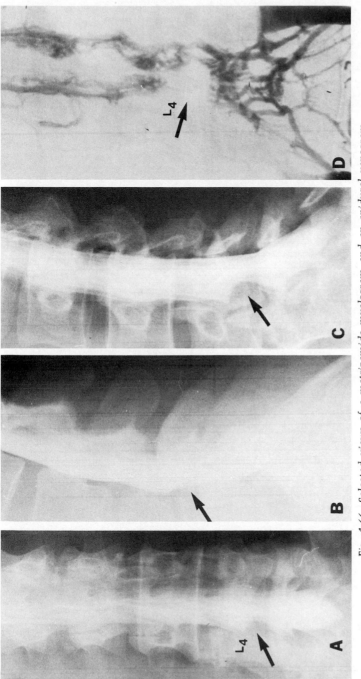

Fig. 4-66. *Selected views of a metrizamide myelogram and an epidural venogram showing evidence for large right L4 disc abnormality (**arrows**).*

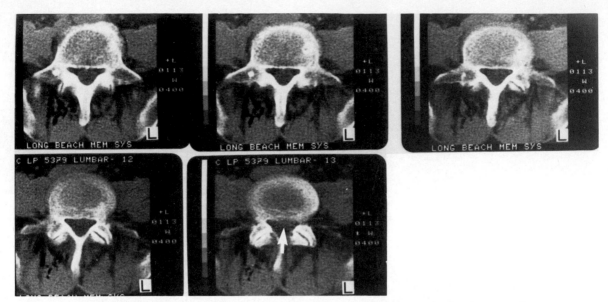

Fig. 4-67. Transverse sections (8-mm thick) taken at 3-mm intervals showing central L4 disc bulge on only two images **(arrows).**

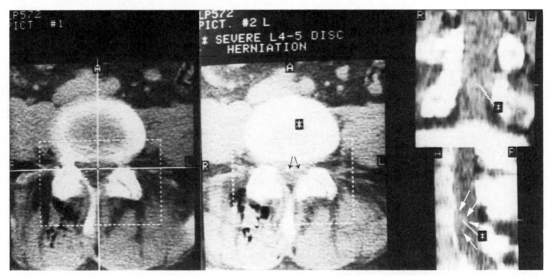

Fig. 4-68. MPD views showing large central and bilateral L4 disc bulge best seen in the sagittal view. Note excellent correspondence of sagittal image with lateral myelographic view in Fig. 4-69.

ries of sagittal images from medial to lateral. On occasion, we have missed significant foraminal encroachment by not reviewing sagittal images through the lateral portions of the nerve canals.

The reassuring CBT-myelographic correlations shown for lumbar disc abnormalities earlier in this chapter are also illustrated with degenerative disease and spondylolisthesis. In Figure 4-86, the CBT findings of posterior canal encroachment and spinal stenosis at both L3 and L4, plus a mild L4–5 spondylolisthesis, correlate with myelographic findings shown in Figure 4-87. The

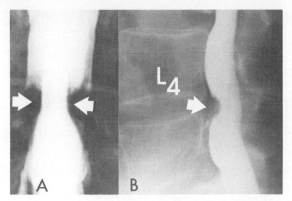

Fig. 4-69. Anteroposterior and lateral myelogram views showing large central and bilateral L4 disc bulge.

stenosis resulting from an L4–5 spondylolisthesis, in which the canal is comprised anteriorly by the vertebral body step-off and posteriorly by the displaced inferior articular processes (here primarily unilateral on the left) of the higher vertebral body. The severe stenosis predicted from CBT corresponds to a complete block on the myelogram in Figure 4-92.

Postoperative Evaluation Cases

The case illustrated in Figures 4-93 and 4-94 was that of a woman with a history of seven previous back operations. The CBT examination was the last step in her preoperative workup. The extradural defects shown on the myelogram in Figure 4-94 were interpreted as arachnoiditis or scarring from previous back surgery, and the decision was made not to offer this patient another surgical procedure. The findings of the CBT examination (definite posterior bony encroachment, rather than soft-tissue or scar encroachment, of the canal) reversed that decision. The patient subsequently underwent surgery, and showed improvement during the short-term postoperative period. Long-term followup is not available.

sagittal CBT corresponds closely with the lateral myelogram view. In another case of severe stenosis and degenerative disease, the bilateral bony encroachment (seen on the reconstructed coronal image in Figure 4-88) compares favorably with the anteroposterior myelographic presentation in Figure 4-89. Similarly, the sagittal CBT demonstration of grade I spondylolisthesis with anterior and posterior bony encroachment at the L4 disc space level (Fig. 4-90) corresponds with the lateral myelogram view in Figure 4-89. Figures 4-91 and 4-92 show the severe spinal

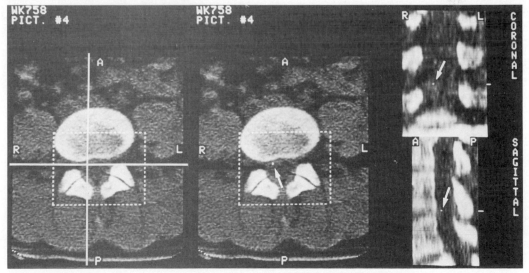

Fig. 4-70. MPD views interpreted as mild to moderate, right-sided, L4 disc bulge (arrows).

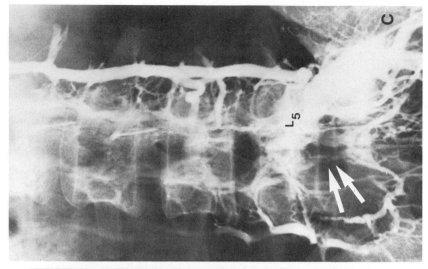

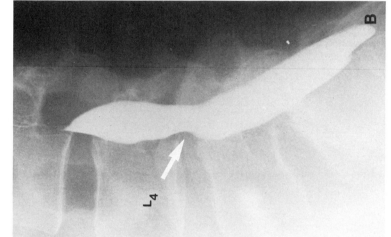

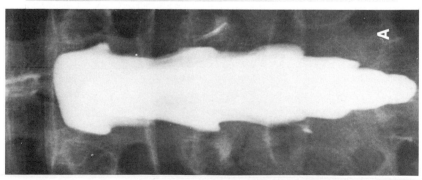

Fig. 4-71. AP and lateral myelographic views plus AP view of epidural venogram. The myelogram was interpreted as a central and bilateral L4 disc abnormality (**arrow**). The epidural venogram, however, was interpreted as showing a right-sided disc abnormality one level lower at L5–S1 (**double arrow**).

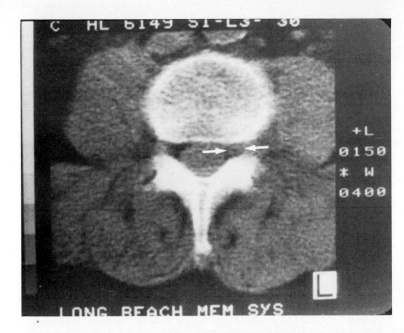

*Fig. 4-72. Transverse CBT section through upper margin of L3 disc and lower margin of L3 body showing replacement of left anterior epidural fat by small soft tissue density **(arrows)**.*

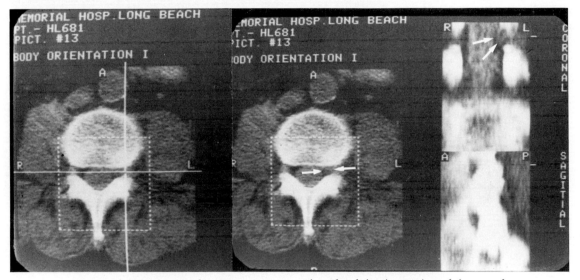

*Fig. 4-73. MPD views showing asymmetry of epidural fat **(arrows)** on left at and immediately above the L3 disc space. Coronal asymmetry was particularly convincing. Findings interpreted as swollen left L3 nerve root, laterally extruded disc fragment, or both.*

The case of acquired stenosis illustrated in Figures 4-95 to 4-97 is a particularly good example of the blinking-dot localizing facility provided with the MPD format. The large protrusion of bone into the right L5 canal (see transverse image of Fig. 4-95) corresponds to the large right extradural anter- posterior myleographic defect in Figure 4-97. The same right lateral bony overgrowth on the transverse image can be identified on the coronal and sagittal images of Figure 4-95. On the sagittal view it appears as a posterior mass of bone, which corresponds to the large posterior extradural defect on

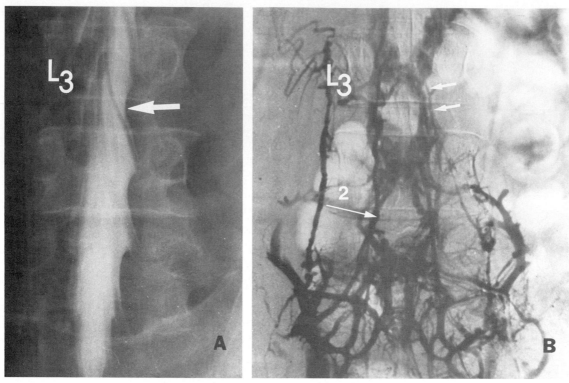

Fig. 4-74. *Cross-table, decubitus myelogram view (left side down) shows a smooth lateral extradural defect on the left at L3 (arrows). The anteroposterior subtraction view of the epidural venogram was interpreted as abnormal on the right at L4 due to nonfilling of the anterior epidural veins (single arrow). Changes laterally on the left at L3 (double arrows) were noted in retrospect following results of a CBT examination.*

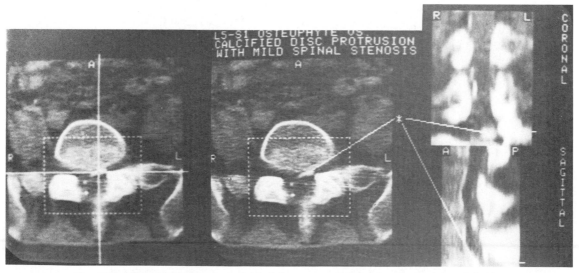

Fig. 4-75. *MPD views showing calcified disc or annulus (or disc fragment) on left (*) at L5–S1. A previous laminectomy defect is also noted on the right.*

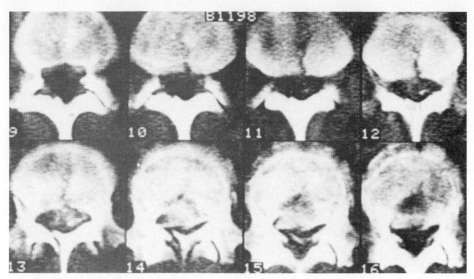

Fig. 4-76. Sequential 8-mm transverse images obtained at 3-mm intervals showing superior end-plate compression fracture of L2 with extrusion of the bone almost obliterating the upper lumbar canal.

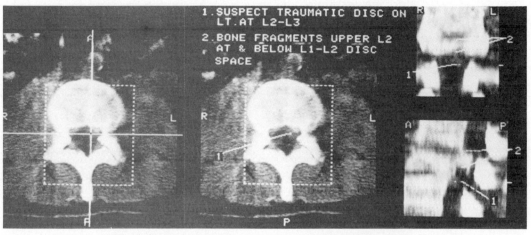

Fig. 4-77. MPD of the L2 fracture shown in Fig. 4-76. Note the sagittal appearance of extruded bone material and the sagittal demonstration of a soft-tissue abnormality, probably representing a traumatic L2 disc herniation one level below the bone fragments. This finding was identified only from the sagittal view.

the lateral myelographic view of Figure 4-97. The same lateral myelographic view shows a smaller anterior extradural defect from osteophytic lipping of the adjacent L4 and L5 vertebral bodies. The corresponding CBT demonstration of this marginal osteophyte is shown in Figure 4-96.

The case in Figure 4-98 is a good example of how not to perform preoperative CBT evaluation of the spine. The initial study

demonstrated stenotic changes at L5–S1. The patient subsequently underwent an L5 laminectomy with partial improvement of symptoms. The problem, however, was that the initial preoperative CBT examination (at our institution) was of the survey type, with transverse images taken every 1 or 1.5 cm. Because the patient had residual hip pain, the detailed postoperative examination shown in Figure 4-98 was performed; it

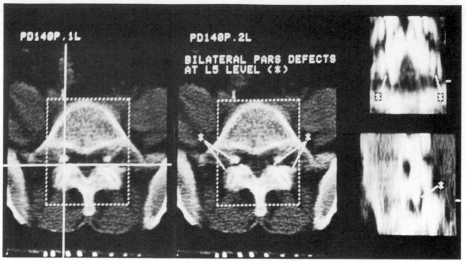

Fig. 4-78. *MPD views showing bilateral L5 pars defects (*). The ridge of bone just anterior to the pars defects on both transverse and sagittal views is typical of patients with this condition. The effect in the sagittal projection is to divide the spinal nerve canal and foramen into anterior and posterior compartments.*

demonstrated a bulging L3 disc with emphasis on the right side, corresponding to the clinical symptoms.

The case shown in Figures 4-99 and 4-100 demonstrates a grade IV L5–S1 spondylolisthesis with a double canal appearance on the transverse images. The midsagittal configuration of the canal shown in Figure 4-99 shows marked constriction due to a very narrow isthmus between the remaining L4 posterior elements (bilateral L5 laminectomy) and the upper posterior margin of S1. The myelogram (Fig. 4-100) demonstrated a narrowing at this level but underestimated the isthmus. Before the sagittal CBT image was seen, it had been decided that this patient was not a candidate for a fifth surgical procedure. The CBT findings reversed this decision, and the patient underwent reoperation for removal of the L4 posterior elements and decompression of the isthmus. There was short-term improvement; long-term followup is not available.

Two cases, shown in Figures 4-101 to 4-104, represent the problem of continued back pain following solid posterior bony fusion and placement of metallic screws. CBT examination in the first case showed a right L4 metallic screw entering the posteroinferior aspect of the right L4 foramen

(Fig. 4-101). While the appearance on the transverse and coronal images is suspicious, the sagittal sections indicated that the right L4 spinal nerve canal and foramen were still open and that the screw probably would not have to be withdrawn. The second case was slightly different, because CBT examination (Fig. 4-103) showed the tip of the screw encroaching on the lateral aspect of the central canal and the medial aspect of the left L4 foramen. Because the epidural venogram (Fig. 4-104) was also positive on the left at L4 near the tip of this screw, the surgeon elected to withdraw this one screw. The patient subsequently improved.

Figures 4-105 to 4-106 show a case with a preoperative myelographic and clinical diagnosis of an L4 disc problem. The myelogram (Fig. 4-107) showed a large anterior extradural defect at L4. The CBT examination was performed after there was no relief of symptoms following surgery. The CBT findings (Figs. 4-105 and 4-106) indicated that surgery had been mistakenly performed at the L3 level and that a large L4 disc problem remained. Figure 4-106 raised the possibility of a small calcified fragment in the anterior aspect of the canal at L3. At this patient's second operation, the original L4

(*Text continues on p. 153.*)

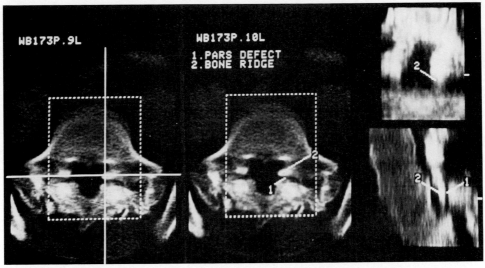

Fig. 4-79. MPD views showing bilateral pars defects and the bone ridge immediately anterior. There is mild lateral encroachment of the L5 canal on the left as shown in both transverse and coronal views. (Hounsfield GN: Computerized transverse axial scanning [tomography]. Part I: Description of system. Br J Radiol 46:1016–1022, 1973; Ambrose J: Computerized transverse scanning [tomography]. Part 2: Clinical applications. Br J Radiol 46:1023–1047, 1973)

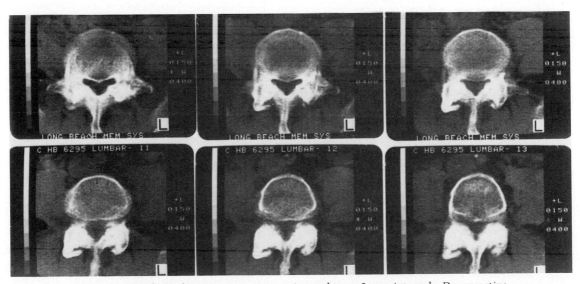

Fig. 4-80. Overlapped 8-mm transverse sections taken at 3-mm intervals. Degenerative changes illustrated include sclerotic bulbous facet joints, laminar thickening, lateral recess stenosis, facet joint osteophytes, and mild central canal stenosis.

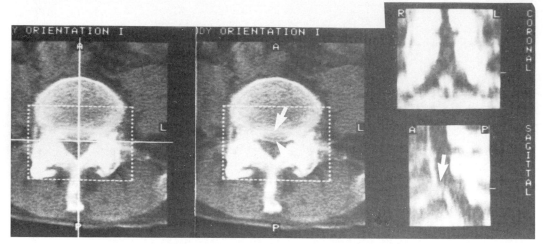

Fig. 4-81. MPD views show mild grade I L4–5 spondylolisthesis (arrows).

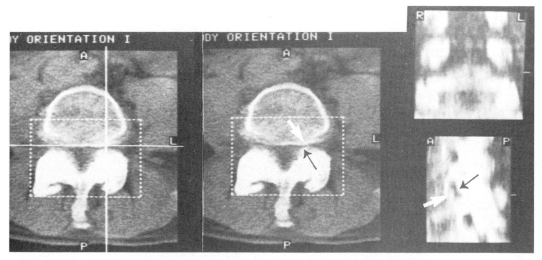

Fig. 4-82. MPD views showing anterior and posterior bony encroachment of the left L4 spinal nerve canal and foramen. The anterior encroachment is caused by a small osteophytic ridge of bone (white arrow) along the posterior margin of the L4 body. The posterior encroachment is caused by a small facet joint osteophyte (black arrow) on the ventral margin of the left L4 inferior articular process.

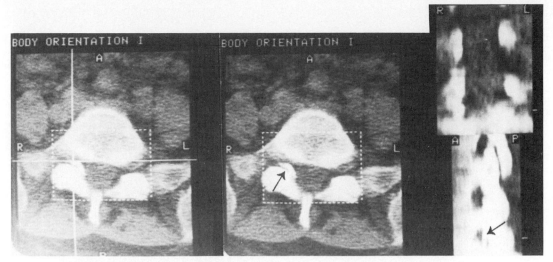

*Fig. 4-83. MPD views showing posterior bony encroachment of right L5 spinal nerve canal and foramen by a facet joint osteophyte **(black arrow).***

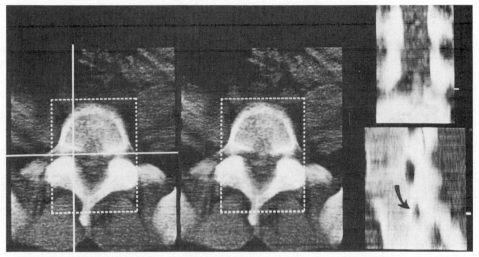

Fig. 4-84. MPD views showing moderate circumferential bony encroachment at the medial aspect of the right L5 spinal nerve canal and foramen.

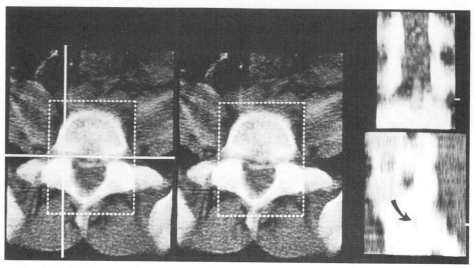

Fig. 4-85. MPD views showing severe bony encroachment of the right L5 spinal nerve canal and foramen. The sagittal image is several millimeters lateral to that shown in Fig. 4-84 and illustrates the often-overlooked need to evaluate the lateral aspect of each spinal nerve canal.

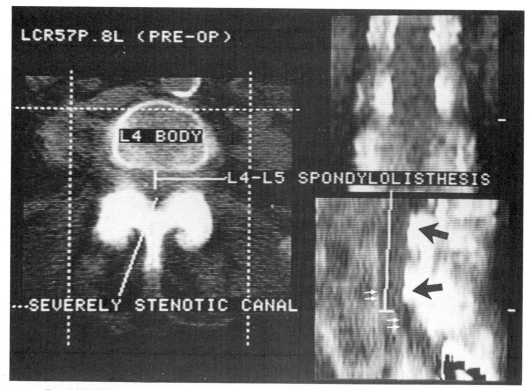

Fig. 4-86. MPD views showing a severe stenotic canal at the L4 level in both transverse and sagittal views. An L4–5 spondylolisthesis is labeled. Posterior bone encroachment **(black arrows)** contributes to severe stenosis at L4 and moderately severe stenosis at L3. This posterior encroachment corresponds to the lateral myelographic view in Fig. 4-87.

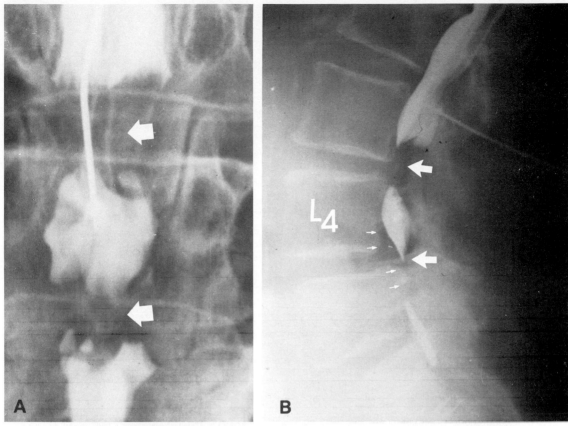

Fig. 4-87. Anteroposterior and lateral myelographic views showing changes of severe spinal stenosis at L3 and L4 (white arrows) and a grade I L4–5 spondylolisthesis (small arrows).

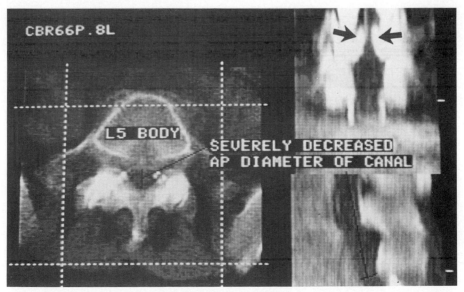

Fig. 4-88. MPD views showing bilateral lateral bony encroachment at the L4 level in the coronal view (black arrows). This appearance corresponds to the bilateral extradural defects seen in the anteroposterior myelographic view of Fig. 4-81.

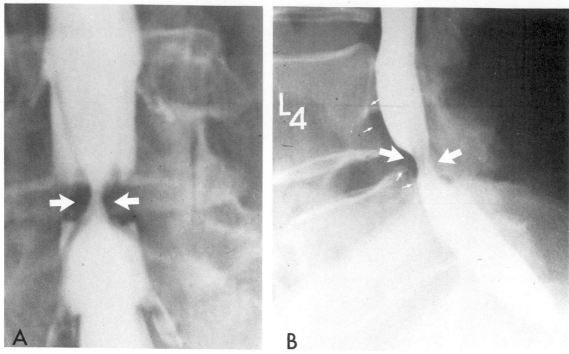

Fig. 4-89. *Anteroposterior and lateral myelographic views showing severe spinal stenosis at L4–5 as a result of both lateral encroachment (anteroposterior view) and anterior and posterior encroachment (lateral view).*

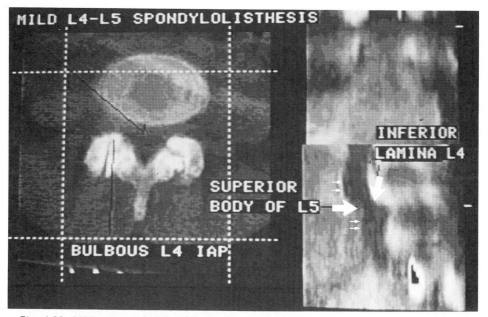

Fig. 4-90. *MPD views showing on the sagittal image evidence for a grade I L4–5 spondylolisthesis* **(small arrows)** *plus anterior and posterior bony encroachment of the canal at the same level* **(large arrows)***. This appearance corresponds to the lateral myelographic view in Fig. 4-89, which demonstrates the same findings.*

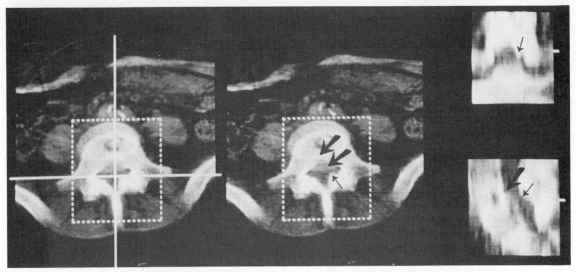

Fig. 4-91. MPD views which show in a patient with spondylolisthesis the anterior L4–5 step-off (large arrows) plus asymmetric anterior inferior displacement of left L4 inferior articular process (small arrow). Anterior displacement is best seen on the transverse image, while inferior displacement is best seen on the coronal section.

disc rupture was confirmed and removed. The L3 level was not reopened; therefore, the possibility of a small anterior fragment at L3 remained unverified. Following the second operation the patient still showed no signs of improvement. Another repeat CBT exam again showed the large L4 disc abnormality. The patient is now better following her third surgical procedure.

Figure 4-108 shows postoperative evaluation of a large, solid posterior fusion. CBT was used to assess the stability of the fusion (solid) and also to evaluate for any possible evidence of spinal stenosis. The fusion overgrowth noted in Figure 4-108 is most likely either scar tissue or hypertrophied ligamentum flavum.

The case in Figures 4-109 and 4-110 shows evidence of extensive posterior decompression for spinal stenosis with residual ligamentum flavum hypertrophy at L3 (Fig. 4-109) and moderately severe bilateral spinal nerve canal and forminal encroachment at L5 (Fig. 4-110).

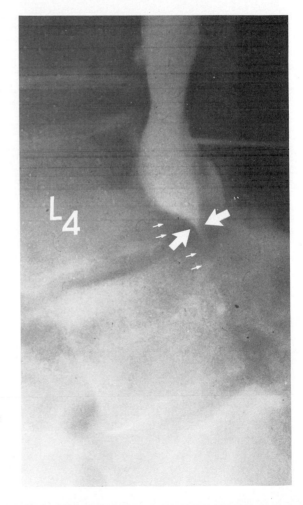

Fig. 4-92. Lateral myelogram view showing a complete block at the L4–5 spondylolisthesis. Note anterior and posterior extradural defect (arrows).

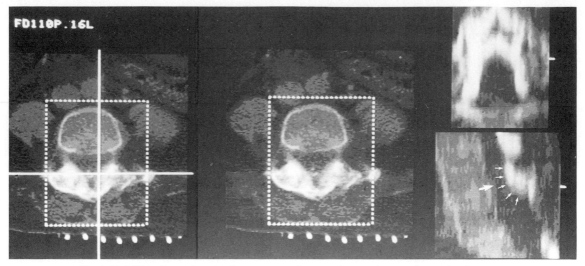

Fig. 4-93. MPD views showing bony encroachment of posterior canal margins best seen on midsagittal view. This posterior indentation corresponds with the lateral myelographic view in Fig. 4-94, but on CBT the indentation can be attributed definitely to bone rather than to scar, or to arachnoiditis.

The last two examples are cases in which both preoperative and postoperative MPD examinations were done. Figures 4-111 to 4-113 illustrate a case of a large calcified or ossified L5 annulus encroaching into the anterior aspect of the lumbar canal. This ossified bony ridge, or annulus, was absent postoperatively in both transverse and sagittal views (Fig. 4-112). In addition, there was posterior decompression and enlargement of the left L5 spinal nerve canal and foramen, as shown in the transverse and sagittal views of Figure 4-113. Figures 4-114 and 4-115 are pre- and postoperative views of the left L1 spinal nerve canal and foramen in a second patient. Following decompression, this patient had complete relief of symptoms (Fig. 4-115).

CBT and Myelography in Lumbosacral Spinal Disease

Although lumbar myelography (LM) has traditionally served as the primary diagnostic imaging method for the lumbosacral spine in the low back pain syndrome, CBT-LS has demonstrated significant advantages over this earlier procedure along three parameters: (1) accuracy (*i.e.*, sensitivity and specificity), (2) risk, and (3) accessibility (*i.e.*, cost, availability, and ease of performance).

Accuracy of CBT-LS is equivalent to LM in both the detection and the prediction of surgically proven lumbar disc disease, according to the results of a recently completed major study within our institution. This study compared the accuracy of both imaging methods in surgically proven cases of lumbosacral spinal disease treated at Long Beach Memorial Hospital between 1977 and 1980.[60] A total of 125 L3, L4, and L5 discs were evaluated by preoperative CBT-LS as well as LM, followed by surgical exploration. Surgically abnormal discs were detected as frequently by CBT (73.4%) as by LM (74.3%). Surgically negative discs were also detected as frequently by CBT (62.8%) as by LM (64.0%). Furthermore, radiographic predictions of abnormal discs were surgically confirmed as frequently for CBT (71.4%) as for LM (72.3%). Thus, both the sensitivity and the specificity of CBT proved equivalent to LM in the radiographic evaluation of lumbar disc disease.

In certain cases, CBT appeared even more sensitive than LM in detecting abnormal

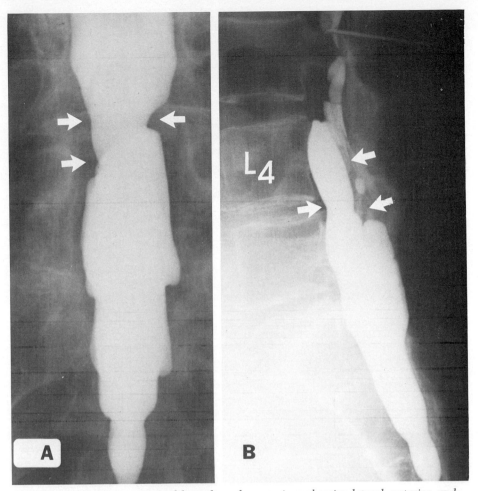

*Fig. 4-94. Anteroposterior and lateral myelogram views showing lateral, anterior, and posterior extradural defects **(arrows)**. Key finding is a distinct posterior indentation seen on the lateral view, with an abrupt change in caliber of the subarachnoid space posteriorly. This was erroneously attributed to arachnoiditis or scar formation in the myelogram report.*

discs. This is especially true in regions such as L5 with a wide anterior epidural space[60,115] or in patients with prior disc surgery whose symptoms reappear owing to scar-induced foraminal stenosis or shift in fixation-screw position.[105] Because LM displays only the contours of the dural sac, its accuracy is quite limited in evaluating the broad spectrum of lesions in the lumbosacral spine.[18,60,152] On the other hand, CBT directly displays all of the tissues surrounding the dural sac (vertebral bodies, discs, articular processes, and laminae), as well as the lateral recesses and nerve root canals. Unlike mye-lography, CBT specifically displays the particular anatomical abnormalities that cause entrapment of neural elements, such as bulging discs, articular process hypertrophy, ligamentum flavum hypertrophy, and postsurgical fusion masses. This ability of CBT has led the Society of Computed Body Tomography to designate CBT as an important, often primary, imaging method for a full range of lumbosacral spinal disorders.[4,65]

The risks of CBT of the spine are substantially lower than the risk of LM for two major reasons. First, LM requires an invasive lumbar puncture. Second, LM requires the

(Text continues on p. 160.)

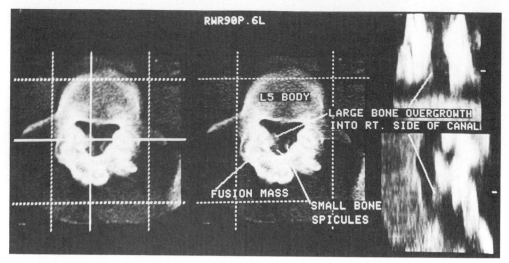

Fig. 4-95. MPD views showing an acquired spinal stenosis caused by postfusion bony overgrowth from the right and posterior aspects of the L5 canal. The large bone overgrowth was identified on the transverse, coronal, and sagittal images with a blinking dot. Note the close correlation of the right lateral bone encroachment with the large, right-sided, extradural defect on anteroposterior myelogram view in Fig. 4-97. The same bone mass viewed here in the sagittal image corresponds to the large posterior extradural defect seen on the lateral myelographic view in Fig. 4-97.

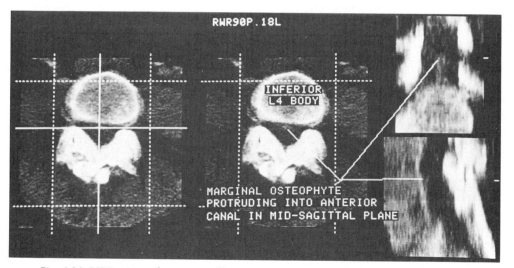

Fig. 4-96. MPD views showing small marginal osteophyte projecting into the anterior aspect of the canal at the L4–5 interspace level. This corresponds with the anterior osteophytic extradural indentation on the lateral myelogram view in Fig. 4-97.

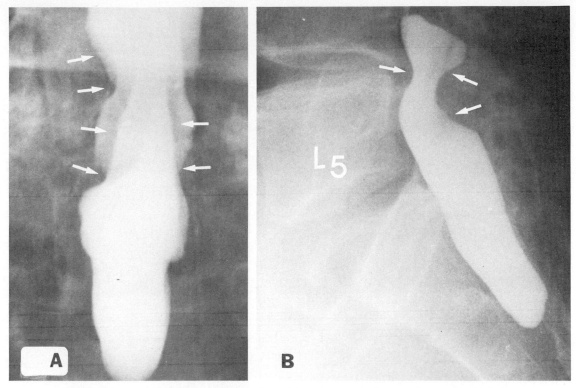

Fig. 4-97. *Anteroposterior and lateral myelographic views showing large right lateral and smaller left lateral extradural defects at L4–5 on the anteroposterior view, and a small anterior and large posterior extradural defect on the lateral view.*

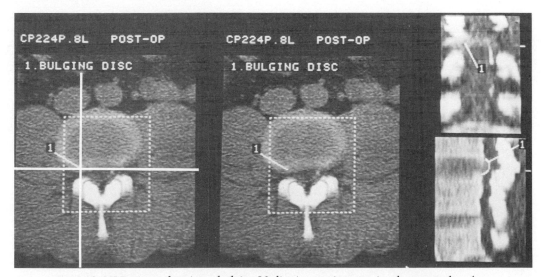

Fig. 4-98. *MPD views showing a bulging L3 disc in a patient previously operated on for L5–S1 spinal stenosis with only partial relief of symptoms. Postoperative complaint was right hip pain, probably caused by the L3 disc, which was not detected prior to surgery because of survey-type preoperative CBT examination, in which images were obtained at 1- to 1.5-cm intervals.*

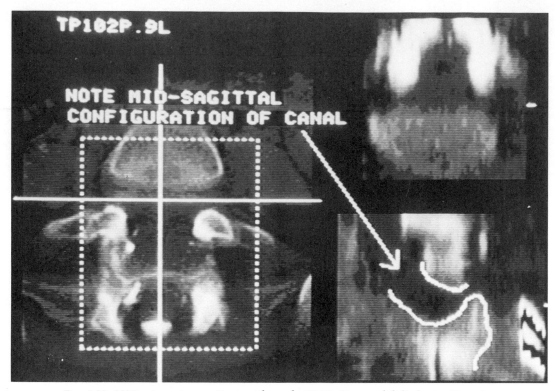

Fig. 4-99. MPD views in a patient with grade IV L5–S1 spondylolisthesis. Note the midsagittal configuration of the canal, and the extremely narrow isthmus between the remaining L4 posterior elements and the upper posterior margin of the sacrum. This single sagittal image was responsible for an important decision in this patient's management (see text).

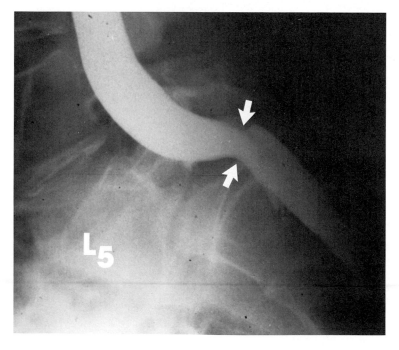

Fig. 4-100. Lateral myelogram view showing isthmus *(arrows)* between L4 posterior elements above and upper posterior sacral margin below. The isthmus was considerably underestimated on this myelogram in comparison with the sagittal CBT view in Fig. 4-99.

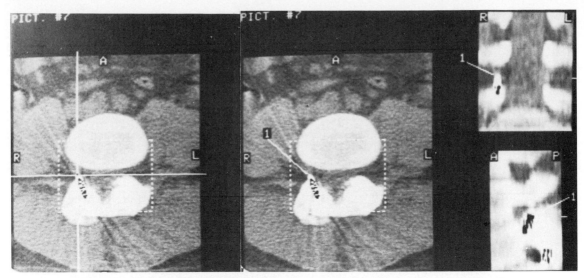

Fig. 4-101. *MPD views showing the point of a metallic stabilizing screw (1) within the posterior inferior aspect of the right L4 spinal nerve canal and foramen. (Hounsfield GN: Computerized transverse axial scanning [tomography]. Part I: Description of system. Br J Radiol 46:1016–1022, 1973)*

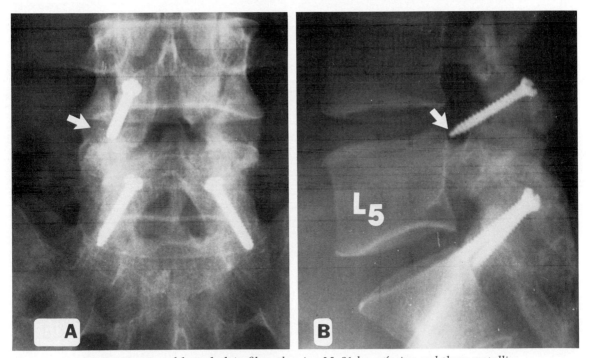

Fig. 4-102. *AP and lateral plain films showing L5–S1 bony fusion and three metallic screws. Exact position of the tip of the right L4 screw* **(arrow)** *was established on CBT examination in Fig. 4-101.*

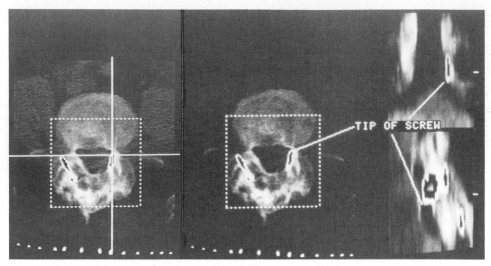

Fig. 4-103. MPD views showing tip of metallic screw on the left at L4 encroaching the medial aspect of the nerve root canal. These findings confirmed the left L4 abnormality seen on the epidural venogram of Fig. 4-104.

introduction of subarachnoid contrast medium.

The inherent side-effects of lumbar puncture have been reviewed in a number of reports,[37,45,58] and these risks are frequently increased when the technique is performed by inexperienced hands such as junior house staff. The introduction of subarachnoid contrast, while associated with a low incidence of immediate reaction, carries a substantial risk of longer-term sequelae owing to the sensitivity of meninges to foreign substances.[99] A number of reports have described several classes of adverse reactions to oil-based contrast agents for LM, including: vascular intravasation of contrast, pulmonary embolism, lipoid granuloma, transection and withdrawal of nerve root filaments, and adhesive arachnoiditis.[7, 10, 11, 14, 16, 17, 19–21, 33, 39–42, 52, 54, 57, 59, 69, 70, 82, 84–86, 90, 92, 94, 107, 109, 110, 112, 113, 116, 117, 120, 124, 129, 145, 149–151, 154–156, 158, 161–162, 164, 170, 174, 175] Even the newer water-soluble contrast agents have been implicated in increasing the incidence of seizure activity and arachnoiditis.[3, 76, 78–81, 127, 173]

Adhesive Arachnoiditis

The complication of adhesive arachnoiditis is a serious problem frequently noted after multiple Pantopaque myelography and back surgery procedures. Multiple procedures in chronic low back pain syndromes are extremely common; one study reports an average of 3.6 surgeries and 3.8 myelographies per patient.[38] Adhesive arachnoiditis is often undetected at operation, because the dural sac generally remains unopened during surgery.[22] Primary symptoms reported in a study of 65 cases include leg pain in 90%, low back pain in 80%, and loss of sphincter control in 25%.[19,21] Both Pantopaque and some of the water-soluble myelographic contrast substances other than Metrizamide have been implicated in adhesive arachnoiditis. This syndrome can also be simulated by spinal stenosis. One study of 93 cases of cauda equina syndrome reported a 65% incidence of patients with spinal stenosis simulating arachnoiditis.[14] It

(Text continues on p. 164.)

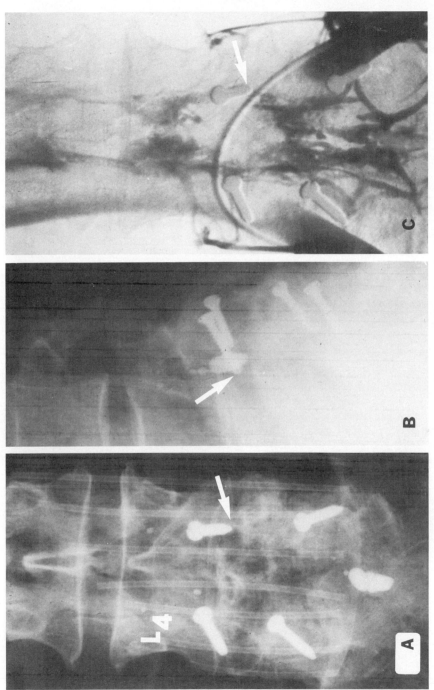

*Fig. 4-104. AP plain film and AP subtraction view of epidural venogram. Note on venogram that there is a lack of filling of the anterior epidural veins on the left at L4 (**arrow**) near the tip of the left L4 screw.*

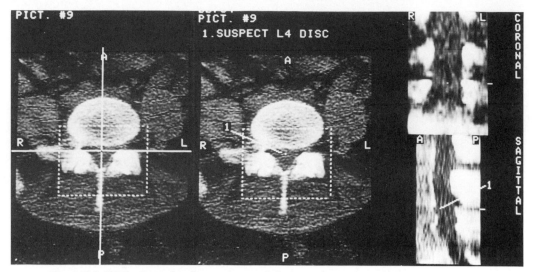

Fig. 4-105. MPD views showing very poor definition of anterior soft tissues within the lumbar canal at the L4–5 disc space. A large L4–5 bulging disc was suspected. (Hounsfield GN: Computerized transverse axial scanning [tomography]. Part I: Description of system. Br J Radiol 46:1016–1022, 1973)

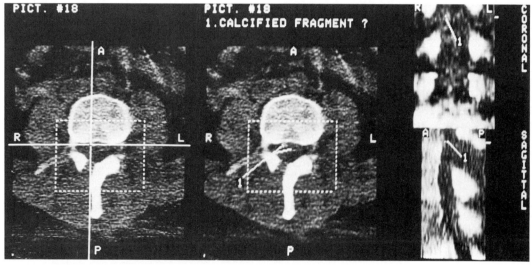

Fig. 4-106. MPD views showing evidence for a right L3 laminectomy and a subtle calcified density along the anterior aspect of the canal adjacent to the L3 body. (Hounsfield GN: Computerized transverse axial scanning [tomography]. Part I: Description of system. Br J Radiol 46:1016–1022, 1973)

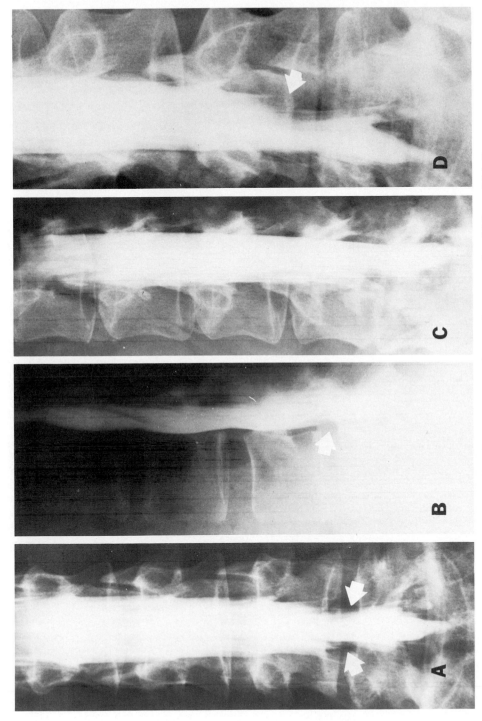

Fig. 4-107. Multiple myelographic views showing large central and bilateral L4 disc abnormality (arrow).

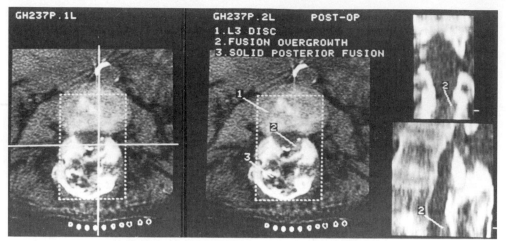

Fig. 4-108. MPD views showing soft tissue fusion overgrowth, thought to represent either scar tissue or hypertrophied ligamentum flavum. Note solid posterior fusion. (Ambrose J: Computerized transverse scanning [tomography]. Part 2: Clinical applications. Br J Radiol 46:1023–1047, 1973; French BN, Maass L: Revolution in neurodiagnosis: Computed tomography of the brain. West J Med 127:231, 1977)

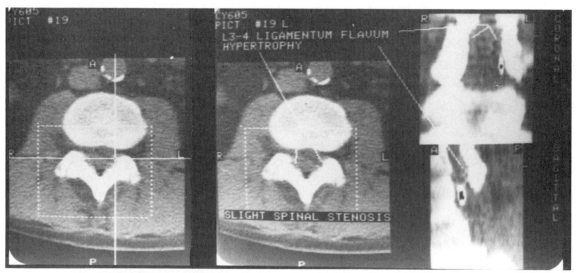

Fig. 4-109. MPD views showing a large previous L4–5 laminectomy (sagittal view) and suspected L3–4 ligamentum flavum hypertrophy.

is expected that CBT both will reduce the incidence of myelography-induced adhesive arachnoiditis and will permit detection of spinal stenosis mimicking this condition.

By comparison with myelography, the risks involved with CBT-LS are minimal. Usually the procedure neither is invasive nor requires contrast. Contrast use in CBT-LS is rare, and Metrizamide is reserved primarily for the evaluation of unusual cases of dysrhaphism or tumor. Furthermore, contrast-enhanced CBT-LS is minimally invasive and requires only a peripheral IV injection of iodinated contrast material.

Current radiation exposure in the course of CBT-LS remains slighly higher than in LM (20 versus 10 rads respectively), although newer techniques and equipment will reduce

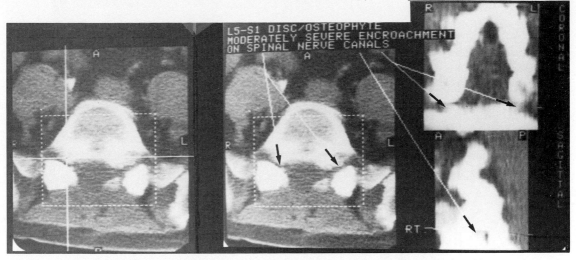

Fig. 4-110. MPD views showing previous L5 laminectomy for spinal stenosis (transverse image) and residual bilateral L5–S1 spinal nerve canal and foraminal encroachment caused by either an L5–S1 disc or an osteophyte.

CBT radiation exposure to under 5 rads.[12,60,65,101,130–132] Examination time in CBT-LS will also be reduced from the current figure of 40 to 50 minutes per scan to a 20 to 25 minute total scan time in the near future.[60] Thus the current radiation-related risks of CBT-LS already compare very favorably with LM, and these risks should decline further in coming years.

Finally, accessibility of CBT-LS exams compares favorably with LM on several indices, including ease of performance, scanner availability, and competitive cost per exam. CBT-LS is easy to perform owing to its noninvasive nature, and it can be handled entirely by a radiological technician. However, data retrieval, image display manipulation, and interpretation require a roentgenographer with some specialized training in computer data manipulation using a relatively straightforward computer program. Standard reporting forms for CBT data on the lumbosacral spine are already available, and a standard CBT-LS programming guide for radiologists is being developed.[61,65]

Availability of CBT scanners has increased dramatically in the past 5 years, with over 750 CBT scanners currently operational in major medical institutions in the United States, from community hospitals to university medical centers. Although newer body scanners incorporate many useful technological advances, older existing systems can be retrofitted at modest expense with the necessary computer capability for spinal studies. The current cost of equipping an existing computer with both increased capacity data storage devices and MPD software is about $60,000 to $80,000.[60,65]

The unit cost of CBT-LS scans, despite the initial high expense of scanner purchase, compares very favorably with LM. AT our institution the current CBT-LS unit cost is $518 per exam compared to $578 for LM (including hospitalization). It is further projected that CBT-LS unit costs will have dropped by 1982 to $400 per exam.[60]

Thus CBT-LS is increasingly displacing myelography as the primary diagnostic method for the evaluation of lumbosacral spine disease, by virtue of its comparable accuracy. Lower risk, and comparable cost. Myelography is being reserved for the selected evaluation of persistent low back pain that remains undiagnosed after initial CBT examinations. A primary role for CBT in the diagnostic evaluation of persistent low back pain syndromes is supported by findings

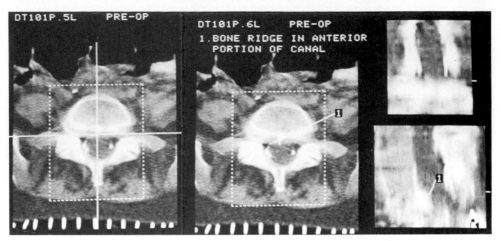

Fig. 4-111. MPD views showing preoperative appearance of a bony ridge representing either a calcified or an ossified L5 disc or annulus. (Hounsfield GN: Computerized transverse axial scanning [tomography]. Part I: Description of system. Br J Radiol 46:1016–1022, 1973)

from a number of studies over the past 2 years.[23,61,65,77,115,134–138]

At our institution, there has been a continual increase in the absolute number of CBT scans performed since 1977. Spinal column studies currently represent no less than 50% of all CBT scans performed, and there has been a consistent increase in the number of CBT-LS scans to about 80 to 85 cases per month at the current time. This trend reflects the increasingly accepted use of CBT-LS exams at Long Beach Memorial Hospital.

Low Back Pain Syndrome and CBT

Low back pain syndrome is a remarkably common presenting complaint in surgical and medical practice; there is an enormous patient population afflicted with this disease.[48–50] The problem of low back pain may be discussed in terms of prevalence, social effects, individual effects, and medical intervention efforts.

Prevalence of Low Back Pain

The prevalence of low back pain is almost universal, especially in advancing age, affecting 80% of adult humans at some point

in their lifetimes.[172] The natural history of low back pain syndrome features a 90% recovery rate within 2 months of initial onset, regardless of treatment approach. Many patients suffer from a common, self-limited, benign form of low back pain syndrome. However, fully 50% of patients with initial low back pain symptoms will have a subsequent recurrence, and approximately 12% will eventually prove to have a herniated nucleus pulposus. This latter group represents a population of well over 10 million patients in the United States requiring diagnostic evaluation for possible surgical intervention.

Social Effects

Staggering social effects of recurrent low back pain syndrome have long been reported in many industrialized nations, in terms of lost productivity, industrial compensation claims, individual morbidity, and medical costs. In England, low back pain is responsible for a greater proportion of work days lost (3.6%) than are strikes.[114] In Sweden, 4% of the employed population misses work some time in any given year because of back pain, and the duration of most of these absences exceeds 3 weeks.[114] In the United States, one major corporation recently re-

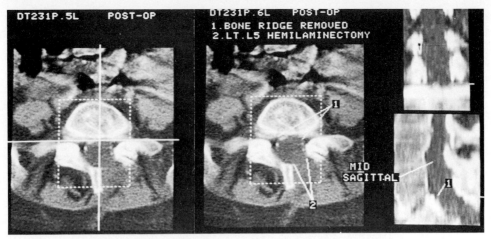

Fig. 4-112. MPD views examination showing postoperative removal of calcified or ossified disc or annulus. A laminectomy defect is seen on the left at L5. (Hounsfield GN: Computerized transverse axial scanning [tomography]. Part I: Description of system. Br J Radiol 46:1016–1022, 1973; (Ambrose J: Computerized transverse scanning [tomography]. Part 2: Clinical applications. Br J Radiol 46:1023–1047, 1973)

ported that low back pain was the second most frequent cause of employee absenteeism, after common respiratory infections.[114]

Industrial compensation claims for low back pain are generally known to present enormous social costs every year. The National Safety Council in the United States reported 400,000 claims per year for low back pain disabilities in recent years. In Ontario, Canada, over 2000 claims for low back pain related disabilities are received annually.[172]

Individual Effects

Individual morbidity in chronic low back pain patients frequently deteriorates into chronic disability. Over 60% of chronic low back pain patients are alcohol abusers, 78% are obese, and a majority develop dependence upon analgesic medications.[172] Psychological coping skills often show a major decline in chronic low back pain patients, who may become increasingly depressed, dependent, hypochondriacal, and even sociopathic. The development of such serious psychiatric symptoms often impedes accurate clinical evaluation of chronic low back pain patients for surgical and medical intervention. Fur-

thermore, chronic low back pain patients with significant functional overlay are notoriously reluctant to accept psychiatric referral, and many show as little lasting improvement with psychotherapy as they do with other medical and surgical therapies.

Medical Intervention Efforts

The medical costs of low back pain syndromes are as colossal as the other social costs. A recent HEW report states that more than 7 million requests for low pack pain treatment were processed in the United States during a single year.[17] In California, low back pain comprises the most costly Workmen's Compensation disability treated.[172] In 13 Western states, low back pain is the primary cause of hospitalization covered by Workmen's Compensation.[172] Each year several hundred thousand low back operations are performed in the United States, primarily on patients with low back pain syndrome.[20]

Despite large-scale medical efforts in relation to chronic low back pain, the proportion of suboptimal therapeutic outcomes remains disappointingly high. A particularly troublesome issue for the surgical community is the high incidence of failed back surgeries noted in the treatment of low back pain syndrome. This unfortunate response to a wide spectrum of costly medical and surgical treatments reflects at least two basic problems in low back pain syndrome:

1. The incentives for remaining disabled provided by compensation systems to chronic low back pain patients
2. The difficulty of assessing accurately the frequently coexisting physical and psychiatric abnormalities in chronic low back pain patients

This second problem hampers both the selection of optimal treatment modalities and the accurate assessment of treatment results. Orthopedic surgeons frequently face formidable problems, both in deciding on surgical intervention and in evaluating the results of prior surgery on chronic low back pain patients. At least part of the orthopedist's problem is shared by the consultant radiologist, has traditionally relied upon imaging techniques that are incapable of visualizing a variety of symptom-causing abnormalities in the lumbosacral spine. Anatomical lesions have been missed, because traditional imaging techniques were too indirect to visualize precisely the subtle yet significant bony and soft tissue abnormalities. LM, for example, is limited to displaying the outline of the contrast-filled dural sac; it cannot display the nature of lesions encroaching upon the sac. Nor can compressed nerve roots within stenotic lateral recesses or foramina be clearly imaged by this procedure. Epidural venography is even more indirect than myelography and permits visualization only of displaced epidural veins. Thus, only a massive lateral disc herniation causing substantial displacement of epidural veins is detectable by epidural venography.

The direct visualization of physical abnormalities in all the bony and soft tissue structures of the lumbosacral spine has only become available with the advent of CBT. It is anticipated that this vastly increased capability for direct imaging of abnormalities will significantly promote the accurate anatomical evaluation of patients with low back pain syndrome.

CBT and Surgical Intervention in Lumbosacral Spine Disease

Patient Selection Criteria

Optimal selection of surgical candidates from the large pool of patients presenting with complaints of chronic low back pain poses difficult orthopedic decisions, owing to compensation benefits, coexistence of anatomical and psychiatric abnormalities, and limitations of indirect imaging methods for visualizing abnormalities. Erroneous decisions about surgical candidate selection based on inadequate anatomical information result in two unfortunate types of therapeutic intervention: (1) surgical treatment of chronic low back pain patients without resectable lesions, and (2) medical and psychiatric therapy applied to chronic low back patients with surgically resectable lesions. In the first instance, the surgeon faces professional criticism and potential litigation for unneeded surgery; in the second, an opportunity is lost to offer the benefits of potentially curative surgery to the patient. In both instances, the patient generally suffers by failing to show lasting improvement.

The detailed visualization of anatomical structures offered by CBT-LS should clearly promote a significant increase in the detection rate of surgically correctable lesions. Soft tissue encroachments on the cord itself due to ligamentum flavum hypertrophy, and compression of individual nerve roots due to foraminal stenosis exemplify two types of resectable lesions commonly missed on myelographic examination but reliably detected by CBT-LS. Chronic low back patients with resectable lesions now detected by CBT-LS may thus be offered the benefits of highly selective surgical intervention, rather

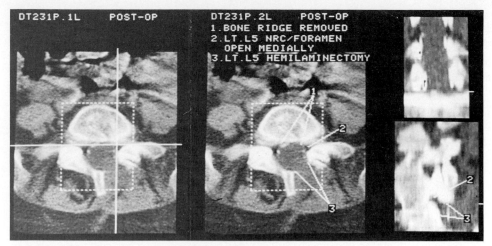

Fig. 4-113. MPD views showing postoperative enlargement and decompression of the left L5 spinal nerve canal and foramen. The preoperative views showed complete obliteration.

than being referred for ineffective medical therapy or dismissed as malingerers. This should help to increase the absolute number of positive surgical outcomes in chronic low back pain patients.

Conversely, patients with low back pain complaints and wholly negative CBT scans of the lumbosacral spine can be spared inappropriate surgery and treated with other modalities. The resulting decline of ineffectual surgery should serve to improve the operative result statistics of surgeons and contribute to a gradual reduction in the previously high incidence of failed back surgery. An absolute decrease in the number of negative surgical outcomes should also serve to discourage litigation against surgeons whose operative selections are guided by the exacting anatomical images provided by CBT scans. Furthermore, surgeons armed with precise preoperative CBT scan radiographs will possess excellent objective evidence in defending themselves against inappropriate and unwarranted malpractice litigation. These considerations support a role for CBT-LS as a primary radiographic screening approach to selection of surgical candidates.

In planning an optimal surgical approach to resectable lesions in the lumbosacral spine, the direct visualization of lesions on

CBT scans could prove invaluable to the surgeon. The detailed thin-slice anatomical images in the variety of planes offered by CBT should enable the surgeon to know ahead of time not only what the locus of a given cord or root compression is, but also precisely which structures are causing the compression and require resection. No longer will such decision have to made primarily during the course of surgical exploration.

Not infrequently a coexisting but subtle secondary lesion (*e.g.*, foraminal stenosis) remains undetectable both on myelography and during the initial surgical resection of a gross primary lesion, only to result in a gradual recrudescence of symptoms and eventual reexploration. The detection of subtle but clinically significant secondary lesions on CBT scans will provide the surgeon with the option of resecting these abnormalities immediately on initial exploration. The use of CBT scans in planning operative procedures can be expected to increase the number of positive surgical outcomes.

The evaluation of prior surgical outcomes by CBT scans will prove particularly helpful in reducing many common postsurgical problems. The largest number of cases potentially requiring such evaluation consists of patients with failed back surgery. Failed

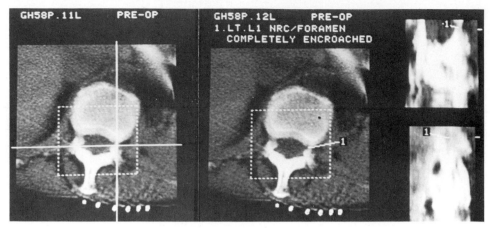

Fig. 4-114. *MPD views showing complete preoperative encroachment of the left L1 spinal nerve canal and foramen.*

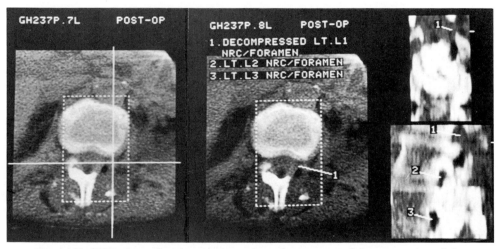

Fig. 4-115. *MPD views showing postoperative enlargement and decompression of the previously obliterated left L1 spinal nerve canal and foramen. It now has an appearance similar to the open left L2 and L3 foramina. (Hounsfield GN: Computerized transverse axial scanning [tomography]. Part I: Description of system. Br J Radiol 46:1016–1022, 1973; (Ambrose J: Computerized transverse scanning [tomography]. Part 2: Clinical applications. Br J Radiol 46:1023–1047, 1973; French BN, Maass L: Revolution in neurodiagnosis: Computed tomography of the brain. West J Med 127:231, 1977)*

back surgery patients are usually defined as patients who suffer long-term functional disability or who require reoperation. The incidence of failed back surgery cases following initial surgery is estimated to be as high as 10% to 40%; in recent studies, a 37% rate has been reported following surgery without fusion, and a 30% rate following surgery with fusion.[17,55,56,128] Repeat surgeries are often multiple, with 50% of patients requiring from two to seven repeat surgical procedures, according to one source.[26]

Many of these back surgery cases fail owing to nerve root entrapment in stenotic lateral recesses and foramina. Such stenosis may be idiopathic and go undetected on initial explorations, or it may be iatrogenic and caused by postsurgical fusion overgrowth, scar tissue, ligamentum flavum hypertrophy, articular facet subluxation, osteophyte formation, or positional change in fixation screws.[128]

Although inadequate decompression of stenotic lesions causing nerve root entrapment is frequently regarded as a primary cause of failed back surgery, myelography has generally proven inadequate in detecting these abnormalities.[105] CBT, on the other hand, permits direct display of all the involved structures and thus promises both an inncreased rate of initial detection and the development of quantitative criteria for diagnosing the gamut of these stenotic lesions.

Noncontributory Anatomical Variants

The exquisite anatomical detail displayed by CBT images carries the risk that symptomatically irrelevant anatomical variants may be erroneously considered for surgical resection. Furthermore, the complex display capacities of CBT scanners, particularly those with MPD options, provide a large amount of anatomical detail to be reviewed for each case. Both the volume of image data and the problems of distinguishing contributory from noncontributory anatomical abnormalities will require a close collaboration between radiologists and orthopedists in coming years, in order to optimize assessment for surgical intervention. Much is to be learned by both groups about the optimal display modes for visualizing important anatomical details on CBT scans, as well as about the pathophysiological significance of the various structures and variants encountered on CBT-LS images.

References for Part 1

1. Epstein BS: The Spine: A Radiological Test and Atlas, ed 3, Philadelphia, Lea & Febiger, 1969
2. Ford L, Goodman FG: X-ray studies of the lumbosacral spine. South Med J, 10:1123, 1966
3. Horal J: The clinical appearance of low back disorders in the city of Gothenberg, Sweden. Acta Orthop Scand, Suppl 118, 1969
4. Hult L: The Munk Fors investigation. Acta Orthop Scand, Suppl 16, 1954
5. Splitoff CA: Roentgenographic comparison of patients with and without backache. JAMA, 152:1610, 1953

References for Part 3

1. Ahlgren P: Long-term side-effects after myelography with water soluble contrast media—Conturex, Conray Meglumine 282, and Dimer X. Neuroradiology, p:206, 1973
2. Allen WE, VanGilder JC, Collins WF: Evaulation of the neurotoxicity of water soluble myelographic contrast agents by electrophysiologic monitors. Radiology 188:89–95, 1976
3. Arnell S, Lidstrom F: Myelography with Skiodan (Abrodil). Acta Radiol (Diagn) 12:287–88, 1931
4. Batson OV: The function of the vertebral veins and their role in the spread of metastases. Ann Surg 112:138–149, 1940
5. Bergquist-Ullman M: Acute low back pain in industry. Acta Orth Scan, (Suppl) 170, 1977
6. Bingel A: Intralumbale Lufteinbläsung zur Hohendiagnose intraduraler extramedullarer Prozesse und zur differential Diagnose gegenüber intramedullarer Prozessen. Deutsche Ztochr, f. nervenhlk, 72:359, 1921
7. Bonneau R, Morris J: Complications of water-soluble contrast lumbar myelography. Spine 3:343–345, 1978
8. Brahme F, Sova M, Powell H, Long DM: Perfluorocarbon bromides as contrast media in radiography of the central nervous system. Acta Radiol (Suppl) 347, 1975
9. Brodsky AE, Binder WF: Lumbar discography: Its value in diagnosis and treatment of lumbar disc lesions. Spine, 4, 2:110–120, 1979
10. Campbell RL, Campbell JA, Heimburger RF, Halsbeck JE, Mealey J Jr: Ventriculography and myelography with absorbable radiopaque medium. Radiology 82:286–289, 1964
11. Cuatico W, Gannon W, Samoukos E: A needle designed for myelography. J Neurosurg, 28:87, 1968
12. Cloward RB: Anterior herniation of ruptured lumbar intervertebral discs: Comments on diagnostic value discogram. Arch Surg 64:457–563, 1952
13. ———: Cervical diskography: Technique, indications and use in diagnosis of ruptured cervical disks. Am J Roentgenol 79:563–574, 1958
14. Cloward RB, Buzaid LL: Discography: Technique, indications and evaluation of normal and abnormal intervertebral disc. Am J Roentgenol 68:552–564, 1952
15. Dandy WE: Roentgenography of the brain

after the injection of air into the spinal canal. Ann Surg 70:397, 1919

16. Drasin GF, Daffner RH, Sexton RF, Cheatham WC: Epidural venography: Diagnosis of herniated lumbar intervertebral disc and other disease of the epidural space. Am F Roentgenol 126:1010–1016, 1976

17. Epstein BS: The Spine: A Radiological Test and Atlas, ed 3, Philadelphia, Lea & Febiger, 1969

18. Erickson TC, Van Baaren JJ: Late meningeal reaction to ethyl iodophenylundecylate, used in myelography: Report of a case that terminated fatally. JAMA, 153:636, 1953

19. Erlacher, PR: Nucleography. J Bone Joint Surg, 34B:204, 1952

20. Finneson BE: Diagnosis and Management of Pain Syndromes, ed 2, Philadelphia, WB Saunders, 1969

21. Finney LA, Gargano FP, Buermann A: Intraosseous verebral venography in the diagnosis of lumbar disk disease. Amer J Roentgen 92:1282–1292, 1964

22. Gargano FP, Meyer JD, Sheldon JJ: Transfemoral ascending lumbar catheterization of the epidural veins in lumbar disk disease. Neuroradiology May:329–336, 1974

23. Gershater R, Holgate RC: Lumbar epidural venography in the diagnosis of disc herniations. Am F Roentgenol 126:992–1002, 1976

24. Gonsette R: An experimental and clinical assessment of water-soluble contrast media in neuroradiology: A new medium—Dimer-X. Clin Radiol 22:44–56, 1971

25. Grainger RG, Grumpet J, Sharpe DM, Carson J: Water-soluble lumbar radiculography: A clinical trial of Dimer-X—A new contrast medium. Clin Radiol 22:57–62, 1971

26. Gresham JL, Miller R: Evaluation of the lumbar spine by diskography. Orthop Clin, 67:29, 1969

27. Hanraets TRMJ: The Degenerative Back and its Differential Diagnosis. Amsterdam, Elsevier Publishing Co, 1959

28. Hilal SK: Hemodynamic changes associated with the intra-arterial injection of contrast material: New toxicity test and a new experimental contrast medium. Radiology 86:615–633, 1966

29. Hilal SK, Dauth GW, Hess KH, Gilman S: Development and evaluation of a new water-soluble iodinated myelographic contrast medium with markedly reduced convulsive effects. Radiology, 126:417–422, 1978

30. Hitselberger WE, Witten RM: Abnormal myelograms in asymptomatic patients. Journal of Neurosurgery, 28:204–206, 1968

31. Jacobaeus HD: On insufflation of air into the spinal canal for diagnostic purposes in cases of tumors in the spinal canal. Acta Med Scan, 55:555, 1921

32. Kieffer S, Binet E, Esquerra J, Hantman R, Gross C: Contrast agents for myelography: Clinical and radiological evaluation of Amipaque and Pantopaque. Radiology 129:695–705, 1978

33. Kodama JK, Butler WM, Tusing TW, Hallett FP: Iothelamate, a new intravascular radiopaque medium with unusual pharmacotoxic inertness. Exp Mol Pathol (Suppl) 2:65–80, 1963

34. Lang JH, Lasser EC: Nonspecific inhibition on enzymes by organic contrast media. J Med Chem, 14:233, 1971

35. Lang JH, Lasser EC, Kolb WP: Activation of serum complement by contrast media. Inv Rad, 11:303–308, 1976

36. Lasègue C: Considerations sur la sciatique. Arch Gen de Meil 24:558, 1864

37. Lindblom L: Diagnostic puncture of intervertebral discs in sciatica. Acta Orthop Scan, 17:231, 1948

38. Lindblom L: Acta Radiol, 22:711, 1941

39. Mason MS, Raaf J: Complications of pantopaque myelography. Case report and review. J Neurosurg, 19:302, 1962

40. Metrizamide, a nonionic water-soluble contrast medium. Acta Radiol (Suppl) 335, 1973

41. Nachemson AL: The lumbar spine, an orthopedic challenge. Spine 1:1, 59–71, 1976

42. Oftedal SI, Kayed K: Epileptogenic effect of water-soluble contrast media: An experimental investigation in rabbits. Acta Radiol (Suppl) 335:45–55, 1973

43. Praestholm J: Experimental evaluation of water-soluble contrast media for myelograph. Neuroradiology 13:25–35, 1977

44. Sackett JF, Strother CM, Quaglieri CE, Javid MJ, Levin AB, Duff TA: Metrizamide—CSF contrast medium: Analysis of clinical application in 215 patients. Radiology, 123:779–782, 1977

45. Schobinger RA: Intraosseous Venography. New York, Grune & Stratton, 1960

46. Schobinger RA, Krueger EG, Sobel GL: Comparison of intraosseous vertebral venography and Pantopaque myelography in the diagnosis of surgical conditions of the lumbar spine and nerve roots. Radiology 77:376–397, 1961

47. Schobinger RA, Krueger EG: Intraosseous epidural venography in the diagnosis of surgical diseases of the lumbar spine. Acta Radiol 1:763–776, 1963

48. Scoville WB, Moretz WH, Hankins WD: Discrepancies in myelography: Statistical survey of 200 operative cases undergoing Pantopaque myelography. Surg Gynec Obstet 86:559–564, 1948

49. Sicard JA, Forestier J: Method radiographique d'exploration de la cavite epidurale par le lipiodol. Rev Neurol, 37:1264, 1921

50. Sovak M, Nahlovsky B, Lang JH, Lasser EC: Preliminary evaluation of diiodoephenyltriglucoside: An approach to the design of nonionic water-soluble radiographic contrast media. Radiology, 117:717, 1975

51. Sovak M, Ranganathan RS, Lang JH, Lasser EC: Concepts in design of improved intravascular agents. Ann Radiol, 21:4, 1978

52. Steinhausen TB, Dungan CE, Furst JB, Plati JT, Smith SW, Darling AP, Wolcott EC Jr, Warren SL, Strain, WH: Iodinated organic compounds as contrast medicine for radiographic diagnosis. III. Experimental and clinical myelography and ethyl iodophenylundecylate (Pantopaque). Radiology, 43:230, 1944

53. Tarlov IM: Pantopaque meningitis disclosed at operation. JAMA, 129:1014, 1945

54. Wideroe S: On intraspinal luftinjektion ogom dens diagnostiske betydning ver rygmervslidelser, saerlig ved svulster. Norsk Mag f Laegevidensk, 32:49, 1921

55. Wise RE, Weford EC: X-ray visualization of intervertebral disc: Report of case. Cleveland Clinic Quarterly 18:127, 1951

References for Part 4

1. Aaro S, Dahlborn M, Svensson L: Estimation of vertebral rotation in structural scoliosis by computer tomography. Acta Radiologica Diag, 19:990–992, 1978.

2. Abrams HL, McNeil BJ: Medical implementations of computed tomography (CT scanning). N Engl J Med, 298(5):255–261 and 298(6):310–318, 1978

3. Ahlgren P: Amipaque myelography without late adhesive arrachnoid changes. Neuroradiology, 14:231–233, 1973

4. Alfidi RJ, et al: Special report: New indications for computerized body tomography. Am J Roentg, 133:115–119, 1979

5. Ambrose J: Computerized transverse scanning (tomography). Part 2: Clinical applications. Br J Radiol, 46:1023–1047, 1973

6. Ambrose J, Gooding MR, Uttley D: EMI scan in the management of head injuries. Lancet, 1:847–848, 1976

7. Auld AW: Chronic spinal arachnoiditis, a postoperative syndrome that may signal its onset. Spine, 3(1):88–91, 1978

8. Axelbaum SP, Schellinger D, Gomes MN, et al: Computer tomographic evaluation of aortic aneurysms. Am J Roentgenol, 127:75–78, 1976

9. Baker HL Jr: The impact of computed tomography on neuroradiologic practice. Radiology, 116:637–640, 1975

10. Benner B, Ehni M: Spinal arachnoiditis, the postoperative variety in particular. Spine, 3(1):40–43, 1978

11. Bergeron RT, Rambaugh CL, Fang H, et al: Experimental Pantopaque arachnoiditis in the monkey. Radiology, 99:95–101, 1971

12. Bloomfeld. In Post, reference 125.

13. Boyd H: Iatrogenic intraspinal epidermoid. Report of a case. J Neurosurg, 24:105, 1966

14. Brodsky A: Cauda equina arachnoiditis, a correlative clinical and roentgenologic study. Spine, 3(1):51–60, 1978

15. Brugman E, Palmers Y, Staelens B: Congenital absence of a pedicle in the cervical spine: A new approach with CT scan. Neuroradiology, 17:121–125, 1979

16. Burton CV: Guest Editor Reply, Spine, 4(1):93–94, 1979

17. Burton CV: Lumbosacral arachnoiditis. Spine, 3(1):24–30, 1978

18. Burton CV, Heithoff KB, Kirkaldy-Willis W, et al: Computed tomographic scanning and the lumbar spine. Part II: Clinical considerations. Spine, 4:356–368, 1979

19. Burton CV, Wiltse LL: Editorial: Summary statement on myelographic media from a round table symposium on arachnoiditis. Spine, 3(1):32, 1978

20. Burton CV, Wiltse LL: Guest Editor Comment. Symposium on lumbar arachnoiditis nomenclature, etiology, and pathology. Spine, 3(1):23, 1978

21. Burton CV, Wiltse LL: Summary statement on myelographic media from a round table symposium on arachnoiditis. Neurosurg, 1:171–172, 1977

22. Burton CV, Wiltse LL (eds): Symposium on lumbar arachnoiditis: Nomenclature, etiology, and pathology. Spine, 3:21–91, 1978

23. Carrera GF, Houghton VM, Syvertsen A, et al: Computed tomography of the lumbar facet joints. Radiology, 134:145–148, 1980

24. Carter BL, Ignatow SB: Computed body tomography, how useful is it? Postgraduate Medicine, 63(5):66–80, 1978

25. Carter BL, Kahn PC, Wolpert SM, et al: Unusual pelvic masses: A comparison of computed tomographic scanning and ultrasonography. Radiology, 121:383–390, 1976

26. Cauchoix J, Ficat C, Girard B: Repeat surgery after disc excision. Spine, 3(3):256–259, 1978

27. Coin CG, Chan YS, Keranen V, et al: Computer assisted myelography in disc disease. J Comput Assist Tomogr, 1:398–404, 1977

28. Coin CG: Computed tomography of the spine. Chapter 15 in reference 125.

29. Coin C, Keranen VJ, Pennink J, *et al:* Computerized tomography of the spine and its contents. Neuroradiology, 16:275–278, 1978

30. Coin CG, Keranen VJ, Pennink M, *et al:* Evidence of CSF enhancement in the spinal subarachnoid space after intravenous contrast medium administration: Is intravenous computer assisted myelography possible? J Comput Assist Tomogr, 3(2):267–269, 1979

31. Coin CG, Pennink M, Ahmad WD, *et al:* Diving-type injury of the cervical spine: Contribution of computed tomography to management. J Comput Assist Tomogr, 3(39:362–372, 1979)

32. Colley DP, Dunsker SB: Traumatic narrowing of the dorsolumbar spinal canal demonstrated by computed tomography. Radiol, 129:95–98, 1978

33. Davis FL: Effect of unabsorbed radiographic contrast media in the central nervous system. Lancet, 2:747–748, 1956

34. Di Chiro G, Axelbaum SP, Schellinger D, *et al:* Computerized axial tomography in syringomyelia. N Engl J Med, 292:13–16, 1975

35. Di Chiro G, Doppman JL, Wener L: Computed tomography of spinal cord arteriovenous malformations. Radiology, 123:351–354, 1977

36. Di Chiro G, Schellinger D: Computed tomography of spinal cord after lumbar intrathecal introduction of Metrizamide (computer-assisted myelography). Radiology, 120:101–104, 1976

37. Drips RD, Vandam LD: Hazards of Lumbar puncture. JAMA, 147:1118, 1951

38. Dujovny M, Barrionuevo PJ, Kossovsky N, *et al:* Effects of contrast media on the canine subarachnoid space. Spine, 3(1):31–35, 1978

39. Epstein BS, Epstein JA: The cineroentgenographic observations of Pantopaque intravasation during myelography. Am J Roentgenol, 94:576, 1965.

40. Epstein JA: Obliterative arachnoiditis, a complication of spinal stenosis. Spine, 3(1):83, 1978

41. Erickson D: Letter to the Editor. Spine, 4(3):279–280, 1979

42. Erickson TC, van Baaren HJ: Late meningeal reaction to ethyl iodophenylundecylate used in myelography: Report of a case that terminated fatally. JAMA, 153:636–639, 1953

43. Ethier R, King DG, Melancon D, *et al:* Development of high resolution computed tomography of the spinal cord. J Comput Assist Tomogr, 3(4):433–438, 1979

44. Evens RG, Alfidi RJ, Haage JR, *et al:* Body computed tomography: A clinically important and efficacious radiologic procedure. Radiology, 123:239–240, 1977

45. Everett AD: Lumbar puncture injuries. Proc Roy Soc Med, 35:208, 1942

46. Faerber, EN, Wolpert SM, Scott RM, *et al:* Computed tomography of spinal fractures. J Comput Assist Tomogr, 3(5):657–661, 1979

47. Fielding JW, Stillwell WT, Chynn KY, *et al:* Use of computed tomography for the diagnosis of atlanto-axial rotatory fixation. JBJS, 60–1(8):1102–1104, 1978

48. Finneson BE, Low Back Pain. Philadelphia, JB Lippincott, 1973

49. Finneson BE, Diagnosis and Management of Pain Syndrome, 2 ed. Philadelphia, WB Saunders, 1969

50. Finneson BE, Low Back Pain, 2 ed. Philadelphia, JB Lippincott, 1980

51. Forbes WSC, Isherwood I: Computed tomography in syringomyelia and the associated Arnold-Chiari type I malformation. Neuroradiology, 15:73–78, 1978

52. Ford LT, Key JA: An evaluation of myelography in the diagnosis of intervertebral-disc lesions in the low back. J Bone Jt Surg, 32A:257–266, 1950

53. French BN, Maass L: Revolution in neurodiagnosis: Computed tomography of the brain. West J Med, 127:231, 1977

54. French JD: Clinical manifestations of lumbar spinal arachnoiditis: A report of thirteen cases. Surgery, 20:718–729, 1946

55. Frymoyer JW, Hanley E, Howe J, *et al:* Disc excision and spine fusion in the management of lumbar disc disease. Spine, 3(1):1–6, 1978

56. Frymoyer JW, Matteri RE, Hanley EN, *et al:* Failed Lumbar disc surgery requiring second operation. Spine, 3(1):7–11, 1978.

57. Fullenlove IM: Venous intravasation during myelography. Radiology, 53:410–412, 1949

58. Gellman M: Injury to intervertebral discs during spinal puncture. J Bone Jt Surg, 22:980, 1940

59. Ginsburg LB, Skorneck AB: Pantopaque pulmonary embolism: a complication of myelography. Amer J Roentg, 73:27–31, 1955

60. Glenn WV, Brown BM, Murphy RM, Rhodes ML, *et al:* Computerized Body Tomography (CBT) and the Lumbar Spine. Part I: CBT as a Substitute for Lumbar Myelography in Disc Disease, submitted for publication, August 1980

61. Glenn WV, Rhodes ML, Altschuler EL, *et*

al: Multiplanar CBT applications in lumbar disc disease: The proponent's viewpoint. Chapter 5 in reference 125.

62. Glenn WV Jr, Davis KR, Dwyer SJ: Alternative display formats for computed tomography (CT) data. Current concepts in radiology. EJ Potchen (ed). 3, 1977

63. Glenn WV Jr, Johnston RJ, Morton PE, *et al:* Further investigation and initial clinical use of advanced CI display capability. Invest Radiol, 10:479–489, 1975

64. Glenn WV Jr, Johnston RJ, Morton PE, *et al:* Image generation and display techniques for CT scan data: Thin transverse and reconstructed coronal and sagittal planes. Invest Radiol, 10:403–416, 1975

65. Glenn WV Jr, Rhodes ML, Altschuler EL, *et al:* Multiplanar display (MPD) computerized body tomography applications in the lumbar spine. Spine, 4:282–352, 1979

66. Glenn WV Jr, Lancourt JE, Wiltse LL: Multiplanar CT applications in the spine: Early clinical experience. In Korobkin M (ed): Proceedings of CT Conference, San Francisco, California, 1978

67. Glenn WV Jr, Taveras JM, Johnston RJ, *et al:* Clinical feasibility of reconstructing coronal, sagittal and thin transverse sections from overlapped 8.0mm CT scans. In Ter-Pogussian MM, Phelps ME, Brownell GL (eds): Workshop on Reconstruction Tomography in Diagnostic Radiology and Nuclear Medicine. New York, University Park Press, 1975

68. Goitein M, Wittenberg J, Ferrucci J, *et al:* Prospective study of the value of CT scanning in radiation therapy treatment planning. J Comput Assist Tomogr, 1:372, 1977

69. Grainger RG: Letter to the Editor. Chronic spinal arachnoiditis. British Med J, Nov 4, 94, 1978

70. Grieg JH, Wignall N: A case of arachnoiditis associated with "Pantopaque" myelography. J Canad A Radiologists, 17:198, 1966

71. Grossman ZD, Wistow BW, Wallinga HA, *et al:* Recognition of verebtral abnormalities in computed tomography of the chest and abdomen. Radiology, 121:369–373, 1976

72. Haaga JR, Alfidi RJ, Havrilla TR, *et al:* CT detection and aspiration of abdominal abscesses. Am J Roentgenoal, 128:465–474, 1977

73. Haaga JR, Alfidi RJ, Havrilla TR, *et al:* Definitive role of CT scanning of the pancreas: The second year's experience. Radiology, 124:723–730, 1977

74. Hammerschlag SB, Wolpert SM, Carter BL: Computed tomography of the spinal canal. Radiology, 121:361–367, 1976

75. Handel SF, Twiford TW, Reigel DH, *et al:* Posterior lumbar apophyseal fractures. Radiology, 130:629–633, 1979

76. Hansen BEB, Fahrenkrug A, Praestholm J: Late meningeal effects of myelographic contrast media with special reference to metrizamide. British J of Radiol, 51(605):321–327, 1978

77. Harwood–Nash DCF, Fitz CR, Resjo M, *et al:* Congenital spinal and cord lesions in children and computed tomographic metrizamide myelography. Neuroradiology, 16:79–70, 1978

78. Haughton RM, Ho KC, Larson SJ, *et al:* Comparison of arachnoiditis produced by meglumine locarmate and metrizamide myelography in an animal model. Am J of Roentgenology, 131:129–132, 1978

79. Haughton VG, Ho KC, Unger GF: Arachnoiditis following myelography with water-soluble agents. Radiology, 125:731–733, 1977

80. Haughton VM, Eldevik OP, Ho KC, *et al:* Arachnoiditis from experimental myelography with aqueous contrast media. Spine, 3(1):65–69, 1978

81. Hilal SK, Dauth Gw, Hess KH, et al: Development and evaluation of a new water-soluble iodinated myelographic contrast medium with markedly reduced convulsive effects. Radiology, 126:417–422, 1978

82. Hinkel CL: The entrance of Pantopaque into the venous system during myelography. Amer J Roentg, 54:230–233, 1945

83. Hounsfield GN: Computerized transverse axial scanning (tomography). Part I: Description of system. Br J Radiol, 46:1016–1022, 1973

84. Howland WJ, Curry JL: Experimental studies of pantopaque arachnoiditis. Radiology, 87:253–261, 1966.

85. Howland WJ, Curry JL: Pantopaque arachnoiditis: Experimental study of blood as a potentiating agent and corticosteroids as an ameliorating agent. Acta Radiol [Diagn] (Stockholm), 5:1032–1041, 1966

86. Hurteau EF, Baird WC, Sinclair E: Arachnoiditis following the use of iodized oil. J Bone Jt Surg, 36A, 393–400, 1954

87. Hyman RA, Merten CW, Liebeskind AL, *et al:* Computed tomography in ossificiation of the posterior longitudinal spinal ligament. Nueroradiology, 13:227–228, 1977

88. Isherwood I, Fawcitt RA, Nettle JRL, *et al:* Computed tomography of the spine: A preliminary report. In du Boulay GH, Mosely IF (eds): Computerized Axial Tomography in Clinical Practice, pp 322–335, Berlin, Springer Verlag, 1977

89. Isherwood I, Rutherford RA, Pullen BR: Computerized tomography of brain. Br Med J, 2:746–747, 1975

90. Jaeger R: Irritating effect of iodized vegetable oils on brain and spinal cord when divided into small particles. Arch Neurol Psychiat, 64:715–719, 1950

91. James HE, Oliff M: Computed tomography in spinal dysraphism. J Comput Assist Tomogr, 1:391–397, 1977

92. Johnston JDH, Matheny JB: Microscopic lysis of lumbar adhesive arachnoiditis. Spine, 3(1):36–39, 1978

93. Kadoya S, Nakamura T, Tada A: Neuroradiology of ossification of the posterior longitudinal spinal ligament. Comparative studies with computer tomography. Neuroradiology, 16:357–358, 1978

94. Keats TE: Pantopaque pulmonary embolism. Radiology, 67:748–750, 1956

95. Kershner MS, Goodman GA, Perlmutter GS: Computed tomography in the diagnosis of an atlas fracture. Am J Roentgenol, 128:688–689, 1977

96. Kirkaldy-Willis WH, Heithoff K, Bowen CVA: Pathological anatomy of lumbar spondylosis and stenosis, correlated with the CT scan. Chapter 2 in reference 125.

97. Klinger A, Rhodes ML, Glenn WV Jr: General view imagery from paralled image planes. Proceedings San Diego Biomedical Symposium, Feb 1–3, 1978, pp 387–391

98. Kramer LD, Krouth GJ: Computerized tomography. An adjunct to early diagnosis in the cauda equina syndrome of ankylosing spondylitis. Arch Neurol, 35:116–118, 1978

99. Krol G, Khomeini R, Deck MF: CT of the spine. Neuroradiology, 16:362–363, 1978

100. Kuo YM, Rhodes ML, Glenn WV: Elements of a comparative data base for structured measurement in computerized tomography. In Proceedings from Conference on Computer-Aided Analysis of Radiological Images, Newport Beach, June 1979, pp. 334–340

101. Kwoh YS, Reed IS, Truong TK: A generalized w-filter for 3–D reconstruction. IEEE Trans Nucl Science NS-24, 1977

102. Lancourt JE, Glenn WV Jr, Wiltse LL: Multiplanar CT applications in the spine: A gross anatomic-computerized tomographic correlation. Spine, 4:379–390, 1979

103. Larsen GN, Glenn WV Jr, Kishore PRS, *et al:* Computer processing of CT images: Advances and prospects. J Neurosurg, 1(1), 1977

104. Lee BCP, Kazam E, Newman AD: Computed tomography of the spine and spinal cord. Radiol, 128:95–102, 1978

105. Lee CK, Hansen HT, Weiss AB: Development of Lumbar spinal stenosis. Pathology and surgical treatment. Spine, 3(3):246–255, 1978

106. Lipson SJ, Mazur J: Anteroposterior spondyloschisis of the atlas revealed by computerized tomography scanning. JBJS, 60A:1108–1109, 1978

107. Luce JC, Leith W, Burrage WS: Pantopaque meningitis due to hypersensitivity. Radiology, 57:878–881, 1951

108. MacGee EE: Osteochondroma of the cervical spine: A cause of transient quadriplegia. Neurosurgery, 4(3):2659–2660, 1979

109. Mann NJ, Uihlein A, Kernohan JW: Intraspinal epidermoids. J Neurosurg, 19:754, 1962

110. Martin CM: Myelography with sodium diatrizoate (Hypaque). Report of a case of inadvertent use complicated by acute renal failure. California Med, 115:57, 1971

111. Martin K, Krastel A, Hamer J, *et al:* Symptomatology and diagnosis of diastematomyelia of children. Neuroradiology, 16:89–90, 1978

112. Mason MS, Raaf J: Complications of Pantopaque myelography: Case report and review. J Neurosurg, 19:302–311, 1962

113. Mayher WE, Daniel EF, Allen MB: Acute meningeal reaction following pantopaque myelography. J Neurosurg, 34–396, 1977

114. McNab I: *Backache*, Williams and Wilkins Co., Baltimore, 1977

115. Meyer GA, Haughton VM, Williams AL: Diagnosis of herniated lumbar disk with computed tomography. The New England Journal of Medicine, 301(21):1166–1167, 1979

116. Miller DS: Post-myelographic coccygodynia. Am J Proctol, 18:292, 1967

117. Morretin LB, Wilson M: Severe reflex algodystrophy (Sudek's atrophy) as a complication of myelography. Report of two cases. Am J Roentgenol, 110:156, 1970

118. Muhm JR, Brown LR, Crowe JK: Detection of pulmonary nodules by computed tomography. Am J Roentgenol, 128:267–270, 1977

119. Naidich TP, Moran CJ, Pudlowski RM, *et al:* Advances in diagnosis: Cranial and spinal computed tomography. Med Clinics of North America 63(1):849–895, 1979

120. Nainkin, L: Arachnoiditis ossificans, report of a case. Spine, 3(1):83–88, 1978

121. Nakagawa H, Huang YP, Malis LI, *et al:* Computed tomography of intraspinal and paraspinal neoplasms. J Comput Assist Tomogr, 1(4):377–390, 1977

122. Nykamp PW, Levy JM, Christensen F, *et al:*

Computed tomography for a bursting fracture of the lumbar spine. JBJS 60-A (8):1108–1109, 1978

123. Oberson R, Azam F: CAT of the spine and spinal cord. Neuroradiology, 16:369–379, 1978

124. Peacher WG, Robertson RCL: Pantopaque myelography: Results, comparison of contrast media, and spinal fluid reaction. J Neurosurg, 2:220–231, 1945

125. Post MJD (ed): Radiographic Evaluation of the Spine: Current Advances with Emphasis on CT. New York, Masson, 1980

126. Post MJD, Gargano FP, Vining DQ, et al: A comparison of radiographic methods of diagnosing constrictive lesions of the spinal canal. Toshiba unit vs CT scanner. J Neurosurg, 48:360–368, 1978

127. Praestholm J: Experimental evaluation of watersoluble contrast media for myelography. Neuroradiology, 13:25–35, 1977

128. Quencer RM, Murtagh FR, Post MJD, et al: Postoperative bony stenosis of the lumbar spinal canal: Evaluation of 164 symptomatic patients with axial radiography. Am J Roentgenol, 131:1059–1064, 1978

129. Quiles M, Marshisello PJ, Tsairis P: Lumbar adhesive arachnoiditis, etiologic and pathologic aspects. Spine, 3(1):45–50, 1978

130. Reed IS, Glenn WV Jr, Chang CM, et al: Dose reduction in x-ray computed tomography using a generalized filter. IEEE Trans Nucl Science NS-26(2):2904–2909, 1979

131. Reed IS, Glenn WV, Chang CM, et al: The optimum filtering of successive overlapping sections of an x-ray reconstruction. IEEE Trans Biomedical Engineering. BME 27(2), Feb 1980

132. Reed IS, Glenn WV Jr, Truong TK, et al: The x-ray reconstruction of spinal cord using bone suppression. IEEE Trans Biomedical Engineering BME 27(6):293–298, 1980

133. Reese DF, Carney JA, Gisvold JJ, et al: Computerized reconstructive tomography applied to breast pathology. Am J Roentgenol, 126:406–412, 1976

134. Resjo IM, Harwood-Nash DC, Fitz CR, et al: Computed tomographic metrizamide myelography (CTMM) in intraspinal and paraspinal neoplasms in infants and children. Am J Roentgenol 132:367–372, 1979

135. Resjo IM, Harwood-Nash DC, Fitz CR, et al: Computed tomographic metrizamide myelography in spinal dysraphism in infants and children. J Comput Assist Tomogr, 2:549–558, 1978

136. Resjo IM, Harwood-Nash DC, Fitz CR: Computed tomographic metrizamide myelography in syringohydromyelia. Radiology, 131:405–407, 1979

137. Resjo IM, Harwood-Nash DC, Fitz CR, et al: CT metrizamide myelography for intraspinal and paraspinal neoplasms in infants and children. AJR 132:367–372, 1979

138. Resjo IM, Harwood-Nash DC, Fitz CR, et al: Normal cord in infants and children examined with computed tomographic metrizamide myelogram (CTMM). Radiology 130:691–696, 1979

139. Rhodes ML, Glenn WV, Awazzi YM: "Extracting Oblique Planes from Serial Section." To be published in JCAT, 1980

140. Rhodes ML, Glenn WV Jr: Fast general view display for CT image data. IEEE Trans Biomed Eng. To be published in JCAT, 1980

141. Rinaldi I, Kopp JE, Harris WO, Jr, et al: Computer assisted tomography in syringomyelia. J Comput Assist Tomogr, 2:633–635, 1978

142. Rinaldi I, Mullins WJ, Delaney WF, et al: Computerized tomographic demonstration of rotational atlanto-axial fixation. J Neurosurg, 50:115–119, 1979

143. Roub LW, Drayer BP: Spinal computed tomography: Limitations and applications. AJR, 133:267–273, 1979

144. Rozario RA, Levine H, Stein BM: Cervical myelopathy and radiculopathy secondary to ossification of the posterior longitudinal ligament. Surg Neurology, 10:17–20, 1978

145. Sarkisian SS: Spinal cord pseudotumor: A complication of Pantopaque myelography. US Armed Forces Med J, 7:1683–1686, 1956

146. Scatliff JH, Bidgood WD, Jr, Killebre K: Computed tomography and spinal dysraphia: Clinical and phantom studies. Neuroradiology, 17:71–75, 1979

147. Schaner EG, Chang AE, Doppman JL, et al: Comparison of computed and conventional whole lung tomography in the detection of pulmonary metastases. J Comput Assist Tomogr, 1:363, 1977

148. Schaner EG, Head GL, Doppman JL, et al: Computed tomography in the diagnosis, staging, and management of abdominal lymphoma. J Comput Assist Tomogr, 1:176–180, 1977

149. Schultz EC, Miller JH: Intravasation of opaque media during myelography: 3 cases. J Neurosurg, 18:610, 1961

150. Schurr PH, McLaurin RL, Ingraham FD: Experimental studies on the circulation of the cerebrospinal fluid and methods of producing communicating hydrocephalus in the dog. J Neurosurg, 10:515–525, 1953

151. Shapiro R: Myelography. Chicago, Year Book Medical Publishers, 1975

152. Sheldon JJ, Leborgne JM: Computed tomography of the lumbar vertebral column. Chapter 3 in reference 125.

153. Sheldon JJ, Sersland T, Leborgne J: Computed tomography of the lower lumbar vertebral column. Radiology, 124:113–118, 1977

154. Skalpe IO: Adhesive arachnoiditis following lumbar myelography. Spine, 3(1):61–64, 1978

155. Steinbach HL, Hill WB: Pantopaque pulmonary embolism during myelography. Radiology, 56:735–738, 1951

156. Steinhausen TB, Dungan CE, Furst JB, et al: Iodinated organic compounds as contrast media for radiographic diagnoses. III. Experimental and clinical myelography with ethyl iodophenylundecylate (Pantopaque). Radiology, 43:230–234, 1944

157. Stephens DH, Sheedy PF II, Hattery RR, et al: Computed tomography of the liver. Am J Roentgenol, 128:579–590, 1977

158. Tabaddor K: Unusual complication of iophendylate injection myelography. Arch Neurol, 29:435, 1973

159. Tadmor R, Davis KR, Roberson GH, et al: Computed tomographic evaluation of traumatic spinal injuries. Radiol, 127:825–827, 1978

160. Tadmor R, Davis KR, Roberson GH, et al: The diagnosis of diastematomyelia by computed tomography. Surg Neurol, 8:434–436, 1977

161. Tainter EG, Grayson CE: Large volume myelography. Ann NY Acad Science, 78:956–965, 1959

162. Tarlov IM: Pantopaque meningitis disclosed at operation. JAMA, 129:1014–1016, 1945

163. Thijssen HOM, Keyser, A, Horstink MWM, et al: Morphology of the cervical spinal cord on computed myelography. Neuroradiology, 18:57–62, 1979

164. Todd EM, Gardner WJ: Pantopaque intravasation (embolization) during myelography. J Neurosurg, 14:230–234, 1957

165. Ullrich CG, Binel EF, Saneuci NG, et al: Quantitative assessment of the lumbar spinal canal by computed tomography. Radiology, 134:137–143, 1980

166. Verbiest H: The significance and principles of computerized axial tomography in idopathic developmental stenosis of the bony lumbar vertebral canal. Spine 4(4):369–378, 1979

167. Vinocur CD, Dinn WM, Dudgeon DL: Computed tomographic scanning in children. J Pediatric Surg, 12(6):847–856, 1977

168. Weinstein MA, Rothner AD, Duchesneau P, et al: Computed tomography in diastematomyelia. Radiology, 118:609–611, 1975

169. Whalen JP, Watson RC: The potential role of computerized tomography in bone diseases. Proceedings of the Conference on Computerized Tomography in Radiology, St. Louis, U. of Missouri, 1976, pp 25–28

170. Winkelman NW, Gotten N, Scheibert D: Localized adhesive spinal arachnoiditis. A study of twenty-five cases with reference to etiology. Trans Am Neurol Assoc, 15–17, 1953

171. Wolpert SM, Scott RM, Carter BL: Computed tomography in spinal dysraphism. Surg Neurol, 8:199–206, 1977

172. Wood, KM: New approaches to treatment of back pain. West J Med, 130:394–398, 1979

173. Wray AR, Templeton J, Laird JD: Seizure following lumbar myelography with metrizamide. British Medical Journal, 23–30, 1978

174. Young DA, Burney RE: Complication of myelography-transection and withdrawal of a nerve root filament by the needle. NEJM, 285:156–157, 1971

175. Zito JL, Schellinger D: Nontraumatic intravasation of myelographic contrast medium. American Journal Roentgenology, 132:795–797, 1979

Psychology of Low Back Dysfunction 5

Psychology of Pain

The greatest handicap a low back pain physician can have is lack of interest in and awareness of the psychosocial environment of the patient. Two patients may describe their low back symptoms in almost identical terms, yet the terms may have very dissimilar meanings. An appreciation of this difference is most important. Only with an adequate understanding of what the patient is trying to tell us are we able to provide appropriate treatment.

Pain may be defined as a psychobiologic phenomenon with both physical and emotional components. This dual aspect of pain is linked to the distinction between perception and reaction. Perception of pain may be evaluated in terms of quality and intensity, while reaction to pain is manifested by such symptoms as tachycardia, anxiety, fear, panic, and prostration.

Physicians may emphasize the anatomic pathways, the physiologic mechanisms, the neurochemical reactions or other important components involved in pain. But their understanding of these elements does not mean they can claim to have defined pain, any more than engineers who construct a TV transmitter or repairmen who fix TV receivers are specifically qualified to comment on the news as it is being reported on the screen. Sir Thomas Lewis stated: "Pain, like similar subjective sensations, is known to us by experience and described by illustration. Reflection tells me that I am so far from being able satisfactorily to define pain, that the attempt would serve no useful purpose." With or without a satisfactory definition of pain, it remains the province of the clinician to work out a practical solution consistent with the needs of the patient.

Organic Pain and "Imaginary" Pain

In the practice of clinical medicine, emotional factors are often not considered part of a pain syndrome unless the pain is labeled imaginary or the patient is identified as a malingerer. Most patients complaining of pain usually have at least some physiological basis for their complaints, although neurotic mechanisms may greatly exaggerate their suffering. The very term **psychosomatic medicine** epitomizes the dual nature of the mind and body concept. The constant effort we physicians make to separate the purely physiologic from the purely psychologic and to label symptoms as either organic or functional has a certain futility about it.

The use of "organic" phraseology to depict an emotional or psychologic state is often encountered in the expressions used in daily conversations, such as, "You are a pain in the neck," or "You make me sick," or, "That job is a headache." That such symbolic uses of organic expressions are com-

179

pletely understood and require no explanation indicates that the merging of mind and body is indeed a natural one; and it is only the "trained" mind of the physician that often creates a false problem in attempting to separate the two when there is no actual division. For example, if an individual states that a certain job is a headache, no one would consider treating this condition medically. But when a patient with a backache of emotional etiology is seen in the office, it is much easier to treat him medically than to attempt to evaluate and to deal with the etiology of his backache. Thus, as physicians, we are always called on to make a "value judgment" regarding the organicity of pain.

If we decide that the pain is actually organic, it is either because we can identify the etiology of the pain or because the characteristics of the pain fall into a known or readily classifiable pattern. When we are able to identify a pain successfully as organic in nature, we then carry out the appropriate therapeutic measures. If we are unable to diagnose the patient's pain as organic, we do not feel as comfortable in managing the patient. Because of our own frame of reference with regard to nonorganic symptoms, which in part results from our background and training, we are inclined to consider this pain response somewhat inappropriate. When we label a symptom as functional or psychogenic we are, to some extent, making light of it.

Pain and the Doctor-Patient Relationship

Whenever a physician is dealing with a pain problem, he must bear in mind the relationship he has with the patient and the patient's attitude toward him. It is my experience that the vast majority of patients have a high regard for their physicians, and it gives them considerable regret if they are not significantly improved by treatment administered. Most patients rarely say that any particular method of treatment is completely ineffective. The physician is more likely to get the guarded response: "It's only a little better."

Because of the normal tendency to prefer praise to blame, we tend to become frustrated or even antagonistic, and are apt to label the pain problem as functional when the patient does not improve. Most of us have had the expereince of treating a symptom complex that we would ordinarily expect to improve with our method of therapy, and of developing a somewhat hostile attitude toward the patient when the expected satisfactory result does not occur. Although we are sometimes able to assess adequately our own feelings toward the patient, we must also remain aware that the patient's feelings toward us often play a significant role in determining the success of therapy. In some instances, the patient may develop hostility toward the physician and announce with triumph at each visit, "Your medicine doesn't do a thing for me." The patient may not feel that he is able to complain overtly to his physician, but his continued suffering despite treatment is a form of covert criticism, which renders the physician powerless to respond.

This example of hostility between doctor and patient is somewhat oversimplified, and, of course, persistent pain invariably has many more ramifications than described in this primitive psychological schema. But it is often with a sense of punishment that the patient is referred to a psychiatrist or other specialist. The patient feels that he has annoyed the physician, and in many cases he truly has. When this is true, the patient often feels banished to a psychiatrist for symptoms he feels are certainly not imaginary. It is my own impression that probably 50% of all psychiatric referrals in a general hospital can be classified, at least in part, as pain syndromes.

Reactions to Pain

EMOTIONS

There are no really satisfactory and universally accepted methods for gauging pain intensity, but studies based on the techniques currently available to us provide some information on individual "pain thresholds." The patient with a prefrontal lobotomy may have a normal threshold for pain and acknowledge pain on direct inquiry, but will manifest a decreased reaction to a painful stimulus.

A number of factors influence the reaction to pain. Conditioning experience and emotions may either increase or decrease the reaction. When a child who is ordered to go upstairs to bed, barks his shin as he is sulkily climbing the stairs, he howls with pain. An identical injury suffered by the same child while climbing to a stadium seat to see a ball game may go unnoticed. The pain of a superficial laceration is easily tolerated by most adults, but apprehension and inexperience will cause a child with the same wound to experience a much amplified reaction. Conversely, a dull pain over the left anterior chest wall in an adult may provoke considerable apprehension and alarm. The child under identical stimulus will probably not interrupt his play.

The patient harboring malignant disease, whose suffering is almost always most intense in the gloom of night after all routine activities have ceased and he is alone with his thoughts, illustrates the role of emotions in increasing the reaction to pain. The testimony of prizefighters is often cited to indicate the effect of emotions in decreasing appreciation of pain. During the course of a bout, they may be cruelly battered and yet not notice any pain. This experience shared by soldiers in combat who state that their wounds do not become painful until they are evacuated from the dangers of the combat area, is probably only partly due to emotional influences.

Initial absence of pain is a common phenomenon accompanying sudden trauma. For example, a bullet wound that shatters the tibia may be appreciated as a heavy but painless blow to the shin. The observation has been made that if a man cries out noisily when wounded during combat it is likely that the wound is not a severe one. Although high-speed projectile wounds are more often mentioned in this connection, stab wounds are often first noticed when blood trickles down the skin, producing a sensation of wetness.

ADAPTATION

If a stimulus to a sensory receptor is maintained at a constant intensity, the frequency of discharge from this receptor gradually diminishes. This phenomenon is called **adaptation,** and the rapidity with which different receptor organs adapt varies. The proprioceptors, which are concerned with the automatic maintenance of posture and knowledge of the position of the limb segments of the body, adapt quite slowly, as is necessary in order to sustain positional attitudes and reflexes. Touch receptors, on the other hand, adapt very rapidly, which is compatible with the innocuous nature of the stimulus and yet allows the receptor to remain ready to receive new impressions. Pain receptors adapt very little and continue to generate pain impulses for the duration of the painful stimulus. This is consistent with the protective function of pain.

Under special circumstances the phenomenon of adaptation to pain may come into play and create permanent elevation of pain thresholds. This was the case in a number of Allied prisoners of war subjected to three years of imprisonment and torture during World War II. Some of these survivors had varying degrees of persistent anesthesia, and one had complete insensitivity to all sensations except those on the cornea.

SOCIOECONOMIC AND CULTURAL FACTORS

Social, economic, and cultural, in addition to situational and environmental, factors may produce alterations in reaction to pain. An interesting project in this regard was carried out by Richard A. Sternbach and Bernard Tursky, in the Department of Psychiatry, Harvard Medical School. They attempted to determine whether the tolerance for pain was different for various ethnic groups. They obtained their subjects in response to classified advertising in local papers. All the subjects were housewives who had at least one child of school age, so that the process of transmitting attitudes toward pain could be explored in interviews. Ethnic membership was defined as follows: Yankees were Protestants of British descent whose parents and grandparents were born in this country; Irish, Italians, and Jews were those whose parents came to this country as immigrants, were Roman Catholic in the case of the Irish and Italians, and Orthodox or conservative in the case of Jews. Each subject participated in an interview lasting about an hour in which the purpose of the study was explained, family history was gathered, and the specific incidence of reactions to injuries was collected. The pain stimulus was produced by electrical stimulation delivered through an annular disc electrode on the treated dorsal surface of the left forearm. Standard psychophysical procedures were employed, including a notation of the level at which the subject asked that stimulation be stopped in response to the instruction, "We will gradually make it stronger until you tell us you don't want any more." This level was referred to as the **unmotivated upper threshold.** Then some subjects who asked to stop before a certain current had been reached were coaxed to try higher levels referred to as the **motivated upper threshold.** The mean upper (unmotivated and motivated) thresholds for the four ethnic groups were as follows:[3]

Response	Yankee	Irish	Jewish	Italian
Unmotivated upper threshold	9.74	8.68	8.83	6.12
Motivated upper threshold	10.23	9.35	10.16	7.11

Subjects also performed a "magnitude estimation" test as follows. Given a measured stimulation, they were told to call this stimulus "10" and to assign appropriate numbers to other intensities according to their subjective impression of each.

The findings of this study were correlated with and tended to support certain hypotheses regarding the attitudinal dissimilarities among those subcultural groups. It is felt that each group has its own configuration of attitudes toward painful stimuli and toward the expression or response to pain.

The fact that the Italian women showed significantly lower pain thresholds (and that fewer of them would accept the full range of stimuli) is quite consistent with the finding of a present-day orientation in this group with respect to pain, a focusing on the immediacy of the pain itself. This concern may be constrasted with that of the Jewish subjects, who similarly display distress when in pain, but whose distress is due to concern for the implications of the noxious stimulati. In our laboratory situation, where the stimuli carried no implication of future impairment, no activation of this concern would be expected for the Jewish group, and therefore no difference would be expected between them and the Yankees and Irish, who tend to be undemonstrative with respect to pain. But one would expect the Italian group, who are primarily concerned with the avoidance of the unpleasant stimuli, to be reluctant to accept the stronger intensities.[3]

The relatively undemonstrative Yankees had an adapting matter-of-fact orientation toward pain, but the similarly undemonstrative Irish subjects considered a painful stimulus a burden to be endured and suffered in silence.

Thus, the similar demonstrativeness of the Italians and Jews in response to pain arises from dissimilar attitudes, as does the similar undemonstrativeness of the Yankees and Irish.

ATHLETICS

Another attempt to evaluate reaction to pain was carried out by Ryan and Kovacic from the University of California, who attempted to measure pain tolerance and athletic participation.

From observation of everyday experiences in athletics, it would be expected that ability to withstand pain should be related to participation in certain types of athletic events. In many sports, such as football or boxing, the ability to withstand pain appears to be essential to successful performance, while in sports such as tennis or golf, the ability to withstand pain would be less important. Thus, it is not inconceivable that an individual's ability or inability to tolerate pain may well determine the category of participation he selects. An individual with a high pain threshold might be oblivious to bumps and bruises received in a football game, whereas the individual with a low pain threshold might avoid such contact.[2]

For this reason, pain threshold and pain tolerance were studied in three groups of subjects: contact athletes, noncontact athletes, and nonathletes. That the study was related to athletic participation was not known by the subjects.

Three methods were used to deliver controlled pain:

1. Radiant heat was focused on the subject's forehead, and the time of radiation was used to measure the subject's pain threshold.
2. Gross pressure was used to measure pain tolerance by means of a plastic aluminum-tipped football cleat secured to a curved fiber plate and fitted to the leg. The cleat was placed against the anterior border of the tibia, midway between the ankle and the knee, and a sphygmomanometer was used to secure the cleat properly in place. Cleat pressure was obtained by inflating the sphygmomanometer armlet at a slow constant rate until the subject indicated verbally that he was no longer willing to endure the pain.
3. Muscle ischemia was the third method of evaluating pain tolerance. After the sphygmomanometer cuff was applied to the upper arm and the pressure elevated to 300 mm of mercury, the subject opened and closed his fist once per second until he was unwilling to proceed.

Each test was carried out twice. After the first trial, the examiner remarked to each of the subjects that the score was quite a bit lower than the average of the group tested and the subject was asked to take the test a second time and do better, if possible.

Examination of the results indicated a definite relationship between the subject's willingness or ability to tolerate pain and the type of athletic activity in which he chooses to participate. The contact athlete . . . tolerated more pain than the athlete who participated only in noncontact sports such as tennis or golf, and both groups of athletes are willing to tolerate more pain than the nonathlete. In addition, after being told that his initial effort was poor, the contact athlete showed marked improvement on the second attempt, while the noncontact athlete improved some, but the nonathlete tolerated less pain than on the first attempt.

The question of cause and effect—whether a boy learns to tolerate pain because he engages in contact sports, whether he engages in contact sports because he can more easily tolerate pain (either for physiological or psychological reasons) . . . is unanswered by these data.[2]

BODY AREA

The body area of the pain is sometimes a factor in determining the patient's reaction. For example, many patients are reluctant to complain about rectal pain or genital pain. Headache is more popularly considered a socially acceptable form of discomfort. In this respect, I recall a patient who had been referred to me in the late 1950s, when I still practiced general neurosurgery. Because of the intractable nature of his headaches, this patient was eventually hospitalized for a complete neurological work-up. In the course of a complete physical examination carried out by the intern, very severely thrombosed hemorrhoids were noted. I saw this on the chart and asked the patient about his hemorrhoids. After some equivocation, he admitted that he had suffered quite severely from rectal pain for more than a year, and despite the fact that he was going to a physician at regular intervals for headaches, he had never mentioned the rectal pain. The reason given was that he was "ashamed of having a painful rectum" but considered the headache socially acceptable. Obvious psychosexual mechanisms may be involved here with the patient having a great reluctance to submit this area of his body to probing and assessment.

PSYCHOSIS

Most psychotic patients do not differ from sane patients in their reactions to pain. However, many of them complain of severe pain in various portions of their anatomy as a part of their mental illness. On the other hand, some schizophrenic patients have amputated their genitals, fingers, or ears, or have extensively mutilated themselves in other ways without expressing a reaction to pain.

Absence of Pain

A number of papers have described persons born without a sense of pain. In spite of this lack these rare individuals usually are able to cope with the routine problems of daily living and to avoid burns and other injuries, which the adult who develops syringomyelia (which causes loss of pain and temperature sensations) is likely to incur. Because absence of pain is extremely uncommon and postmortem confirmation is not readily available, the site of any possible organic lesion is not clearly documented. Some workers believe that this condition represents a form of sensory agnosia or an aphasialike inability to formulate an appreciation of pain.

Pain and Sensory Deprivation

At one time the ability to withstand pain was considered a factor in evaluating men for future space travel. One of the potential problems of prolonged travel in space is a form of sensory deprivation resulting from isolation and confinement. Studies of persons subjected to prolonged sensory deprivation have demonstrated a deterioration in performance capabilities, due to the improverished sensory environment. In addition, a number of personality aberrations have resulted from experimental sensory deprivations, such as increased anxiety, feelings of insecurity, and in some cases, hallucinations. In all cases, motor coordination and precision of motor performance are impaired.

Because pain is a sensory phenomenon, one might speculate that those persons who were hypersensitive to pain and had low pain thresholds were extremely sensitive to all sensory stimuli. With this presumed hypersensitivity, such individuals should have a less detrimental reaction to prolonged sensory deprivation. An analogy of this concept is that of a powerful (hypersensitive) radio receiver picking up the faint signals of a distant broadcast (sensory deprivation) while the ordinary low power (hyposensitive) set would not register the signal.

This hypothesis was advanced by Dr. A. Petrie, who postualted that sensitivity to pain is the reverse of sensory deprivation sensitivity. To carry this hypothesis further, since there might be a negative relationship between insensitivity to pain and performance under reduced sensory input conditions, astronauts who are most sensitive to pain ought to be selected for prolonged space travel because they would be able to endure reduced sensory input conditions for a longer time without degradation in performance. On the other hand, those with higher pain thresholds would not be able to endure reduced sensory input conditions and would manifest an inferior performance.

Studies were carried out by Dr. J. Peters and his associates of the Space Environment and Life Sciences Laboratory of the Republic Aviation Corporation in Farmingdale, Long Island, on a number of volunteers who were first tested for their ability to tolerate pain. After this had been established, the subjects were then placed in an environment of sensory deprivation.

Each volunteer rested on a contour couch in a full scale model of a multiman space capsule.

The subjects could communicate with the observer at any time during the experiment, but the observer only responded when a subject requested termination of his stay in the cabin. Each subject donned ear defender headsets with built-in ear phones such as are typically worn by workers at airfields. "White" noise was fed into the headsets at a low decibel load sufficiently above ambient noise to shut out any orientation to the world outside, yet the subject obviously had monotonous and continuous hearing stimulation. The subject wore goggles modified to allow light to come through translucent but not transparent lens surfaces. Thus, the subjects were visually stimulated by incandescent light which always illuminated the cabin, but the illumination was unchanging and unpatterned. The subjects wore heavy leather gloves, similar to those worn by electric arc-welders, and they were instructed to keep the gloves on at all times. Thus, sensations normally received by the fingers and hands were diminished, and the threshold for discernable patterns of sensation was raised. This tended to make the sensory input from the hands monotonous. Similarly, the subjects wore heavy wool socks to diminish sensory input from the feet. Because of the attached sensors and wires, the movement of the subjects was restricted. They were instructed not to leave their contour chairs and advised that the electronic wiring allowed only limited movement. Thus, the subjects would only turn from side to side, flex and unflex their limbs, and sit up or lie down. The food, Sustagen, was a bland, high caloric liquid, neither markedly pleasant nor unpleasant in taste. The subjects were encouraged to take nourishment whenever they desired, but when they did so, to take a least several ounces of the liquid. Thus, oral stimulation tended to be minimized.[1]

This study seemed to indicate a direct and positive correlation between the ability to endure pain and the ability to endure reduced sensory input conditions. The original idea that there is a negative relationship between the ability to endure pain and the ability to endure reduces sensory input conditions was not supported. The evidence suggested that subjects who were most able to endure pain were better able to tolerate reduced sensory input conditions, suffered less anxiety with attendant headaches and nausea, and remained in good functional condition for longer periods of time than those who were least able to endure pain.

Evaluation of Pain

From time to time most well-adjusted persons will experience aches or pains in various areas of their bodies which will not interfere with activities of daily living. The psychoneurotic person is often prone to seize upon such a nidus of pain and so distort and exaggerate it that the major symptom complex he eventually manifests can hardly be recognized in relationship to the original pain. The various psychologic mechanisms at work in creating this type of distorted clinical picture vary greatly and should always be considered when the symptoms are inconsistent with the findings on examination.

DIFFICULTIES IN DIAGNOSIS

The evaluation of pain for treatment is made difficult by the fact that pain is an almost entirely subjective phenomenon. It is especially difficult to differentiate organic from psychic factors. The problem is further complicated because in most, if not all patients, both factors contribute to the final expression of pain. Furthermore, the proportion of contribution by the somatic and psychic spheres changes constantly. It is in this area of diagnosis that the "art" of the physician is most severely challenged and is almost impossible to subject to quantitative evaluation and criticism. Estimation of the intensity of pain is likewise difficult for the physician. Nevertheless, he must evaluate the intensity in order to determine what therapy is justified for relief of pain. Such questions as the constancy of pain, its interference with performance of duties, and how it affects vital functions such as sleep, must be answered and evaluated clearly by the examiner.

A careful history is the principal basis for establishing a diagnosis of the pain syndrome and its severity. It often requires considerable time and patience to elicit findings that permit the diagnosis of a specific organic syndrome, or to demonstrate that none exists.

An understanding of a patient's personal conception of the workings of his body or of his medical idiosyncrasies can be instrumental in evaluating the clinical picture. A patient with a spinal cord tumor had been hospitalized on two previous occasions for a complaint of pain radiating into the epigastrium. Because this patient experienced temporary relief of pain following enemas, he was thought to have gastrointestinal disease. It was not until he developed long-tract signs with weakness of both lower extremities that disease of the spinal cord was considered. Subsequent questioning revealed that the patient held to an "auto-intoxication" theory and believed that most body ills were related to chronic constipation.

The patient with a medical history of multiple surgical procedures, frequent hospitalizations, and short tryouts of a parade of physicians should increase the physician's caution in diagnosing organic disease. In a large number of pain problems the factor of litigation and secondary gain is present and must be evaluated as a possible motivating force. As a general rule, it is necessary to rest an organic diagnosis upon clear objective changes or on the conformity of the complaints to a known syndrome. Again, only a careful, and often time-consuming, history and examination by an unprejudiced observer will permit a true evaluation of the patient's complaints. Often the behavior of the patient is so bizarre that a firm opinion regarding the existence of any underlying pathologic change cannot be offered. In such instances it is generally wise not to initiate therapy that may cause permanent changes and to avoid an iatrogenic contribution to the clinical picture.

Management of Pain

OVERTREATMENT

The most important principle in the management of pain is avoidance of overtreatment. This pitfall is a great source of danger and often tests the physician's critical judgment. The aphorism, "Excess always carries its own retribution," is particularly relevant to the management of low back pain, for violation of this principle may have unfortunate results.

One unfortunate man is a monument in my memory to the hazards of overtreatment. This patient had originally complained of severe pain in the low back and lower extremity for which he was subjected to six myelograms and three lumbar laminectomies. Each successive diagnostic and surgical procedure served only to increase the original pain. The diagnosis of adhesive arachnoiditis of the cauda equina, secondary to the multiple myelograms and surgery, was made, and an alcohol block of several lumbar roots was performed to control nerve root pain. As a complication of this procedure the patient became paraplegic but continued to complain of his original pain. By this time, the patient was a confirmed narcotics addict. In an effort to control the addiction and to alleviate his pain, a prefrontal lobotomy was carried out. A craniotomy wound infection developed, necessitating removal of the entire frontal bone flap before healing could occur. This extensive bony defect involved the upper half of the forehead and resulted in a particularly unfortunate cosmetic result. The patient then developed severe crossed adductor spasms involving his lower extremities. These were a form of the "mass reflex" involving bladder and bowels, so often seen in paraplegia. Because these spasms prevented him from sitting in a wheelchair and in other ways interfered with his general nursing care, a decision was made to section all the lumbar and sacral nerve roots. It was at this stage, when I was a neurosurgery resident in 1950, that I first saw the patient and, in fact, performed this last operative procedure. After the massive rhizotomy, the mass reflex spasms improved but his original pain persisted.

This patient's history revealed that each ofhis operative procedures was performed by a different surgeon, with the exception of the first and third lumbar laminectomies. There is no question that these physicians were not only well-intentioned but also of outstanding professional competence. Obviously, each was convinced that the patient's symptoms were nonorganic after he had performed surgery and seen the results. Then another surgeon would be besieged until he was convinced that the patient "deserved another look." The phrase, "We must do something for this suffering patient," has often led to a result much worse than the original ailment.

TARGET FIXATION

In World War II, some of the bravest and most courageous young men this country has ever produced were selected for training as fighter pilots. When these fledglings engaged in their first few "dog fights," they sometimes so riveted their attention on the enemy that even after the object of their pursuit had been destroyed they were unable to collect themselves in time to veer from a midair collision; they sometimes followed close on the tail of their victim as he crashed into the ground. This phenomenon was called target fixation. With experience, pilots learned to maintain that important sense of objectivity even while in the heat of deadly combat, so that this catastrophe could be avoided.

In his desire to relieve suffering, no matter what the source, the physician sometimes develops a form of target fixation. He becomes enmeshed and entangled in the demands of the patient for relief of a symptom which is associated with an ever-increasing nonorganic component and eventually involves major psychologic dysfunction. This physician-patient entrapment may progress from drugs of increasing potency, through a variety of physiotherapeutic measures, and sometimes to surgery. If the physician is able to view the problem objectively, he is more apt to be of benefit; whereas if he manages such a problem improperly, he may only compound the progressive nature of the symptoms and cause additional suffering.

Placebos and the Placebo Effect

I was once called in consultation to see a low back pain problem and, upon asking about the efficacy of placebos, I was told by the attending physician that this type of deception was never practiced on his patients. The physician who made this statement was extremely able and conscientious, and because of his obvious sincerity and concern for the health of his patients, he enjoyed their trust and confidence to an unusually high degree. It is certain that whatever medications he prescribed, the results were frequently augmented by a placebo effect based on his splendid personality.

Viewed realistically, many types of treatment, other than the traditional capsule filled with lactose, can create the placebo effect, since it is based upon trust in the physician and faith in medicine generally. We have all seen patients whose intractable pain from malignant disease was temporarily relieved by an injection of sterile water. This is completely in accordance with our present understanding of psychosomatic medicine and the interrelationships of the mind and somatic illness. It has been shown that placebos can actually cause changes in laboratory data, such as the sedimentation rate, carbon dioxide combining power, and the white blood cell count. The faith of the prescribing physician in a drug may have a definite effect on its action.

DOUBLE-BLIND TEST

Knowledge of the placebo effect has led to the use of the double-blind method of testing drugs, in which the physician as well as the patient is unaware whether the drug being administered is a placebo or the medication being tested. Just as the best sales personnel are not necessarily the brightest people but those who are the most enthusiastic about the product, so the physician who actually believes in the curative properties of the drug may create a greater effect than the doctor who is uncertain about the merits of the medicine prescribed. In addition to drugs, physical measures including diathermy and massage create a positive psychologic effect which is sometimes the basis for the cures achieved by many healing cults.

Probably surgery has the most potent placebo effect that can be exercised in medicine. The detailed preliminaries, the rendering unconscious by anesthesia, and the removal or manipulation of vital organs within the body all create a profound and almost mystic emotional effect on the patient. This effect, of course, varies greatly from patient to patient. But in evaluating the results of any large series of surgical procedures, this placebo effect must certainly be considered. A well-known physician, an outstanding pioneer in the field of neurosurgery, when faced with a problem case of low back pain which he believed to be nonorganic in etiology, occasionally had the patient prepared and anesthetized for laminectomy and merely made the skin incision, which he then promptly sutured. Although several cases were reportedly "cured" by this method, I would guess that the long-term results were not uniformly happy.

MECHANISM OF ACTION

How can we explain the action of a placebo? The explanation most commonly accepted is that the patient's faith in the physician and in the medicine he prescribes is responsible for placebo action. Somewhat allied to this explanation is the staunch conviction that many patients entertain regarding the necessity for active treatment of their symptoms making the placebo a sort of required precondition of improvement.

Also responsible for many placebo effects noted in clinical medicine are the spontaneous remissions characteristic of most illnesses. Any drug given at an opportune time may coincide with symptomatic improvement which would have eventuated regardless of treatment; this improvement is attributed by both patient and physician to the medication. Such symptom fluctuations, implicit in the natural history of most disease states, emphasize the importance of evaluating a new drug not only with a placebo-receiving group but also with a separate control group receiving no treatment.

Most experienced clinicians are aware of the deliberately falsified response as a factor which must be considered in the evaluation of all drug effects including placebo effects. Reasons for such deliberate falsification vary, but they most often relate to the patient's desire to please the physician by giving the desired response.

"PLACEBO-REACTOR TYPE": FACT OR FANCY?

Are some patients likely to respond to placebos with consistency while others respond only to the pharmacologic actions of medications, or is reaction to placebos a factor potentially possessed by all, depending upon the particular environment and the personal predisposition present at the time the placebo is administered?

Considerable discussion has been directed toward this question and evidence has been cited both for and against the concept of a placebo-reactor type. The bulk of informed opinion at this time considers placebo reactivity a tendency that can be exhibited by anyone and is not a specific attribute possessed by some but not by others.

A USEFUL TOOL

In the early 1950s the double-blind method of assessing drugs became a mandatory step in routine testing procedure. The effort of devising such careful controls to eliminate the placebo effect created a somewhat negative or unfavorable connotation for placebos. This discreditable aura has been augmented by our medical training, which encourages therapy based on validly developed, updated scientific data.

Rather than ignore and disdain this potential source of comfort and well-being to our patients, it might be advisable to learn more about the placebo phenomenon so that we can utilize its effects appropriately. Since it is based on the patient's confidence and trust in the physician, the doctor-patient relationship must be given thought and consideration. Interactions expressing human concern and a cautiously hopeful outlook remain an essential aspect of medical care that is easily overlooked in this day of great scientific advances.

Secondary Loss and Secondary Gain

An adequate evaluation of any pain problem requires an understanding of the effect the pain is producing upon the patient's total lifestyle in terms of secondary loss as well as secondary gain. If the low back dysfunction prevents gainful employment, threatens the family's standard of living, or makes the patient dependent upon others, the usual response is depression and anxiety. When dealing with such secondary loss, the physician must be on the alert for denial of existing symptoms in the patient who is strongly motivated to recover.

Secondary gain factors may exist if the pain gratifies some deep seated need to suffer or to be dependent on and cared for by others; if financial gain is a consideration; or if the low back dysfunction removes the patient from a disliked job.

PROLONGATION OF SYMPTOMS AND SECONDARY GAIN

Prolongation of symptoms in the face of secondary gain is a fact acknowledged by all physicians. At one time, I believed that such prolongation of symptoms was entirely due to malingering, but in the past 20 years I have gradually reversed my opinion. When these patients have been observed surreptitiously, many of them continue to exhibit signs of low back dysfunction. I am convinced that a significant number of these patients have prolonged symptoms owing to psychological conditioning resulting from the secondary gain situation. Previously published statistics from the Crozer-Chester Medical Center Low Back Pain Clinic demonstrate this fact. The Center carried out an analysis of 623 patients with low back pain who were successfully treated by nonsurgical measures. Of this number, 324 patients without secondary gain averaged a total disability interval of 16 days for the specific episode. The 281 secondary gain patients averaged 36 days of total disability. These statistics, which refer only to the single episode of pain, do not take into account the recurrence rate, which presumably would be higher in the secondary gain cases. Seventy-two of 1000 surgically treated patients with herniated lumbar discs were classified as having had unsatisfactory results. This broke down to 657 nonsecondary gain patients, with 34 (or 5%) unsatisfactory results; and 343 secondary gain patients, with 38 (or 11%) unsatisfactory results.

The factors involved are complex and vary from case to case. In work-connected injuries where compensation is involved, all the underlying resentment of an employee toward the employer (company) may surface in the course of the illness. Particularly in large organizations, many workers tend to feel that their labors are undervalued and unappreciated. Any overtime or extra duties they have performed in the past may not have been sufficiently acknowledged.

Having incurred a physical injury in the course of their work, they may feel that the plant physician turns a deaf ear to their complaints and is unsympathetic to their suffering. The injury may have occurred as the result of someone else's carelessness or somewhat inadequate safety controls on the job site, and this further intensifies their resentment. The injury-producing job may be unpleasant or hazardous, and until the time of the accident the patient had no valid mechanism for reacting against it. Prolongation of symptoms provides the patient with an honorable and sociably acceptable retreat from a vexatious task, without scorn or criticism from either fellow workers or the family. He may attempt to utilize his symptoms to get work under less hazardous circumstances and more comfortable surroundings.

Although a significant percentage of compensation-related low back patients consciously prolong their symptoms for self-serving purposes, a greater proportion are unaware of the psychological mechanisms associated with their persistent symptoms. Confronted with such a schema, most patients would react with genuine astonishment and indignation. Explanations of this nature only tend to increase patient resentment and exasperation over their plight and also to increase their feeling of abandonment. Rather than pursuing this elucidative approach, a generous "lump sum" early settlement may be more effective in terminating the undue prolongation of symptoms. From an industrial compensation point of view, an early settlement of this nature might well be less costly.

A similar secondary gain situation associated with prolongation of symptoms is seen with low back problems which result from vehicular accidents. An interminable legal contest often results with the defense hard at work minimizing and deprecating the symptoms, and the plaintiff-patient repeatedly documenting a persisting disability. Such prolonged legal sparring, which often involves an attack on the patient's validity, may serve to create a more firmly fixed symptom complex than would occur in a nonadversary situation. Those states in which the so-called no fault vehicular insurance plans are in operation have reduced the number of cases brought to adversary proceedings and have demonstrated a significant reduction in duration of symptoms.

Nonorganic Backache

Apocryphal Diagnosis

A large percentage of patients complaining of low back pain have symptoms which are recognized as nonorganic or functional, but for a number of reasons the physician is hesitant to label the patient with such a diagnosis. In off-the-record conversations, most doctors will readily admit the frequency of this type of symptom in their practice but shy away from imparting their clinical impressions to the patient. It would be enlightening to examine the reasons for the reticence of physicians on this subject.

1. Often both patient and family will not readily accept a diagnosis of nonorganic disease. Frequently, when such a diagnosis is proposed, the patient does not return and will seek medical opinion and aid elsewhere.

2. When a diagnosis of nonorganic low back pain is submitted, under the present insurance system the cost of evaluating and managing the problem may not be completely underwritten. When an incident occurring during work was the alleged cause of low back symptoms, the workman's compensation carrier may attempt to avoid payment of the hospital and doctor bills. When industrial compensation is not a factor, many hospitalization insurance plans may object to accepting the cost of hospitalization with a final diagnosis of functional low back pain.

3. In medicolegal problems, mention of nonorganic symptoms is anathema to the patient's attorney, since this will weaken his bargaining position at settlement or in court.

4. Most doctors are concerned about er-

roneously considering the patient's complaint as nonorganic in the presence of organic disease. An obviously neurotic patient can also be organically ill, and in many instances it is difficult to separate the organic from the nonorganic.

Proper patient management of a suspected nonorganic backache demands a thorough and, in some instances, an exhaustive evaluation. Every experienced physician is able to recall a number of patients initially identified as neurotics who turned out to have hidden organic disease causing their symptoms. Before committing a patient to a diagnosis of functional illness, every effort is made to uncover organic disease. In most cases, hospitalization for some portion of this investigation is necessary.

Hypochondriac and Malingerer

It is usually possible to identify the hypochondriac or malingerer with a nonorganic low back syndrome. Sometimes the zone of demarcation between these separate entities is indistinct and preplexing, but there are distinguishing features which may be helpful in attempting to establish a working differential diagnosis.

HYPOCHONDRIAC

These persons are often intelligent and may be subjected to considerable tension at work and in their home life as well. They may be involved in high pressure work that requires unusual abilities, and can be successful in their occupational endeavors.

The history of most hypochondriacs is distinctive. They have usually seen many physicians in the past and have a tendency to be rather critical of each one in turn. They will discuss their previous physician's deficiencies at some length without much urging.

Previous hospitalizations have been necessary for a variety of complaints, often for symptoms involving different anatomical systems, the three most common being gastrointestinal, cardiac or chest, and musculoskeletal. Objective findings are rare, and results of tests and studies performed during previous hospitalizations and on an outpatient basis are nonrevealing or inconclusive.

As symptoms from one system clear, symptoms from a new system will appear after a short period of time.

Each doctor they have seen, in turn, will prescribe a new medication and none of these seems to be particularly helpful. They are familiar with the names of the medications and are aware of their action, "Oh yes, I have tried Butazolidin alka." "No, the Valium was not helpful." They are not unhappy to be hospitalized, and gladly undergo all sorts of tests and studies and are eager to try out all varieties of treatment. The latest ultrasonic or fancy new diathermy machine will be eagerly used and may have some short-term beneficial effect. Occasionally, the patient may buy his own diathermy machine.

In many cases, the spouse, either husband or wife, enters completely into the spirit of the exercise and is just as conversant with the symptoms as the patient. During the taking of the history, they will sit eagerly by the side of the patients and prompt them, interject with a forgotten symptom, correct them on dates, and, in general, take an active role. One such husband of a hypochondriac wife, who was not particularly wealthy, fitted out his entire basement with a variety of mechanical devices, including a diathermy machine and a traction apparatus, so that it resembled the physiotherpy department of a small hospital.

In addition to backache, the hypochondriac usually manifests symptoms of irritability and nervousness, such as excessive perspiration or tremor of the hands. A telephone ring or an intercom buzzer may produce a striking startled reaction.

Other illustrative symptoms are the tension type of headache with a sensation of "a tight band around my head," "difficulty swallowing," a "constant lump in my throat." There may be voice changes with inability to speak above a whisper. Gastrointestinal symptoms are common and may be categorized as an "irritable colon" or "spastic colitis." Insomnia is a frequent complaint as is shortness of breath, and any or all of these may be aggravated by increased intensity of the backache.

Some of these patients have had a number of surgical procedures carried out for indications which were less than classical. They may be willing to submit to surgery, and this may alleviate their symptoms for several months.

MALINGERER

This condition is not possible without involvement of secondary gain in some form. Secondary gain does not necessarily have to be financial. It may involve changes in work status. These commonly include less physically strenuous work and in the case of salesmen, jobs that involve less traveling. This could also include less hazardous work such as for a police officer, an inside job rather than patroling a "beat." Sometimes these changes may be so subtle and may seem so unimportant to the physician that he may not be aware that he is dealing with a secondary gain situation. I recall such a patient who complained of back pain, which was not particularly severe and did not prevent him from working. I was not able to "cure" this patient until the third visit, when it was revealed to me that he was acutely concerned with his car parking privileges. He had developed an emotional need to park in a small parking lot close to the factory which was reserved for higher ranking personnel, and not in the larger parking lot for the rest of the employees which was a greater distance away. After he was satisfied that he could continue to park his car in the closer lot, his symptoms improved to the point where I did not have to see him again. There is no specific type of personality or character makeup that relates to this syndrome.

There is no relationship whatsoever between the severity of the injury and the intensity or duration of symptoms. I recall a middle-aged secretary who was struck in the midlumbar region by a gum eraser tossed playfully by a young secretary who meant to hit another young office worker. The intended victim had ducked, causing this small missle to strike my patient. The prolonged duration and intensity of her symptoms prevented her from returning to work for five months and were probably nurtured, in part, by the unconscious resentment and hostility she had for her prankish younger fellow workers.

The symptoms, as a rule, are somewhat vague and usually variable, changing from time to time. It is wise to document the symptoms carefully and in the patient's own words as much as possible. Several weeks later the symptoms may be quite different, and oftentimes the patient denies having stated what was recorded in the first session.

The characteristics of the low back pain may be unusual in several respects. That improvement came with bed rest or inactivity is denied, which is somewhat unusual since most backaches do improve with rest and inactivity. The area of pain is often nonphysiologic, and complaints will be heard of pain that runs "from the bottom of my spine up to the top of my neck," or that radiates forward through the umbilicus or extends into the inguinal areas causing severe genital discomfort. If the pain extends into the lower extremities, the patient is very vague when attempting to point out the exact course or distribution of the pain as it radiates down the leg. Most patients with valid root compression syndromes are quite specific about the course of their pain; if the physician acts as though he did not understand and points to the lateral aspect of the thigh when the patient had indicated the pain coursing down the posterior thigh, and states, "You mean it hurts here?" the patient with organic pain will almost always correct the physician. The malingerer is more likely to accept the different site suggested by the physician with the thought that perhaps this is the spot that "should be hurting." If you ask, "Which leg hurts?" the answer may be vague and all-encompassing with generalized bilateral leg pain. Their description of the pain may be unusual, and terms such as "like a shock of electricity" or "sharp, like a knife" are often heard.

A differentiating characteristic between malingering and hypochondria is that the malingerer tends to emphasize symptoms related to the injured area and is not as likely to press what are thought to be irrelevant symptoms.

The malingerer in a work-connected accident is often reticent to resume the job at which the accident occurred; this may be realistic, particularly if it was a somewhat hazardous occupation. A frequent source of symptom prolongation is a valid concern over being fired if he goes back to work. In the meantime, he has a "sure thing," with his compensation check coming in every week. If layoffs are occurring and his job seniority is such that he is afraid of being laid off, he may continue to see the physician when his symptoms subside and he is pronounced fit to go back to work. The physician then will experience some difficulty in curing him.

A serious sign, and possibly the onset of a pattern that may be difficult to deal with, occurs when a man's wife who has never previously worked outside the home takes a job to supplement the loss of income caused by his disability. She may make a fairly good salary, and he may get used to doing a little housework. When his disability check is combined with her pay, this gives them a fairly adequate income and may leave a lot of time for fishing, "visiting the boys at the volunteer firehouse," and other such activities. After a time his friends may get used to his carrying on various time-consuming nonpaying duties in civic and social organizations, and an irrevocable way of life has become established.

Oftentimes, the malinger has been given a low back support, which he claims to need

very desperately and which he has supposedly been wearing constantly for the past year. Yet, if this appliance is closely examined, relatively little wear may be noted.

Physical examination of a malingerer claiming low back pain is often helpful and revealing.

Gait changes may be significant. Prior to the formal examination, the patient may walk into the office without noticeable dysfunction, but when asked to walk during the examination, an obvious and striking abnormality may develop.

Inspection of the lumbar spine may reveal a **relaxed lumbar lordosis,** whereas in the presence of persistent low back pain one would expect some paraspinal muscle spasm with flattening of the normal lumbar curvature. Minimal stimuli, such as light pressure over the lumbar musculature, will cause **intense discomfort,** and trifling, inconsequential touches may cause some patients to jump with pain. The patient will often be **unable to bend** more than 5 degrees forward, despite the absence of paraspinal muscle spasm to digital palpation. (In the absence of muscle spasm, patients with practically complete lumbar fusions can bend forward to the point where they may touch their toes, since considerable rotation at the hips is possible despite almost total lack of mobility of the lumbar spine.) **Tenderness** to pressure may be elicited **over the sacrum,** rarely a tender site unless there is an underlying sacral malignancy or cyst. Sacroiliac compression may be very painful. **Straight leg raising** may be limited while lying supine on the table. If this is noted, one should attempt the same maneuver with the patient seated. In the seated position, 90 degrees elevation may be painlessly achieved. If straight leg raising is painful, the physician should first flex the knee and then the hip. If 90 degree hip flexion causes the same degree of pain with the knee flexed, sciatic radiation is eliminated, and the pain is explainable either by hip disease or nonorganic symptoms. In performing voluntary straight leg raising, the development of tremors or "spastic jerking" of the elevated leg is usually indicative of functional disease.

Sensory changes are often very helpful in evaluation of functional backache. A frequently encountered form of nonorganic sensory change in the lower extremity is the **stocking type of hypesthesia.**

Testing of motor strength is often quite revealing. Lower extremity weakness of long-standing duration is invariably associated with some objective evidence of atrophy or loss of muscle tone. When testing some muscle strength, if the patient is resisting against the opposing arm or finger of the physician, a quick unexpected release of opposing pressure will cause even a weakened muscle to rebound immediately. If the patient is not resisting with full strength, the tested member will not rebound.

Complaints of a weak, tender, numb leg in the face of **normal reflexes and no atrophy** or loss of muscle tone are of questionable organic significance.

Bizarre reactions to drugs may be seen in both malingers and hypochondriacs. They may be tranquilized by stimulants or vice versa. Both may also have unhappy reactions to injection therapy, "I was pretty good until you stuck those needles in my back, and now I can't even get out of bed."

Both male malingerers and hypochondriacs are likely to complain of **sexual dysfunction.** Normal sexual functions "have been impossible since that accident, doctor."

Management

It must be recognized that the management of this type of patient often requires more time and thought than of one with average organic low back problem. I believe it is helpful in every regard to get these patients back to work as soon as possible. Return to a work program and resumption of the normal activities of daily living is often associated with improvement, both physically and mentally. Intractable problems of functional low back pain may require psychiatric guidance.

INSIGHT

Physicians seem to have little difficulty in perceiving the lack of insight manifested by their psychologically skewed low back pain patients, but they may be less perspicacious in gauging their own presumptions and biases. Most of us who are involved in the management of low back pain soon learn to identify the several most common syndromes causing back pain. It doesn't take long to develop an effective treatment program to deal with each of these conditions. Our skill in identifying and alleviating the pain caused by these organic syndromes is usually rewarded by the esteem and approbation of our patients. It follows that we like to see a patient who presents a clearly definable organic syndrome that is likely to respond to treatment. We may be understandably reluctant to see a low back patient with a nonorganic syndrome. This patient is much less likely to respond to treatment, and we are likely to incur reproach rather than esteem, despite our best efforts. Some physicians may develop an actual animosity toward this type of patient. Those who have the self-awareness to recognize this aversion will realize that they are not suitable physicians for nonorganic problems. Since a significant portion of low back pain patients do present with a varying degree of nonorganic factors, a physician who is in this field has two choices. He can find some acceptable method of treating the organic problems and shunting the nonorganic ones out of his practice, or he can prepare himself for recurrent frustrating and fretful intervals in his existence.

USEFUL MANAGEMENT REMINDERS

Psychogenic Backache.

1. The doctor should bear in mind that, from the patient's point of view, there is no such thing as a psychogenic backache. Patients are completely satisfied that the longstanding pain which brings them to your

office was caused by "that accident," and they take for granted that you will support them in their belief.

2. The physician should appreciate the judgmental nature of the word psychogenic: "You mean I'm a fake," or "You think I'm just imagining this pain."

3. One should avoid a blunt confrontation. "You are a neurotic," is almost never helpful.

4. During a discussion describing how emotions may influence low back symptoms, it is important not to become upset or rankled when you see an expression of incredulity on your patient's face.

Compensation.

1. Our present workmen's compensation system does augment pain, and many patients are forced to utilize this augmented pain to solve their needs. They often have no practical alternative.

2. An explanation of how the psychological mechanisms involved in a secondary gain situation prolong symptoms, or a discussion of the statistics demonstrating the increased duration of symptoms with secondary gain, will almost invariably be considered by patients as somewhat irrelevant to their specific problem. They will expect you to recognize that "these facts and numbers are interesting, but this case is different."

3. Defining an existing secondary gain situation is advisable, but clearly expressing a judgment that the secondary gain is the primary cause of pain prolongation is not usually helpful.

4. In dealing with a compensation problem, under certain circumstances accommodation and not necessarily cure may be the proper goal. For example, if lighter work with less pay is available, some sort of settlement, with the establishment of a partial disability, may be the appropriate treatment.

5. An integral part of the rehabilitation effort involves some mechanism permitting vindication of patients' behavior so they can believe in themselves when they return to work. This vindication can occur in a variety of forms and include biofeedback, hypnosis, acupuncture, nerve blocks, electrical stimulation, drugs, placebos, PT, traction, hospitalization, and occupational therapy. The primary concern is to avoid an irreversible and potentially destructive form of therapy such as unwarranted surgery.

Malingering.

1. Accurate detective work on malingering is brutal. Malingering is always very difficult to prove or disprove, probably because very few malingerers are totally without either some nidus of pain or some fear of pain recurrence. In addition, some have an element of conversion hysteria while others present sociopathic manifestations. Since very few things in medicine are absolute, we can expect to find very few absolutely pure malingerers.

2. If a physician arrives at the conclusion that the patient is a malingerer, no benefit, to either patient or physicain, is gained by continued treatment. If he is in error, the patient is better served by a different physician who may bring a more positive approach to therapy. If the physician's opinion is valid, continued therapy is a sham.

Limitations of Management. It is helpful to recognize certain situations in which we as physicians are not likely to provide an adequate solution.

1. Financial impoverishment, where the patient anticipates a continued existence based on his income before he developed low back dysfunction. He is unable and unwilling to alter his lifestyle in accordance with his limited physical condition and reduced earning capacity. In the patient's struggle to regain what he considers his due and rightful financial level he may find it necessary to employ a variety of legal, workmen's-compansation, and insurance maneuvers. The physician who by his nature is inclined to

support his patient in all aspects of his health care must guard against the tendency to assume so partisan a role that his medical reports and statements exceed the bounds of truth and reason.

2. Primary personality dysfunction, when the "problem" of low back pain is really the solution. The existence of such a mechanism is apparent in the addicted patient or certain types of passive dependent or passive aggressive patients.

3. The medicolegal problem, in which the patient comes to a physician under the guise of treatment. The prime intent of the patient, however, is to establish the reality of the pain and document the level of disability. This may present a complex management situation with a number of obvious difficulties.

Psychiatry. The role of psychiatry and psychology in the active treatment of this problem is not clearly established. Unless the psychiatrist has a special interest in pain problems or is involved in a pain clinic utilizing a team approach, his efforts are likely to be disappointing. Often the patient who is referred to a psychiatrist will have several sessions. Then they seem to lose faith in each other. The psychiatrist may find the patient naïve in not wanting to deal with insights and the patient may not want to acknowledge them since they mean accepting a negative self-judgment. The patient may solve this dilemma by avoiding it, stating, "I am not worried about being nervous. I just want my back to feel better."

Psychological Tests. A variety of psychological tests are available which deal primarily with interpersonal, social, and vocational areas. Only a few tests have a significant amount of item content dealing with physical concerns. The Minnesota Multiphasic Personality Inventory (MMPI) is by far the most commonly used test delineating the psychological involvement in various medical syndromes.

The first three scales of the MMPI are most specifically helpful in relating to medical problems. The first scale is identified as **Hypochondriasis** and is based on a series of patients having multiple somatic complaints without a sufficient organic basis. The item content of this scale relates almost entirely to preoccupation with one's physical health. The second scale is called **Depression** and this scale is essentially a depressed mood scale. The third scale is called **Hysteria** and in the original criteria group used in the development of the MMPI, the predominant symptom was that of pain lacking a sufficient organic basis. These three scales, when charted, can assume various meaningful patterns and configurations. For example, many psychiatric patients have a particularly high depression score creating an sort of mountain peak effect in comparison with the lower hypochondriasis and hysteria scales on either side.

Another significant pattern is the so-called hypochondriasis–hysteria V (or valley). In this syndrome the first and third scales, which are somatically oriented, are quite elevated, and the second (depression) scale is fairly low. This particular configuration is predictive of a poor response to any medical treatment including surgical intervention. This conforms to the classic psychological pattern of the patient manifesting "la belle indifference" (lack of appropriate distress) in the face of severe complaints. Services providing MMPI computer printout narrative reports are available and are certainly the least costly method of this type of screening. However, clinicians who find this study most helpful work in close conjunction with a pain-oriented psychologist.

Psychological Problems and Surgery. The patient who has positive surgical indications in association with evidence of a psychological disorder is a difficult problem. Theoretically, the ideal solution is to refer the patient for psychiatric or psychological counseling and to operate after clearance from a specialist. Such a decision requires deep reflection to avoid converting a difficult problem into an impossible one.

A Reminder. One may occasionally feel deficient in the assessment and management of a nonorganic low back pain syndrome. At these times, allow the history of medicine to raise your flagging spirits. Until the 19th century the physician had very little to offer in the way of organic treatment, and the benefits he brought to his patient were largely personal. Despite this lack, the physician has somehow managed to retain his respected position throughout the ages.

References

1. Peters J, Benjamin FB, Helvey WM, Albright GA: Study of sensory deprivation, pain and personality relationships for space travel. Aerosp Med 34:830, 1963
2. Ryan ED, Kovacic CR: Pain tolerance and athletic participation. Percep Mot Skills 22:383, 1966
3. Sternbach RA, Tursky B: Ethnic differences among housewives in psychophysical and skin potential responses to electric shock. Psychophysiology 1:243, 1965

Conservative Treatment 6

PART I

Nonsurgical Management of Low Back Pain and Sciatica

Certain basic principles can be applied to the conservative management of most lumbar-sciatic syndromes. An understanding of these principles and the mechanisms by which they provide symptomatic relief is essential to proper treatment.

Rest

Limited Activity Program

Patients who have low back discomfort from almost any cause will instinctively attempt to avoid activity and will rest. The method and extent of rest largely depends upon the severity and nature of the symptoms. Patients suffering from mild low back discomfort may be well served by a limited activity program, which prohibits heavy lifting, prolonged forward bending, excessive stooping, or long auto trips. Activity can be further reduced by eliminating prolonged standing, extensive walking and frequent stair climbing. When climbing stairs is unavoidable, the patient is instructed to "baby walk" the stairs by placing both feet on the same step before advancing to the next. If such a limited activity program does not provide adequate relief of symptoms, bed rest must be considered.

Mattress

A firm mattress is most important for rest of the patient which low back symptoms. Some physicians strongly advocate a mattress with no springs, consisting of hair stuffing, firm kapok, or foam rubber padding. There seems to be no significant clinical advantage resulting from the use of any of these special mattresses other than reasonable firmness. If the mattress does sag when supporting the weight of a body, boards in the form of either individual slats or three-quarter inch plywood between the mattress and the box spring are helpful.

Bed Rest

Whether bed rest is to be carried out at home or in the hospital may be the patient's choice. The flat supine position maintains the lumbar lordosis and is less effective in affording symptomatic relief than is a position of slight lumbar flexion (Fig. 6-1). This flexion can be achieved if the hospital bed is adjusted to a 30 degree elevation of the

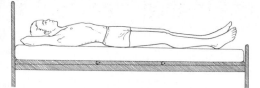

Fig. 6-1. Bed rest in the flat supine position maintains the lumbar lordosis.

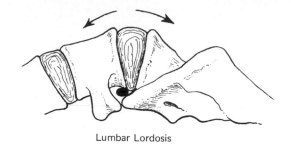

Lumbar Lordosis

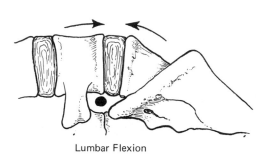

Lumbar Flexion

Fig. 6-3. Altered relationship of annulus, nerve root, and intervertebral foramina in lumbar lordosis and lumbar flexion.

head and slight flexion of the knee break (Figs. 6-2 and 6-3). The elevated head allows the patient to read, watch TV, and greet visitors, making bed confinement more tolerable. The position can be varied by assuming the modified supine position with elevation of the legs above the head or a side lying position, keeping the hips and knees flexed (Figs. 6-4 and 6-5). The modern electrical hospital bed has a great advantage in allowing the patient to change the bed configuration without leaving the bed, reducing the need for outside help.

Meals are served to the patient and bed rest is strictly enforced, with the exception of toilet privileges. The use of a bedpan produces at least the same, if not a greater, degree of mechanical stress upon the lumbar spine as allowing the patient to go to the bathroom once or twice daily, and the patient is invariably more satisfied with this arrangement. If a toilet is not reasonably close to the bed, the use of a bedside commode may be helpful.

Many patients prefer to be treated at home, and yet, strict bed rest is less likely to be adhered to in a home situation. Most patients who are not observed tend to get out of bed for a variety of reasons, such as

answering the doorbell, taking care of children, or general restlessness. The more controlled hospital environment, with meals served at the bed, the use of an electric bed, and the usually firmer mattress are all more conducive to symptomatic improvement. If the patient does elect to be treated with bed rest at home, an electric hospital bed should be rented.

In prescribing prolonged bed rest it must be recognized that as a result of lack of activity and muscle disuse a certain degree of muscle atrophy will occur. In addition, there may be loss of calcium from the bones, loss of protein, and certain circulatory changes which may give rise to light-headedness and (in some cases) syncope once the erect position is resumed. An appreciation

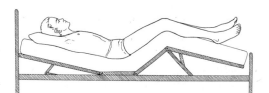

Fig. 6-2. Adjustment of the hospital bed to provide a position of slight lumbar flexion is helpful in affording symptomatic relief.

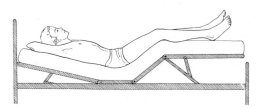

Fig. 6-4. Modified supine position.

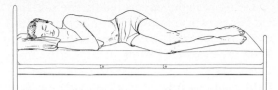

Fig. 6-5. Lateral position, with hips and knees flexed.

of these adverse effects of prolonged bed rest will allow the physician to estimate properly the total period of management. After pain relief has been achieved, the patient may require a period of strengthening activities, including exercises and gradually progressive mobilization procedures, before returning to a normal existence. In addition to repairing the adverse effects of prolonged bed rest, some of these measures are important in preventing recurrence of the original symptoms.

It may be necessary to stage the mobilization to the point where total bed rest is reduced to several hours daily in addition to the usual night-time rest. When the patient is out of bed, a low back support may be necessary. If this program is successful, progressive mobilization can continue until the patient is no longer at bed rest except during hours of sleep.

Traction

Traction is a time-honored procedure, having been used in the conservative manage-

ment of low back dysfunction for more than 50 years. The earlier forms, such as Buck's or Russel's traction, employed the pull directly upon the lower extremities. The most popular form of traction for low back dysfunction at this time is pelvic traction, which employs a snug canvas girdle encircling the pelvis and hips, with traction straps leading from this girdle to weights hung at the foot of the bed.

The benefits of traction were originally attributed to a distraction or separation of the vertebrae, permitting a protruding disc to "slip back into place." It is contrary to all reasonable expectation that leg traction, which must transmit a force through the knee and hip joints before involving the lumbar intervertebral joints, should be effective (Fig. 6-6). Pelvic traction, when utilized on the patient maintained in the flat supine position, requires a tremendous weight (40 to 70 pounds) to produce separation of the vertebrae (Fig. 6-7).

When traction is employed on a patient in slight lumbar flexion, it can be adjusted to exert a lever action on the spine to promote further lumbar flexion (Figs. 6-8 and 6-9). Theoretically, the increased mechanical effect of leverage will distract the posterior elements of the vertebral column, reducing compression upon the posterior portion of the annulus fibrosis and increasing the aperture of the intervertebral foramina.

In addition to the possible mechanical benefits, pelvic traction, which the patient can apply and remove at will, may alleviate

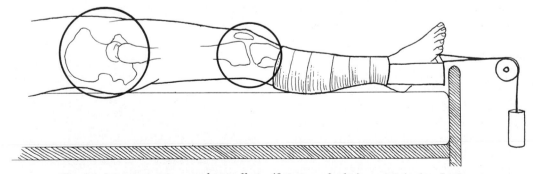

Fig. 6-6. Leg traction is a mechanically inefficient method of traction for low back pain, since the traction force must be transmitted through the knee and hip joints before affecting the low back.

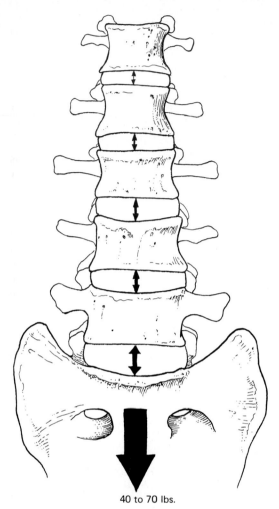

Fig. 6-7. In the flat supine position, a load of 40 to 70 lbs is necessary to produce distraction of the lumbar intervertebral joints. Traction effect upon the intervertebral discs progressively diminishes in a cephalad direction.

the monotony of enforced bed rest and be of some psychological advantage in imparting to the patient a sense of active therapy. If confined to bed without traction, the complaint, "Nothing is being done for me," is frequently voiced. Pelvic traction using 15 to 30 pounds allows the patient to move the lower extremities and also to turn freely from side to side while in bed, so that there is no additional risk of thrombophlebitis. Any form of traction employing the pull directly upon the lower extremities does increase the risk of thrombophlebitis.

Setting placebo effects aside, the mechanical benefits of traction are conjectural. However, an unbeatable combination of patient demand, hospitalization insurance requirements for "active conservative management," and acquiescent physicians has kept this form of therapy in high usage.

Trigger Points

Patients with long-standing chronic and recurrent muscle pain develop tender, tense areas in the painful muscles. These tender sites occasionally can be palpated as nodules, the exact nature of which is speculative. Some investigators have reported microscopic changes including increased fibrous tissue, waxy degeneration of muscle fibers, destruction of fibrils, and increase in number of nuclei of muscle fibers and fatty infiltration. To refute the claims by some that these nodules are essentially areas of localized muscle spasm, some investigators report that the nodules do not change even when the patient is under general anesthesia and, in fact, remain unchanged after death. Somewhat similar local hardened areas are produced in animal experimentation by tetanic stimulation of the leg of a rabbit and by local freezing of animal muscles.

The existence of areas of tender nodules is generally accepted, but most investigators have been unable to confirm the histologic changes in these areas. Whatever the exact nature of these lesions, it seems certain that they constitute a clinical entity character-

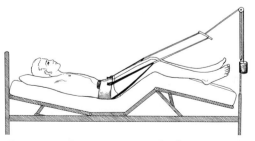

Fig. 6-8. Pelvic traction with the patient in moderate lumbar flexion.

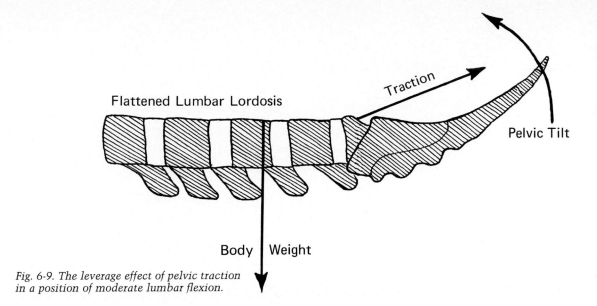

Flattened Lumbar Lordosis

Traction

Pelvic Tilt

Body Weight

Fig. 6-9. The leverage effect of pelvic traction in a position of moderate lumbar flexion.

ized by the presence of painful, tender areas situated either in the muscle belly or at the ligamentous attachment of the muscle. Exposure to cold and exertion are factors in producing these lesions, and emotional tension seems to augment their formation. In palpating the relaxed muscles of the low back, one can often feel small hard nodules which, when pressed upon, will produce either local or radiating pain. Occasionally, ultrasound current over these areas may produce localized pain and will help identify these trigger points, although the examiner's experienced hand is more reliable. They are found often in the sacrospinal muscles from the lower thoracic region to the sacrum. Ligamentous trigger points are sometimes palpated at the spinous processes of the lumbar spine, the sacroiliac joint, iliac crest, and greater trochanter.

Although a number of nodules may be palpated in examining the muscles of the low back, they should not be considered true trigger points if pressure upon them does not produce pain; injection of these sites is not indicated.

To inject these trigger point nodules approximately 10 cc of Xylocaine is used and one can sometimes feel an increased resistance when the needle enters the nodule. If after injection of one or two trigger points the patient appreciates significant relief of pain, it may be helpful to repeat the injection two or three times.

PART II

Modalities in the Treatment of Acute and Chronic Low Back Pain

ROBERT H. CONDON

Physical medicine and rehabilitation are an important part of the treatment of the patient with low back pain. The treatment program generally involves the use of therapeutic heat, cold, and exercise. The modalities most commonly used to provide therapeutic cold and heat include ice, infrared radiant heat, hydrocollator packs, whirlpool, and ultrasound. All of these have in common the capability of reducing pain and muscle spasm and thereby increasing patient mobility. The transcutaneous nerve stimulator is also quite effective in short-term use for increasing patient mobility, owing to its very portable nature. A strengthening program follows when pain and spasm have been controlled. All treatment programs have a significant placebo effect, and it is important to use this to the best advantage of the patient. More specifically, prior to the initiation of any modality program, it should be discussed with the patient especially as to its beneficial effects. Also utilize the patient's impressions as to what modalities have been effective in the past. There are specific contraindications for each of the modalities which will be discussed later, but in general it is important to keep in mind

the possible need for more definitive treatment when a malignancy exists or when the patient fails to improve with a neurological deficit.

Acute Low Back Pain

Acute low back pain will be defined as present less than 3 days. It may be confined to the low back region or in addition involve a radicular component.

Therapeutic Cold

Therapeutic cold is most effective in acute low back pain. Physiologic cooling is associated with a decrease in the tissue metabolic rate and a vasoconstriction of the arterial system. The vasoconstriction leads to an effect that penetrates tissues deeper than does heat. Anesthesia is produced, probably in relation to nerve fiber block secondary to cold. While therapeutic cold is especially helpful in reducing pain, swelling, and muscle spasm related to the acute phase, there are several contraindications which must be kept in mind. First, anyone with hypersensitivity to cold such as seen in Raynaud's phenomenon is best not treated with cold. Secondly, patients with rheumatoid arthritis often tolerate cold poorly; however, in these cases a therapeutic trial might be indicated, as some patients do respond well. Thirdly, a significant increase in systolic blood pressure might be seen, but this is most common when cooling is more generalized. Finally, the skin must be observed closely so that excessive cooling does not result in tissue damage. There are several methods of therapeutic cooling including immersion, cold packs, fluromethane spray, and ice massage. The last, in general, is most effective and is accomplished by using an ice stick. This can be made simply by placing a tongue blade into a paper cup filled with water and putting it into the freezer until the ice is solid (Fig. 6-10). The paper cup is then removed from the ice, and the tongue blade serves as a handle in applying the ice to the patient (Fig. 6-11). The **ice massage** is performed over the affected area for 10 to 12 minutes. In approximately 3 to 4 minutes the patient usually experiences a burning sensation. It is important to continue past this to obtain significant relief of pain and muscle spasm. If the patient cannot tolerate this, it may be helpful to treat the patient initially with a cold pack for 10 to 15 minutes and then apply the ice massage. The cold pack is not placed in direct contact with the skin but wrapped in a moist towel. The duration of relief from pain and spasm is significantly longer with cold than with superficial heat. However, some patients do not tolerate therapeutic cold and, therefore, superficial heat is indicated.

Superficial Heat

Superficial heat is effective in the treatment of low back problems because of its analgesic effect. It also, however, produces a vasodilatation which can promote swelling. In the patient with acute low back pain

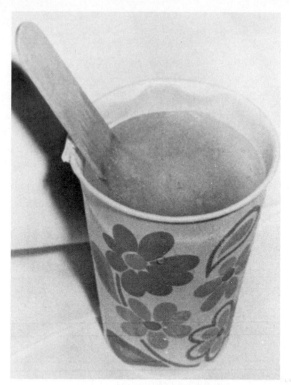

Fig. 6-10. Ice stick made in paper cup.

secondary to trauma who may have tissue disruption, this tendency to produce swelling contraindicates its use. Other contraindications to superficial heating include impaired circulation as with scar tissue. In this case, the blood supply is not adequate to dissipate the heat being applied, and a burn may result. In any patient with decreased sensation the administration of heat must be monitored very closely. The three most common methods for utilizing superficial heat include hydrocollator packs, infrared or radiant heating, and whirlpool. A **hydrocollator pack** is a method of conductive heating (Fig. 6-12). It is wrapped in towels to prevent excessive heating and placed on the affected back area for 30 minutes with the patient prone (Fig. 6-13). Again, the patient must be watched closely for any signs of thermal injury. **Infrared heating,** unlike the hydrocollator pack, enables the therapist to observe the area being treated. An incandescent bulb with a reflector is an effective means of providing this modality.

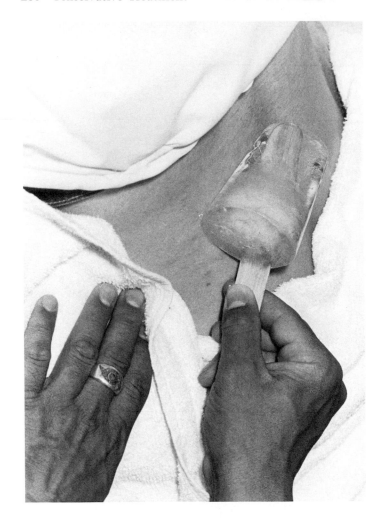

Fig. 6-11. Use of ice stick in ice massage.

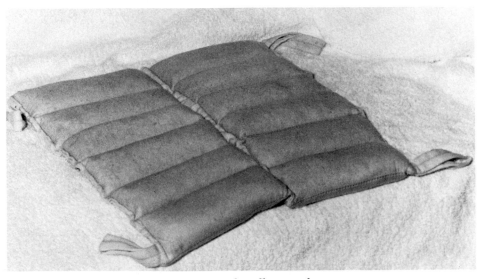

Fig. 6-12. Hydrocollator pack.

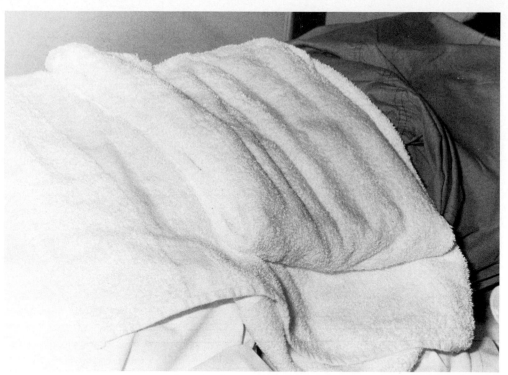

Fig. 6-13. Hydrocollator pack with towel wrapping applied to patient in prone position.

The intensity of the heat is controlled by the wattage of the bulb and the distance from the skin. Again, close observation is necessary; an average treatment time is 30 minutes. The **whirlpool bath** is a method of convective heating. It is not an efficient way of treating low back pain, since it either requires a patient with impaired mobility to climb into a small tank or ties up an entire Hubbard tank. Also, the patient's cardiovascular status must be carefully assessed as core temperature is raised upon immersion in water above body temperature. Gentle kneading massage may be used to supplement either the heat or the cold in relief of muscle spasm.

Ultrasound is a method of providing heat to deeper tissues. It is generally not indicated in the acute phase, owing to the tendency of heat to produce swelling. It will be considered in more detail in the discussion of chronic low back pain. Also rare in the acute phase is the use of transcutaneous electrical nerve stimulation, as bed rest generally pro-

vides adequate pain relief. This, therefore, will also be discussed when considering the more chronic phase of low back pain.

In summary, then, ice is generally the most effective treatment for the patient with acute low back pain. Superficial heat is used when the patient cannot tolerate cold.

Chronic Low Back Pain

Chronic low back pain can be defined as that which is present for more than 3 days. It may or may not have a radicular component. Icing, which was useful in the acute stage, may be effective in the chronic phase as well, especially when muscle spasm is prominent. Superficial heat is also helpful in this phase and may facilitate breaking the pain spasm cycle. As previously mentioned, both can be complemented with the use of a gentle, deep kneading massage.

Ultrasound

Several deep heating modalities are available for chronic low back pain, including shortwave and microwave diathermy and ultrasound. Shortwave and microwave diathermy generally heat the subcutaneous tissues and the more superficial musculature. The more commonly used therapy is ultrasound, which produces a high frequency vibration and heats primarily the deeper musculature and the bone and joint tissues. Absorption is directly related to the protein content of the tissue. Ultrasound is applied by moving the applicator head back and forth in short strokes in a coupling medium covering the skin (Fig. 6-14). It is important to monitor the temperature of both the coupling medium and the skin. To avoid high skin or applicator temperatures, ultrasound should be used prior to application of hot packs, and the applicator should be dipped in cool tap water for a minute after each field of application. Therapeutic intensities range from one to four watts per centimeter squared, with the most commonly used intensities being 1.5 to 2 watts per centimeter squared. Pain due to periosteal irritation can be used as an indication of excessive temperature and the need to lower the intensity. The treatment should be applied to any given area for 7 to 10

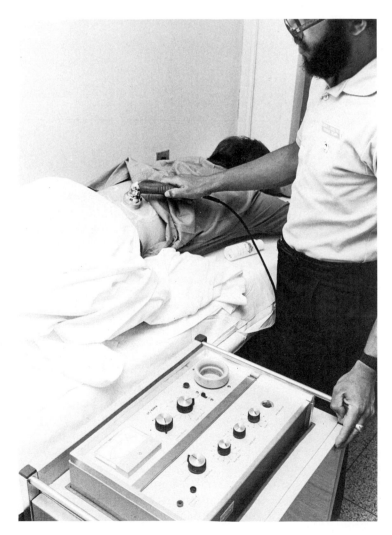

Fig. 6-14. Application of ultrasound to the low back.

minutes. Relative contraindications include treating an area of the spinal column where a laminectomy has been done, and treating a documented radiculopathy, because swelling could increase pressure on a nerve root and intensify the patient's pain. It should not be used in areas where there is vascular insufficiency, sensory impairment, or an underlying malignancy. It is also contraindicated in bleeding disorders.

Transcutaneous Electrical Nerve Stimulation

Transcutaneous electrical nerve stimulation (TENS) is a therapy in which a small electrical current passes through the skin. This current produces depolarization of sensory nerves and affects peripheral and central pain mechanisms which as yet are not fully clarified. Melzack and Wall's gate control hypothesis or the action of endorphines are two possible explanations for the pain inhibition. The great advantage of the TENS

unit is that it is easily carried by the patient and therefore permits mobilization with relief of pain. Use at home enables the patient to resume typical daily activities gradually, with little pain, and therefore with normal body mechanics. Most TENS units have controls for amplitude, rate of pulsation, and pulse width. When the electrodes are attached all controls should be at the lowest setting. Then the amplitude is increased until the patient feels a strong but not uncomfortable sensation. The rate is then adjusted to give the best pain relief, lowering the amplitude if necessary to accommodate this rate. Finally, the pulse width is adjusted, again lowering the amplitude if necessary till a comfortable setting is achieved. In general, four surface electrodes are used either through a two-channel device or one channel expanded with the use of Y cables (Fig. 6-15). There are no fixed body locations which provide maximal pain relief. A trial-and-error method of electrode attachment is most effective for maximal pain relief. In

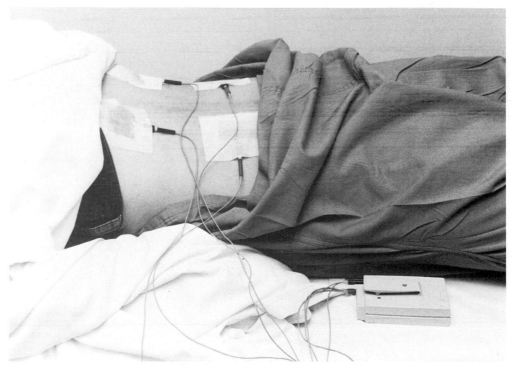

Fig. 6-15. Transcutaneous electrical nerve stimulation unit with Y cable electrodes attached to low back bilaterally.

general, when treating lumbosacral pain with radiculopathy, two electrodes on the trunk and two more distally on the extremity are used. Typical areas treated would be the paraspinal muscles, the sciatic notch, and the posterior thigh. The TENS unit should not be used with cardiac pacemakers and should be used with care in patients operating potentially dangerous machinery, the latter because loosening of the electrode can cause an unpleasant shock which could distract the patient. If skin irritation occurs at the electrode site it should be moved to another location.

The effectiveness of TENS and the proper electrode placement for a particular patient may be determined in the therapy department. It then can be used as part of a therapy program including other modalities such as ultrasound; or arrangements can be made for rental, with the patient using it at home. The latter has the advantage of availability for use most of the day, and in general this produces more satisfactory pain relief. After 1 or 2 months of use it is often possible to wean the patient from the device, especially if an effective exercise program has been started.

PART III

Further Conservative Treatments

Medication

The basic policy in prescribing analgesic medication for the isolated acute pain syndrome is to give an amount commensurate with the patient's pain. A common error is to dole out sparing doses of drugs, particularly narcotics. Oftentimes, one or two substantial doses of Demerol or morphine will be sufficient to alleviate a severe paraspinal muscle spasm which is exacerbating the pain, after which a less potent, nonaddictive drug will maintain the patient in reasonable comfort. Low back pain associated with muscle spasm may give rise to a pain cycle in which the muscle spasm produces pain and pain increased the severity of muscle spasm. Interruption of such a cycle may require potent analgesic medication.

If the initial pain is severe, have no hesitation about giving the patient a strong analgesic drug such as Demerol or morphine and then gradually reducing this analgesic medication until none is necessary. The quicker one can interrupt the muscle spasm pain cycle, the more efficacious will be the improvement in the overall pain complex.

In contrast, when dealing with the unremitting and protracted pain of the chronic low back syndrome, the use of analgesic medication for an indefinitely prolonged interval is ill-advised, and we attempt to substitute pain-relieving physical measures.

MORPHINE

Morphine, the principal alkaloid of opium, remains the standard to which other analgesics are compared. However, because of its undesirable qualities it has lost the preeminent status which it long enjoyed.

Action. Morphine relieves pain, causes euphoria, and in large doses may induce sleep. In therapeutic doses, it depresses the respiration and constricts the pupils. The action of morphine consists mainly in a descending depression of the central nervous system. Its apparent stimulant effects are attributable to depression of inhibitory mechanisms, but its emetic action is caused by stimulation of the chemoreceptor trigger zones of the vomiting center. Morphine exerts its analgesic action not only by increasing the pain threshold (*i.e.,* the magnitude of the stimulus necessary to evoke pain), but also by dulling the sensibility (*i.e.*, the reaction to pain).

Side-Effects. Side-effects associated with the use of morphine include nausea and emesis, itching, particularly of the nose and cheeks, and constipation. Morphine also slows the heart, increases the tone of smooth muscle, inhibits the secretion of the gastrointestinal tract and, in susceptible individuals, may induce convulsions, excitement, and delirium. The most serious drawback to the use of morphine is its tendency to induce tolerance, necessitating the increase of the dose to attain a therapeutic response, and to develop addiction, a liability shared by all morphinelike analgesics.

Therapeutic Use. Morphine is a reliable analgesic when given parenterally, although considerably less effective by mouth. No other established drug equals its analgesic capacity and at the same time is free of undesirable qualities. The analgesic dose-response curve for morphine reaches a plateau at about 10 mg for a 70 kg person, and this represents the optimal dose. A dose of 15 mg provides somewhat longer relief of pain but also brings about a significant increase in side-effects. The interval between the subcutaneous injection and the onset of some degree of pain relief is 10 minutes, and the duration of analgesia about 4 hours.

SYNTHETIC DERIVATIVES OF MORPHINE

Hydromorphone (Dilaudid). Hydromorphone is five to ten times as potent as morphine, but its duration of action is less than that of morphine and it is also more toxic. It is used in the same manner as morphine but in smaller doses (1 to 2 mg) for acute pain of short duration. It is administered by injection, orally, or as a rectal suppository.

Oxymorphone (Numorphan). A 1 mg injection of oxymorphone is equal to 10 mg of morphine as an analgesic. But at this dose oxymorphone is at least as likely as, and

perhaps more likely than, morphine to produce untoward effects.

Levorphanol (Levo-Dromoran) Tartrate. Levorphanol tartrate resembles morphine in action but is somewhat longer acting and is less likely to cause constipation than morphine. It is administered in doses of 2 to 3 mg (for adults) orally or subcutaneously for the relief of severe pain. As with most morphine substitutes, doses several times larger are required orally than by injection to attain the same analgesic effect.

CODEINE

Codeine, one of the most widely used of all analgesics, is an effective analgesic when used in adequate dosage. It is less effective when administered orally than parenterally. When given in the ordinary dose of 32 mg by mouth, it is slightly more effective than the usual dose of aspirin (650 mg) in relieving pain. In fact, for short-term use in musculo-skeletal syndromes, it would appear that aspirin is more reliable and effective. When either drug alone is ineffective, the combination of codeine plus aspirin is often quite effective. There is a summation of effect when 32 mg of codeine is combined with 600 mg of aspirin. Codeine by injection in doses of 60 mg approaches, but is not equal to, 10 mg of morphine and also possesses most of the disadvantages of morphine. Hence, when used parenterally, 10 mg of morphine is superior.

Codeine rarely causes addiction. It depresses respiration and causes other undesirable morphinelike symptoms such as constipation, nausea, and itching.

SYNTHETIC ADDICTING ANALGESICS

A number of synthetic compounds have been prepared as substitutes for morphine and its derivatives in the hope that such compounds might be devoid of the undesirable actions of morphine, particularly its addictive property. Like morphine, they are not only potent analgesics but also highly addictive.

Meperidine (Demerol). Meperidine in doses of 60 to 80 mg parenterally can be substituted for 10 mg of morphine as an analgesic, but in equianalgesic doses it produces many of the side-effects seen with morphine, including respiratory depression.

Meperidine at one time was prescribed by physicians instead of morphine under the mistaken assumption that it was less addictive. Experience has shown that this is not the case and that addiction to meperidine is far less amenable to cure than addiction to morphine.

Methadone (Dolophine). When used in comparable analgesic doses, methadone is as toxic as morphine, exerting the same depressing effects on the circulation and respiration. Methadone is addictive, but because withdrawal symptoms following prolonged administration of the drug come on more slowly and are of lesser intensity, it has proved useful in the treatment of morphine and heroin addiction. For this purpose, methadone is substituted for the latter drugs and subsequently withdrawn. Its use in narcotic detoxification or maintenance efforts is limited to those programs approved by the Food and Drug Administration and the designated state authority. In equianalgesic doses, the occurrence of side-effects is similar to morphine.

Methadone is an effective analgesic for most forms of moderate to severe pain. It is administered orally in doses of 2.5 to 10 mg every 3 to 4 hours. When oral administration is undesirable, the drug may be injected subcutaneously or intramuscularly, but it should not be given intravenously.

Alphaprodine Hydrochloride (Nisentil). Alphaprodine hydrochloride acts promptly and is a potent, short-acting narcotic useful in intense pain of brief duration. It can be used prior to low back manipulative therapy.

Alphaprodine is administered by subcutaneous injection in doses of 40 to 60 mg, depending upon the weight of the patient. Analgesia is induced within 5 minutes and lasts for about 2 hours. Overdose may be counteracted by nalorphine. Alphaprodine may also be administered intravenously in doses of 20 to 30 mg (when very rapid and brief analgesia is desired). Analgesia is produced within a few minutes and lasts from half an hour to an hour.

Anileridine (Leritine). Anileridine is intermediate in analgesic potency between meperidine and morphine. Like meperidine, it exerts mild antihistaminic and spasmolytic actions but lacks the constipating action of the opiates. Its sedative and hypnotic actions resemble those of meperidine.

From 30 to 60 mg of anileridine can be substituted for 100 mg of meperidine and equivalent doses of morphine in most clinical situations. It has one advantage, namely, that it is more efficacious by the oral route in comparison to its parenteral potency than morphine and many of the morphine substitutes. Milligram by milligram, however, it is not as potent by mouth as by injection. In doses of 30 to 60 mg it has significant pain-relieving capacity by either route of administration. In other respects the drug has no superiority over older drugs, and side-effects may possibly be greater than those of equianalgesic doses of other agents.

Anileridine hydrochloride is administered orally in the form of 25 mg tablets every 6 hours, but dosages up to 50 mg may be used at more frequent intervals in cases of severe pain. Anileridine phosphate is administered by subcutaneous, intramuscular, or intravenous injection in dosages of 25 to 50 mg (1 to 2 ml) at intervals of 4 to 6 hours.

Oxycodone (Percodan). Oxycodone is most available with aspirin, phenacetin, and caffeine. This combination is called Percodan and is an extremely effective oral analgesic. It may produce psychic dependence, physical dependence, and tolerance upon repeated administration, and so should be prescribed with caution. Because of its highly addictive tendencies, it should never be utilized for the patient with a chronic low back syndrome.

NON-NARCOTIC ANALGESICS

Analgesics which are nonaddictive and relatively nontoxic have been available for many years, and, being procurable without prescription, are used widely for low back pain not requiring the attention of a physician. These drugs exert an antirheumatic action, which renders them particularly valuable as analgesics in many low back dysfunctions.

Aspirin. Aspirin is one of the most widely used of all drugs, as evidenced by the fact that over 60 million pounds are consumed annually throughout the world. It is versatile in its actions, being an effective antipyretic, analgesic, and antirheumatic; it exerts a specific therapeutic effect in rheumatic fever; in large doses, it exerts antiallergic, cholesterol-lowering, uricosuric, hypoglycemic, litholytic, anticoagulant, and other actions. The mechanism responsible for so wide a spectrum of activity is unknown.

The effectiveness of aspirin in painful states has been demonstrated repeatedly and it is particularly suited for use as a universal analgesic. It is absorbed from the stomach, but for the most part from the small intestine. Peak blood levels are reached within two hours, at which time it exerts its maximum analgesic action. It is one of the safest of all drugs, but potentially dangerous allergic reactions may attend its use in patients sensitive to the drug. True aspirin allergy is relatively unusual, and in most cases the patient will mean that his gastrointestinal tract is intolerant to aspirin. This can usually be countered by enteric-coated forms or by accompanying antacid medication. Hematemesis and melena may occur when aspirin is taken in large doses for prolonged periods.

Aspirin, administered in doses of 300 to 600 mg every 2 to 4 hours, preferably after meals, is effective for mild and moderate degrees of low back pain. Combined with phenacetin, caffeine, or codeine, it exerts a synergistic action. Various combinations of these drugs are marketed, as in the APC (aspirin, phenacetin, caffeine) formulation, to which codeine and other analgesic, antihistaminic, or tranquilizing drugs are also added.

Anti-inflammatory doses are higher than those needed for analgesia and usually have to be given in a range of 900 to 1200 mg every 4 hours, depending upon the size of the individual. A good rule-of-thumb to obtain maximal beneficial anti-inflammatory effects without severe toxicity from side-effects is to give the patient a total daily dosage of ½ to ¾ grain per pound of body weight in divided dosages administered every 4 hours. One should attempt to obtain a serum salicylate level of 20 to 25 mg per 100 ml for full anti-inflammatory activity. In most instances, exceeding this therapeutic level will cause unpleasant side-effects such as tinnitus, partial deafness, vertigo, nausea, vomiting, diarrhea, and occasionally both auditory and visual hallucinations. Aspirin may be used as the plain aspirin tablet, an enteric-coated form, or as a timed-release preparation, the latter two causing less local gastric irritation.

An extremely effective public advertising program has extolled the benefits of adding buffering agents to aspirin. Although this combination does increase the rate of absorption slightly, it does not diminish gastric intolerance.

Other Salicylic Acid Derivatives. A number of other derivatives of salicylic acid are also available for use as analgesics. Sodium salicylate resembles aspirin in action. Methyl salicylate (oil of wintergreen) is used externally as a rubefacient over surface areas of low back pain.

A timed-release preparation of aspirin (Measurin) is also available, which claims to have a prolonged analgesic effect and less adverse gastric effects than aspirin.

The use of salicylates is contraindicated in patients with severe renal disease and should be used with caution in patients with a history of allergic reactions.

Phenacetin (Acetophenetidin). The use of phenacetin and mixtures containing the drug has come under scrutiny during recent years as a possible cause of certain cases of pyelonephritis. The etiologic role of phenacetin in renal disease remains unproven.

Phenacetin is rarely used alone but is usually administered in combination with aspirin and caffeine to which codeine and other drugs are at times also added.

Propoxyphene (Darvon). Chemically, propoxyphene is most closely related to methadone, and in high doses it has all of the adverse effects of any narcotic. It can produce drug dependence characterized by psychic dependence and, less frequently, physical dependence and tolerance. High doses taken orally (as in suicide attempts) will cause respiratory depression, convulsions, and overall central nervous system depression. When introduced, this drug was designated as a non-controlled substance by the Food and Drug Administration, but because of toxic effects and fatalities following overdose, it is now listed as a controlled drug. Propoxyphene is available as propoxyphene hydrochloride (Darvon) or as the napsylate salt (Darvon-N).

Darvon is manufactured in unmixed form, in combination with aspirin (Darvon with ASA), or with aspirin, phenacetin, and caffeine (Darvon compound). Darvon-N is manufactured in unmixed form, in combination with aspirin (Darvon-N with ASA), or with acetaminophen (Darvocet-N). The usual dosage is one every 4 hours as needed. It is less effective then codeine and more effective than aspirin. Despite some statements to the contrary, it is a satisfactory oral analgesic.

Ethoheptazine Citrate (Zactane). Ethoheptazine citrate is available as a two-layered tablet (Zactirin Cpound-100), which contains 100 mg ethoheptazine citrate, 227 mg aspirin, 162 mg phenacetin, and 32.4 mg caffeine. One tablet of the drug is administered orally three or four times daily for low back pain and sciatica. Side-effects include nausea, with or without vomiting, epigastric distress, and dizziness, but these symptoms are rarely observed.

Methotrimeprazine (Levoprome). Methotrimeprazine is a potent, nonaddicting analgesic, comparing favorably with morphine and meperidine. In doses of 20 mg it is equal in analgesic action to 10 mg of morphine or 75 mg of meperidine and equals these drugs in speed and duration of action. Tolerance to the analgesic effects of the drug has not been reported.

Addiction has not been noted, and the drug is therefore not subject to the restrictions of the Harrison Narcotic Act. In normal subjects it does not depress the respiration as the narcotics do. Excessive sedation, orthostatic hypotension, dizziness, and fainting constitute the major side-effects of the drug and restrict its use to nonambulatory patients. Other adverse effects noted with phenothiazine derivatives should be considered when the drug is used for a month or longer.

Methotrimeprazine is available only for intramuscular injection in a solution containing 20 mg per ml. The initial dose in adults is 10 to 15 mg and may be increased for greater relief of pain, if tolerated. The drug is indicated especially for severe pain in addiction-prone patients where sedation is desirable and depression of respiration is to be avoided. The drug should not be used concurrently with antihypertensive drugs or depressants of the central nervous system in patients with clinically significant hypotension, or in patients under 14 years of age.

In addition to hypotension, other adverse reactions occasionally encountered include amnesia, disorientation, dizziness, drowsiness, excessive sedation, weakness, slurring of speech, abdominal discomfort, nausea and vomiting, dry mouth, nasal congestion, difficulty in urination, chills, uterine inertia, and pain at the site of injection. As with other phenothiazines, the possibility of blood dyscrasias, hepatotoxicity, and extrapyramidal effects should be considered possible ractions. Administration for more than 30 days is not advised.

Pentazocine (Talwin). This drug manifests potent analgesia with minimal addictive properties. Most of the cases of addiction to this drug are patients with a previous history of addiction to other drugs. True primary addiction rarely occurs. Pentazocine is not subject to narcotic controls. Unlike morphine, tolerance to the drug does not develope. Side-effects to pentazocine consist of nausea, which occurs in about 5% of patients, and to a lesser degree, vertigo, dizziness, vomiting, and euphoria. Hallucinations, disorientation, and confusion occur rarely. Respiratory depression is noted in about 1% of patients. Pentazocine is relatively free from the severe respiratory depression, urinary retention, and constipation associated with the use of morphine.

Pentazocine is used in place of morphine and other narcotic analgesics. The recommended dose is 30 mg by intramuscular, subcutaneous, or intravenous routes, repeated, if necessary, every 3 to 4 hours. It is manufactured in 50 mg tablets for oral dosage of one tablet every 3 or 4 hours as needed. The drug should be used with caution in patients with myocardial infarction who have nausea or vomiting, in patients with impaired renal or hepatic function, and in patients with respiratory depression. It has the pharmacologic action of antagonizing the analgesic effects of narcotics, so it should not be used in conjunction with drugs such as morphine or meperidine.

Mefenamic Acid (Ponstel). Mefenamic acid is a non-narcotic analgesic for oral administration. It is indicated for short-term administration for the relief of back pain. Its use is contraindicated in patients with intestinal ulceration, in women of childbearing potential, and in children under 14 years of age. Patients with diarrhea must have the drug promptly discontinued and are usually unable to tolerate the drug thereafter. The drug should also be administered with caution in patients with abnormal renal function or inflammatory disease of the gastrointestinal tract, and should be withdrawn promptly if rash or diarrhea occurs. It should also be used with caution in asthmatics.

Mefenamic acid is administered orally in capsules of 250 mg in doses of 500 mg initially, followed by 250 mg every 6 hours as needed. It should not be used for periods exceeding 1 week. Adverse reactions most frequently observed are drowsiness, nausea, dizziness, nervousness, gastrointestinal discomfort, and headache.

ANTI-INFLAMMATORY DRUGS

Phenylbutazone (Butazolidin). Both phenylbutazone and its derivative, oxyphen-butazone (Tandearil), are effective anti-inflammatory agents. Both drugs, however, must be administered with care, since potential toxicity (gastrointestinal tract bleeding, agranulocytosis, decrease in red cell count aplastic anemia, nausea, vomiting, and skin rash) is great. An advantage is that they are usually more easily tolerated than an equivalent pharmacologic dose of silicylates.

In 1954, initial reports were published indicating that phenylbutazone produced bone marrow depression, leading in some cases to complete agranulocytosis. Prior to these reports, doses of up to 1200 mg daily were often used for relatively prolonged durations. After this knowledge was disseminated, the use of phenyl-butazone was greatly diminished for several years until it became apparent that the bone marrow reaction was dose-related and that limited amounts could be effective and reasonably safe. For low back syndromes, it is most frequently administered in a loading dose of 400 to 800 mg daily for 1 to 2 days, then reduced to 100 mg three times daily for an additional 4 to 6 days.

Indomethacin (Indocin). Indomethacin also has antipyretic and analgesic effects. The drug is given in a dosage range of 75 to 100 mg per day in 3 to 4 divided doses. Its primary side-effects are gastrointestinal: the drug is capable of causing peptic ulcers and associated gastrointestinal bleeding. In addition, it may cause severe headaches that are unresponsive to aspirin, as well as nausea, vomiting, rashes, vertigo, and rarely, hematologic and hepatic reactions. During the 10 years of its clinical use, there has been frequent controversy regarding the effectiveness of this drug.

In terms of anti-inflammatory activity, indomethacin lies between salicylates and phenylbutazone when all are used in appropriate pharmacologic doses. Patients using the drug for long-term therapy may develop a tolerance to it, and so its initial effectiveness may be lost. As with other drugs in this category, when it is taken on a relatively full stomach, the gastric symptoms are decreased.

Four more recent anti-inflammatory agents are ibuprofen (Motrin), released in 1974, and naproxen (Naprosyn), fenoprofen calcium (Nalfon), and tolmetin (Tolectin), released in 1975.

Ibuprofen (Motrin). This anti-inflammatory agent does not have the analgesic potency of phenylbutazone but has received wide acceptance and use because of its infrequent production of serious side-effects. It may be helpful for long-term use in those patients who are unable to tolerate the gastrointestinal side-effects of the other anti-inflammatory medications. It is available in 300 and 400 mg tablets for oral administration. For low back syndromes 300 or 400 mg t.i.d. or q.i.d. is the usual dosage.

Naproxen (Naprosyn). This drug has a fairly high incidence of adverse reactions related to the gastrointestinal tract. Nausea and abdominal pain have been reported, as well as gastrointestinal bleeding which was not always preceded by premonitory gastrointestinal symptoms. This bleeding has occasionally reached serious levels with a number of fatalities reported. Naproxen is available in 250 mg tablets. A dosage of 250 mg b.i.d. is recommended.

Fenoprofen Calcium (Nalfon). Food decreases the levels of Nalfon in the blood, so the drug should be given 4 hour before or 2 hours after meals. The most common side-effects are nausea, dyspepsia, headache, somnolence, pruritus, and tinnitus. Fenoprofen calcium is available in 300 mg pulvules and 600 mg tablets. The recommended dosage is 600 mg q.i.d. Nalfon is an effective anti-inflammatory agent.

Tolmetin (Tolectin). This effective anti-inflammatory drug differs from the other three newer agents since Motrin, Naprosyn, and Nalfon are all phenylalkanoic acids while the pyrrole structure of this drug relates it to indomethacin. Despite its different basic structure, this agent produces similar side-effects to the other new anti-inflammatory drugs. The most common are gastrointestinal distress and headaches. It is available in 200 mg tablets. The recommended dosage is 400 mg t.i.d.

Corticosteroids

MEMBRANE STABILIZATION

Corticosteroids can truly be considered the wonder drug of the 20th century. Dr. Hench first demonstrated the powerful anti-inflammatory effects of cortisol, and steroid chemists subsequently manipulated the basic corticosteroid structure to create a diminution of the mineral activity and an increased potency of the glucosteroid effect.

The exact mechanism of corticosteroid action is still unknown, but its effects on generalized membrane stabilization would explain many of the most significant features of the anti-inflammatory activity. It diminishes vascular permeability and inhibits leukocyte migration. A wide variety of corticosteroid preparations of variable potency and toxicity is available.

The panorama of potential side-effects of corticosteroids can be frightening. The incidence of such unwanted effects is largely dose-dependent; the higher the dose and the longer the duration of treatment, the more likely one is to develop some complication from the drug.

RATIONALE FOR USE

The inflammatory response of nerves is receiving increasing attention in our attempts to explain the mechanisms responsible for low back pain syndromes. The two nerve systems primarily involved are the nerve roots and the smaller, more anatomically variable, less completely understood complex identified as the sinuvertebral nerves. In some instances, an irreversible fibrosis of these neural tissues may eventually occur in association with ischemic changes. The rationale for corticosteroid use is that it provides a mechanism which will reverse the inflammatory response and hopefully avoid neural fibrosis.

NOT A LONG-TERM SOLUTION

Because of the adverse effects associated with prolonged use of this drug, it is reserved for the management of the isolated, acutely painful episode and not as a long-term solution for chronic low back dysfunction. By providing pain relief of the acute attack, it will reduce the need for hospitalization and facilitate rehabilitation.

DIAGNOSTIC BENEFIT

Occasionally, the local injection of steroids may be helpful in the differential diagnosis of a pain syndrome. When an epidural steroid injection is performed on a patient with low back and sciatic pain (assuming the injection was technically satisfactory), one could reasonably expect at least some temporary remission of symptoms. If no improvement occurs, further thinking about the etiology of the syndrome is in order.

MODE OF ADMINISTRATION

Corticosteroids are available in every conceivable form and in conjunction with a wide variety of medications; almost any mode of administration is possible. The question that must be answered when treating low back dysfunction is whether to administer the drug systemically or locally, intrathecally, epidurally, or into the facets.

Because of the adverse effects of systemic steroid medication, and since we are dealing with an anatomically limited condition, local injections are justified. Conversely, an adverse tissue reaction to the medication being instilled into and adjacent to delicate and sensitive neural structures is a serious hazard of local injection. Because of the dangers of adhesive arachnoiditis, we no longer recommend intrathecal injection of steroids. We presently favor the epidural instillation of steroids, on the assumption that the dura will behave as an adequate natural barrier and prevent injury to the neural elements.

Occasionally, the patient who suffers a very acute episode of pain will benefit from a 1-week course of systemic steroid therapy. Prednisone 20 mg b.i.d. for 3 or 4 days followed by a tapering dose may be used. This is often as effective as a local injection. If the pain recurs following oral steroids, we would not repeat the systemic treatment but would be more likely to consider a local injection. Prolonged delay of anti-inflammatory agents and exclusive reliance on analgesic medications may not be advisable if one accepts the rationale for the use of steroids in preventing development of an irreversible neurofibrosis with ischemic changes.

DOES USE OF CORTICOSTEROIDS REDUCE THE NEED FOR SURGERY?

A number of patients with acute low back and sciatic pain syndromes will benefit by either systemic or local use of corticosteroids. Approximately half of those so benefited will have an excellent post-treatment course and consider themselves "cured." The other half will improve for only a relatively short interval and, because of persisting pain and incapacity, will require surgery. Those surgeons who list persisting incapacity for a significant duration as one of their criteria for surgery would probably conclude that the use of corticosteroids does not reduce the need for surgery.

The technique of lumbar epidural and caudal injections is described in the chapter on analgesic blocks.

MUSCLE RELAXANTS

As a general group, the orally prescribed muscle relaxants are not very potent. Most of them induce muscle relaxation by creating a calming or tranquilizing effect.

Diazepam (Valium) is the most frequently utilized muscle relaxant. It is not suitable for treatment of the patient with chronic long term low back dysfunction because prolonged usage can lead to physical and psychological dependence. In addition, it acts as a mood depressant which is not helpful when dealing with a chronic pain situation.

ANTI-DEPRESSANTS

Amitriptyline HCl (Elavil) is a tricyclic anti-depressant drug and is the most commonly used drug of its category for chronic pain problems. For ambulatory patients it is often used in a nightly dose of 50 to 100 mg as a "sleeping pill" at bedtime. A sedative effect will be apparent before the anti-depressant effect is noted. An adequate anti-depressant effect may take as long as 30 days to develop.

Fluphenazine hydrochloride (Prolixin) is a phenothiazine derivative commonly used in the management of psychotic disorders. This drug is often used in conjunction with Elavil for the chronic low back pain problem (1 mg t.i.d.).

Occupational Changes

In the management of low back dysfunction it is most important to delve carefully into the patient's work history. Oftentimes a patient can relate low back symptoms to specific activities performed either at work or in activities of daily living. Occasionally, a modification of such activities may serve to alleviate or improve symptoms to the point where more intensive management is not necessary.

Potential Side-Effects of Corticosteroids

Glucocorticoid action
—Hyperglycemia
—Polyuria
Mineral corticoid action
—Hypokalemia
—Metabolic alkalosis
—Fluid retention and edema
—Cardiac failure
—Hypertension
Protein metabolism
—Muscle atrophy
—Myopathy
Bone
—Osteoporosis
—Retarded growth
—Fractures
—Avascular necrosis
Endocrine
—Hirsutism
—Acne
—Menstrual irregularities
—Premature menopause
Metabolism
Fat and deposition
—Moon facies
—Buffalo hump
—Supraclavicular fat pad
—Increased abdominal girth
—Hyperlipidemia
Host defense
—Staphylococcal infection
—Tuberculosis spread
—Fungal infection
Gastrointestinal tract
—Dyspepsia
—Bowel perforation
—Peptic ulcer
—Esophagitis
—Hypersatiety
—Pancreatitis

Katz WA: *Rheumatic Diseases, Diagnosis and Management*, p. 887. JB Lippincott Co, 1977.

One must keep in mind that it is often the patient's activities that precipitate low back dysfunction so that treatment is necessary. Such activities should be modified for the future. If a patient has had long-standing low back dysfunction and is performing heavy activities which involve great stress on the low back, treatment of the presenting symptoms without attempting to modify the stress-producing activities is unrealistic. When the patient is free of pain following treatment, it is a bit shortsighted to allow him to return to the same conditions that originally produced the pain.

Psychotherapy and Hypnotherapy

The daily psychic stresses from family problems and work may generate emotional tension and aggravate low back pain involving muscle spasm. Sometimes emotional guidance may be helpful, but with few exceptions psychotherapy is neither necessary nor helpful. Occasionally in very refractory cases hypnosis has been effective. Hypnotherapy is most effective in those individuals complaining of an anatomically limited specific area of persisting pain. A generalized intermittent low back ache is not as receptive to this form of management.

Activities of Daily Living and Faulty Posture

The fundamental principle of treating faulty posture and physical activities productive of low back pain is directed toward the goal of reducing the lumbar lordosis (Fig. 6-16). Since increased lordosis primarily depends upon the lumbosacral angle that relates to the pelvic position, our endeavors are directed toward education of the patient in attainment of decreased pelvic angle. This involves alteration of habitual postural patterns which are well established and not easily altered (Fig. 6-17).

Such a retraining program involves a combination of corrective exercises in association with altered postural attitudes, but it has many pitfalls and is not easily achieved. The corrective exercises are time-consuming and require diligence on the part of the patient, who may not possess the psychological resources for this task. If the patient is capable and willing to devote an adequate period of time to these exercises, the manner in which they are performed may require checking at intervals by the physician. Patients occasionally modify or embellish the exercise program, in some cases producing an adverse effect. When the patient is faithful

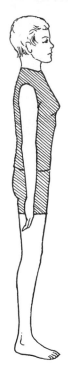

Fig. 6-16. A satisfactory flattened low back, erect posture.

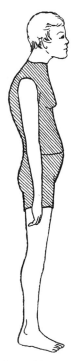

Fig. 6-17. A posture of increased lumbar lordosis.

in the performance of the corrective exercises, but in the remainder of the day continues to maintain a position of increased lumbar lordosis during activities of daily living, no decrease in low back dysfunction will be realized. (Description of low back exercises later in this chapter.)

All activities involving daily living must be carefully reviewed with an appreciation of the body mechanics involved, in an effort to avoid excessive stress on the low back.

Standing and Walking

Standing and walking should be done in an erect position with the chest uplifted so that it, rather than the abdomen, becomes the most anterior portion of the trunk. In an effort to decrease lumbar hyperlordosis, women should be dissuaded from wearing high heels, particularly for prolonged periods of standing or walking, since this results in a compensatory increase in the lumbar lordosis (Fig. 6-18).

The patient can practice proper erect posture by standing against a wall and pressing the belt line against the wall but not the head and shoulders, so that the lumbar spine is as close to the vertical plane as is comfortably possible (Fig. 6-19).

When initially performing this exercise, the patient is instructed to place the feet a foot from the wall, facilitating flattening of the lumbar spine against the wall. With time, lumbar flattening can be accomplished with less effort and the feet can be positioned closer to the wall.

The patient should occasionally check his posture in front of a full-length mirror, viewing the body position from the side as a reminder to avoid the protruding abdomen and substitute the uplifted chest.

Individuals with occupations involving prolonged standing may achieve comfortable flattening of the lumbar lordosis by placing one foot on a low stool 6 to 8 inches high (Fig. 6-20). Such a posture, which flexes one

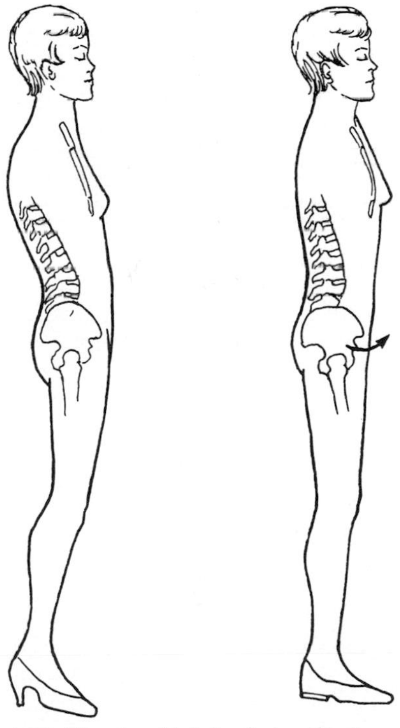

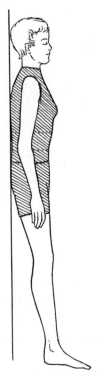

Fig. 6-18. Wearing high heels results in a compensatory increase in lumbar lordosis.

Fig. 6-19. Proper erect posture can be practiced by flattening the low back against a wall.

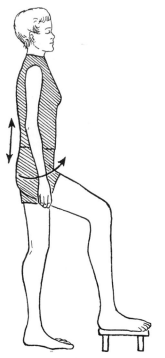

Fig. 6-20. Resting one foot on a low stool will flex the hip, reduce iliopsoas, and result in reduction of lumbar lordosis.

hip, reducing iliopsoas and hip flexor pull upon the lumbar spine, results in a relaxed reduction of lumbar lordosis. The flexed hip should be alternated from time to time. Tavern keepers, whose livelihood is directly related to the length of time their clientele remain standing at a bar, have intuitively appreciated this postural truth for the past century. The well-known "brass rail" permits their patrons to stand comfortably at the bar for many hours.

It is sometimes difficult to convey to patients the concept of maintaining a flattened lumbar spine in the erect position. They may flatten their lumbar spine against a wall and immediately upon withdrawing from this firm surface will resume the lumbar lordotic position. Such terms as "tuck in the pelvis" may be meaningless to patients, and they are unable to grasp what is desired. Occasionally, it is helpful to have the patient place one hand on the symphysis pubis and the other on the xyphoid and attempt to bring both hands closer together,

which will result in an upward tilt of the pelvis (Fig. 6-21).

Another teaching aid is to have the patient imagine that he must hold a coin between the buttocks by squeezing them together. Such a maneuver will also result in an upward pelvic tilt and a reduction of the lumbar lordosis.

Sitting

Sitting is done by first flexing the lumbar spine and then performing a flexion in both the hips and knees. When sitting, the lumbar spine should be slightly flexed; if the chair is too high to sit in this fashion, a short stool may be necessary beneath the feet. Because of the shorter height of most women, chairs are often a bit too high to sit in this position and a compensatory correction may be achieved by crossing the knees (Figs. 6-22 through 6-26).

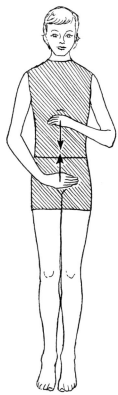

Fig. 6-21. The patient places one hand on the symphysis pubis, the other on the xiphoid, and attempts to bring the hands closer together.

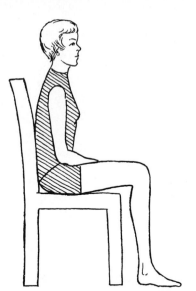

Fig. 6-22. *Good flat-backed sitting position in chair of satisfactory height with a firm seat and back.*

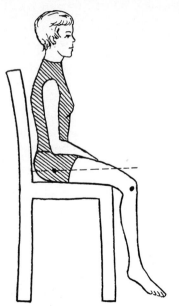

Fig. 6-23. *An excessively high chair allows the feet to dangle, causing the knees to be lower than the hip joints. This will increase lumbar lordosis.*

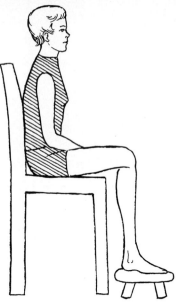

Fig. 6-24. *Correction of excessively high chair with a short stool beneath the feet.*

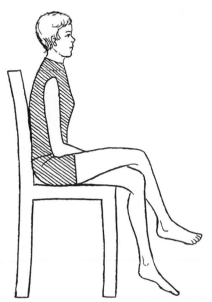

Fig. 6-25. *Correction of excessively high chair by crossing the knees.*

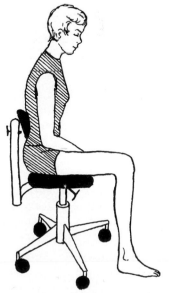

Fig. 6-26. *Poorly constructed typist's chair with a narrow back rest produces increased lumbar lordosis.*

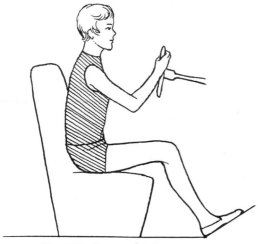

Fig. 6-27. Correct driving posture.

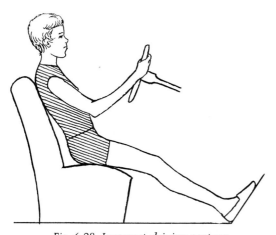

Fig. 6-28. Incorrect driving posture.

Driving

When driving, the seat should be advanced forward so that the knees are at a slightly higher level than the hips; this tends to reduce lumbar lordosis (Figs. 6-27 and 6-28). The car seat should not be pushed so far back that the knees are lowered with extension of the lower extremities, resulting a compensatory increased lumbar lordosis.

Lifting

Lifting any significant load is done with a slight flexion of the hips and knees and a flexion of the lumbosacral spine. The load should not be lifted with the knees and lumbosacral spine in extension (Fig. 6-29).

Sleeping

The patient with low back dysfunction should sleep on the side with hips and knees in flexion (see Fig. 6-5). If sleeping on the back is habitual, a sizable blanket roll beneath the mattress at the level of the knees is advisable, since a pillow placed in that position will become displaced from normal movements occurring during sleep (Fig. 6-30). Sleeping on the abdomen tends to increase the lumbosacral angle and often causes increased discomfort (Fig. 6-31). It is best avoided.

With long-standing low back dysfunction, it may be necessary for a patient to obtain a hospital bed with the various adjustments available for proper sleeping position.

Establishing Proper Habits

Every task the patient does, from household chores, such as using a broom or carpet

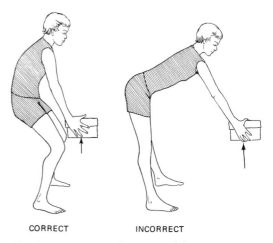

CORRECT   INCORRECT

Fig. 6-29. Correct and incorrect lifting postures.

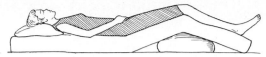

Fig. 6-30. *If sleeping in a supine position is habitual, a blanket roll beneath the mattress at the level of the knees will decrease the lumbar lordosis.*

sweeper, or getting in and out of a car, must be analyzed in terms of body mechanics. The patient must practice these defensive and protective movements until they become second nature.

A frequent deficiency in the management of a conservative treatment program is that the physician will prescribe a low back support shortly after pain has subsided. The patient will wear this support for an indefinite period of time without any specific instruction or corrective exercises.

The greatest barrier to a satisfactory end result is the formidable task of convincing a patient who is no longer suffering from severe pain to carry out an ongoing exercise and a daily living program which will permit resumption of activities with reasonable expectation that the future will not be marred by recurrent attacks of low back dysfunction.

In many cases the patient has a protuberant abdomen with inadequate abdominal and lumbar musculature. The program will be directed toward reducing obesity with a combination of diet and exercise, in addition to improving lumbar mobility by progressive stretching and elongation of the hamstring muscles and hip flexors so that a well-distributed but not excessively lordotic curvature of the lumbar spine may eventually be achieved. Most physicians must take time to stress the advantages of this program to

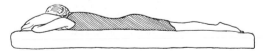

Fig. 6-31. *Sleeping on the abdomen increases lumbar lordosis.*

the patient, recounting the potential evils of what may occur in the future if such a regimen is not followed.

Low Back Exercises

Purpose

Many physicians, including those who devote considerable time and interest to patients with low back dysfunction, may not clearly appreciate the intended purpose of a low back corrective exercise program. The word exercise, in this regard, may be misleading, giving rise to images of gymnastics or strenuous athletics. Although there is certainly no objection to the improvement of general body muscle tone and rehabilitation of an overweight person to a more suitable habitus, this is not our specific object. The fact is that many patients suffering from low back dysfunction are quite trim and may be splendid tennis players or golfers with no need to be built up physically. It must be constantly borne in mind that the express intention of the exercises is to help achieve an improvement of the mechanical dysfunction which is productive of low back pain.

Many patients manifesting chronic, recurrent back pains often exhibit an increased lumbar lordosis and require an exercise program designed to produce a flattened or reduced lumbar lordosis. Dr. Paul C. Williams, a pioneer in the field of low back pain, originally introduced the concept of reducing an excessive lumbar lordosis by means of a corrective exercise program. The Williams lumbar flexion exercises have been incorporated into almost every low back rehabilitative program. A second commonly encountered finding on examination is reduced elasticity of the lumbar paraspinal muscle groupings. Such a lack of suppleness tends to make the patient vulnerable to recurrent back pains following lumbar flexion or torsion movements. A number of the exercises are designed to improve suppleness and elasticity.

Exercises Adapted to the Patient's Specific Needs

Often a standard set of "back exercises" may be handed to the patient with little instruction, and he is left to devise his own regimen. Sometimes, the entire exercise program is turned over to a therapist who may have been trained to give the same set of exercises to all "low back problems." As in any low back therapy, whether it be rest, the wearing of a low back support, or medication, exercises must be in keeping with the patient's individual needs.

In planning a low back exercise program, an understanding of the role played by the principal muscle groupings upon the lumbar spine is mandatory (Fig. 6-32). To meet the individual needs of the patient, four factors must be considered:

1. The specific postural impairment manifested by the patient.
2. Preexercise evaluation of the strength and flexibility of the principal muscle groupings.
3. The special action each of the various exercises exerts upon the principal muscle groupings.
4. The degree of muscle strength and flexibility demanded by each exercise in accordance with the limitations imposed by the patient's present clinical status.

When to Start Low Back Exercises

The program is instituted as soon as pain relief has been achieved with bed rest. Relaxation of muscle spasm can be helped along with several sessions of massage and diathermy; to both the abdominal and low back musculature, in preparation for exercises which can be initially carried out on a flattened bed. When compatible with the patient's condition, a firmer surface, such as

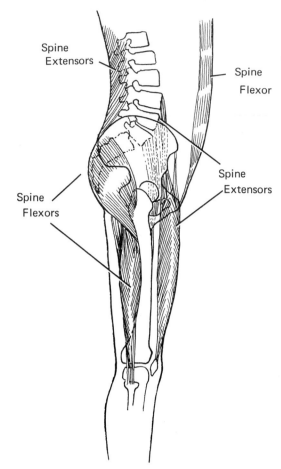

Fig. 6-32. *Diagrammatic illustration of the principle muscle groupings involved in flexion (lordosis) and extension (flattening) of the lumbar spine. The spine extensors (erector spinae, etc.) and the iliopsoas muscles extend the spine by direct action. The gluteal and hamstring muscles flex the spine, and the quadriceps extends the spine, by tilting the pelvis. The abdominal muscles flex the spine by decreasing the distance between the anterior thoracic cage and the pelvis, thereby tilting the pelvis also.*

mat- or rug-covered floor, is preferable because it provides easier maneuverability and permits greater awareness of points of body contact.

Establishing an Exercise Program

The exercises should not be performed during a period of acute pain. When pain has subsided, however, the patient must establish a habit of performing the low back exercises twice daily. It should be emphasized that even in days that involve considerable emotional stress or increased work activity, time should be set aside for these exercises. It is probably in such times of increased stress that the exercises are most helpful. An erratic exercise program is ineffectual.

Relaxation Exercises

Low back exercise programs should include relaxation and limbering exercises. The following exercises are described in the form of instructions to the patient:

1. While lying on the floor, raise your arms slowly over your head as you inhale deeply; then exhale as you allow your arms to return slowly to the floor. Repeat 10 times and with each exhalation allow your arms and legs, head and shoulders to rest limply on the floor, making your entire body as flaccid as possible.
2. Breathe deeply again and with each slow inhalation, bring your legs and feet tightly together, arms tightly at your sides, make tight fists, tighten the muscles of your body, tighten your buttocks; with each exhalation relax as completely as possible allowing your arms and legs to drift away from your body. Close your eyes and allow your jaw to sag. Repeat 10 times.

Alternating muscle contractions with relaxation is a helpful device to emphasize and accentuate relaxation by directing the patient's attention to the difference between muscle tension and muscle relaxation. If done properly, each succeeding period of relaxation is a bit more profound and produced total physical and mental relaxation prior to starting the low back exercises.

Promote Elasticity

Almost all patients with chronic recurrent low back pain demonstrate lack of suppleness of the lumbar paraspinal muscle groupings. This reduced elasticity is the reason that a lumbar flexion or torsion movement may tug and overly stretch a tendon or muscle, setting up a low back pain cycle. An identical body movement in an individual with normally elastic tissues will be easily tolerated and produce no symptoms.

The first five stretching exercises of phase 1 are given to almost all patients who have chronic intermittent low back dysfunction. The most common error made by most patients when doing low back exercises is to perform them too rapidly. To quote Dr. George Skeehan, all muscle stretching exercises must be done "with the speed of a glacier and the patience of a guru." The following exercises are graded into 2 phases on the basis of mechanical stress.

PHASE 1

These exercises are prescribed to patients who have recently recovered from a bout of low back pain.

Exercise 1 (Fig. 6-33). Lie flat on your back, flex your knees, and slowly allow them to fall to the floor in an extended position, limp and relaxed. Repeat 5 times. Purpose: To promote lumbar and hamstring elasticity.

Exercise 2 (Fig. 6-34). Lie on your back,

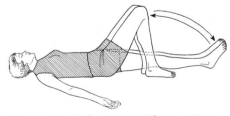

Fig. 6-33. Low Back Exercise. Phase 1, Exercise 1.

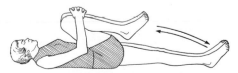

Fig. 6-34. Phase 1, Exercise 2.

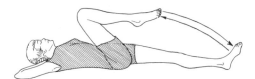

Fig. 6-35. Phase 1, Exercise 3.

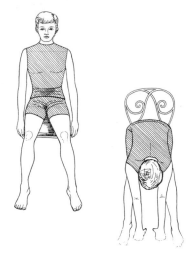

Fig. 6-37. Phase 1, Exercise 5.

flex your knees. Then bring both knees up to your chest, and with your hands clasped pull your knees toward your chest. Hold this position for a count of 10 and then return your legs to the starting position of lower extremity extension. Repeat this exercise 3 times. Purpose: To promote lumbar and hamstring elasticity.

Exercise 3 (Fig. 6-35). Lying on your back with legs flat on the floor, hands clasped behind your neck, raise one knee up as far as you can toward your chest. Maintain this position to the count of 10. Return the flexed leg to the neutral position and repeat the movement with the opposite leg until each leg has been flexed 5 times. Purpose: To promote lumbar, hamstring, and iliopsoas elasticity; to increase lower abdominal muscle strength.

Exercise 4 (Fig. 6-36). Lie on your back with your arms above your head and your knees bent. Flatten your back against the mat; at the same time contract the abdominal muscles. Maintain this position for a count of 10 and repeat 5 times. Purpose: To increase upper and lower abdominal muscle strength.

Exercise 5 (Fig. 6-37). Sit in a chair with your hands at your sides, drop your head down between your knees, and allow your hands to rest on the floor. Maintain this

position for a count of 3. Bring your body back up into a sitting position. Relax. Repeat the exercise 5 times. Purpose: To promote lumbar and hamstring elasticity; to increase lower back muscle strength.

Phase 1 exercises should be done twice daily for a period of 4 weeks. If, at the end of that period of time, no difficulty is encountered in carrying out the exercises, the patient may add on the next set of exercises in Phase 2.

PHASE 2

Exercise 1 (Fig. 6-38). Lying on the back, bring both knees up to a bent position with

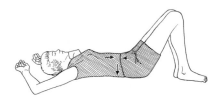

Fig. 6-36. Phase 1, Exercise 4.

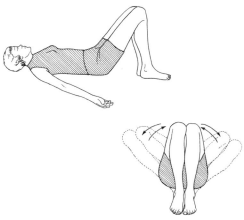

Fig. 6-38. Phase 2, Exercise 1.

feet resting on the floor. Rotate the pelvis and legs to the right and then to the left side of the body. Repeat 5 times. Purpose: To promote lumbar and hamstring elasticity.

Exercise 2 (Fig. 6-39). Lying on the back, raise feet 12 inches from the floor. Maintain this for a count of 10. Then slowly lower feet to the floor. Repeat 5 times. Purpose: To increase lower abdominal muscle strength.

Exercise 3 (Fig. 6-40). Stand erect while holding onto a table or chair. Squat down, straighten up again. Repeat 5 times. The table or chair should be used merely to maintain balance, not to help pull the body up into the erect position. Purpose: To increase quadriceps and muscle strength.

Exercise 4 (Fig. 6-41). Lying on the back with legs outstretched, straight leg raise one leg as far as possible without producing discomfort. Lower it slowly to the floor and straight leg raise the opposite leg. Repeat 5 times with each leg. Purpose: To promote lumbar, hamstring, and iliopsoas elasticity.

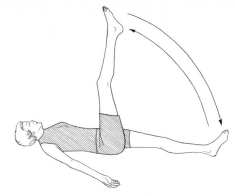

Fig. 6-41. Phase 2, Exercise 4.

Exercise 5 (Fig. 6-42). Lying on the back with both legs extended, bring the right foot up to the left knee, resting the heel and sole of the foot on the knee. Slowly rotate the flexed knee laterally as far as is comfortable, and then rotate the knee medially as far as is comfortable. Repeat the exercise with the opposite leg, alternating sides until the exercise has been done 5 times with each leg. Purpose: To promote hip rotator elasticity.

Exercise 6 (Fig. 6-43). Stand erect, relax your body by inhaling and exhaling deeply. Slowly flex the head and neck and allow the trunk to bend slowly forward from the hips with the knees straight. Try to touch the floor with your fingertips. Repeat 5 times. Purpose: To promote lumbar and hamstring elasticity.

Exercise 7 (Fig. 6-44). Kneel on one knee, place the opposite leg forward in a position of hip and knee flexion, and position both hands on the floor in front of the flexed leg.

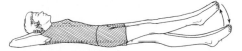

Fig. 6-39. Phase 2, Exercise 2.

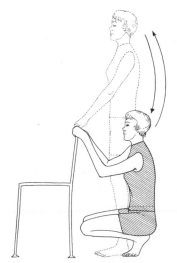

Fig. 6-40. Phase 2, Exercise 3.

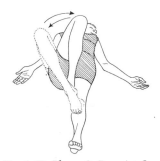

Fig. 6-42. Phase 2, Exercise 5.

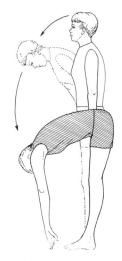

Fig. 6-43. Phase 2, Exercise 6.

Using the hands for balance, completely extend the posterior leg and rock back and forth 10 times. Repeat, alternating legs. The stretched hip flexors are those on the side of the extended leg.

The extent to which the iliopsoas stretching exercises are performed should be modified in accordance with the patient's clinical status.

The exercises in Phase 2 should be done twice daily for 4 months. At the end of that time, if these exercises can be done comfortably, the patient may go on to Phase 3.

"Pelvic Uptilt"

"Pelvic uptilt" maneuvers are an essential element in the Williams flexion exercises. These are a necessary and important part of

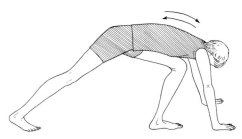

Fig. 6-44. Phase 2, Exercise 7.

the rehabilitative low back program when the patient manifests symptoms that are related to an increased lumbar lordosis. The patient who is not in need of lumbar flattening exercises is not likely to derive any benefit and may possibly suffer aggravation of pain resulting from these maneuvers. The following types of patients may be helped by lumbar flexion exercises:

1. The patient with marked increase in lumbar lordosis demonstrated by physical examination and roentgenograms.

2. The grossly obese patient with protuberant abdomen which tends to increase lumbar lordosis.

3. The patient in whom ambulation in a stooped-forward position of lumbar flexion is comfortable and an erect position is uncomfortable.

4. The patient for whom lying in a flat supine or prone position is painful and lying on the side with hips and knees flexed is not.

5. When testing lumbar mobility, the patient in whom lumbar flexion is less painful and more freely performed than lumbar extension, which is more painful and limited.

If the patient is confined to bed for the treatment of an acute attack of low back pain, the exercise may be initially performed in bed after the low back pain and muscle spasm have eased. As soon as the clinical status permits, the maneuver should be carried out on a firmer surface. After the "pelvic tuck" has been mastered in a supine position, it is practiced in the erect position, keeping in mind that the eventual object of the exercise is to flatten the lumbar lordosis.

The exercise is performed in a supine position with a pillow beneath the patient's head. When first practiced the hip and knees are well flexed, both feet flat on the floor, with the heels fairly close to the buttocks. The patient then presses his lumbar spine firmly against the floor by contracting the gluteal and abdominal muscles. After the lumbar spine is pressed against the floor, the pelvis is "tucked" or "uptilted" by raising the buttocks off the floor but maintaining the pressure of the lumbar spine against the floor (Fig. 6-45).

The most common patient error in this exercise is to elevate the lumbar spine from the floor along with the buttocks, thus effecting an adverse position of lumbar extension (lordosis) rather than the desired flexion (flattening). This maneuver should be performed 10 times twice daily and in time the number of tucks should be gradually increased until a fatigue plateau is reached. Patients over 50 years of age should have no difficulty doing 20 tucks 2 times daily. Younger patients may be able to do 40 tucks twice daily.

Gradually, over a variable period of time, the hip and knee flexion is reduced until complete extension of both legs is achieved. Extension of the lower extremities increases the lumbar extension action of the iliopsoas. As a result of the necessity to overcome this muscle antagonist, not only is greater exertion required to perform the exercise, but also a lesser degree of lumbar flexion is achieved than is possible in the flexed leg position. Only after the exercise has been performed with extended lower extremities for at least 4 weeks should it be practiced in the upright position.

When performing this maneuver in the upright position, most individuals prefer to press the lumbar spine against a wall to provide an area of body contact on which to measure the degree of lumbar flattening. Initially, this is best done with the feet 12 inches away from the wall to sufficiently reduce the opposing pull of the iliopsoas. With practice, the feet can usually be moved progressively closer to the wall until the heels are in direct contact with the wall.

PHASE 3. RECREATIONAL ACTIVITIES

Some years ago we had a phase 3 exercise program consisting of several relatively strenuous exercises which were selectively prescribed. In the past 5 years this has been abandoned in favor of encouraging the patient to participate in a suitable recreational or sporting activity of personal preference. The patient is more likely to continue with a gratifying activity in contrast to an exercise program, which is usually discontinued after the recollection of low back pain fades from memory.

Horseback riding and sport weightlifting are discouraged as being the two most detrimental activities for an individual with preexisting low back dysfunction. Golf and bowling, although not quite as inadvisable as riding or weightlifting, remain high on the list of sports best avoided. Enthusiasm for both of these recreations, especially golf, is often quite high, so the physician may be obliged to compromise, allowing the patient to participate while wearing a lumbosacral support. Tennis, which is a much more physically vigorous sport than either golf or bowling, seems to be more easily tolerated by the low back patient. Some speculate that tennis involves more stress upon the shoulder and upper extremity complex in comparison to the direct forceful lumbar torsion required by golf and bowling. Jogging for distances greater than a mile or two tends to bring to the fore symptoms of a preexisting musculoskeletal asymmetry or weakness. If the patient desires, it may be given a trial, but often it is not a particularly satisfactory sport for individuals with chronic low back dysfunction.

Swimming is often cited as the perfect sport for back pain patients because it is unique in being non-weightbearing. This is

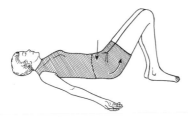

Fig. 6-45. "Pelvic uptilt." 1: Supine position, flex hips and knees. 2. Press lumbar spine firmly to the floor. 3. Maintaining pressure of the lumbar spine upon the floor, elevate the buttocks, uptilting the pelvis.

often a good choice and proves satisfactory. However, the body position assumed by some swimmers involves an increased lumbar lordosis, so a significant number of patients who turn to swimming as a cure for their backaches find that this activity produces an exacerbation of pain.

Bicycle riding is often well tolerated. Care should be taken to adjust the bicycle seat to achieve a slight lumbar flexion body position. Both ice and roller skating are often well tolerated, as is skiing.

All of the above recreational activities are to be started at a very minimal level and gradually increased. The minute anatomical variations characteristic of all individuals make any of these choices haphazard at best, so a cautious approach is advisable.

Low Back Supports and Braces

The use of low back supports in the form of braces or corsets must certainly extend beyond the limits of recorded history. It is almost instinctive for those who carry out heavy activities to wear heavy leather belts or to use other supporting measures. The Colorado State Hospital Museum in Denver contains a tree bark corset dating to about A.D. 900, originating from the pre-Columbian Indian cliff dwellings (Fig. 6-46).

The earliest spinal braces were cumbersome, but by the 12th century surgeons of the Bolognese school of Italy had constructed fairly effective spinal supports of simple design made of wood and metal.

During the past 150 years a voluminous literature has detailed a great number of braces and corsets made of a variety of materials.[1] In the 19th century, braces were designed in this country for the two most widely prevalent diseases of the spine: Pott's disease and scoliosis. The best-known spinal brace of American origin was designed by Charles Fayette Taylor in 1863, and was popularly referred to in that time as the "spinal assistant." The basic design and function of this brace is still utilized in various modifications in a number of braces

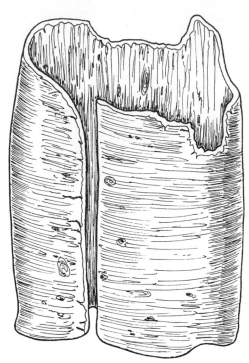

Fig. 6-46. Drawing of tree bark corset found in pre-Columbian Indian cliff dwellings. (Colorado State Historical Museum, Denver)

today. He utilized the now familiar three-point principle of support to produce hyperextension of the spine by exerting force backward at the hip and shoulders and forward in the middle of the back. Another commonly used brace of American origin is that designed by James Knight in 1884. This brace was originally designed as a supporting brace for tuberculosis; a later modification of this brace was used by Knight for treatment of scoliosis. The Taylor brace was one which produced hyperextension of the spine, while the Knight brace provided lateral support, preventing lateral and rotary movements and, therefore, is widely used for support of the lower lumbar spine. There are many modern modifications of this brace, and it is designated by various names. It is often referred to as the "chair back brace."

General Principles in the Use of Low Back Supports

A large proportion of those patients seen in our clinic who have had braces or corsets previously prescribed for them fall into two distinct categories. The "brown paper baggers" are those who employ paper sacks in which to carry the appliance, which may be of variable vintage but often reveals few signs of wear. As a rule, the corset is brought in by this category of patient primarily for the purpose of demonstrating what was not beneficial to them in the past and to indicate that they are not especially interested in receiving another support in the future. The other extreme is the patient who wears a frayed, dilapidated corset and upon removing it, displays permanent cutaneous signs of long-standing appliance wear. It is this second category of patient who often states, "I can't get along without my brace," and their primary purpose is to obtain a replacement for their threadbare and weatherbeaten support. If it appears that such a renewal will make the patient happy, and the patient is over the age of 50, order it. Conversely if the patient objects to wearing a corset or brace don't order one.

This advice will seem somewhat sophomoric and simplistic but may be helpful. All back supports are to some degree irksome. A patient who states an objection to a low back support in advance is likely to find it excessively vexing and will not wear it. The second category of patient who is physically and psychologically dependent on a low back support should theoretically be placed on a rehabilitative exercise program to improve muscle tone so that the support can be eliminated. My experience with this approach has been disappointing with the older individual. When such a patient is weaned away from the support, the incidence of incapacitating exacerbations increases.

LOW BACK MECHANICS

The spine stripped of its musculature may be considered a modified elastic rod. It has an intrinsic stability resulting from the pressure of the nucleus pulposus pushing the vertebral bodies apart and opposed by the annulus which holds the bodies together.

When the isolated spine is maintained in the erect position, the heaviest load it can sustain without buckling is 4 or 5 pounds. This is illustrated by the anesthetized patient who cannot maintain a sitting position unless externally supported. The spine, thus, cannot function without the extrinsic stability provided by the paraspinal and abdominal musculature.

Compression tests have been carried out on isolated spinal segments. In a young adult, the intervertebral disc will yield and be deformed at pressures exceeding 1400 pounds and in older individuals will yield at about 350 pounds. The vertebral body of a young adult will yield at a compressive force of between 1000 and 1300 pounds, whereas in the elderly, failure can occur at only 300 pounds. Vertebral body fracture will take place before failure of the intervertebral disc.

These tests clearly demonstrate that single severe stresses subjecting the spine to a compressive force of 300 to 1000 pounds are likely to produce vertebral body fracture. Yet with strenuous activity, forces theoretically far exceeding 1400 pounds may be applied to the lower lumbar vertebral bodies and intervertebral discs. An understanding of the mechanism whereby the spine can withstand these forces derives from study of the trunk musculature. By increasing the pressures within the thoracic and abdominal cavities during strenuous activities, trunk muscle contraction can convert the trunk into a fairly rigid cylinder. With the accompanying increase in intercavitary pressure, the load on the lower lumbar intervertebral discs is diminished by at least 30%. Based on the same principle, the load on the low lumbar spine can be reduced drastically by wearing a tight abdominal corset.

Electrical activity of trunk musculature studied during lifting. Muscle contraction and intercavitary pressure are found to increase proportionately with the load being lifted. However, when wearing a corset results in abdominal compression, the electrical activity of the abdominal muscles markedly decreases. This would indicate diminished contraction of the abdominal muscles in the presence of external support. It may also be true that prolonged wearing of such a support will result in muscle atrophy. This suggests that a proper program for a patient with low back dysfunction should include abdominal and postural exercises with the corset being considered a temporary expedient to be ultimately supplanted by the strengthened abdominal and trunk muscles.

IMMOBILIZATION—FACT OR FANCY

A spinal support exerts some immobolizing effects upon the spinal segment which it contains. However, Norton and Brown have shown that motion tends to be increased in the segments adjacent to the ends of the appliance. They further demonstrated increased lumbosacral motion in some subjects when a long spinal brace was worn.[3] It follows that the use of a brace following lumbosacral fusion may actually increase motion at a site where immobilization is being sought. In an effort to hold down this compensatory increase in motion, supports have been designed to extend well down onto the pelvis and to grip it firmly. This is an important consideration in prescribing an appliance for lumbosacral pathology.

The lower the lumbar spine lesion, the greater the problem involved in splinting that lesion. The lowest level of the brace is limited since we must allow hip joint immobility and permit the patient to sit. It is essential that the inferior border of the brace extend as far below the lumbosacial joint as possible so that the steel paravertebral supports do not produce an adverse leverage on this specific joint.

FITTING SUPPORTS

In fitting supports consideration should be given to comfort, convenience, and patient acceptance. Pressure is necessary in order to achieve the effects desired. The discomfort of pressure can be lessened by reducing its force or by increasing the surface area on which it acts. Bony prominences and superficial structures should be avoided or carefully padded. An appliance should be contour-fitted so that no sharp edge concentrates compression. The effects of pressure should be evaluated during motion as well as rest. Sliding movements of spinal supports which apply sheer forces and may produce tension on underlying tissues or produce skin abrasion can be minimized by proper contour and fit. The use of low friction materials or the wearing of the support over some clothing is helpful. Moisture adds to the undesirable effects of friction and can be minimized by the use of a brace rather than a corset, and by the use of perforated or absorbent material. An appliance should be designed to permit easy application and removal. Buckles and straps used today are of improved design. The increasing use of Velcro to fasten the apron of the brace permits easy removal for laundering. Materials should be lightweight and durable as well as easy to keep clean and odor-free. The patient should be carefully instructed in the application and removal of the appliance, as well as in how to clean it.

Cosmetic considerations deserve attention in the design so that the appliance will be as inconspicuous as possible. Female patients in particular may either refuse to wear a brace or wear it only sporadically unless it is cosmetically acceptable.

PURPOSES OF A SPINAL SUPPORT

A spinal support is designed to:

1. Limit spinal motion.
2. Correct posture.
3. Diminish mechanical stress on lower lumbar spine.

A corset or brace is indicated when it is desired to achieve one or more of these effects.

BRACE VERSUS CORSET

A brace differs from a corset only in having horizontal rigid elements. In all other respects they are similar. Corsets may be made fairly rigid by the addition of paraspinal steels. A brace and a corset may be combined to obtain the advantages of both.

Advantages of a brace:

1. Limits motion to a greater degree.
2. Allows better lumbar positional control.
3. Limits lateral and rotary motion.

Advantages of a corset:

1. More acceptable cosmetically, especially under a dress.
2. Better control over obesity; improved support when patient is obese.
3. Usually lighter than a brace.
4. Thought, by some, to be less likely to weaken muscles with long-term use.
5. Often more acceptable to elderly patients.
6. More likely to provide abdominal compression.

Although both devices may benefit the same condition, it should be recognized that the beneficial effects of each are created by dissimilar mechanisms. The brace acts principally by limiting spinal mobility, and the corset by creating an abdominal binder effect (Fig. 6-47). The binder not only increases

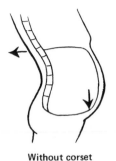 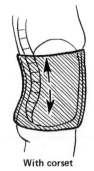

Without corset   With corset

Fig. 6-47. The abdominal binder effect of a corset flattens out the protuberant abdomen.

intra-abdominal pressure which will diminish the weightbearing load on the intervertebral disc, but it also flattens out the protuberant abdomen; this mechanical action will reduce the lumbar lordosis.

Selection of the proper device must be based on both the condition to be treated and the patient's somatotype (Fig. 6-48). The obese patient with a protuberant abdomen is best treated with a corset. The narrow-waisted individual with wide iliac crests and a flared-out rib cage will not receive an adequate abdominal binder effect with a corset and is better served with a brace.

A consideration of the characteristics of specific braces and corsets in relation to the particular low back dysfunction and the type of patient will permit selection of the proper appliance. The four most commonly prescribed appliances are the lumbosacral support, Knight spinal brace, Williams brace, and the Knight-Taylor brace.

Braces

"THREE-POINT PRESSURE" PRINCIPLE

Braces designed to support the lumbar spine are constructed in accordance with the three-point pressure principle described by Henry H. Jordan in his text, "Orthopedic Appliances."[2] He proposed that the supporting forces of an effective brace must be applied from three directions (Fig. 6-49). For example, the three forces may consist of: (a) a backward thrust against the pelvis anteriorly, (b) a backward thrust against the thoracic cage anteriorly, (c) a forward thrust over the lumbar spine posteriorly.

The particular location of the three forces may vary. In the Williams lordosis brace, for example, the components are reversed with two forces posteriorly at the (a) low thoracic level, and the (b) sacral region, opposing the single force anteriorly at the (c) lower abdomen (Fig. 6-50).

In all instances, however, the sum of the two forces should be equal to the single

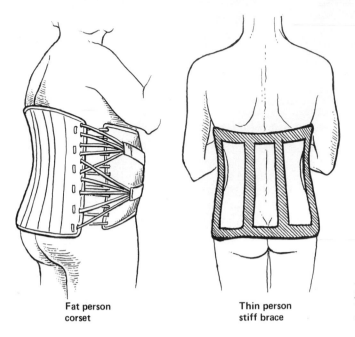

Fat person corset

Thin person stiff brace

Fig. 6-48. The obese patient benefits most from a corset. The narrow-waisted individual with wide iliac crests and a flared-out rib cage benefits most from a brace.

force, which should be located approximately midway between the two opposing forces.

KNIGHT SPINAL BRACE

The Knight spinal brace, currently the most widely used brace, is a metal frame made up of two lumbar posterior and two lateral uprights attached to a pelvic band below and a thoracic band above (Fig. 6-51). It has an abdominal apron fastened with three pairs of straps. The Knight spinal brace limits flexion, extension, and lateral trunk motion, as well as providing abdominal compression.

WILLIAMS BRACE

The Williams brace, also called the Williams Lordosis Brace, consists of a pelvic band, a thoracic band, a pair of lateral uprights pivoting on the thoracic band, and a pair of oblique lateral uprights pivoting on the vertical lateral uprights and rigidly attached to the pelvic band (Fig. 6-52). There is an abdominal or corset front and a pelvic strap. This rather unusual support limits lumbar lordosis or extension and lateral tilt. The adjustable three-point pressure system restrictively diminishes the lumbar lordosis, and the corset front increases the intra-abdominal pressure. Unlike most spinal braces which are primarily supportive in nature, the Williams brace is specifically designed to "exert a constant corrective force on the lumbar spine" by restrictively reducing the lumbar lordosis.

TAYLOR BRACE

The Taylor brace is made up of two thoracolumbar posterior uprights attached to a pelvic band (Fig. 6-53). The uprights are secured by an intrascapular bar to which axillary straps are attached. There is a corset or abdominal front. This is a hyperextension brace which limits trunk flexion in the thoracolumbar area and slightly in the lumbar area.

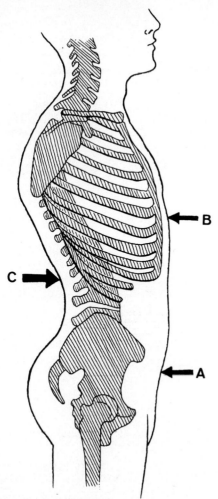

Fig. 6-49. Diagrammatic illustration of the three-point-pressure principle in design of spinal braces.

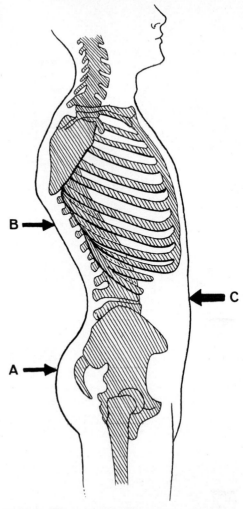

Fig. 6-50. Diagrammatic illustration of the three-point-pressure principle in design of the Williams lordosis brace.

Corsets

Corsets are constructed of fabric reinforced with flexible or rigid stays. They are adjusted by side or back lacing. Side lacing provides firmer back support and permits the addition of heavy steels posteriorly for contouring and reinforcement. The lacing should be capable of being securely tightened with some reserve reamining. A properly fitted corset does not require perineal straps to hold it in place.

TROCHANTER BELT

The trochanter belt ranges from 1 to 3 inches in width and is worn within the iliac crest and the greater trochanter (Figs. 6-54 and 6-55). It acts to support the sacroiliac joints by strengthening the pelvic ring and preventing excessive stress. Some believe it tilts the pelvis forward. The wearing of such an appliance, or a similarly fitting snug leather belt, has long been a practice of laborers. (*Text continues on p. 240.*)

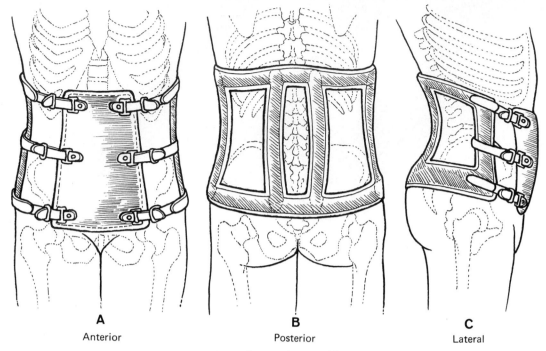

A
Anterior

B
Posterior

C
Lateral

Fig. 6-51. The Knight spinal brace.

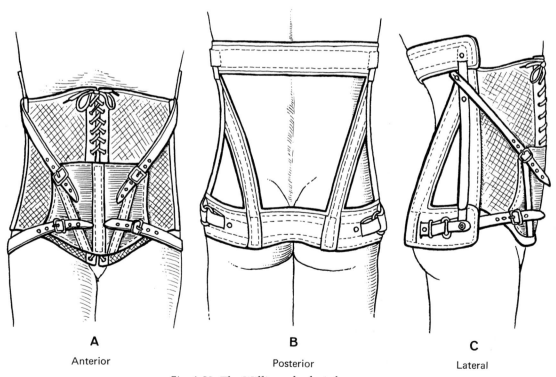

A
Anterior

B
Posterior

C
Lateral

Fig. 6-52. The Williams lordosis brace.

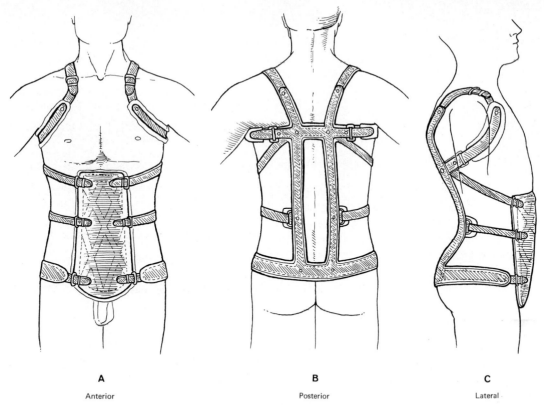

A	B	C
Anterior	Posterior	Lateral

Fig. 6-53. The Taylor spinal brace.

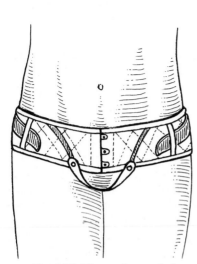

Fig. 6-54. The trochanter belt.

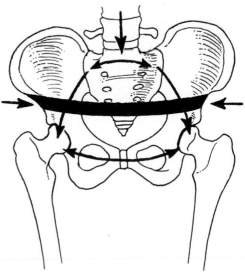

Fig. 6-55. Pelvic arch support furnished by the "hoop action" of an encircling belt about the pelvis.

SACROILIAC CORSET

The sacroiliac corset is somewhat wider but serves much the same purpose as a trochanter belt (Fig. 6-56).

LUMBOSACRAL CORSET

The lumbosacral corset is the most commonly used of all appliances (Fig. 6-57). It should extend well above the dorsal lumbar junction in the back, be contoured to the upper buttocks below and extend down to the upper thighs in women. Side lacing is preferred together with paravertebral steels to diminish the lumbar lordosis.'

Most of the lumbosacral supports are reinforced with two steel posterior stays which are not flexibile. These are uniformly shaped to follow the spinal configuration of a normal lumbar lordosis. The patients who are in need of this appliance usually have considerable alteration of the normal spinal curvature, demonstrating some degree of lumbar flattening or a lumbar scoliosis in association with severe paraspinal muscle

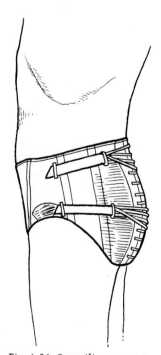

Fig. 6-56. Sacroiliac support.

spasm. The pressure of these unyielding curved stays on the somewhat tender, spastic paraspinal muscles may be an added source of discomfort. Rather than molding the lumbar spine into the desired normal configuration, quite the reverse may be accomplished. However, many patients who have been unable to tolerate a reinforced lumbosacral support are surprised by the relief this garment provides after the rigid posterior stays have been removed. I usually order a nonreinforced lumbosacral support with flexible plastic stays posteriorly. These function primarily to maintain the shape of the garment, preventing it from rolling down on itself.

DORSOLUMBAR CORSET

The dorsolumbar corset is similar in construction to the sacroiliac corset (Fig. 6-58). It extends up the back over the scapulae and is additionally secured by shoulder straps.

Less Frequently Used Supports

Less frequently used supports are those molded of leather, plastic of paris, or plastic materials. These have the advantages or precise fit, the widest possible distribution of pressure, light weight, and, in the case of plastics, ease of cleaning. The molded leather jacket has the disadvantage, however, of absorbing perspiration (with attendant odor) and of being difficult to clean.

PLASTER BODY JACKET

Twenty or 30 years ago the plaster body jacket was used with greater frequency than is the case today (Fig. 6-59). It is not an easy plaster to apply, and either a low back support or bed rest will approximate most of its benefits. Possibly a properly applied cast will provide greater immobilization of the lumbar spine and may be of use in the refractory situation.

The plaster body jacket should fit snugly

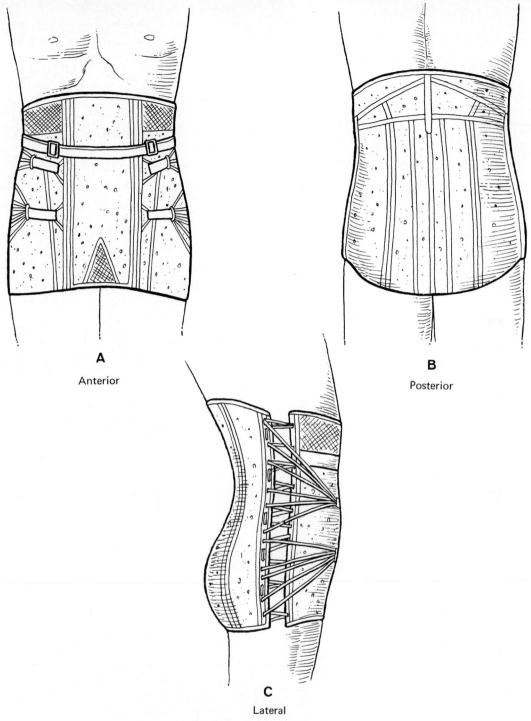

A

Anterior

B

Posterior

C

Lateral

Fig. 6-57. Lumbosacral support.

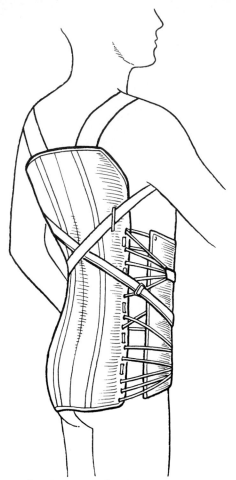

Fig. 6-58. Dorsolumbar support.

with all pressure points well protected. During application, the lumbar lordosis is flattened by having the patient stand with one foot elevated on a short stool. To prevent the jacket from sliding up and down when the patient changes position, it should fit snugly over the iliac crest and the inferior margin of the rib cage. The plaster should be contoured against the anterior abdominal wall, so that by increasing the abdominal pressure, a reduction in weightbearing stress on the spine will occur.

Negative Effects of a Low Back Support

When utilizing a brace or corset we should be aware of the adverse effects that can be created by such an appliance.

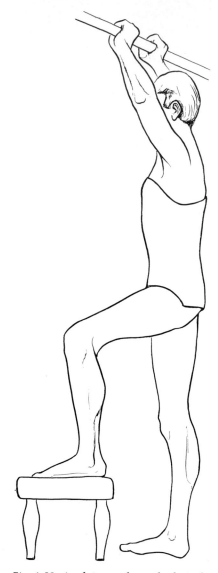

Fig. 6-59. Applying a plaster body jacket.

1. Muscle weakness and atrophy of disuse may result from reduced functional demands.

2. The limitations of mobility imposed by the various appliances may reduce the suppleness and elasticity of the muscles and tendons relating to the integrity of the spine. Such soft tissue contracture may give rise to a new source of pain.

3. Psychological dependence on a low back support may persist long beyond the mechanical need for the appliance. Since

both muscle weakness and soft tissue contractures are related to duration of use, this nonorganic reaction can eventually lead to organic changes.

With the above three adverse effects in mind, every device should be prescribed with a plan to eliminate it. This treatment plan should incorporate all of the rehabilitative measures necessary for satisfactory low back hygiene.

Suggested Readings for Part 2

1. Cailliet R: Low Back Pain Syndrome. Philadelphia, FA Davis, 1968

2. Krusen FH, Kottke FJ, Ellwood TM: Handbook of Physical Medicine and Rehabilitation. Philadelphia, WB Saunders, 1971
3. Licht S (ed): Therapeutic Heat and Cold. New Haven, Elicabeth Licht, 1965

References to Part 3

1. Edward JW: Orthopaedic Appliances Atlas. I. Ann Arbor, American Academy of Orthopaedic Surgeons, 1952
2. Jordan HH: Orthopedic Appliances. New York, Oxford University Press, 1939
3. Norton PL, Brown T: The immobilizing efficiency of back braces. J Bone Joint Surg 39A (1), 1957

Spinal Manipulative Therapy in the Management of Low Back Pain

7

Scott Haldeman

Spinal Manipulative Therapy (SMT), also referred to as manipulation, manual therapy, or manual medicine, can be broadly defined as including all procedures where the hands are used to mobilize, adjust, manipulate, apply traction, massage, stimulate or otherwise influence the spine and paraspinal tissues with the aim of influencing the patient's health. Some form of spinal manipulation has been utilized by clinicians since ancient times and has been referred to in the writings of such prominent physicians as Hippocrates (400 B.C.), Galen (130–120 B.C.), Avicenna (980–1037), Ambriose Pare (1510–1590), Percivall Pott (1715–1788), Sir James Paget (1844–1899), and many others.[54,75] Primitive forms of manipulation of the spine appear to have been available and widely used by almost every society in recorded history, from the ancient Romans, Greeks, Japanese, and South American civilizations, through the Middle Ages, including the folk medicines of India, Egypt, Bohemia, China, and Finland, to modern times.[28,54,74,75] Throughout history and in almost every society, there has been a physician with the interest and skill to provide spinal manipulation as a service.

In modern times these services are provided by chiropractors, osteopathic physicians and a small but growing number of medically trained physicians and physical therapists. There has been, and presumably will continue to be, some conflict between practitioners of different training. There continue to be differences in the skill, standards of practice, and theoretical emphasis among clinicians who practice SMT. However, the trend over the past decade has been towards investigating the clinical efficacy of SMT and determining its mechanism of action. This has led to a better understanding of the relative value of the various theories and techniques of manipulation and to a convergence of opinions, although by no means total agreement, on its role in health care.

Clinical Efficacy

Over 90,000,000 patient visits are made each year in the United States to chiropractors by an estimated 3.6 to 5.5% of the population.[16,36] This figure increases significantly if other practitioners of manipulation are included. Over 50% of these office visits are for low back pain.[5,84] It is not unexpected, therefore, that the main thrust of clinical research into the effectiveness of SMT has been in the area of low back pain.

The reports from uncontrolled prospective and retrospective case studies have been difficult to interpret.[37,61,63] The percentage of patients with low back pain who respond favorably to spinal manipulation varies from 51% in patients hospitalized for low back pain to over 90% in patients seen in a private

245

practitioner's office.[3,12,24] The relative importance of manipulative skills and patient selection in explaining this difference is not clear.[37]

However, a number of recently conducted controlled clinical trials have been published which compare the results of manipulation to a number of placebo treatments for low back pain. These trials have been summarized in Table 7-1 where the most optimistic results from the various papers have been quoted. In many cases, these results were not seen on reexamination of patients after different periods of treatment,[7,19] In others, only certain populations of patients with back pain responded this well.[21,31] For specific criticisms of this research, one can refer to papers by Nachemson, Haldeman, and Greenland and associates.[35,37,63]

Detuned ultrasound has been considered the most viable placebo by both Glover and colleagues and Bergquist-Ullman and Larsson.[1,31] In the former study, manipulation was significantly more effective than the placebo only in those paitents who had their pain for less than 7 days. This disappointing result may have been due to the use of a relatively crude long lever manipulation in these trials. The results of Bergquist-Ullman and Larsson, on the other hand, showed significant improvement in the clinical results observed with the use of more specific articulating and mobilization techniques when compared to a placebo treatment. The patients who received manipulation complained of less pain after 6 weeks, required less sick leave following treatment, and had a decreased tendency to change their occupation. Manipulation combined with physiotherapy, however, was not found to be significantly more effective than a very sophisticated and well-organized patient education program or back school. It would be interesting to see whether manipulation combined with the back school (the more logical approach) would improve on the results of each applied separately. When compared to bedrest an analgesia, analgesia alone, short wave therapy, or heat, exercise and massage, manipulation appears to be a significantly more effective method of treating low back pain.[15,21,23,71] The only study in which the authors felt that there was no significant difference between the effectiveness of manipulation and the other conservative forms of treatment for low back pain is that by Doran and Newell.[19] At least one reevaluation of their statistics has suggested that manipulation was indeed significantly more effective than the other treatment modalities after 3 weeks.[35]

The study by Buerger and associates has helped to rule out the psychological effect of laying on of hands.[6,7] By selecting patients who were unable to tell the difference between a manipulative thrust and simple massage, it was possible to demonstrate that there is something intrinsic to the manipulation which can cause improvement of symptoms in patients with low back pain.

Indications for Manipulation

One of the difficulties most clinicians experience is the selection of patients who might benefit from manipulative therapy. This difficulty is due, in part, to the current poor understanding of the pathogenesis of back pain and the unsophisticated techniques available for examining the spine. Many authorities feel that the breakdown of back pain into numerous different diagnostic categories is not valid.[62] Nonetheless, practitioners of manipulation have found varying results in patients diagnosed as having different symptom complexes or specifically diagnosed origins of their pain. Table 7-2 lists a few of the proposed causes of low back pain thought to respond to spinal manipulation.

Uncomplicated Low Back Pain

This nonspecific diagnostic category is used to include those patients with low back pain of recent onset in the absence of leg pain or radicular signs. It is this category of

Table 7-1. COMPARATIVE AND CONTROLLED TRIALS ON THE EFFECTIVENESS OF MANIPULATION IN PATIENTS WITH LOW BACK PAIN (% IMPROVED)

Author	Time Period	Manip- ulation	Analgesia + Bedrest	Heat Massage Exercise	(+) or (−) Short Wave	Physio- therapy	Back- school	Massage	Corsets	Comments
Coyer and Curwen (1955)	1 week / 6 weeks	55% / 88%	27% / 72%							no statistics
Rasmussen (1979)	2 weeks	92%			25%					$p < 0.01$
Evans et al (1978)	3 weeks	60%	18%							$p < 0.05$
Edwards (1969)	not mentioned	84%		68%						aggregate of results
Doran and Newell (1975)	3 weeks / 3 months	64% / 71%	49% / 56%			52% / 67%			49% / 68%	$p = 0.5$ N.S.
Glover et al (1947)	immediate / 7 days	43% / 85%			12% / 70%					$p < 0.05$ N.S.
Sims-Williams et al (1978)	1 month	90%			73%					$p < 0.1$
Buerger et al (1979)	immediate effect	83%						67%		$p < 0.003$
Bergquist-Ullman and Larsson (1977)	1 year	40%			29%		36%			% without recurrence

Where different types of assessment or multiple assessments at different times periods were done, the most favorable results from manipulation are quoted. References should be checked for details.

Table 7-2. THE INDICATIONS FOR
MANIPULATION IN PATIENTS WITH
LOW BACK PAIN

Patients Reported to Respond to SMT

Uncomplicated low back pain (lumbago)
Sciatica without neurological deficit
Uncomplicated chronic low back pain
Post surgical chronic low back pain
Intervertebral disc degeneration, type IV, bulging disc
Intervertebral disc degeneration, type V, sequestered
  fragment
Posterior facet syndrome
Scaroiliac syndrome
Sacroiliac strain
Piriformis syndrome
Psoas syndrome
Spondylolisthesis
Spinal stenosis: central stenosis and lateral entrapment

patients which Glover and associates found to be significantly more responsive to a single long lever rotatory manipulation than to a placebo treatment.[31] The significance was most noticeable immediately after the manipulation was given. The patients who responded to manipulation in the trial by Bergquist-Ulllman and Larsson had a median duration of symptoms of less than 9 days prior to entering their trial.[1] Potter similarly noted that patients with acute back pain had the highest response rate, with 93% of such patients either fully recovered or much improved following manipulation.[68] The classic comic strip or TV characterization of spinal manipulation, where an individual with an acute catch in his back is "straightened" with immediate relief, falls under this heading.

Complicated Acute Low Back Pain

These patients complain of low back pain of recent onset with either leg pain or neurological deficits. Leg pain or sciatica appears to respond very well to spinal manipulation.[26,55] Both Potter and Edwards found that over 75% of patients with pain radiating into the buttock or down the leg recovered or improved considerably following spinal manipulation.[21,68] Painful limited straight leg raising was one of the objective parameters shown to improve following spinal

manipulation in the blinded clinical trial by Buerger.[6] When frank neurological deficit is present, many practitioners of manipulation become much more cautious.[17,26] Most of the trials quoted earlier excluded patients with such deficits. Where patients with acute neurological deficit have been subjected to spinal manipulation, the results have been less rewarding.[12,68]

Uncomplicated Chronic Low Back Pain

The only report which compares the results of SMT in patients with acute and chronic back pain is that by Potter.[68] His conclusion, that chronic pain is less responsive than acute pain, is not surprising. He did, however, claim that 71% of patients classified as having uncomplicated chronic low back pain showed improvement of their symptoms. Similarly, Riches claims that 86% of patients diagnosed as having chronic back strain improved following manipulation.[73] The results of SMT on patients referred to a university hospital for chronic back pain reported by Kirkaldy-Willis and Cassidy varied greatly depending on the pathogenetic diagnosis, but in all cases over 65% of patients showed some degree of improvement.[44] It should be remembered that this group of patients, by defintion, was not recovering spontaneously.

Complicated Chronic Low Back Pain

The comments made concerning patients with acute low back pain complicated by leg pain or neurological deficit apply equally well to the patient with chronic back pain. Potter found that chronic leg pain improved in approximately 70% of patients treated with SMT; the number of successes decreased considerably when neurological signs were present.[68] One interesting aspect of this study was the observation that previous back surgery did not significantly alter the results and therefore did not serve as a contraindication to manipulation.

Disc Degeneration or Herniation

The effect of spinal manipulation on intervertebral disc disease is a controversial one. Cyriax feels that the primary effect of manipulation is the reduction of nuclear protrusions in the disc.[17] Matthews and Yates claim to have demonstrated the reduction of disc prolapses by epidurography.[57] On the other hand, Chrisman and associates found the results of manipulation in patients with disc protrusion demonstrable by myelography to be much poorer than in patients with normal myelograms.[12] They were unable to demonstrate any reduction in positive myelogram findings following manipulation. Kirkaldy-Willis and Cassidy were similarly unimpressed with the results of manipulation in patients with demonstrable nucleus pulposis herniation.[44] Nonetheless, manipulation is being widely recommended for patients diagnosed as having intervertebral disc degeneration without frank herniation or neurological deficit.[17,78,85]

Posterior Facet Syndrome

Mennell, Lewit, and Gillet are among the many practitioners of spinal manipulation who believe that the primary effect of manipulation is the mobilization of "fixated" or "blocked" posterior facet joints.[29,51,59] The basis for this supposition is the mostly subjective impression that there is an increase in the mobility of the spine following manipulation. In the differentiation of patients with chronic back pain by Kirkaldy-Willis and Cassidy, 72% of patients diagnosed as having posterior facet syndrome improved following manipulation.[44]

Sacroiliac Syndromes

Some of the best results from spinal manipulation have been reported in patients where the diagnosis of sacroiliac syndrome has been made. Both Kirkaldy-Willis and Cassidy and Riches claim that over 90% of patients with this diagnosis show improvement in their back pain following manipulation.[44,73] Many practitioners of manipulation place a great deal of emphasis on the analysis of sacroiliac motion and position and choose their manipulation technique according to these findings.[30,33,53] If one makes the diagnosis of sacroiliac syndrome, manipulation appears to be a very effective method of treatment.

Muscle Syndromes

A variety of muscles have been implicated in the genesis of back pain including piriformis, psoas, quadratus lumborum, and the long paraspinal muscles.[58,83] Specific manipulation techniques have been developed with the aim of stretching or manually massaging these muscles in an attempt to relax them. The importance of these muscle syndromes in the genesis of back pain remains speculative. Still, when diagnosed, the treatment of choice is either manipulation or the injection of a local anesthetic.

Spondylolisthesis

Back pain associated with spondylolisthesis was found to improve through spinal manipulation in 85% of cases reviewed by Kirkaldy-Willis and Cassidy and Cassidy and colleagues.[10,44] These authors made it quite clear that no claim was being made that spinal manipulation influenced the spondylolisthesis itself. Instead, they speculated that in most cases the spondylolisthesis was an incidental finding. Care was taken by these clinicians to avoid any direct force at the area of slippage. Manipulations were, instead, directed at the sacroiliac joint or the posterior joints above the level of slippage. The one point which appears to arise from this observation is that spondylolisthesis is not a contraindication to nontraumatic specific short level manipulations in skilled hands.

Spinal Stenosis

As one would expect, the results of manipulation in patients whose low back pain is diagnosed as being due to spinal stenosis is not good. What is surprising is that any such patients respond. Kirkaldy-Willis and Cassidy and Potter reported that a significant number of patients with either lateral spinal nerve entrapment or central spinal stenosis showed some improvement following manipulation.[44,69] Very few of these patients, however, became symptom free. Further case reports on the beneficial effects of manipulation in patients with neurogenic claudication thought to be due to spinal stenosis have been presented by Henderson.[39] The relief these patients obtain from SMT is usually only temporary.

Contraindications to Manipulation

Spinal manipulative therapy should not be considered a totally innocuous procedure. Although there are less than 100 reported cases where serious complications of manipulative therapy have occurred, these complications are often quite devastating.[46,52] Extreme care should therefore be taken in the selection of patients and the choice of manipulative techniques in order to minimize their occurrence.

By far the major portion of severe complications arises from injury to the cerebral circulation or spinal cord following cervical manipulation.[2,46,79] Injuries from lumbar spine manipulation are much less common. The most frequent complication is the prolapse of a herniated intervertebral disc resulting in a cauda equina syndrome.[41,72,78] These complications are probably due to the use of long-lever, high force rotational manipulative techniques in the side lying position.[46] The other commonly encountered complication of lumbar rotational or thoracic manipulation is spraining of the costovertebral or costochondral joints. These

Table 7-3. THE CONTRAINDICATIONS FOR MANIPULATION OF THE LUMBAR SPINE

Contraindications for High Velocity Manipulation Techniques

Unstable fractures
Severe osteoporosis
Multiple myeloma
Osteomyelitis
Primary bone tumors
Metastatic bone tumors
Paget's disease
Any progressive neurological deficit
Spinal cord tumors
Cauda equina compression
Central intervertebral disc herniations
Hypermobile joints
Rheumatoid arthritis
Inflammatory phase of ankylosing spondylitis
Psoriatic arthritis
Reiter's syndrome
Anticoagulant therapy
Congenital bleeding disorders
Acquired bleeding disorders
Inadequate physical and spinal examination
Poor manipulative skills

Under certain circumstances soft tissue, nonforce manipulation or mobilization procedures may still be possible.

painful incidents are again usually due to poor technique.[46,55]

The contraindications for manipulation of the lumbar spine, as listed in Table 7-3, for the most part are based on common sense. They include the following symptoms or disorders.

Weakening of Bone Structure

Unstable fractures, severe osteoporosis, osteomyelitis, multiple myeloma, bony tumors, or any other disorder which results in weakened bone structure is the most obvious contraindication to spinal manipulation.

Severe or Progressive Neurological Deficits

There is some debate as to whether or not spinal manipulation should be applied to patients showing minor stable signs of radicular injury. However, many practitioners of manipulation would not be inhibited from using light mobilization or traction maneuvers in such patients. Patients with signs of progressive neurological loss, acute cauda equina compression, or a spinal cord lesion, on the other hand, may require immediate surgical intervention and should not be subjected to any form of manipulative therapy until fully evaluated.

Acute Inflammatory Joint Disease

The forceful manipulation of any joint which is acutely inflamed can be very painful. This is also true of the sacroiliac and posterior spinal articulations. For this reason, patients with such disorders as rheumatoid arthritis, ankylosing spondylitis, psoriatic arthritis, or Reiter's disease should be carefully evaluated for any sign of acute inflammation of the spinal joints before manipulation is attempted. The ligamentous laxity and joint instability that can result from these disorders may also serve as contraindications to manipulation in the dormant stage of the arthritis, especially when this occurs in the cervical spine.[46]

Bleeding Disorders

Manipulation of patients on anticoagulant therapy can cause intraspinal hematoma formation.[18] Therefore, patients who are on anticoagulant therapy or who have a clotting abnormality, either inherited or acquired (e.g., liver disease) should not be subjected to any forceful manipulations.

Inadequate Examination or Manipulative Skills

Perhaps one of the greatest problems in manipulation today is the attempt by clinicians to apply these techniques without any formal training. The reading of a textbook or attendance at a weekend course does not convert an untrained clinician into a skilled practitioner of SMT. Many of the reported injuries following spinal manipulation can be attributed to inadequate examination to rule out contraindications or

the use of crude, long-lever, high force techniques. In the same way, many of the disappointing results from manipulation which have been reported were with the use of primitive, nonspecific manipulation techniques. Like any other skilled procedure, the expected results and number of complications is dependent on the ability of the clinician. Lack of examination and manipulative skills should therefore be considered a contraindication to SMT.

The Manipulable Spinal Lesion

Both practitioners and critics of manipulation have shown extreme ingenuity in the formulation of theories which might explain the clinical results of SMT. In the past, and to a lesser extent even today, practitioners of SMT could be separated into different schools (or professions) depending on the particular theory which was followed. The major theories on which manipulation is based include the reduction of disc prolapse, the correction of posterior joint dysfunction, the mobilization of fixated or blocked vertebral joints, the reduction of nerve root compression, the normalizations of reflex activity, and the relaxation of muscles.[17,29,48,51,56,59,66,67] These theories have been the subject of debate at a number of recent conferences.[8,32,38,49] These references can be referred to for details. It is sufficient here to state that, at this point, the mechanism by which manipulation relieves pain is unknown.

One way of reviewing the principles on which spinal manipulation is based is to look at the clinical characteristics of the lesion to which the manipulation is applied. Despite the wide variation in the theorized mechanism of action of SMT, there is an amazing amount of agreement on the clinical nature of the manipulable spinal lesion. This lesion, also referred to as the "subluxation," "osteopathic lesion," "vertebral fixation or blockage," or "area of spinal or somatic dysfunction," has the five characteristics described below.

Vertebral Malposition

Repeated studies on large groups of patients have shown that there is no relationship between vertebral malposition and low back pain.[50,60] Nevertheless, many practitioners of manipulation continue to make fine measurements of vertebral positional relationships prior to manipulation. The prime reason for determining these relationships, in practice, is to determine the direction in which the manipulative thrust should be given, rather than to determine the level of pathology. If the slope of the facets and the position of the vertebrae are known, a much smaller, less traumatic force can be given to correct the manipulable lesion.

The so-called "listing" of the position of a vertebra is determined by measuring the direction in which the disc is wedged and noting the position of the spinous process in relation to its body.[33,77] Figure 7-1 illustrates four of the classic spinal listings and demonstrates how such a listing might influence the direction in which a manipulation would be given. The significance and importance of these listings have yet to be evaluated. However, clinicians who take into account structural relationships of the vertebrae are convinced that this makes them capable of administering a more specific manipulation with greater ease and less trauma to the patient.

Abnormal Vertebral Motion

Perhaps the most widely held view on the primary effect of manipulation is that it

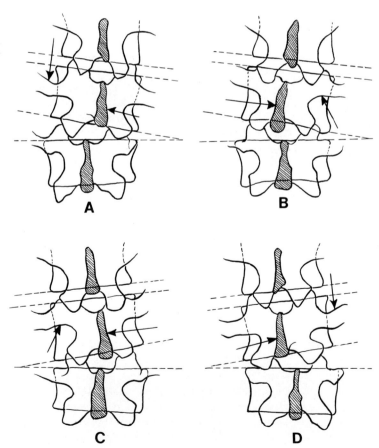

Fig. 7-1. Four examples of the more classic method of "listing" vertebral position according to the direction of intervertebral disc wedging and the position of the spinous process in relation to the vertebral body. The arrows indicate the direction in which an adjustive thrust may be administered in each case. (A) Right disc wedge with right rotation of the spinous process. (B) Right disc wedge with left rotation of the spinous process. (C) Left disc wedge with right rotation of the spinous process. (D) Left disc wedge with left rotation of the spinous process.

increases the range of motion at a joint.[29,30,51,56,59,78] There are at least two reports where increased vertebral movement following manipulation of the cervical spine has been noted on pre- and postmanipulation roentgenograms.[40,42] Similar studies have yet to be done in the lumbar spine and sacroiliac joint. The major criterion for the manipulable lesion by clinicians who adhere to this point of view is, therefore, a restriction, fixation, or blockage of motion at a specific joint in the spine. The location and characteristics of the fixation must be determined before a manipulation can be given. The primary technique for this evaluation is the palpation of motion in the various joints of the spine.

PALPATION OF THE SACROILIAC JOINT AND LUMBAR SPINE

There is a multitude of techniques for palpating motion at the sacroiliac joint.[29,30,45,78] The following three-step procedure is one of the simpler methods.

Step 1. The examiner stands behind the patient and places his thumbs on the patient's posterior superior iliac spines on each side, gripping the iliac wings with his or her fingers (Fig. 7-2A). The patient is asked to elevate and flex one knee as high as possible. Normally this maneuver will cause the ilium on the side of the flexed leg to rotate posterior, causing the posterior superior iliac spine on that side to dip inferior relative to the opposite side (Fig. 7-2B). Fixation of both sacroiliac joints will prevent this movement of one ilium relative to the other.

Step 2. In the same position, with the thumb of one hand, the examiner palpates the posterior superior iliac spine, first the left and then the right side, while placing the thumb of the other hand on the second sacral tubercle (Fig. 7-2C). The patient is asked to elevate the knee as high as possible on the side where the iliac spine is being palpated. With normal sacroiliac movement, the iliac spine will again be felt to dip

posterior and inferior relative to the sacrum (Fig. 7-2D). Failure to perceive this movement is considered indicative of fixation of the upper portion of the sacroiliac joint on the side being palpated.

Step 3. The examiner can now attempt to palpate motion in the lower half of the sacroiliac joint by placing one thumb on the ischium as close to the inferior aspect of the sacroiliac joint as possible (Fig. 7-2E). The thumb of the other hand is placed on the apex or tip of the sacrum. The patient once again elevates his or her knee as high as possible. The ischial contact point will normally be felt to move anterior, superior, and lateral relative to the sacral apex (Fig. 7-2F). Fixation of the inferior sacroiliac joint will prevent this movement.

Numerous variations of these palpation methods as well as techniques for determining movement of the sacroiliac joint during spinal flexion and lateral bending have been described.

The palpation of motion between segments of the lumbar spine is best perceived with the patient sitting.[11,30,55] Each of the normal movements of the lumbar spine may be palpated individually.

1. Flexion-extension motion can be perceived by palpating the interspinous space using the fingers or hand. The examiner's nonpalpating arm is used to grip the patient's shoulders and to move the lumbar spine into flexion and extension. A smooth opening and closing of the interspinous spaces can be felt if normal motion is present (Fig. 7-3).

2. Lateral flexion motion is determined in a similar manner. The relative position of two adjacent spinous processes is determined by hooking the lower spinous process with one finger and pushing the upper spinous process with the other. The clinician assists the patient into lateral flexion by moving the patient's shoulders (Fig. 7-4). Movement of the upper spinous process over the lower one can be perceived, and absence of this movement is suggestive of a lateral bending fixation at that level.

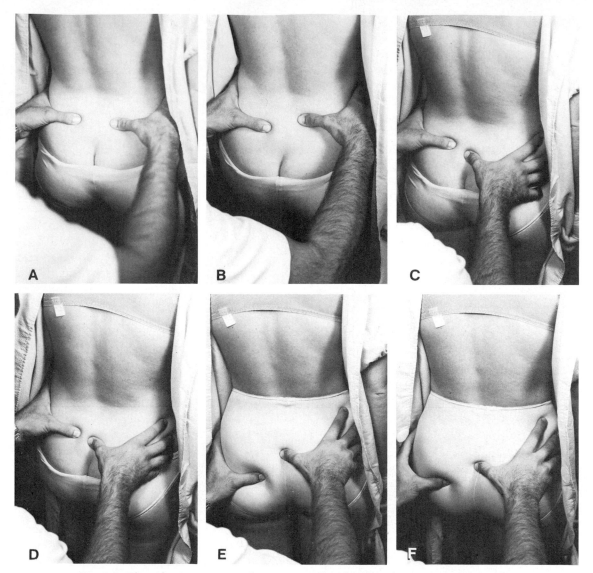

*Fig. 7-2. Three basic motion palpation tests for the sacroiliac joint. **Test 1.** The examiner's thumbs are placed on the posterior superior iliac spines (PSIS) bilaterally **(A)**. On elevation of the left leg, the left PSIS moves inferior **(B)**. **Test 2.** One thumb is placed on the left PSIS, the other on the second sacral tubercle **(C)**. On elevation of the left leg, the PSIS on that side moves inferior **(D)**. **Test 3.** One thumb is placed on the left ischium, the other is placed on the sacral apex **(E)**. On elevation of the left leg, the ischium moves anterior and lateral **(F)**.*

3. In order to examine rotational movement, the examiner palpates two adjacent spinous processes and guides the patient's trunk into rotation (Fig. 7-5). Movement of the superior spinous process over the inferior one should be perceived and would give the feeling of a step at the limit of rotation.

Lack of Joint Play

Springing of a joint and the determination of joint play and end-feel is an integral part of the premanipulation spinal examination.[55,59]

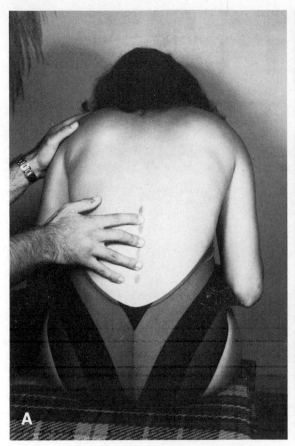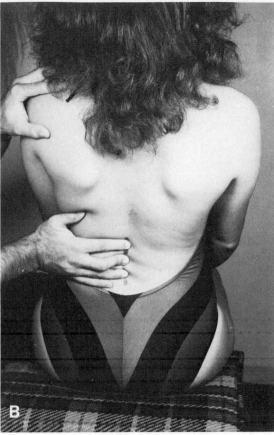

Fig. 7-3. A method for palpating flexion and extension movement in the lumbar spine. The fingertips are placed between the spinous processes, and the patient is moved into flexion and extension.

Neutral or static joint play is determined by springing each vertebra in the neutral position in both flexion-extension and rotation-lateral flexion directions. The patient is placed in the prone position with the abdomen supported. Lateral pressure is exerted over the spinous processes from each side using the examiner's thumb (Fig. 7-6). Counterpressure on the spinous process above or below with the thumb of the other hand can help localize the direction in which the vertebra is being stressed. Normally a pain-free spongy or "springy" movement can be perceived. Extreme tenderness with hard resistance to this pressure is considered an important indicator of a clinically significant manipulable lesion.[55,59] Joint springing in the flexion-extension direction is accomplished by pressing over the transverse processes of the lumbar vertebrae unilaterally or bilaterally (Fig. 7-7). Similarly, compression and flaring of the sacroiliac joints by exerting pressure bilaterally over the iliac crests can be carried out to evaluate play at these joints.

The evaluation of "end play" or end-feel is achieved through the same technique as that used for motion palpation. The vertebral joint being tested is placed at the limit of its passive range of motion and then stressed slightly beyond this limit (Fig. 7-8). A soft, springy, painless end-feel at the limit of each motion should be palpable. The presence of pain or the feeling of solid resistance at the limit of motion is considered abnormal.[30,55,59]

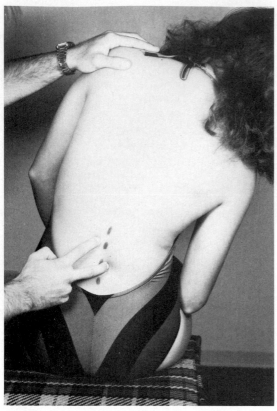

Fig. 7-4. A method for palpating lateral flexion motion in the lumbar spine.

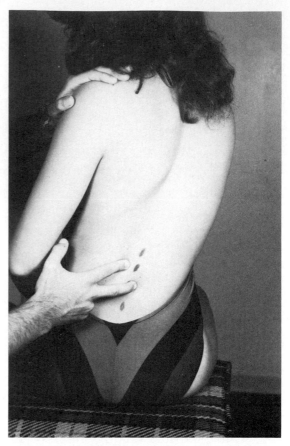

Fig. 7-5. A method for palpating rotational motion in the lumbar spine.

Palpable Soft Tissue Changes

On palpation of the paraspinal tissues it is possible to feel areas of subcutaneous tissue thickening or muscle contraction which are exquisitely tender. These "taut and tender fibers" or trigger points can be found in the long paraspinal muscles, shoulder girdle muscles (infraspinatus, supraspinatus, trapezius, rhomboids, levator scapulae), the pelvis (iliopsoas, piriformis, quadratus lumborum, glutei, tensor fascia lata), spinal ligaments (iliolumbar, anterior and posterior sacroiliac, interspinous, supraspinous, fascia lata), and bony prominences (posterior superior iliac spines, spinous processes, femoral trochanter). In the absence of a destructive lesion, these soft tissue changes are considered important indicators of the lesion which may respond to manipulation.[55,59]

Muscle Contraction or Imbalance

One of the goals common to many manipulative procedures is to stretch or stimulate contracted muscles.[58,78,83] The determination of muscular function is therefore an important part of the premanipulation spinal examination. The muscles which are most commonly evaluated for tender contraction in patients with low back pain include the piriformis, iliopsoas, quadratus lumborum, glutei, and erector spinae. The following examples will serve to illustrate how muscle imbalance is determined.

The so-called "piriformis syndrome" presents as back pain with or without leg pain, external rotation of the leg at rest (Fig. 7-9), limited internal rotation of the leg with the hip extended, and extreme tenderness on

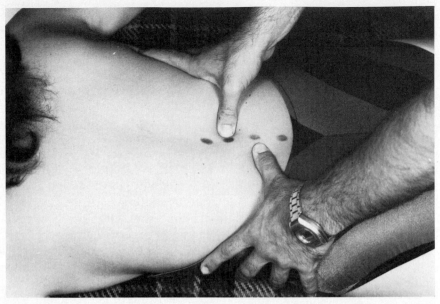

Fig. 7-6. The palpation of neutral joint play between the spinous processes of two lumbar vertebrae.

palpation of the muscle at its insertion above the acetabulum or over the belly on palpation through the rectum.[45,58]

The importance of the quadratus lumborum muscles in lateral flexion of the lumbar spine has been described and a possible role in some forms of scoliosis proposed.[47,65] Since a number of manipulative techniques are aimed partly at stretching this muscle group, it should be examined. This is done by observing any restriction in lateral flexion of the lumbar spine and any

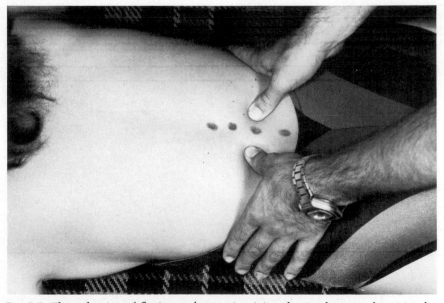

Fig. 7-7. The palpation of flexion and extension joint play in the neutral position by springing one segment of the lumbar spine.

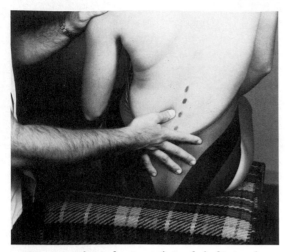

Fig. 7-8. The palpation of "end feel" in the lumbar spine on lateral flexion.

tenderness on palpation over the muscle just lateral to the erector spinae muscles (Fig. 7-10).[82]

Painful limitation of straight leg raising which is not accompanied by motor, sensory, or reflex changes, is not aggravated by dorsiflexion of the foot, and has no bowstring sign, may be due to stretching of tight hamstring muscles or restricted movement in the hip or sacroiliac joints rather than to sciatic nerve irritation. Buerger and associates and Fisk have shown that straight leg raising increases immediately after spinal manipulation when pelvis tilt is used as the end point for limited straight leg raising (Fig. 7-11).[8,25] In the absence of sciatic nerve irritation, this maneuver first brings tension on the hip extensors, then tilts the pelvis and flattens the lumbar lordosis.

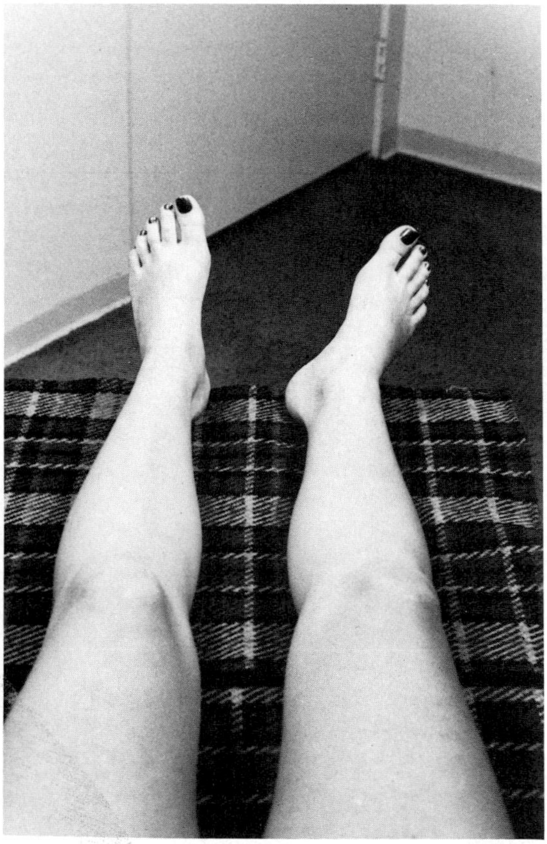

Fig. 7-9. The position of the legs in the supine position at rest in a patient with piriformis syndrome. Note the external rotation of the right leg thought to be caused by muscle imbalance.

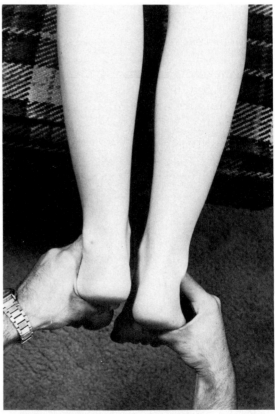

Fig. 7-10. Illustration of a functional short leg on the left in the absence of anatomical leg length deficiency. The shortening of the leg is thought to be secondary to paraspinal muscle imbalance.

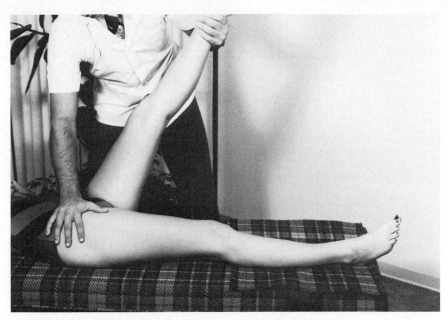

Fig. 7-11. The method for palpating pelvic tilt during straight leg raising.

Manipulative Techniques

The therapeutic goal of spinal manipulative therapy is to correct the manipulable lesion (subluxation, osteopathic lesion, somatic dysfunction, etc.) in the hope that this, in turn, will benefit the patient. Since the exact mechanism of action of the spinal manipulation and the nature of the lesion on which it has its effect is unknown, every manipulation must be considered a therapeutic trial. The effectiveness of any specific manipulative technique is therefore determined by its ability to correct the components of the manipulable lesion with the least amount of force and discomfort to the patient. The ideal manipulative procedure should take into account the structural relationship and facet facings of the vertebrae being manipulated, as well as any structural asymmetries. It should mobilize the areas of restricted or fixated joint movement, reduce painful or abnormal joint play or end-feel, eliminate palpable soft tissue taut or tender fibers, and correct areas of muscle spasm or imbalance. These goals should be achieved without traumatizing the spinal or paraspinal tissues and with a minimum of pain.

There are a multitude of techniques which have been developed over the years to manipulate the spine. Each basic technique, in turn, has numerous variations and refinements. There has been a tendency for practitioners of manipulation to form groups or factions under the leadership of a single teacher who has developed, perfected, and taught a particular system of techniques. Thus, there are currently practitioners of techniques as taught by Cyriax, others with techniques taught by Mennell, Lewit, Maigne, Paris, Kaltenbourn, Maitland, Palmer, Gonstead, DeJarnette, Toftness, Kimberly, Stoddard, or Mitchell. The relative effectiveness of one technique as compared with another has yet to be evaluated, so the choice of manipulative technique continues to be based, to a large extent, on the skills a clinician has developed rather than on a rational understanding of the role of each manipulative procedure.

Although the adherents of many of these technique systems claim to have unique approaches to manipulation, the various techniques have much in common. It is possible to classify all spinal manipulative procedures into six subgroups. The remainder of this chapter will be devoted to a discussion of these six classes of manipulation. Examples have been chosen which illustrate the basic principles of each subgroup. It is impossible to describe every technique in detail. For further information, the textbooks and notes which have been published on the topic, many of which are listed in the bibliography, should be reviewed.

Nonspecific Long Lever Manipulations

This class of manipulation includes all those procedures in which a high velocity force is exerted on a part of the body some distance from the area where it is expected to have its beneficial effect. The long levers used for this type of manipulation include the leg, shoulder, pelvis, and thoracic spine.[14,17,31] Although these manipulations have been widely used, they are generally considered to be the most crude and the least effective of the manipulative techniques. The long lever makes it very diffi-

cult, although not impossible, to make this type of manipulation specific to a particular segment. The force, instead, is exerted into a region of the spine. The vertebral level which receives most of the mobilization is often the one which is already hypermobile rather than the one at which motion is restricted. It is this type of manipulation which is most likely to result in the herniation of degenerated intervertebral discs and damage to soft tissues.

The most commonly used long lever technique for the lumbar spine is the rotational manipulation described by Cyriax and Coplans.[14,17] The patient is placed in the lateral side lying position with the symptomatic side up. The hip and knee of the superior leg are flexed, while the inferior leg is held in extension. The clinician stands in front of the patient and steadies the shoulder with his superior hand, pushing it down to the table. With the other (inferior) hand, he contacts the pelvis or buttock and rolls the patient's pelvis towards him while letting the flexed leg hang over the side of the table (Fig. 7-12). The rotational slack is taken up with the inferior hand and a sharp controlled thrust is given to the pelvis or leg in the

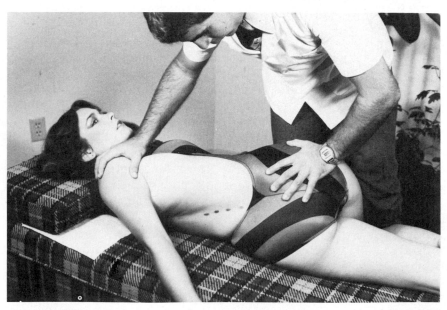

Fig. 7-12. The basic nonspecific long lever rotational manipulation of the lumbar spine.

direction of rotation (downward and laterally).

There are a great number of variations on this technique.

1. It is possible to hook the foot of the patient's superior flexed leg into the popliteal fossa of the inferior leg. This allows the clinician to exert a force through the femur, creating a longer, more powerful lever (Fig. 7-13A).

2. The patient can be placed in the prone position on his or her back with hips flexed and knees crossed. Both knees are twisted towards the clinician while the shoulders are kept flat on the table. The clinician holds the shoulders down with his superior hand while applying force through both legs at the knee. This forces rotation during lumbar side flexion (Fig. 7-13B).

3. A reversed long lever rotational manip-

ulation can be achieved by placing the patient in the side lying position with the clinician standing behind the patient. The thorax is rotated forwards and the pelvis backwards. The examiner forces the rotation by pressing simultaneously on the shoulder and pelvis (Fig. 7-13C).

A second group of nonspecific manipulations are those that force extension of the lumbar spine. For most of these maneuvers, the patient is asked to lie prone on the couch or table. The hands are placed either unilaterally or bilaterally alongside the spinous processes. The patient is asked to relax, the slack in the lumbar spine is taken up, and a high velocity thrust forces the lumbar spine into extension. Considerably greater force can be exerted if one leg is elevated in extension and either used as a lever or simply held in maximum extension with one hand

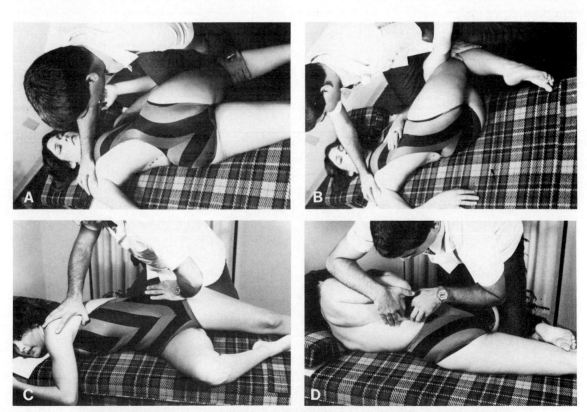

Fig. 7-13. Four variations of the basic nonspecific rotational manipulation of the lumbar spine. The technique shown in Part D, where the spine is palpated during the procedure, can be fairly specific.

while the thrust is given with the other hand to the lumbar spine (Fig. 7-14).

It should be reiterated that these long lever manipulations are crude, nonspecific, and potentially dangerous. Most experienced practitioners of manipulation do not utilize them. They are included here simply for completeness.

Specific Short Lever High Velocity Spinal Adjustment

The manipulative procedure which is most widely used by trained practitioners of SMT is the short lever, high velocity thrust directed specifically at the manipulable lesion (subluxation, osteopathic lesion, etc.). In order to practice this technique, it is essential that a clinician have some basic understanding of spinal mechanics, have the palpatory skills to diagnose the clinically significant manipulable lesion, and develop, through experience, the ability to direct the adjustive thrust to one vertebral segment in a specific direction.

Once the clinically significant manipulable lesion has been found, the direction in which motion is lost has been determined, and the facet facings and structural relationship between the vertebrae is known, it is possible to work out a technique which will theoretically correct the lesion. The patient is placed in a position which will allow movement of the vertebra in the desired direction. Contact is made with a relatively small portion of one hand (thumb, finger, pisiform). The spinal segments, either above or below the segment being manipulated, are locked by moving the spine to the limit of their passive range of motion.[51,55] A high velocity, small amplitude thrust is then delivered through the contact arm and hand to the short vertebral lever (transverse process or spinous process) in the direction which will correct the segmental fixation.

Once again, it is impossible to list the numerous techniques and variations which have been developed to adjust the lumbar spine and sacroiliac joint. Such adjustments may be made with the patient in the prone, supine, side lying, or sitting positions and by using a variety of specially designed adjusting tables, blocks, and traction devices. The following four examples with variations

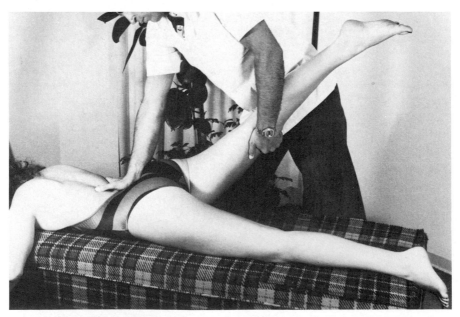

Fig. 7-14. The long lever extension manipulation of the lumbar spine.

hopefully will serve to illustrate a few of the principles of lumbosacral adjusting.

1. Adjustment of the sacroiliac joint is most frequently carried out with the patient in the side lying position.[30,33] The side which is to be adjusted is placed up. The inferior leg is straight and the superior leg flexed. This brings the lumbar spine to its neutral position with the shoulders and hips vertically above each other. The inferior arm is drawn rostrally from under the patient with a minimum of spinal rotation and placed across the chest. The clinician's superior hand is placed on the patient's shoulder and pressure is exerted rostrally with only that amount of spinal rotation and lateral flexion which is necessary to lock the spine down to the segment being manipulated. The pisiform eminence of the clinician's inferior hand is used to contact either the posterior superior iliac spine (for a flexion fixation of the sacroiliac joint) or the ischial tuberosity (for an extension fixation). The inferior leg is flexed to the point where resistance is felt in the sacroiliac joint (approximately 75 degrees for flexion fixations, 90 degrees for extension fixations). Traction is applied to the spine as the patient takes a deep breath and then slowly exhales and relaxes. A high velocity, low amplitude thrust is delivered through the clinician's inferior arm and hand while the superior arm simply stabilizes the trunk and spine. The direction of thrust is determined by the listing of the pelvis. For example, if the iliac spine is felt to have moved posterior and inferior, the thrust is rostral and anterior towards the patient's shoulder (Fig. 7-15A). If the superior ilium is felt to have rotated internally onto the sacrum, the direction of thrust is anterior towards the superior femur in an attempt to open the sacroiliac joint (Fig. 7-15B). The thrust on the ischium for an extension fixation is towards the patient's lower shoulder (Fig. 7-16).[30]

Manipulation of the lumbar spine can be carried out using a very similar technique. The patient is placed in the same position. The spine is locked down to the segment being manipulated through traction and slight rotation of the shoulder. The thrust is delivered to a transverse process or by hooking a spinous process.

With proper placement of the patient, it is seldom necessary to put weight on the femur or to maximally rotate the spine, thus reducing the chance of traumatizing the rib cage, hip joint, or intervertebral disc.

2. The adjustment of the lumbar spine for an extension fixation or posterior segment can best be achieved with the patient prone.[33,34,77] A flat couch, however, does not allow for sufficient extension of the lumbar spine to achieve specific localization of the adjustive force. A number of adjusting tables have been developed to overcome this problem. The segmental table (Fig. 7-17) has a pelvic support that elevates and an abdominal support that drops away. This allows the pelvis to be locked while the lumbar spine is hanging in extension.

Another, much less costly piece of equipment, the knee posture table, similarly allows for locking of the pelvis (on the femurs) with maximal extension of the lumbar spine. The position of pelvis locking can be varied by changing the body femur angle from a perpendicular 90 degrees to 80 degrees or 100 degrees. This is achieved by moving the knees forward or backward. Contact is made over the transverse processes of the segment being adjusted either unilaterally or bilaterally (Fig. 7-18). The clinician may use either his thumbs or pisiform to make the contact. The use of thenar or hypothenar eminences is less effective since it tends to dissipate the force over a number of segments, thus reducing the specificity of the procedure.

The ability to deliver a very sharp, low amplitude thrust is necessary for this procedure. A single "thud" can often be heard and felt over the articulation being adjusted if the procedure is executed properly. Any excessive force or depth to the thrust can be painful. The decision as to whether the thrust should be given unilaterally or bilaterally and the exact direction for the thrust is dependent on the listing, the facet facings,

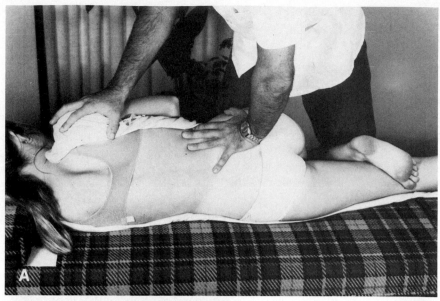

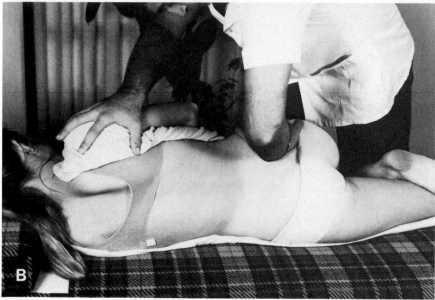

Fig. 7-15. Two methods for delivering a specific spinal adjustment to the sacroiliac joint which is thought to be fixated in flexion. Note the different position of the clinician's hand and arm when used to deliver the thrust. (A) Position for adjusting the sacroiliac joint where the ilium has moved posterior and inferior. (B) Position for adjusting the sacroiliac joint where the ilium has rotated internally on the sacrum.

and whether the fixation is unilateral or bilateral.

3. Sitting rotary and lateral flexion manipulations can be quite specific. The clinician has the advantage of being able to maneuver the patient's spine in all three planes of motion prior to delivering the adjustive thrust.[43,55] The main drawback is the inability to achieve segmental traction.

The patient straddles the edge of the adjusting table and clasps both hands across his or her chest on opposite shoulders or behind the neck. The clinician gains control of the trunk by grasping the patient's shoul-

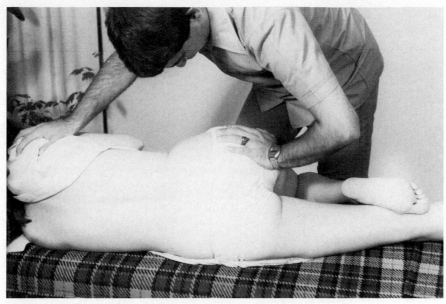

Fig. 7-16. The specific adjustment for an extension fixation of the sacroiliac joint.

ders or arms with one hand. The clinician's other hand is free to make contact in the lumbar spine. The patient can be maneuvered into flexion, extension, rotation, lateral bending, or any combination of these positions. The thrust is delivered to the transverse or spinous process of the lumbar segment being adjusted (Fig. 7-19). The position of the patient prior to giving the thrust and the direction of the thrust are, once again, dependent on the listing and the direction in which the segment is fixated. The thrust is an exaggerated movement of the trunk, with localization being directed

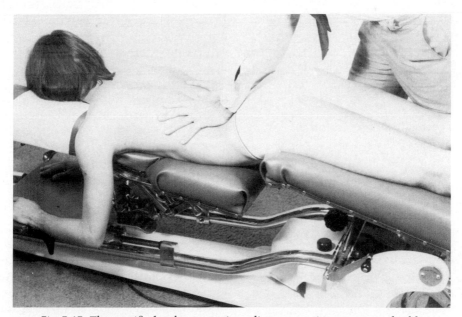

Fig. 7-17. The specific lumbar extension adjustment using a segmental table.

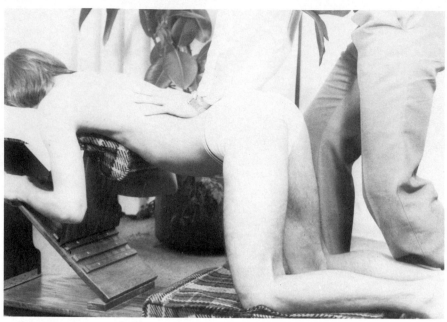

Fig. 7-18. *The specific lumbar extension adjustment using the knee posture table.*

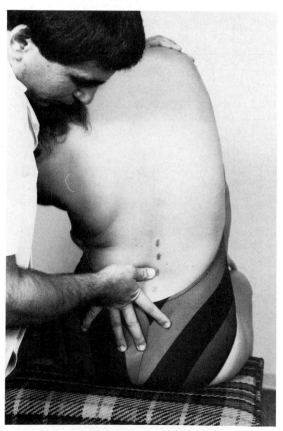

Fig. 7-19. *The rotation-lateral flexion adjustment in the sitting position.*

through the contact point in the lumbar spine.

4. There is a wide variety of specific adjusting procedures which do not utilize a high velocity thrust. These techniques (along with mobilizing procedures) are particularly useful in the management of elderly patients where it may be advantageous not to use heavy force. Kimberly describes a number of so-called "muscle energy" and "respiratory force" procedures.[43] These procedures utilize the patient's own muscles to achieve the correction of a specific fixation. The basic principle of these techniques is to position the patient at the limit of a specific range of motion in the direction of the vertebral fixation. The segment being adjusted is fixed with one hand. The clinician's other arm is used to give resistance in a direction opposite to the direction of fixation. The patient is then asked to exert isometric contraction against this resistance while the segment being adjusted is held firm. When the patient relaxes, the slack created by the isometric contraction is taken up. In this way, the passive range of motion of the segment which was held is increased. This process is repeated a number of times

until movement is felt in the vertebra being adjusted. Muscle energy techniques have been developed in the sitting, prone, and supine positions for almost every direction of movement fixation. Patient positioning is very similar to that used for the high velocity, low amplitude thrust techniques. It is the use of the patient's own muscles rather than a dynamic thrust which is the distinguishing feature.

A simple example of this technique is that described by Kimberly for a restricted or fixated sacroiliac joint where the posterior superior iliac crest is felt to have moved posterior and inferior (Fig. 7-20).[43] The patient is placed prone with the clinician standing on the side opposite to that being adjusted. The clinician elevates the leg on the affected side with one hand and places the other hand on the iliac crest slightly above the posterior superior iliac spine. The leg is elevated in extension and pressure is exerted on the iliac crest until the restrictive barrier at the limit of the passive range of motion is engaged. The patient is then instructed to pull the leg downward toward the table against the resistance of the clinician's hand.

The patient relaxes and the additional slack in the joint motion is taken up until the new restrictive barrier is engaged. The process is repeated 2 to 3 times until the fixation is corrected.

Vertebral Mobilization or Articulation

The procedures generally included under the term mobilization are those in which a joint is manipulated within its physiological passive range of motion. There is no attempt to force the joint beyond its restrictive barrier.[13,56,64] These techniques are extremely valuable in patients with acutely painful joints or where there is some inherent danger to high velocity adjusting techniques (e.g., osteoporosis).

Four grades of mobilization are classically described (Fig. 7-21). A "grade 1" mobilization starts at the neutral position and has only very small excursion. A "grade 2" mobilization begins at the neutral position and has deeper excursion into the normal range of motion of the joint but does not attempt to reach the limit of passive motion. A

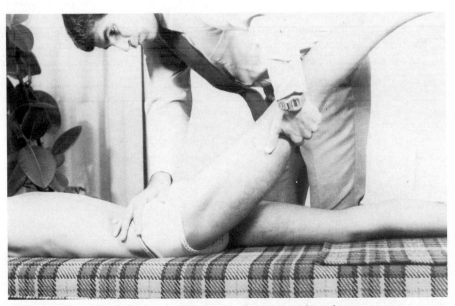

Fig. 7-20. An example of the muscle-energy adjustment. This adjustment is to correct a fixated sacroiliac joint with posterior-inferior misalignment of the ilium. The direction of the patient's muscle force is down towards the table.

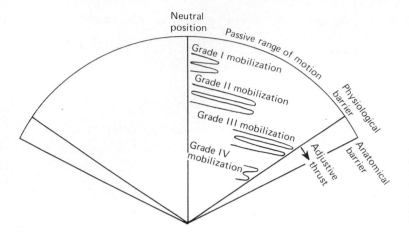

Fig. 7-21. An illustration of the relationship between the four grades of mobilization to the normal passive range of motion of a joint. The adjustment takes place between the physiological and anatomical limits of joint movement.

"grade 3" mobilization begins approximately halfway into the normal motion of the joint and carries through to the physiological barrier of the joint. A "grade 4" mobilization has only short excursion at the limit of the passive motion of the joint.

Mobilization can be either specific to a single vertebral joint or nonspecific to the entire spine or a large segment of the spine. It can be accomplished in flexion, extension, rotation, lateral flexion, or any combination of these movements. The positioning of the patient varies only slightly from that used in nonspecific manipulation and the specific spinal adjustment. It is the degree of movement and the lack of a thrust which distinguishes mobilization from these procedures.

In addition, mobilization can be performed in the neutral position by springing a joint in a specific direction. These neutral mobilizations are identical to the techniques used for determining neutral joint play. In this case, however, the goal is treatment rather than diagnosis. The springing of a joint is repeated a number of times, often with increasing depth (or grades of mobilization) until the full range of motion is achieved and is pain free. This may require repeated mobilizations over a number of days. Figure 7-22 illustrates specific rotation mobilization of a lumbar vertebra in the neutral position by lateral pressure over a spinous process. Figure 7-23 is an example of a technique for specific springing of the lumbar spine in extension.

Manual Traction or Muscle Stretching

The manual application of traction to the legs, arms, head, or trunk falls within the broad definition of spinal manipulative therapy. These techniques are nonspecific for any one vertebral level of joint, the traction being applied to the entire spine. The major advantages of manual over mechanical traction are that the clinician can monitor the amount of traction being given, change the direction of traction by altering the position of the leg or arm which is being pulled, and change the rhythm of intermittent traction.

There are two types of manual traction which have been described for the lumbar spine. The vertical traction technique begins with the patient and clinician standing back to back.[59,78] The patient grasps his or her own shoulders and the clinician reaches behind him to grasp the patient's elbows. The clinician then bends forward, holding the patient's elbows rigid and lifts the patient from the ground. The patient is asked to flex his or her neck. The clinician, after taking up the ligamentous slack in the spine, gives the patient a sharp shake by lifting the patient suddenly higher. This causes straight extension of the spine. It is a clumsy maneuver, but can be effective if vertebral traction and extension is required.

The application of traction to one or both legs has been used in an attempt to open the sacroiliac and posterior joints of the lumbar spine and to stretch the paraspinal mus-

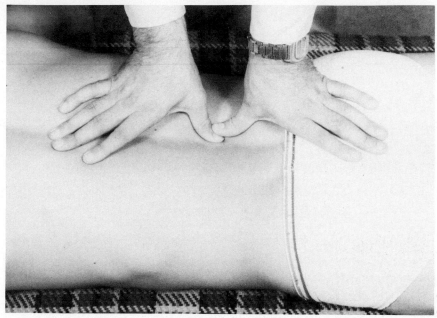

Fig. 7-22. A specific rotational mobilization technique in the neutral position.

cles.[4,30,56] This can take the form of sustained traction on the leg, a short tug on the leg, or a movement from the flexed leg position to the extended position followed by traction (Fig. 7-24). Bourdillon recommends internal rotation of the leg prior to applying the leg tug.

The spray and stretch techniques developed by Travell for the treatment of specific trigger points also fall under this heading.[80,81]

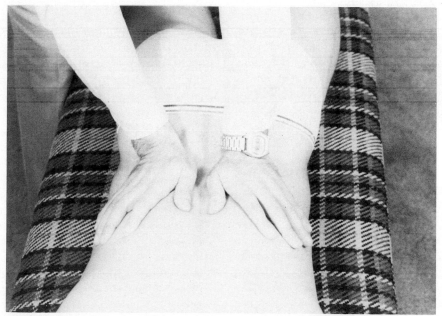

Fig. 7-23. An extension mobilization technique in the neutral position (springing of the lumbar spine).

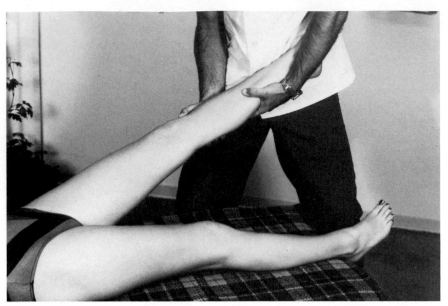

Fig. 7-24. *An example of a traction manipulation using the leg. The force may be gradual, intermittent, or in the form of a sharp tug.*

In this case, traction is applied to muscles rather than to a joint. Travell describes the myofascial trigger points as palpable tender firm bands of muscle which refer pain in a specific pattern, often some distance from the trigger point. The trigger points which are considered important in low back and leg pain are those within the iliocostalis, gluteus medius, longissimus, multifides, gluteus minimus, adductor longus, piriformis, and quadratus lumborum muscles. When a trigger point in a specific muscle is found in a patient with the appropriate pain pattern, the muscle may be stretched to determine the extent of motion restriction caused by the muscle contraction. While maintaining the muscle in the stretched position, the patient is asked to relax the muscle voluntarily, and a stream of vapocoolant spray (fluorimethane) is directed at the muscle. The spray is applied in one direction from the trigger point towards its reference zone in slow, even sweeps over the skin. During the spraying, passive stretch is applied to the muscle with steady, gradually increasing force. The stretch is held at a tolerably painful point which does not result in any contraction or guarding of the muscle.

The trigger point should disappear if the procedure is carried out properly. Figure 7-25 illustrates the technique for spraying and stretching of the hamstring muscles.

Soft Tissue Massage

All forms of massage fall under the definition of manipulative therapy and are often referred to as manipulations.[20,70] The massage techniques can be broken down into superficial stroking or effleurage, deep kneading or friction massage, and the various hacking and clapping procedures.

Two types of massage deserve special mention in a discussion of low back pain. **Connective tissue massage** is a deep stroking massage which utilizes a twisting movement of the fingertips along specific planes of the back. The stroking is sufficiently deep to cause discomfort to the patient and marked hyperemia of the skin. Claims of effective management of back pain have been made for this procedure.[20,27] **Deep transverse friction massage** is the specific focal application of massage across an injured tender muscle, tendon, or ligament.[17] The theoretical basis of this procedure is to break

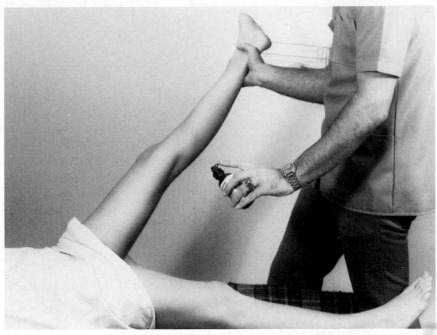

Fig. 7-25. An example of the spray-and-stretch manipulations described by Travell and Mennell. The hamstring muscles are stretched after applying vapocoolant spray.

down scar tissue and increase circulation. The massage is given over a very small area and at right angles to the muscle or ligamentous fibers. Although this technique is usually recommended for known areas of soft tissue injury in the extremities, it is also being used to manipulate trigger points around the spine.

Point Pressure Manipulation

Many of the muscle syndromes considered to be associated with low back pain are said to respond to deep point pressure without any movement of the joint or massage of the muscle. The piriformis syndrome is the most commonly quoted example. The manipulative procedure recommended by Maxwell and Edwards utilizes constant heavy pressure over the piriformis muscle using the thumb or elbow for approximately 30 seconds or until spasm in the muscle is released.[22,58] The easiest way to find the muscle is to have the patient in the lateral recumbant position with the affected side up. The tender contracted muscle can be felt just above the acetabulum when the patient's hip is flexed and adducted (Fig. 7-26).

A variety of practitioners of spinal manipulation claim to be able to change symptoms, increase muscle strength, and influence health by exerting pressure over certain mapped points on the body. The procedures, which have been referred to under such titles as Rolfing, muscle balancing massage, acupressure, and applied kinesiology, recommend the application of deep point pressure over specific points on the body surface, often on an acupuncture meridian or over the same trigger points described by Travell. These procedures have as yet to be discussed in any peer-reviewed journal. They are often couched in farfetched, unsubstantiated theories and claims of success and only deserve mention because of their growing popularity and repeated mention in the popular press.

Spinal manipulative therapy, as currently practiced, is both a diagnostic and treatment approach to spinal disorders. Each of the manipulative procedures is directed at spe-

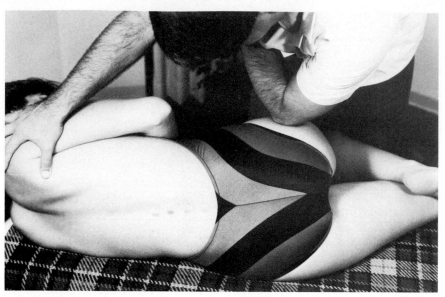

Fig. 7-26. *An example of point pressure manipulation. In this case the piriformis muscle is being manipulated.*

cific physical findings which, at least subjectively, appear to change after a successful manipulation. The choice of manipulation is dependent on a proper diagnosis or analysis of spinal biomechanical aberrations. To practice spinal manipulation without perfecting the palpating diagnostic skills is to assume knowledge of the ultimate effect of the manipulation on the lesion causing back pain. Such an assumption cannot be substantiated for any of the presumptive causes of low back pain. Critics of SMT have shown scepticism of the subjective nature of much of the reported results and the complex theoretical dogma which so often accompanies this approach to spinal disorders. Were it not for the documented results and millions of patients who swear by this form of treatment, this scepticism would be justified. Greater understanding of the relative effectiveness of the various forms of spinal manipulative therapy, its theoretical mechanism of action, the accuracy of the palpatory diagnostic techniques, and the prognosis one can expect after a patient is manipulated awaits further research. Fortunately, practitioners of SMT are no longer as isolated from the mainstream of scientific

medicine as has been true in the past. As the communication gap between practitioners and critics of SMT narrows, the amount of research into the theory and practice of SMT has increased. The final answer to the role of spinal manipulative therapy in the management of patients with low back pain must wait for this research.

References

1. Bergquist-Ullman M, Larsson U: Acute low back pain in industry. Acta Orthoped Scan (Suppl) 170:1–117, 1977
2. Blaine ES: Manipulative (chiropractic) dislocation of the axis. JAMA 85:1356–1358, 1925
3. Bosshard R: The treatment of acute lumbago and sciatica. Ann Swiss Chiropractor's Assn, 50–61, 1961
4. Bourdillon JF: Spinal Manipulation. William Heineman Medical Books, London, 1970
5. Breen AC: Chiropractors and the treatment of back pain. Rheumatol Rehabil 16:46–53, 1977
6. Buerger AA: A clinical trial of rotational manipulation. Pain Abstracts 1:248. Second World Congress on Pain. International Association for the Study of Pain. Montreal, Canada, 1978
7. Buerger AA: A clinical trial of spinal manipulation. Fed Proc 38:1250, 1979

8. Buerger AA, Tobis JS (eds) Approaches to the Validation of Manipulation Therapy. Charles C. Thomas, Springfield, 1977

9. Buerger AA. In The Manipulation Project. A controlled trial of rotational manipulation in low back pain. Submitted for publication— Manuelle Medizin, 1979

10. Cassidy JD, Potter GE, Kirkaldy-Willis WH: Manipulative management of back pain in patients with spondylolisthesis. J Canad Chiropractic Assn 22 (1):15–20, 1978

11. Cassidy JD, Potter GE: Motion examination of the lumbar spine. J Manip Physiol Therapeut 2:151–158, 1979

12. Chrisman OD, Mittnacht A, Snook GA: A study of the results following rotatory manipulation in the lumbar intervertebral disc syndrome. J Bone Joint Surg 46A:517–524, 1964

13. Cookson J: Orthopedic manual therapy—An overview. Part II. The spine. Physical Therapy 59:259–267, 1979

14. Coplans CW: The conservative treatment of low back pain. In Helfet AJ, Gruebel Lee DM (eds) Disorders of the Lumbar Spine. JB Lippincott, Philadelphia, 1978

15. Coyer, AB, Curwen IHM: Low back pain treated by manipulation: A controlled series. Brit Med J, March 19:705–707, 1955

16. Croner CM: The nation's use of health resources, 1976 ed. DHEW Publication No. (HRA) 77–1240, 1976

17. Cyriax J: Textbook of orthopaedic medicine. Vol 2. 8th ed. Bailliere-Tindall, London, 1971

18. Dabbert O: Spinal meningeal hematoma, warfarin therapy and chiropractic adjustment. JAMA 214:11, 1970

19. Doran DML, Newell DJ: Manipulation in treatment of low back pain: A multicentre study. Brit Med J 2:161–164, 1975

20. Ebner M: Connective tissue massage. Physiotherapy 64:208–210, 1978

21. Edwards BC: Low back pain and pain resulting from lumbar spine conditions: A comparison of treatment results. Austral J Physiotherapy 15 (3):104–110, 1969

22. Edwards FO: Pyriformis syndrome. Academy of Applied Osteopathy Yearbook, 39–41, 1962

23. Evans DP, Burke MS, Lloyd KN, Roberts EE, Roberts GM: Lumbar spinal manipulation on trial. Part I. Clinical assessment. Rheum Rehabil 17:46–53, 1978

24. Fisk JW: Manipulation in general practice. N. Z. Med J 74:172–175, 1971

25. Fisk JW: The straight leg raising test: Its relevance to possible disc pathology. NZ Med J 81:557–560, 1975

26. Fisk JW: A practical guide to management of the painful neck and back. Charles C. Thomas, Springfield, 1977

27. Frazer FW: Persistent post-sympathetic pain treated by connective tissue massage. Physiotherapy 64:211–212, 1978

28. Gibbons RW: Chiropractic in America. The historical Conflicts of Cultism and Science. 10th Annual History Forum of Duquesne University, 1976

29. Gillet H, Liekens M: Belgian Chiropractic Research Notes. 10th ed, Brussels, 1973

30. Gitelman R: A chiropractic approach to biomechanical disorders of the lumbar spine and pelvis. In Haldeman S (ed): Modern Developments in the Principles and Practice of Chiropractic. Appleton-Century-Crofts, New York, 1980

31. Glover JR, Morris JG, Khosla T: Back pain: A randomized clinical trial of rotational manipulation of the trunk. Brit J Ind Med 31:59–64, 1974

32. Goldstein M (ed) The Research Status of Spinal Manipulative Therapy. NINCDS Monograph No. 15, DHEW Publication No. (NIH) Bethesda, 76–998, 1975

33. Gonstead CS: Gonstead chiropractic science and art. Sci-Chi Publications, 1968

34. Grecco MA: Chiropractic Technique Illustrated. Jarl Publishing Co, New York, 1953

35. Greenland S, Reisbord L, Haldeman S, Buerger AA: Controlled clinical trials of manipulation. A review and proposal. To be published in J Occup Med, 1980

36. Haldeman S: Chiropractic: A dying cult or a growing profession? Musings Quarterly 1 (3):53–57, 1975

37. Haldeman S: What is meant by manipulation? In Buerger, AA, Tobis JS (eds): Approaches to the Validation of Manipulation Therapy 299–302. Charles C Thomas, Springfield, 1977

38. Haldeman S (ed): Modern Developments in the Principles and Practice of Chiropractic. Appleton-Century-Crofts, New York, 1980

39. Henderson DJ: Intermittent claudication with special reference to its neurogenic form as a diagnostic and management challenge. J Canad Chiropractic Ass 23 (1):9–19, 1979

40. Hviid H: The influence of chiropractic treatment on the rotary mobility of the cervical spine. A kinesiometric and statistical study. Ann Swiss Chiro Ass V:31–44, 1971

41. Jennet WB: A study of 25 cases of compression of the cauda equina by prolapse IVD. J Neurol Neurosurg Psych 19:109–116, 1956

42. Jirout J: The effect of mobilization of the segmental blockade on the sagittal component of the reaction on lateral flexion of the cervical spine. Neuroradiology 3:210–215, 1972

43. Kimberly PE: Outline of Osteopathic Manipulative Procedures. Kirksville College of Osteopathic Medicine, Kirksville, 1979

44. Kirkaldy-Willis WH, Cassidy: Effects of manipulation on chronic low back pain. Presented at a conference on Manipulative Medicine in the Management of Low Back Pain. Sponsored by the University of Southern California and the North American Academy of Manipulative Medicine, Oct 1978

45. Kirkaldy-Willis WH, Hill RJ: A more precise diagnosis for low back pain. Spine 4:102–109, 1979

46. Kleynhans AM: Complications of and contraindications to spinal manipulative therapy. In Haldeman S (ed): Modern Developments in the Principles and Practice of Chiropractic. Appleton-Century-Crofts, New York, 1980

47. Knapp ME: Function of the quadratus lumborum. Arch Phys Med 32:505–507, 1951

48. Korr IM: The spinal cord as organizer of disease processes: Some preliminary prospectives. J Am Osteop Assoc 76:89–99, 1976

49. Korr IM (ed): The Neurobiologic Mechanisms in Manipulative Therapy. Plenum Press, New York, 1978

50. LaRocca H, MacNab I: Value of pre-employment radiographic assessment of the lumbar spine. Can Med Ass J 101: 383–388, 1969

51. Lewit D: Manuelle Medizin. Im Rahmen der Medizinischen Rehabilitation. 2 Auflage. Johann Ambrosius, Leipzig, 1977

52. Livingstone M: Spinal manipulation causing injury. Brit Col Med J 14 (3):78–81, 1972

53. Logan VF, Murray FM (eds): Textbook of Logan Basic Methods. LBM, St. Louis, 1950

54. Lomax E: Manipulative therapy: A historical perspective from ancient times to the modern era. In Goldstein, M (ed): The Research Status of Spinal Manipulative Therapy. NINCDS Monograph No. 15. DHEW Publication No. (NIH) 76–998, 1975

55. Maigne R: Orthopedic Medicine. A New Approach to Vertebral Manipulations. Translated by WT Liberson. Charles C Thomas, Springfield, 1972

56. Maitland GD: Vertebral Manipulation. 3rd ed. Butterworths, London, 1973

57. Matthews JA, Yates DAH: Reduction of lumbar disc prolapse by manipulation. Brit Med J Sept 20:696–699, 1969

58. Maxwell TD: The piriformis muscle and its relation to the long legged sciatic syndrome. J Can Chiropractic Ass 22 (2):51–56, 1978

59. Mennell J: Back Pain. Diagnosis and Treatment Using Manipulative Therapy. Little, Brown and Co, Boston, 1960

60. Nachemson A: A long term follow-up study of non-treated scoliosis. Acta Orthop Scand 39:466–476, 1968

61. Nachemson A: A critical look at the treatment for low back pain. In Goldstein M (ed): The Research Status of Spinal Manipulative Therapy. NINCDS Monograph 15. DHEW Publication No. (NIH) 76–998, 287–293, 1975

62. Nachemson A: The lumbar spine: An orthopedic challenge. Spine. 1:59–71, 1976

63. Nachemson A: Pathophysiology and treatment of back pain: A critical look at the different types of treatment. In Buerger AA, Tobis JS (eds): Approaches to the Validation of Manipulation Therapy, 42–57. Charles C Thomas, Springfield, 1977

64. Nwuga VC: Manipulation of the Spine. Williams and Wilkins, Baltimore, 1976

65. Olsen GA, Allan JH: The lateral stability of the spine. Clin Orthop Related Res 65:143–156, 1969

66. Palmer DD: The Science, Art and Philosophy of Chiropractic. Portland Printing House, Portland, 1910

67. Perl ER: Pain: Spinal and peripheral factors. In Goldstein M (ed): The Research Status of Spinal Manipulative Therapy. NINCDS Monograph No. 15. DHEW Publication No. (NIH) 76–998, 173–182, 1975

68. Potter GE: A study of 744 cases of neck and back pain treated with spinal manipulation. J Can Chiropractic Ass 21 (4):154–156, 1977

69. Potter GE: Chiropractors (letter). Can Med Ass J 121:705–706, 1979

70. Prosser E: Manual of Massage and Movements. London, 1951

71. Rasmussen GG: Manipulation in low back pain: A randomized clinical trial. Manuelle Medizin 1:8–10, 1977

72. Richard J: Disc rupture with cauda equina syndrome after chiropractic adjustment. NY State J Med Sept 15, 2496–2498, 1967

73. Riches EW: End-results of manipulation of the back. Lancet, May 3, 957–960, 1930

74. Schafer RC: Chiropractic Health Care. 2nd ed. Foundation for Chiropractic Education and Research. Des Moines, Iowa, 1976

75. Schiotz, EH: Manipulation treatment of the spinal column from the medical-historical viewpoint. Tidsshr Nor 78:359–372. NIH Library translation, 1958

76. Sims-Williams H, Mayson MIV, Young SMS, Baddeley H, Collins E: Controlled trial of mobilization and manipulation for patients with low back pain in general practice. Brit Med J 2:1338–1340, 1978

77. States AZ: Spinal and Pelvic Technics. Atlas of Chiropractic Technic. 2nd ed. National College of Chiropractic, Lombard, IL, 1968

78. Stoddard, A: Manual of Osteopathic Technique. Hutchison, London, 1959
79. Tissington-Tatlow WFT, Bammer HG: Syndrome of vertebral artery compression. Neurology 7:331–340, 1957
80. Travell J: Symposium on mechanism and management of pain syndromes. Proc Rudolf Virchou Med Society Basel (Switzerland) 16:128–135, 1957
81. Travell J: Myofascial trigger points: Clinical view. Advances in Pain Research and Therapy. 1:919–926, 1976
82. Travell J: The Quadratus Lumborum Muscle: An overlooked Cause of Low Back Pain. Presented at a conference on Manipulative Medicine in the Management of Low Back Pain. Sponsored by University of Southern California and the North American Academy of Manipulative Medicine, Los Angeles, October 1978
83. Travell J, Travell W: Therapy of low back pain by manipulation and of referred pain in the lower extremity by procaine infiltration. Arch Phys Med 27:537–547, 1946
84. Vear HJ: A study into the complaints of patients seeking chiropractic care. J Can Chiropractic Ass October 9–13, 1972
85. White AA, Panjabi MM: Clinical Biomechanics of the Spine. JB Lippincott, Philadelphia, 1979

The valuable advice given by Dr. David Rubin, Dr. Warren Famalaro and my wife, Joan Haldeman, and the assistance with the illustrations by Dr. Warren Famalaro and Barbara Finneson are gratefully acknowledged.

The Sister Kenny Institute, Gravity Lumbar Reduction Therapy Program

8

Charles V. Burton

Axial Traction

Axial traction has been long recognized as an effective means of reducing improperly aligned or displaced vertebral elements as well as their associated intervertebral discs and soft tissues. This application has been best demonstrated in the cervical area where a spectrum of devices, ranging from head halters to cranial tongs, has been employed. Although many attempts have been made to achieve gradual and controlled traction to the lumbar area, the lack of points of fixation and the high degree of force involved have presented significant obstacles.

It became evident to this author in 1972 that the rib cage could serve as a possible site of fixation if the proper distribution of loading were possible. With the assistance of Mr. Wallace Lossing of Lossing Orthopedics, Gail Nida, R.N., and Berkeley Fogelsonger, R.N.T., a polyfoam-Velcro vest and associated traction equipment were developed and clinically introduced with the assistance of the staff of the Sister Kenny Institute Low Back Clinic. In 1974, the Sister Kenny Institute Gravity Lumbar Reduction Therapy Program (GLRTP) was first used in patient care for the conservative management of protruded disc syndromes. Since that time the GLRTP has become a major part of the Clinics conservative treatment program and is presently employed at other institutions from the east to west coasts of the United States.

Therapeutic Method

By grasping the lower border and circumference of the rib cage, the chest harness is able to support body weight, thus allowing the weight of the hips and legs (about 40% of body weight) to exert, by gravity, a reductive force on the lumbar spine. Patients are taught to use this harness and a safety strap system in an electrically operated tilt bed (Fig. 8-1) over a period of days with gradually increasing elevation. Seventy to ninety degrees of traction is considered a necessary goal for patients to be discharged on either a 60 degree or 90 degree maintenance program at home (Fig. 8-2). This program usually consists of 1 hour of traction performed twice a day over a period of 6 to 8 months. Following discharge from the hospital, patients return to normal activity and maintain this throughout the treaments period.

Limitations and Effectiveness

Treatment with GLRTP requires a moderate amount of physical effort on the part of the patient. It is only recommended for medically screened, well-motivated patients whose body size and shape allows this form of treatment. Obesity is the most common

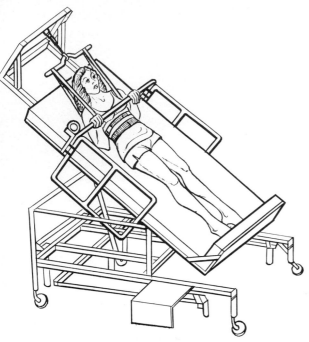

Fig. 8-1. A patient undergoing GLRTP training is shown in an electrically operated tilt bed controlled by the patient. The polyfoam-velcro chest harness is connected to a spreader bar and then connected to the bed through a chain linkage. An important component is a safety strap which is not shown. During acclimitization, the patient will typically hang in traction for about 8 half-hour sessions each day. Traction will start at 30° and increase at 5° to 10° a day to either 70° or 90° depending on tolerance.

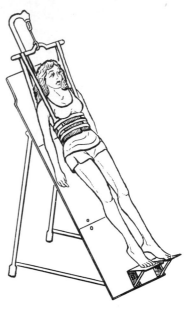

Fig. 8-2. This patient is utilizing a free standing GLRTP maintenance unit which can be set at 60°, 75°, or 90°. This part of the program is intended for 1 hour of traction in the morning and 1 hour at night over a period of time from 6 to 12 months. During the maintenance phase, patients are encouraged to resume normal activities.

reason for exclusion of patients from GLRTP if it is otherwise indicated. The degree of clinical success directly reflects the education and support provided to the patient by the medical and allied professional staff. When used appropriately it has been our observation that GLRTP can serve as the definitive mode of therapy in about 70% of previously screened patients with protruded disc syndromes. The remaining 30% of patients who are not initially improved by GLRTP usually require surgical intervention after appropriate diagnostic procedures have been performed. A recent study at our Institute, performed by Burton and Pelletier, indicated that after 1 year of GLRTP treatment 81% of previously unoperated back patients experienced a significant decrease in the severity of low back pain. It is im-

portant to note that GLRTP is also of value in helping to define surgical candidacy, as patients with advanced discs (i.e. free protrusions) are usually made worse by GLRTP.

A Possible Alternative to Surgery

GLRTP was primarily intended to enhance the conservative treatment options for protruded interverterbral disc syndromes, and this remains its most frequent use. Although back pain problems are now understood to be more complex than previously thought, it is fair to say that until recently too much of the medical profession's therapeutic effort had been directed toward the surgical treatment of disc disease. Unfortunately, the long-term success of surgical intervention has not been consistent with expectations, and for this reason alone there have been compelling incentives to focus more attention on the prevention and conservative management of the lumbar disc syndrome in particular and of back pain in general.

In an era characterized by remarkably high and progressively rising health care costs, it seems appropriate to point out that while low back pain is only the third most common reason for a patient to seek medical help (after emotional-psychiatric needs and headache), back pain is our greatest burden from the purely economic standpoint of loss of worker productivity and of inefficiently applied medical resources leading to an inordinately high liability to the health care system as a whole.

In terms of patient welfare and economics, it is imperative that attention be focused on preventative and conservative means of managing low back pain problems as well as on enhancing the success of cases where surgery is required. GLRTP was developed, and is presently being applied, in the areas noted below, to address some of these needs.

1. Lumbar Disc Herniation (Protrusion). This has been the prime application of GLRTP and is most meaningfully employed in patients who have not experienced previous surgery. It is intended for use only in patients in whom conservative management would ordinarily be considered. When GLRTP significantly accentuates a patients pain or enhances a neurologic deficit, additional diagnostic studies (*i.e.*, water-soluble myelography and computerized tomographic scanning of the lumbar spine) are indicated. This alone has proven to be a valuable provocative test. While logic would tend to support the application of gradually increasing axial traction to the lumbar spine, dynamic studies by Raney have documented that vertebral separation, through the mechanism of pulling the longitudinal ligaments taut, can reduce disc protrusions as seen in full-column myelograms in living subjects.

2. Lumbosacral Strain. GLRTP has shown promise as an initial means of conservative management when used in conjunction with a active program of physical modalities. With the use of GLRTP in an aggressive fashion, injured workers can be rapidly rehabilitated and return to work while also continuing the treatment program.

3. Mechanical Back Syndromes. GLRTP is not recommended for pure mechanical back syndromes. These may be made worse by axial traction and are usually best addressed by manipulation or facet injections or facet nerve blocks.

4. Spondylolisthesis. GLRTP is presently being investigated in the early treatment of spondylolisthesis.

5. Scoliosis. GLRTP has been noted to be beneficial in early cases of scoliosis, particularly in individuals with painful scioliosis of early onset and only after a careful neurologic evaluation has been carried out.

6. Lateral Spinal Stenosis. GLRTP is presently being evaluated as an initial means of conservative treatment. Success rates at this time appear to be less than 50%, but it has been possible to avoid decompressive surgery in a meaningful number of patients.

7. Fusion. While it is illogical and fruitless to utilize GLRTP to produce distraction of fused segments of the lumbar spine, GLRTP appears to have limited value in addressing nerve compression at the transitional vertebral segment between fusion and the normal spine.

8. Postsurgical Management. Recent studies employing computerized tomographic scanning of the lumbar spine have indicated that a common reason for postdiscectomy recurrent nerve compression has related to the development of lateral spinal stenosis secondary to the loss of disc height. GLRTP is presently being employed, in selected patients, as a postoperative measure to address, and thus avoid, this problem. At this time there is no valid data to suggest that this can be accomplished, but this is presently being theorized by the author.

9. Cautions. The primary caution to the use of GLRTP is the presence of a cardiopulmonary medical problem which will be accentuated by mild chest compression. The program is usually contraindicated in patients where obesity prevents the harness from grasping the rib cage. It has been found that some patients with previous abdominal surgery have shown some intolerance. GLRTP clinically accentuates diaphragmatic hernias but also serves as a good provocative test to pick up previously undiagnosed cases. In general, 5% of patients attempting GLRTP cannot tolerate treatment for reasons other than low back or leg pain. The most frequent problem is local tenderness of the inferior rib cage. This can be alleviated by local lotion massage after each episode of traction.

10. Complications. The possibility of device failure with patients in the hanging position always exists. For this reason, use of a safety strap is mandatory at elevations higher than 55 degrees. The patient's toes should never be more than 1 to 2 inches from support when in traction. It can not be emphasized too strongly that only specially designed and clinically tested and proven components should be used for GLRTP.

The diagnosis of lumbosacral strain is probably employed more frequently than any other diagnosis relating to low back dysfunction. Despite this fact, our knowledge of lumbosacral strain is considerably less than of many of the less frequently encountered conditions that give rise to back pain. When dealing with such an ambiguous clinical entity, which often is not authenticated by roentgenogram or laboratory changes, the physician tends to feel unsettled because of his background and training. In many instances, a patient with indeterminate low back dysfunction will be found to have an anatomic or x-ray film abnormality, and the physician will seize upon this finding as the cause of the pain, despite the common existence of such abnormalities in many who are symptom free.

Epidemiology

Lumbosacral strain can occur at any age but is most common between the ages of 25 and 50 years, men being affected approximately twice as frequently as women.

The relationship of this condition to physically strenuous work versus sedentary work is not clear and is subject to definition. However, the patient with a lumbosacral strain who has a physically demanding job is incapacitated, while the sedentary worker with the same condition may be able to function. If absence from work or the allocation of workmen's compensation funds is used as a criterion, then lumbosacral strain is considered much more prevalent with physical workers. At present, however, there is not enough evidence to confirm a causal relationship between lumbosacral strain and specific occupations. It is generally recognized that an increased mechanical load on the patient with lumbosacral strain will produce more pain. No particular somatotype is specifically prone to this disease, with the exception of the grossly obese whose problem is associated with an increased incidence of lumbosacral strain. However, when obese patients reduce their excess weight, low back pain often persists. Though inequality of leg length often is found in persons who have never experienced low back dysfunction, heel lifts are often helpful in compensating for this difference when seen in a patient with lumbosacral strain.

Roentgenographic Abnormalities

(For discussion of lumbosacral strain and x-ray film abnormalities, see Chap. 4.)

Wastebasket Diagnosis?

Many patients who are labeled with a diagnosis of lumbosacral strain, eventually are found to be suffering from a completely different entity. They may have early lumbar disc disease prior to the onset of obvious nerve root signs or symptoms; occult malignancies misdiagnosed before the true nature of the disease process becomes evident; or a host of medical; genitourinary; and gynecological conditions that give rise to low back dysfunction as the presenting symptom. Because of frequent indistinguishable symptoms in the early stages of these other entities, lumbosacral strain is considered by some as a sort of wastebasket diagnosis into which any low back dysfunction which is not readily identified may be placed. Though our factual knowledge of this disease is wanting, and we are not even sure what causes the pain in strain, this condition does exist as a specific entity with special characteristics and findings. It is classified as chronic lumbosacral strain or acute lumbosacral strain.[1]

Chronic Lumbosacral Strain

Chronic lumbosacral strain is the most common low back problem encountered in practice. It is a disease of mechanical stress upon the lower spine owing to a variable combination of unknown factors but often including faulty posture and inadequate musculature. The symptoms are apt to occur after the age of 35 when the spinal ligaments begin to lose their normal elasticity and resiliency and become progressively more fibrous. Prior to that age, the more elastic ligaments of the spine tend to compensate and adjust to the unremitting and strenuous demands which are required in carrying out the normal activities of daily living.

With the passage of time, degenerative changes involving the intervertebral joints will eventually occur, resulting in hypertrophic osteoarthritic degeneration of the vertebrae. These changes may augment preexisting low back dysfunction.

Signs and Symptoms

The symptoms of chronic lumbosacral strain vary greatly in both intensity and periodicity. A prolonged interval of rather mild discomfort may be disrupted by a severe exacerbation of pain of varying duration. At times the mild, persistent pain remains largely in the background and is ignored by the patient who considers his state normal. However, he remains mindful of the potentially latent nature of his pain and may model his physical activities quite defensively in an effort to avoid precipitating a severe and incapacitating flare-up of back pain. This pattern is usually called a chronic recurrent lumbosacral strain. The term chronic in this usage relates to the prolonged history of recurrences rather than to the duration of each specific attack.

The primary complaint is an aching discomfort in the lumbosacral region. The pain often covers a wide area and is not usually of great severity; it is commonly described as "fairly annoying" or even "mild." This discomfort has often been present for a prolonged and somewhat indefinite duration. Although a history of a fall or injury may be elicited, careful questioning usually reveals that some low back discomfort antedated the trauma. Aside from pain, the single most common complaint is fatigue, which is constantly present, despite adequae hours of sleep. Frequently, patients may complain of a "tired feeling" in the back instead of pain. Almost any activity can aggravate the pain, and bed rest may or may not relieve it. The posture and general carriage are usually poor, the patient is often overweight, and the musculature is often generally atonic and flabby. Whether these associated findings are a significant cause of the syndrome or merely an effect of long-standing low back dysfunction is not clear.

Examination may reveal some mild paraspinal muscle spasm in the lumbar area. The lumbar spine is rarely fixed or splinted as a result of spastic paraspinal muscles, and mobility may be fairly good. However, any activity involving repetitive hyperflexion or hyperextension tends to produce moderate aching discomfort, and pressure on the lumbar paraspinal muscles following such activities may be associated with moderate tenderness. A significant increase in the lumbar lordosis may be noted. Reflex, sensation, and straight leg raising tests are usually normal. X-ray films of the spine may reveal an increase of the normal lumbar curvature.

Pathophysiology

The cause or causes of this condition remain uncertain. Constipation, poor diet, inadequate rest, and a host of other poor health habits are frequently elicited in the history. A somewhat flat affect is sometimes considered characteristic. One is less likely to encounter this syndrome in the person who has established a good health regimen. Erect carriage involves a mental as well as a physical state of health.

An individual with a prolonged history of low back pain, seeking refuge from the spectre of increasing pain, may easily fall into a pattern of self-protective maneuvers. Tennis players, golfers, joggers, and other recreational athletes may give up sports which had been a significant part of their life. In an attempt to reduce the physical demands on their low backs, they may make a conscious effort to avoid walking and standing as much as possible, and try to spend more time resting. They will adopt certain antalgic body postures which may involve a slightly slouched position or one that is much more obviously distorted. These defensive measures may eventually produce secondary physical and emotional changes.

Women seem to be more frequently affected by these symptoms, particularly housewives, since the wearing of high heels and girdles may play some role in this syndrome. The routine wearing of high heels requires a compensatory adjustment of the spine in order to maintain erect posture, thus increasing the anterior lumbar curvature which, in the presence of flabby musculature, creates a disproportionate strain upon the lower back. The wearing of a properly fitted corset or girdle could conceivably be of some benefit in lending support to inadequate trunk musculature.

Management

In dealing with a persistent low back problem, a thorough workup is essential. Rectal or pelvic disease must be ruled out. Routine laboratory studies, x-ray films of the lumbar and thoracic spine, and a bone scan are in order. A careful, painstaking evaluation is the first important step in the management of this syndrome, since it gives a certain degree of confidence to the patient and gives the physician the opportunity to rule out a variety of occult conditions. The patient's trust in the physician and a willingness to follow instructions are of prime importance, since the treatment involves many changes in the patient's mode of living. A detailed explanation of basic lumbar spine mechanisms is of great value in securing the patient's confidence and cooperation.

A properly prescribed series of low back exercises designed to increase the strength of the trunk musculature must be regularly performed. (See exercises, Chap. 6.) If the patient is overweight, a gradual weight reduction program is initiated. A moderate decrease in heel length, rather than a sudden shift to a low heel, is advisable in women accustomed to wearing extremely high-heeled shoes. Any abrupt reduction of heel length may aggravate symptoms by placing the shortened Achilles tendon on stretch (Fig. 9-1).

Adequate rest should include 8 hours of sleep at night supplemented by a 1-hour period of bed rest in the afternoon. The mattress should be firm. A plywood board inserted between the spring and the mattress usually corrects a moderate sag. Many pa-

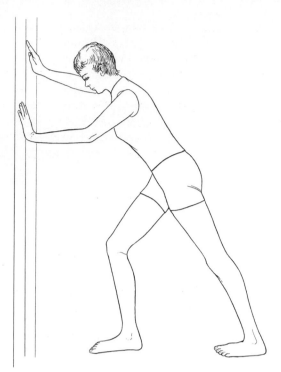

Fig. 9-1. Achilles tendon stretching exercise. When shortening of the Achilles tendons adversely affects proper body position, a corrective exercise is available. This is described in the form of the following directions to the patient: Stand facing the wall, with the palms resting against it. Position one foot 12 in from the wall, the second foot 12 in behind the first. Maintain the heel of the rear foot flat against the floor to stretch the Achilles tendon. Maintain the lumbar spine in slight flexion. Flex the arms and the anterior hip, knee, and ankle to achieve a ryhthmic back-and-forth movement of the body. After 20 rhythmic stretching movements, alternate legs. Perform this exercise twice daily.

tients sleep on bedboards or even buy a special orthopedic mattress, and then sit in overstuffed furniture during their waking hours. Firm, straight chairs support the back best. If a great deal of driving is done, the car seat should be moved forward to reduce the lumbar lordosis.

All of the activities of daily living must be carefully reviewed with the patient in an effort to determine how he may avoid excessive stress on the low back. An explanation describing the body mechanics involved in standing, walking, sitting, lifting, and sleeping is helpful. (See Chap. 6.) Because it is difficult to alter postural habits that

have become established over many years, it usually requires at least 6 months to eliminate symptoms. Initially it is usually necessary to utilize a lumbosacral support designed to sustain the low back and abdominal muscles, but as muscle tone and strength improve, this support can be discarded.

Acute Lumbosacral Strain

This condition can result from injury to the low back, such as from lifting excessive loads, lifting in a mechanically disadvantaged position, direct trauma to the back, or falls in which the low back musculature is strained.

Signs and Symptoms

Precipitating trauma to the low back region invariably causes immediate discomfort. Often, the initial pain is not unduly severe and is appreciated mainly as a stiffness of the low back region due largely to muscle spasm. The patient may continue to work and remain active in the hope that the activity will serve to work away the muscle spasm. Severe acute muscle spasm resulting from trauma frequently worsens with activity, so that the patient may eventually become completely incapacitated. It is not unusual to find the patient lying in bed, or even on the floor, suffering so severely that not only is he unable to move himself, but also the gentlest movement of the stretcher used to transport him to the hospital may cause excruciating discomfort.

The more commonly encountered acute lumbosacral strain syndrome is less severe and is manifested as low back discomfort, usually worse on one side, with the most severe pain often being localized in a rather discrete area.

Examination of the low back reveals severe bilateral or unilateral spasm of the lumbar paraspinal muscles. Forward bending causes increased discomfort with limited mobility of the lumbar spine. If the paraspinal muscle spasm is unilateral, lateral bending of the body away from the side of the spasm is painful, while the same movement toward the muscle spasm is less uncomfortable and may actually relieve the pain. Occasionally, with unilateral muscle spasm, lumbar scoliosis is seen with the concavity toward the side of the spasm. When the spasm is severe and widespread, any body movement, including movement of the lower extremities, may be painful. Reflex and sensory examinations are normal. The x-ray films of the lumbosacral spine are often normal but may reveal some straightening of the normal lumbar curvature; when the muscle spasm is unilateral, lumbar scoliosis may be noted.

Management

A patient who is so incapacitated with an acute lumbosacral strain that he is unable to work should be placed on bed rest. As in all low back problems, a bed board or a firm mattress is necessary. Muscule relaxants are thought by some to be helpful in reducing the muscle spasm, but it may be necessary to use narcotics in fairly substantial dosages if the pain persists despite enforced bed rest. A natural reluctance to use narcotics for a condition which may eventuate in a long, drawn-out, chronic problem may impel the physician to prescribe small doses, which will often be ineffective. Once the physician decides that narcotics are required, 1 or 2 large doses are more effective in relaxing muscle spasm than several smaller doses.

Physiotherapy in the form of heat and gentle massage is often helpful. If muscle spasm persists, in spite of bed rest and medication, infiltration of the paraspinal muscle with a local anesthetic may occasionally provide relief in those patients with discrete localization of pain. This relief hopefully will last beyond the pharmacologic duration of the drug.

Unless an underlying condition is present, such as a herniated disc or a fracture, the muscle spasm will invariably improve with bed rest, medication, and physiotherapy. With the subsidence of muscle spasm, the patient will be comfortable as long as he remains in bed. Before ambulation is permitted, which may aggravate a prompt exacerbation of the muscle spasm, several nonstrenuous low back exercises should be performed while lying in bed. The first three exercises described in the section on low back exercises are suitable. (See Chap. 6, phase 1 exercises.) Exercises 1 and 2 are performed several times daily; if no discomfort is appreciated, exercise 3 is added. After several days of such mobilizing exercises, the patient is ambulated, wearing a lumbosacral support or Knight spinal brace to sustain the low back and abdominal muscles. This support is worn for 6 weeks whenever the patient is out of bed for any activity, including resting in a chair. Activities are increased progressively until the patient is able to resume normal endeavors without discomfort. During the period of convalescence, the patient should be carefully supervised. Excessive exercise may cause exacerbation of the muscle spasm, while excessive rest may not only prolong the recovery period but may also create a so-called "low back neurosis" in which the patient considers himself an invalid. Such a potentially serious situation, if not properly managed, could conceivably progress to permanent disability.

Manipulative therapy to the lower back is occasionally effective in the treatment of the residuals of an acute low back strain. The improvement resulting from manipulation is due chiefly to stretching of muscles and tendons that have become contracted and shortened as a result of spasm. In addition, manipulation may be helpful in stretching the fibrous tissues surrounding the facet joints of the lumbar spine which may have become contracted and may even have developed adhesions after prolonged immobility of the lower back.

For a more detailed discussion regarding treatment, review Nonsurgical Management of Low Back Pain and Sciatica, Low Back

Exercises, and Low Back Supports and Braces in Chapter 6.

References

1. Ford L, Goodman FG: X-ray studies of the lumbosacral spine. South Med J, 10:1123, 1966

2. Horal J: The clinical appearance of low back disorders in the city of Gothenberg, Sweden. Acta Orthop Scand (Suppl) 118, 1969

3. Hult L: The Munk Fords investigation. Acta Orthop Scand (Suppl) 16, 1954

4. Splitoff CA: Roentgenographic comparison of patients with and without backache. JAMA, 152:1610, 1953

Lumbar Disc Disease 10

In properly appraising lumbar disc disease, a searching and deliberative history and examination are required. This information is indispensible for establishing an accurate diagnosis as well as for the medical insight furnished by such an evaluation. Without a complete understanding and knowledge of the patient, a proper and suitable course of management is impossible. Conceivably, a number of medical and surgical conditions exist which can be treated quite adequately with a truncated history and a physical examination limited to the condition under treatment. Lumbar disc disease is not included in this category.

Statistical Analysis

For purposes of statistical analysis of lumbar disc lesions, I have analyzed 1,000 consecutive cases that I personally have operated upon between 1961 and 1970. The advantage of analyzing an even number of cases is that it may offer an explicit statistical mental frame of comparison. When we refer to 643 cases out of 1000, a precise image is imparted that can easily be translated into percentages. All of the patients included in this series were brought to surgery. Using exclusively surgical material will load the statistics toward the more severe disorders, but it does have the advantage of establishing both myelographic and visual verification of each lesion. With regard to evaluating the results of surgery, it is said that "experience teaches slowly and at the cost of mistakes." As I look back, I recognize significant shifts in my judgment and surgical technique.

The patients included in this study ranged in age from 14 to 79 years with a mean age of 42; there were 769 males and 231 females.

Thirty-one patients had midline lesions with no lateralizing preponderance of symptoms. Of those who had lateralizing symptoms, 540 were on the left, and 360 were on the right.

The levels affected were as follows:

L5–S1 = 516
L4–5 = 218
L5–S1 and L4–5 = 243
L3–4 = 16
L2–3 = 3
L1–2 = 2
T12–L1 = 2

Symptoms

Preexisting Backache

Prior to the development of signs and symptoms compatible to a diagnosis of lumbar disc disease, most patients have experienced preexisting low back pain and other symptoms that in retrospect can be related to the ensuing lumbar disc syndrome. For want of a better label these are referred to as "preexisting symptoms." Of 1000 patients subjected to analysis, 643 gave a history of preexisting backache, and 357 denied this symptom. Exactly what produces these preexisting low back symptoms is uncertain. They may represent early changes in the nucleus pulposus, causing force to be transmitted to the annulus fibrosis in an asymmetrical fashion, and, may result in increased tensile stress on the outer layers of the annulus which contain pain fibers.

One of the most characteristic signs of disc disease is intermittency of the pain. Unrelenting and constantly progressive pain must make one alert to neoplasm. Preexisting backaches were classified into 3 groups:

Severe = 192
Moderate = 320
Mild = 131

1. Severe. The 192 patients included in the severe grouping complained of almost constant, varying degrees of low back pain. The pain would fluctuate in severity from "hardly noticeable" to "extremely severe." It often interfered with the activities of daily living and was a source of considerable disruption in their lives. In all instances, they required treatment for this problem, and most of them (164) had been hospitalized for low back pain on one or more occasions. Almost all of these patients had missed periods of time from their occupations. In the case of housewives, the severity of their symptoms at times confined them to bed so that help was needed to carry out their home commitments. The duration of these preexisting symptoms varied from 18 months to 46 years.

2. Moderate. Three hundred and twenty patients were classified as having moderate preexisting symptoms. They had intermittent back pain which was usually associated with strenuous activities but occasionally was spontaneous in onset. Exertion, such as an unusual weekend of sports, gardening,

prolonged stooping, spring housecleaning, or heavy lifting were the types of activities likely to precipitate an exacerbation of backache. As a rule, these episodes of pain improved with rest, and often the patient required no active medical treatment; self-treatment, consisting of a few aspirins and avoidance of strenuous activities, was successful. In many instances, the patient saw a physician for other ailments either on a regular or intermittent basis but rarely saw fit to discuss low back symptoms because the pain was not severe. The general attitude could be summarized by such a statement as, "I got used to the idea of living with my backache." Most of the patients classified as moderate had experienced several attacks of low back pain that they considered severe. They were incapacitated for the duration of these attacks, and 102 of them required previous hospitalizations for treatment of severe backache. The duration of these preexisting backaches was from 6 weeks to 12 years.

3. Mild. Of the 131 patients classified as having mild preexisting backache, most of these had to reflect a bit before stating that they, indeed, did have a history of backache. Terms such as "mild ache," "tired feeling in my back," "a weak back" were used. A number of these patients actually denied having backaches, but when leading questions were asked regarding how they fared when carrying out strenuous tasks such as moving furniture, gardening and so forth, a history of some low back dysfunction was elicited. A typical comment was, "I feel a bit stiff on rising in the morning, but in a half an hour or so, I've limbered up." Mild discomfort on prolonged car trips, necessitating disembarking from the vehicle and strolling about to "ease the stiffness," was also heard.

The duration of these preexisting symptoms was from 8 weeks to 5 years. Four patients had been hospitalized for low back pain, and in 3 of these patients this hospitalization represented the only severe episode of previous backache.

SECONDARY GAIN

Of the 643 patients with a history of preexisting low back symptoms, 57 claimed injury either while working or as the result of an accident with medicolegal involvement.

This factor introduces consideration of possible secondary gain, in the form either of direct financial reward or of time off from work with financial remuneration. The circumstances of this type of arrangement involve some genuine or implied advantages in having all of the symptoms date from the alleged injury, with some motivation on the part of the patient to negate any previous symptoms that could be related to the present condition.

Secondary gain was a potential consideration in 286 of the 357 patients who denied preexisting backache. Approximately 80% of these patients were involved in a secondary gain situation, while less than 9% of patients who gave a history of preexisting back pain were in a position to derive possible secondary gain from their symptoms. To ignore the human element in these statisitcs is to close our eyes to reality.

HISTORY OF TRAUMA

A history of trauma in the etiology of lumbar disc disease was elicited in the majority of patients (764 out of 1000), but the actual clinical significance of this type of information is open to question.

When Harvey Cushing collected statistics on his personal series of meningiomas, he reported a greater than 60% incidence of cerebral trauma in association with the development of this tumor. As a result of these statistics, for years credence was given to trauma as a possible etiology for meningiomas. Of course, trauma to the cranium is a common occurrence, and when questioned carefully, many of his patients could recall instances of varying degrees of cerebral trauma. Since some form of direct or indirect trauma to the low back occurs frequently in

the course of daily living, considerable discretion and imagination are needed to evaluate such information properly.

On the basis of our present understanding of the pathophysiology of lumbar disc disease, a single episode of trauma may be a precipitating, but rarely a causative, factor. Augmenting this line of reasoning, if sufficient stress is applied to the spine, a fracture of the bony elements will occur before any damage is done to the disc (Fig. 10-1). Furthermore, it is often minor episodes of trauma, such as picking a light object up off the floor or bending forward over a sink to wash one's face, that often precipitates a severe attack.

Out of 1000 patients, 764 alleged that trauma was the direct cause of, or played a significant role in, the development of their lumbar disc symptoms; 343 were involved in a possible secondary gain situation, in which they were hoping to derive compensation as restitution for their injuries. Since trauma is implicit in this situation, 100 % of these patients gave a history of trauma. The trauma was classified into 3 categories:

Severe = 24
Moderate = 71
Mild = 248

1. Severe. All of the 24 patients classified as having suffered severe trauma were hospitalized as a result of these injuries. In many instances the initial hospitalization was for treatment of symptoms other than of the lumbar spine (*i.e.*, long bone fractures, severe head injuries, soft tissue injuries). The trauma included falls from ladders or heights over 10 feet, severe vehicular injuries, or direct trauma to the body from falling or propelled objects.

2. Moderate. The 71 patients classified as having suffered moderate trauma experienced fewer associated injuries than the severe group. In addition to falls, direct trauma, and vehicular injuries, a variety of lifting experiences were included. A number of patients reported lifting a heavy object with a partner's help. Either through loss of

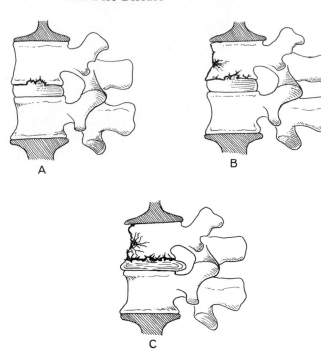

A

B

C

Fig. 10-1. Stress applied directly to the spine will fracture the bony elements before rupturing the intervertebral disc.

footing or inadequate hand purchase, the partner released his portion of the load, placing the increased weight unexpectedly on the patient. Of these patients 18 were hospitalized for treatment of their initial injuries.

3. Mild. The 248 patients in the mild trauma classification displayed the greatest degree of variation. In addition to the usual falls, many patients reported losing their footing on a slippery floor. In preventing themselves from falling, they "twisted" the back. Lifting relatively light objects was cited, as was prolonged stooping or working in a cramped position.

NO SECONDARY GAIN

Of the 657 patients not involved in a secondary gain situation, 236 (36%) gave a history of trauma.

Severe = 12
Moderate = 83
Mild = 141

There is little in the way of differentiation between the severe and moderate categories of the secondary gain patients and those who are not. In the mild classification, the only significant difference is the considerable uncertainty in the mind of the patient who has no secondary gain regarding this mild trauma as a precipitating factor of symptoms. In the secondary gain group, most of the patients were quite certain that the episode of mild trauma was the causative factor.

Primary Symptoms

Of the 756 patients who had backache as an initial symptom, 643 had preexisting intermittent, anatomically diffuse low back pain which varied in severity from rather mild backache to occasionally severe pain; 113 denied a preexisting history of intermittent low back pain prior to the onset of backache which persisted and eventually led to clearly definable lumbar disc symptoms.

Of the 643 patients with preexisting back pain, 448 could relate the onset of backache leading to disc symptoms to some trauma; 57 claimed secondary gain, and 391 had no secondary gain claim. Of the 113 patients without history of preexisting backache, 104 could relate the onset of their symptoms to trauma; 86 were in a secondary gain situation, and 18 had no secondary gain claims.

ABSENCE OF SCIATICA

Of 46 patients who had no significant sciatic symptoms, either bilateral or unilateral backache was the chief complaint. Included in this group are those who complained of numbness or tingling in one or both feet and mild aching or crampy discomfort in one or both calves or in the buttocks. I reserve the term sciatica for those who had symptoms that conformed, at least in part, to the distribution of a lumbar root. Of the 46 patients without sciatica, 31 had midline disc protrusions. Of the remaining 15 cases, the disc protrusions were at the following levels: 2 at the L1–2 interspace, 1 at L2–3 interspace, 7 at the L3–4 interspace, 3 at the L4–5 interspace, and 2 at the L5–S1 interspace.

SCIATICA

Manifesting sciatica, either with or without backache, were 964 patients; 386 noted a marked diminution in the low back pain with onset of sciatica, often appreciated as an extension of low back pain into the hip. The hip pain then began to assume a different character from the low back pain, described in such terms as "tooth-ache-like," rather than like the muscle-spasm type of pain noted in the low back (Fig. 10-2). With extension of the discomfort down the posterior thigh and eventually involvement of the entire course of the nerve root, the low back pain gradually subsided.

Developing sciatica after a bout of backache were 324 patients, and both symptoms remained acute with no significant subsidence of the backache during the entire course of illness; but 208 patients developed sciatica as the primary symptom.

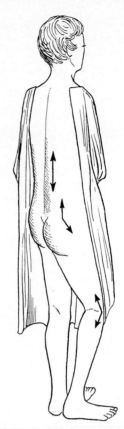

Fig. 10-2. Flattening of the normal lumbar lordosis in association with severe paraspinal muscle spasm.

SCIATIC DISTRIBUTION

It is always an unexpected rarity to encounter a sciatic neuralgia that extends every inch of the way down a specific nerve root dermatome without a hiatus or gap. In fact, such a perfect pattern may cause one to worry about the possibility of malingering. The two most commonly encountered sites of lumbar disc disease are the L5–S1 and the L4–5 levels. If the sciatic pain and paresthesia reaching the foot follow a dermatomal pattern, the specific level affected may be identified. The L5–S1 (S1 root) syndrome extends along the lateral aspect of the foot and usually involves the fourth and fifth toes. The L4–5 (L5 root) syndrome extends over the dorsum of the foot toward the great toe. Unfortunately, the pain and paresthesia of many sciatic syndromes stop at the ankle,

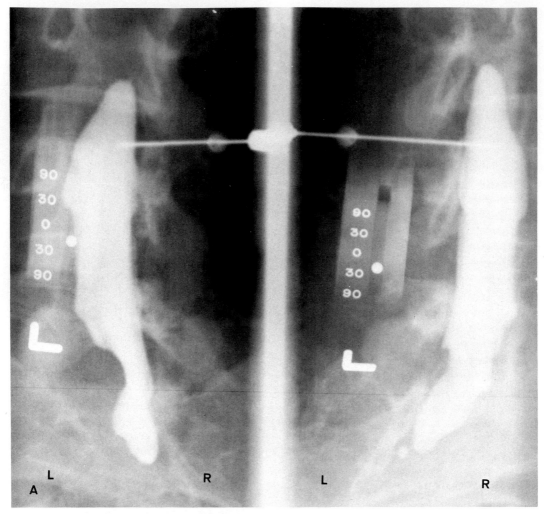

Fig. 10-3. **(A)** *This 36-year-old female complained of long-standing low back and left sciatic pain. Signs and symptoms were compatible with S1 root compression, including an absent left Achilles reflex plus pain and numbness along the lateral border of the foot within the S1 dermatome. She manifested an alternating sciatic scoliosis with concavity to the left when seen in outpatient clinic and concavity to the right 2 weeks later upon hospital admission. On the basis of the alternating sciatic scoliosis, it was presumed that the disc protrusion was in a position beneath the root that would allow*

preventing identification of specific root involvement on the basis of symptoms.

Of the 964 patients with sciatica, 585 had pain and paresthesia within an identifiable nerve root pattern, enabling a correct diagnosis to be established; 171 had a seemingly identifiable distribution of pain, but this clinical localization was incorrect when correlated with the myelogram and operative findings; 208 did not have sufficiently identifiable distribution of pain or paresthesia to

enable a reasonable clinical opinion regarding the involved interspace (Fig. 10-3).

ACTIVITIES AND POSTURE

Most patients with lumbar disc disease appreciate some relief of their discomfort with rest, and increased pain with such activities as prolonged standing or walking, forward bending, stooping, and sitting. Climbing in and out of a car and prolonged

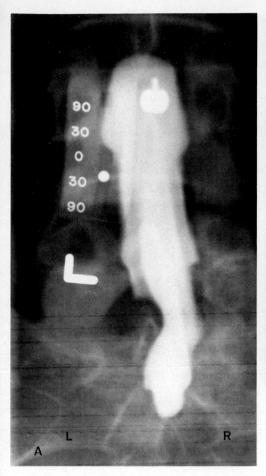

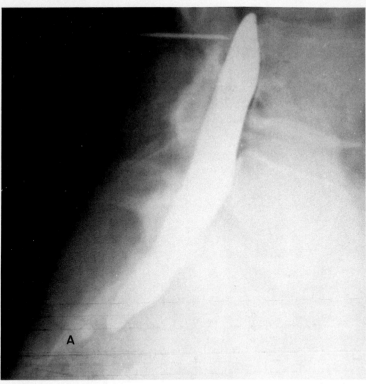

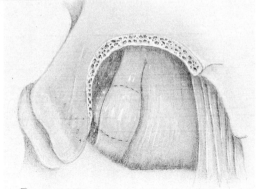

B

(Fig. 10-3, cont.)
*the root to slip to either side of the protrusion. The myelogram revealed a large filling defect seen only on the AP and oblique views, with no defect visualized on the lateral, cross-table view. This is compatible with a lesion directly beneath the root but not producing significant medial elevation of the dural sac. **(B)** Disc protrusion L5–S1 immediately below the S1 nerve root.*

vehicular driving or even riding are often painful. Occasionally, a patient will be seen who states that bed rest aggravates the pain, and the position of least discomfort is standing. This is often related to muscle spasm which may be appreciated after a period of immobility, so that when the patient first arises from bed, he feels extremely stiff and uncomfortable. Many patients who deny any significant improvement in their symptoms with bed rest at home, when maintained at absolute bed rest in the hospital will appre-

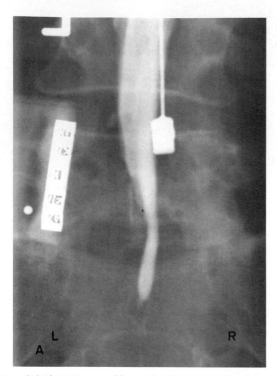

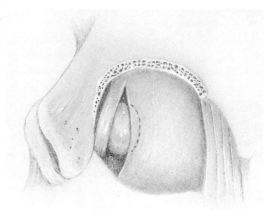

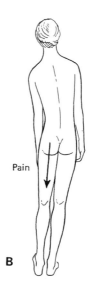

Fig. 10-4. **(A)** *This 35-year-old man had long-standing left sciatica compatible with S1 root compression. He had severe sciatic scoliosis with concavity to the left, which was clinically indicative of "axillary" protrusion. Myelogram reveals nerve root cleavage compatible with free disc fragment between nerve root and dural sac.* **(B)** *Large free fragment of intervetebral disc within axilla of nerve root.*

ciate some definite easing of their pain after 2 or 3 days.

Reactions to coughing and sneezing have often been cited as ways of differentiating disc lesions from lumbosacral strains. The presumption in this case is that the sudden increase in intraspinal pressure resulting from these activities will produce a reflected shock or impulse to be transmitted through the root sleeve to the already irritated nerve root. However, any musculoskeletal pain may be aggravated by the sudden movement of the body caused by coughing or sneezing, so that this cannot be considered a pathognomonic symptom of nerve root pressure. Straining at stool, a type of Valsalva maneuver, seems a more valid test of this principle.

No associated sudden movement of the body occurs with this maneuver to becloud the issue.

RADICULITIS

Exactly what it is that causes the nerve root pain is not clearly understood. It involves more than a simple pressure phenomenon. One can occasionally see a patient with metastatic carcinoma invading the lumbar spine and a multiple nerve root pressure syndrome producing numbness and weakness of an entire lower extremity who yet suffers surprisingly little pain. Why is this type of pressure so often not as painful as the radiculitis produced by a protruding disc? Possibly the combination of root compression and associated inflammatory changes involving the root is productive of the typical nerve root pain associated with lumbar disc disease.

Why is the onset of sciatica so often associated with subsidence of low back pain? The low back pain may be caused by the tensile stress on the outer layers of the annulus which are known to contain pain fibers. Once the annulus has ruptured, these fibers are no longer under the same tension, reducing the stimulus for low back pain.

It is, of course, the material extruding from this site of rupture that does cause compression and irritation of the nerve root creating acute sciatic pain.

MOTOR SYMPTOMS

Occasionally, a patient's chief complaint will be a foot drop with very little, if any, pain. Less frequently, weakness of the quadriceps muscle is produced by a disc protrusion at the L3–4 or L2–3 interspaces, resulting in instability of the knee; this will occasionally cause the leg to buckle without warning. One patient complained of falling and was unable to completely understand the true reason for these attacks. Root compression from disc protrusion rarely causes painless motor dysfunction; usually weakness and pain are associated.

SENSORY SYMPTOMS

There is often a discrepancy between the radicular symptoms relating to pain and those involving sensory impairment. As a rule, the pain is appreciated proximally and gradually diminishes as it progresses more distally, so that the average patient with sciatica will note increased pain in the hip and posterior thigh, with pain of a lesser intensity in the leg and foot. When numbness is noted, it seems to be more distinct distally, and less so proximally. Most patients who complain of numbness seem to be more aware of this symptom in the foot

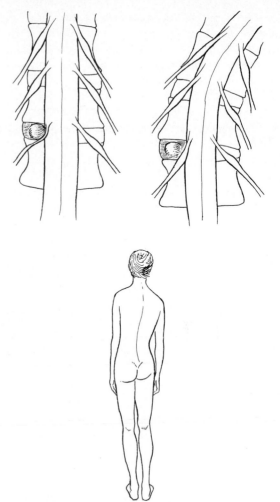

Fig. 10-5. The mechanism of sciatic scoliosis. Decreased root tension may result in decreased sciatic pain.

or leg, and it is unusual for them to appreciate this sensation in the hip or thigh. The same is true of sensory testing, with the examiner more likely to elicit a zone of numbness distally.

SCOLIOSIS AND POSTURE

The position of the nerve root in relationship to the disc protrusion will determine the posture manifested by the patient (Figs 10-4 through 10-8). As a rule, the normal lumbar lordosis is flattened because of paraspinal muscle spasm. In some cases, with very severe muscle spasm, there is reversal of the lumbar lordosis into a position of slight lumbar flexion. Less frequently, in association with flattening of the lumbar lordosis, a scoliosis occurs to one or the other side. It is not that type of long-standing scoliosis that first occurs in childhood and progressively worsens; it is a "sciatic scoliosis" associated with pronounced spasm of the paravertebral muscles and is a protective measure allowing the patient to maintain a posture which provides some degree of pain relief. It is, of course, involuntary on the part of the patient, but sciatic scoliosis does permit reduction of nerve root irritation by decreasing root pressure related to root stretch or tension. If the disc protrusion is on the medial side of the nerve root displacing it laterally, the spine is scoliosed with the concavity toward the side of the lesion in order to afford relief of radicular symptoms. Conversely, if the protrusion is lateral to the nerve root, displacing the root medially, scoliosis with the concavity away from the side of the lesion will provide relief of radicular pain. When the protruded portion of the disc is directly under the root, the scoliosis may shift from one side to the other. Because the splinting of the lumbar spine by protective muscle spasm and spinal distortion are mechanisms to decrease irritation and motion at the involved interspace, it is not uncommon to observe patients who have a striking lumbar scoliosis with severe muscle spasm experiencing relatively little discomfort. When this is the case, any effort to straighten out the low back by traction, manipulation, exercise, or brace may disrupt the patient's protective mechanisms and worsen the pain.

GAIT

The gait of a person suffering from a lumbar disc syndrome has considerable variability. In almost all cases, as a result of the paraspinal muscle spasm in the lumbar region, the gait is stiff and a bit deliberate to avoid increasing pain. When root pain is severe, the patient appreciates increased discomfort, with complete straightening or extension of the affected lower extremity. To walk in comfort, the patient may maintain a position of slight flexion at the hip and knee in an attempt to maintain the trunk as rigid as possible. This produces a characteristic limp with a slight tilting of the entire body toward the side of the pain. In some cases the root pressure is so severe that the foot is maintained in a position of plantar flexion, and the patient is unable to lower his heel to the floor. This is an antalgic protection designed to avoid tension on the sciatic nerve. With exrtmely severe pain the patient is unable to ambulate at all and must remain in a flat position. Any movement, including breathing, will increase the discomfort.

Signs

Mobility of the Spine

Lumbar spine mobility in the presence of lumbar disc protrusion depends on two factors: the degree of paraspinal muscle spasm and subsequent splinting of the lumbar spine, and the severity of nerve root pressure (Table 10-1). Flexion is, as a rule, more restricted than extension. If the patient has a splinted lumbar spine as a result of severe muscle spasm and attempts forward flexion, movement will occur at the hip joints and in the thoracic and cervical spines, but the lumbar spine will be maintained in a fixed position. This is noted visually and also can be checked manually by placing the thumb and forefinger on the lumbar spine and determining if a separation of these fingers occurs with movement. Occasionally, when the spine is completely fixed by muscle spasm, remarkably little pain is produced with forward bending, in view of the splinting action of these muscles. Although flexion is more impaired, extension too will be limited with lumbar disc disease. If extension is attempted at a time when paraspinal

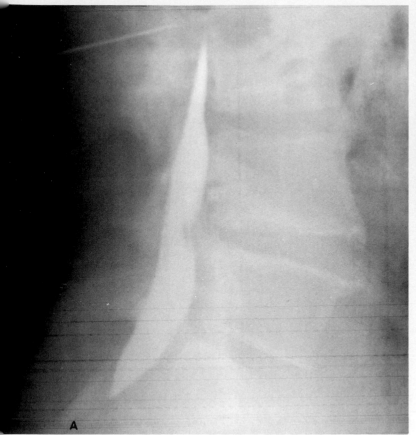

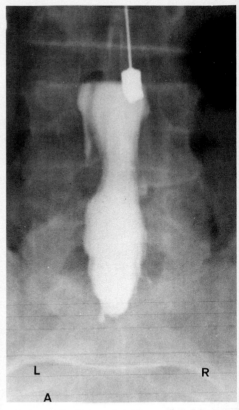

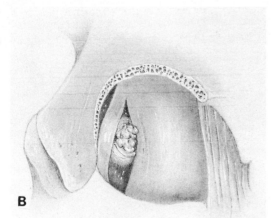

Fig. 10-6. **(A)** *This 55-year-old man complained of long-standing low back and left sciatic pain. In addition to typical signs and symptoms compatible with L5 nerve root compression (including weakness of great toe extensor power and hypesthesia over the dorsum of the left foot within the L5 sensory dermatome) he demonstrated marked and persistent sciatic scoliosis with concavity to the left. A diagnosis was made of disc protrusion at the L4–5 level on the left. In addition, we presumed on the basis of the scoliosis that the protrusion was within the "axilla" of the root and was displacing the nerve root laterally. Myelography demonstrated a disc protrusion at the L4–5 level on the left, with root cleavage indicative of protrusion discernible between the dural sac*
(Legend continues on p. 299.)

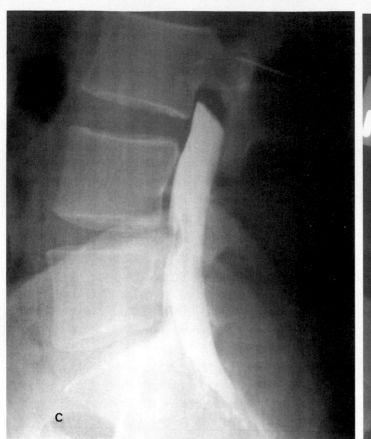

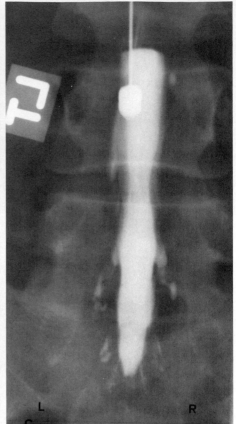

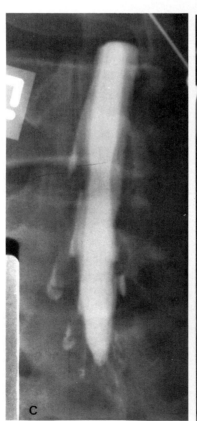

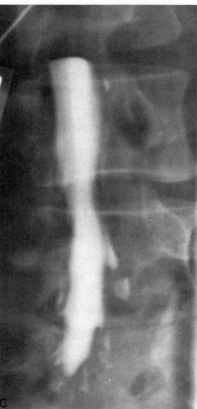

(Fig. 10-6, cont.) and root. Surgery confirmed the protrusion medial to the root within the axilla. (B) Partially extruded disc within axilla. (C and D) This 28-year-old man complained of long-standing low back and right sciatic pain. His signs and symptoms were compatible with L5 nerve root compression, including marked weakness of great toe extensors and hypesthesia over the dorsum of the right foot within the L5 sensory dermatome. He manifested a persistent sciatic scoliosis with the concavity to the left. A diagnosis was made of disc protrusion at the L4–5 level on the right. In addition, on the basis of the scoliosis, the protrusion was thought to be lateral to the nerve root. Myelography demonstrated a lateral disc protrusion at the L4–5 level. Surgery confirmed the lateral position of the protrusion.

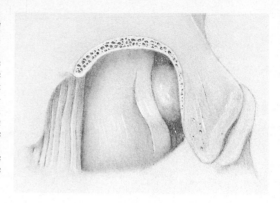

muscle spasm is severe, the entire trunk will tilt backward rather than extending, and a slight extension of the thoracic spine and hyperextension of the cervical spine will occur.

Lateral flexion is tested by having the patient bend laterally to either side and noting the distance the extended fingers reach on the thigh and knee. Normally, the extended fingers are able to reach the knee or a few inches below the knee. Even with relatively severe muscle spasm, the spine has fairly good lateral flexion. In some instances, when the disc protrusion is lateral to the root, lateral flexion toward the painful side increases the radicular pain and so is limited on the side of the lesion. When the lesion is medial to the nerve root, displacing it laterally, root tension is relieved by bending toward the side of the lesion and worsened by lateral flexion away from the lesion. It must be noted, however, that it is the relationship of the protrusion to the root that may hamper lateral flexion and not the paraspinal muscle spasm itself.

Rotation of the spine is determined by having the patient stand erect, with the examiner maintaining the hands on each of the iliac crests, and have the patient turn head and shoulders as far as possible in one direction and then in the other. Normally, the arc of shoulder rotation is a bit less than 90 degrees to either side and may be diminished slightly with severe paraspinal muscle spasm.

The proper way to palpate muscle spasm is to start at the midline, over the spinous

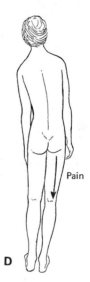

processes, and move laterally to determine the degree of muscle resistance and firmness (Fig. 10-9). This is done gently. It is a common mistake to palpate directly over the muscle mass, which is a less revealing method of evaluating paraspinal muscle spasm and which only determines the grosser degrees of difference.

Reflex Examination

Reflex examination is likely to reveal a diminished or absent Achilles reflex, if the S1 root is compressed from an L5–S1 disc. Reflexes will probably be normal, if the herniation is at the L4–5 level; and hernia-

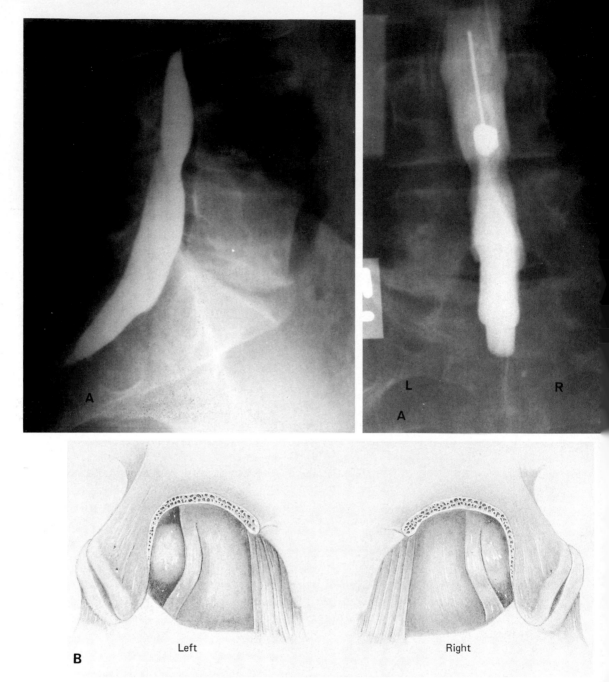

Fig. 10-7. This 53-year-old woman presented a long-standing history of low back pain, which in the past 2 years was associated with left sciatica. Six months prior to admission, she also developed right sciatica. Clinically, she manifested evidence of bilateral L5 nerve root compression. Myelography revealed changes compatible with bilateral disc protrusions at the L4–5 level. Surgery confirmed the presence of laterally positioned protrusions of the L4–5 intervertebral disc, and these lesions were excised via bilateral interlaminar exposures.

Table 10-1. CLINICAL DIFFERENTIATION OF AFFECTED LEVEL

Most patients with lumbar disc disease affecting any level, have back pain which is sensitive to mechanical and postural changes. Clinical differentiation of the specific level is principally determined by the area of pain, site of sensory dysfunction, specific motor dysfunction, reflex changes, and response to straight leg raising. The following table is a summary of the principal differentiating characteristics.

	Area of Pain	Sensory Dysfunction (Subjective and Objective)	Motor Dysfunction	Reflex Changes	Straight Leg Raising Test
L5–S1	Low back, Buttock, Sciatic distribution extending to lateral aspect of foot	Lateral aspect of foot	Minimal plantar flexion foot	Diminished or absent Achilles reflex	Positive
L4–5	Low back, Buttock, Sciatic distribution extending over dorsum of foot toward big toe	Dorsum of foot	Extensor weakness big toe and foot	None	Positive
L3–4	Low back, Lateral buttock and hip, Posterolateral aspect of thigh and anterior tibial area	Posterolateral thigh and anterior tibial area, rarely below upper third of leg	Quadriceps weakness	Diminished patellar reflex	Patients positive 50%
L2–3	Midlumbar area, Lateral hip, Anterolateral thigh (never below knee)	Anterolateral thigh	Quadriceps weakness	Diminished patellar or suprapatellar reflex	Patients negative 80%
L1–2	Midlumbar, Flank, Anterior and medial aspect of upper thigh	Anterior and medial aspect of upper thigh	Slightly weak quadriceps	Slightly diminished suprapatellar reflex	Negative
T12–L1	Inguinal region and medial thigh	Inguinal region and medial thigh	None	None	Negative

tion at the L3–4 or L2–3 level may reveal a diminished patellar or suprapatellar reflex (Fig. 10-10).

In eliciting reflexes, it must be realized that many patients have reflex changes unrelated to nerve root compression. Many persons have hypoactive or completely absent deep tendon reflexes. Bilaterally absent reflexes are often seen in elderly patients with peripheral neuropathy. Long-standing diabetics with peripheral neuropathy commonly have absent Achilles reflexes. If the radicular symptoms are unilateral, one must look for an asymmetrical reflex diminution or absence on the side of the pain before it is considered significant.

Sensory Changes

Various instruments and gadgets are available to test sensation, such as pinwheels, along the circumference of which are multiple points which can be rolled over the surface of the body. After practicing with these instruments, I invariably return to the humble safety pin. In testing sensation with a pin it is best to test a specific area and compare it with the same region in the opposite extremity. Certain sites tend to be more sensitive than others. For example, the fleshy portion of the calf which indents under the pinpoint is less sensitive to pinprick than the unyielding skin over the

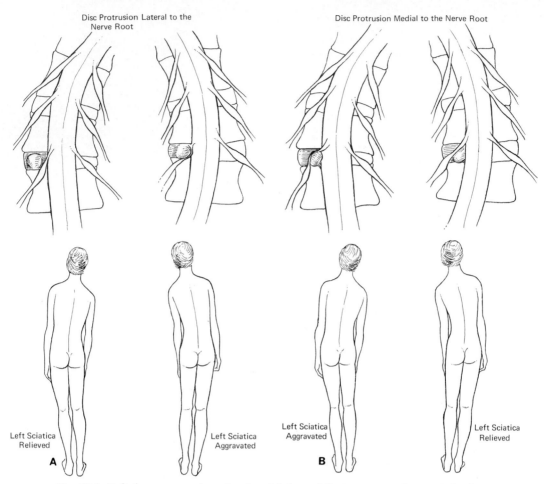

Fig. 10-8. Relief or aggravation of pain with lateral flexion may indicate if the disc protrusion is lateral or medial to the nerve root.

anterior tibial region, despite identical pressure. Because of this difference in anatomical sensitivity, it would be a mistake to compare two different sites. Examination may occasionally elicit sensory changes which do not correlate with the other clinical findings or do not follow a dermatomal pattern. Because of the subjective aspect of sensory testing, an abnormal sensory pattern is considered of clinical significance only if it can be correlated with the other radicular signs and symptoms.

In carrying out a sensory examination it is important to use the same number of pinpricks in comparing opposite limbs, since the physiological principle of summation of stimuli is in effect. Not only each individual pinprick, but the total number of pricks creates an overall sensory impression.

Motor Dysfunction

Another test of motor weakness is the action of muscles under repetitive weight bearing. If there is some slight calf muscle weakness, when a patient walks on his toes, there may be a tendency to drop the heel a little closer to the ground on the weaker side with each step. With weakness of the dorsiflexors of the foot, a slight weakness can be demonstrated by having the patient walk on his heels; the examiner will note a slight tendency for the toes to drop closer to the floor each time weight bearing occurs.

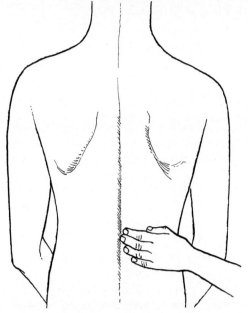

Fig. 10-9. Appreciation of paraspinal muscle spasm is best gained by placing the fingers at the midline and palpating laterally.

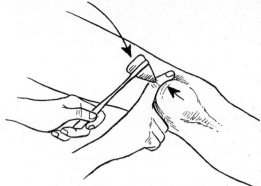

Fig. 10-10. The suprapatellar reflex.

Straight Leg Raising

Pain occurs with straight leg raising on the affected side, and usually the opposite leg can be raised without any great discomfort. Occasionally, straight leg raising on the unaffected side is productive of pain in the affected side. This finding, which occurs in 20% or 30% of disc herniations, is indicative of a large protrusion. It is the single most reliable sign of disc herniation.

FALLIBILITY OF THE NEUROLOGIC EXAMINATION

Neurosurgeons, in comparison to their orthopedic colleagues, are perhaps a bit more prone to rely upon the neurologic examination to identify the level of disc protrusion. There are, of course, certain findings, such as severe paraspinal muscle spasm in the lumbar area or poor mobility of the lumbar spine, which are common to most levels of disc protrusion and which are not considered of localizing value. The Achilles reflex, ex-

tensor weakness of the great toe, and sensory changes involving the foot are generally accepted as the three most useful findings for interspace localization. The following factors may limit the accuracy of localization.

1. Location of Disc Protrusion. The disc fragment may extrude laterally into the foramen so that it compresses the exiting root from the interspace above. Such a laterally placed fragment at the L5–S1 foramen may produce an L4–5 syndrome.

2. Neuroanatomic Changes. A partially lumbarized first sacral segment, which may be dismissed as of no clinical significance, might be associated with a postfixed plexus. In such a situation an L5–S1 disc protrusion may produce great toe weakness and numbness over the dorsum of the foot within the L5 dermatome and might be identified as an L4–5 protrusion on the basis of the neurologic examination.

3. Temporal Changes. As the patient grows older, degenerative changes within the discs occur in a progressively cephalad direction. This is well documented by discography, which demonstrates that degenerative changes usually occur first at the L5–S1 level; some years later they advance to the L4–5 interspace; and with advancing age, they move progressively cephalad. For this reason, an individual over the age of 50, who has severe sciatica associated with an

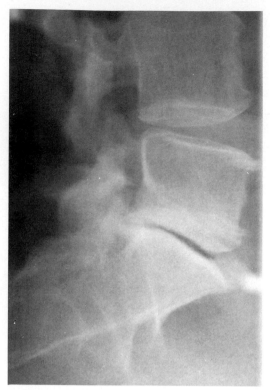

Fig. 10-11. *Vacuum phenomenon L5–S1 intervertebral disc.*

Roentgenographic Findings

X-ray films of the lumbosacral spine are necessary in the evaluation of all patients who are considered to have lumbar disc disease. The chief value of these films is to exclude conditions such as neoplasm, infection, ankylosing spondylitis, and spondylolisthesis, all of which may mimic a lumbar disc syndrome. Several positive X-ray film findings are of possible significance, and although not in themselves diagnostic, they are compatible with lumbar disc disease. The physician should look for intervertebral space narrowing with or without hypertrophic osteoarthritis of the adjacent vertebral bodies. Occasionally, condensation or sclerosis of the subchondral bone of the vertebral bodies above and below the involved disc may be seen. Calcification either in the nucleus pulposus or the annulus fibrosis may be significant.

Vacuum Phenomenon

The vacuum or pneumatization phenomenon should also be looked for, although the actual significance of this finding is uncertain, and it may occur without any significant symptomatology. The vacuum phenomenon is noted on extension and may last for only a short time, so that the x-ray film has to be taken quite promptly. Some authorities imply that this phenomenon indicates gross fissuring of the annulus.

Intervertebral Disc Space Narrowing

Narrowing of the intervertebral disc space is probably the single most valuable plain roentgenographic finding in lumbar disc disease, although it is often difficult to interpret. In some cases, it may be more apparent than real when the angulation of the x-ray tube is such that a false impression is created, with one interspace appearing wider than the other as a result of improper technique (Fig. 10-11). Often, these narrowings

absent Achilles reflex and a narrow L5–S1 disc space, could be suffering from an acute L4–5 lesion. The absent Achilles reflex may be a residual finding from a previously protruded L5–S1 lesion which was fibrosed and is no longer a source of pain; the acute lesion at L4–5 may not have been present long enough to establish definitive neurologic findings.

Consideration of Other Lesions

Any patient with back and leg pain must have evaluation of peripheral vascular status. The posterior tibial and dorsalis pedis arteries are examined, and the skin temperatures in both feet are compared.

One must always be alert to the fact that back and leg pain can occur with metastatic, intra-abdominal and retroperitoneal lesions.

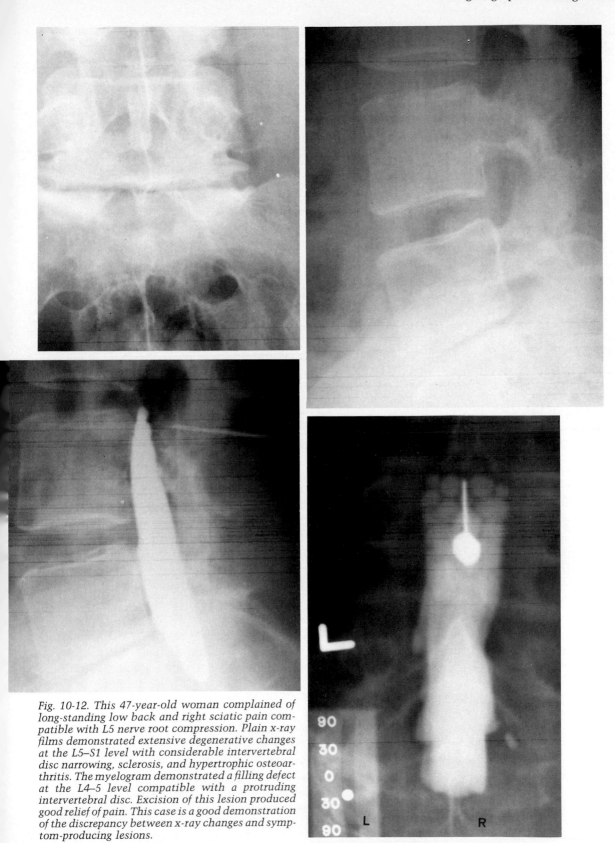

Fig. 10-12. This 47-year-old woman complained of long-standing low back and right sciatic pain compatible with L5 nerve root compression. Plain x-ray films demonstrated extensive degenerative changes at the L5–S1 level with considerable intervertebral disc narrowing, sclerosis, and hypertrophic osteoarthritis. The myelogram demonstrated a filling defect at the L4–5 level compatible with a protruding intervertebral disc. Excision of this lesion produced good relief of pain. This case is a good demonstration of the discrepancy between x-ray changes and symptom-producing lesions.

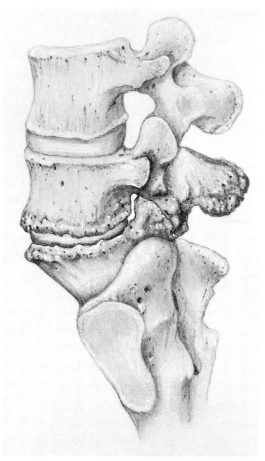

Fig. 10-13. Stenosis of the L5–S1 intervertebral foramen secondary to degenerative changes.

may be quite subtle, and it should further be remembered that the L5–S1 interspace is often narrowed after the age of 35. Therefore, a narrowed interspace may indicate the usual degenerative process occurring with advanced years and not symptom-producing lumbar disc disease. Narrowing will also occur with acute infection, such as pyogenic, infections, or chronic infections, such as TB. Often, such narrowing is related to an old, previously existing infection, which at this time has long since resolved and is not directly related to the presenting symptoms. Other possible indicators of lumbar disc disease, are in addition to narrowing, arthrosis of the intervertebral joints of the lumbar spine with osteophyte formation, sclerosis, and condensation of the subchon-

dral bone. These findings are of greater significance when they are limited to one intervertebral space. In elderly patients such alterations are widespread, involving much of the lumbar spine, and may not be associated with a specific symptom-producing condition.

Vertebral Body Alignment

Changes in alignment of the vertebral bodies may occur when the posterior facets are in an oblique downward and forward plane, allowing the upper vertebrae to settle in a slightly posterior position in relationship to the lower vertebrae. Often backward displacement of L5 occurs at the L5–S1 level; it can also be encountered at the L4–5 and L3–4 levels, but less frequently.

Degenerative Changes

It is rare to see calcification of the nucleus pulposus, but calcification of the anterior portion of the annulus is common, particularly in elderly patients or those who have considerable intervertebral lumbar arthrosis (Fig. 10-12).

On reviewing lumbar spine x-ray films, one can see disc lesions that involve the superior and inferior cartilaginous plates and that sometimes protrude anteriorly. Except as an indication of lumbar disc degeneration, in most cases these lesions are not symptom producing. Symptoms usually occur in association with posterior protrusions of the annulus fibrosus and disc.

Anterior displacement of nuclear material is more common than is generally appreciated, because this lesion is not symptom producing. When extruded nuclear tissue penetrates the anterior fibers of the annulus and comes to lie immediately beneath the anterior longitudinal ligament, an erosion of the centrum at the site of the protrusion may occur. Eventually, this type of lesion will form an anterior osteophyte.

Schmorl described extrusions of nuclear material into the spongiosa of the vertebral bodies. This penetration of nuclear tissue usually occurs just behind the center of the cartilaginous plate where the plate is quite thin and sometimes defective. Reactive formation of a thin layer of dense bone around the displaced material occurs within the spongiosa of the vertebra, allowing diagnosis of this lesion on plain x-ray film. Because of his original description of this condition, these are usually referred to as Schmorl's nodes.

Narrowing and stenosis of the intervertebral foramina is best seen on lateral and oblique views of the lumbar spine (Fig. 10-13). Often, this will be seen at many levels and may not be associated with symptoms. However, if a root is irritated and becomes swollen at a level where there is intervertebral foraminal encroachment, radicular symptoms will likely occur.

Prior to myelography about 50% of the plain x-ray films of patients with suspected lumbar disc disease were interpreted as revealing either significant lumbar interspace narrowing or degenerative changes involving the lumbar vertebrae.

Transitional Lumbosacral Vertebrae and Root Function

Traditional lumbosacral vertebrae occur in approximately 6% of the population as a whole (Fig. 10-14). This implies that the last (fifth) lumbar vertebra assumes the anatomical appearance of the first sacral segment, resulting in only four lumbar vertebrae, or the first sacral vertebra anatomically resembles the last lumbar vertebra resulting in six lumbar vertebrae. A sacralized lumbar vertebra is described as sacralization and a lumbarized sacral vertebra, lumbarization.[9]

In considering identification of root function in the presence of lumbosacral transitional vertebrae, counting down from the last rib is usually a less reliable guide than counting up from the nonsegmented solid sacrum. In other words, a disc protrusion at

the L5–6 interspace will likely be associated with a symptom complex characteristic of an L4–L5 protrusion. However, this is far from an infallible rule and, in the face of transitional vertebrae, root localization will remain uncertain.

Treatment of Lumbar Disc Disease

Selection of proper treatment is related to a number of factors, the duration of symptoms being of foremost importance. The patient who has had recurrent symptoms of lumbar disc disease for a number of years may be a suitable candidate for surgery, while the individual with recently developed back pain and sciatica requires a suitable course of conservative management. The presence of motor dysfunction, in addition to severity of pain, are essential considerations in determining method of management. The patient's ability to tolerate pain, the medication required for pain relief, and the existence of secondary gain all deserve attention in making a decision. The socioeconomic status and the physical requirements of work are also factors. Are we dealing with a patient who is content to rest in bed for an indefinite period of time, hoping that surgery can be avoided? Or, is this a patient with limited resources, who must return to work in a stated period of time; when returning, must he or she be able to perform physically strenuous work for an indefinite period?

If we do elect to treat conservatively with rest and medication, how long should we wait before considering surgery? How long should we wait if there is a partial foot drop? How long before irreversible motor weakness will occur so that, despite eventual decompressive surgery, the dysfunction persists? Many patients manifest a symptom complex presenting clear indications for appropriate management. Others will have a more provisional clinical picture, and only the physician's judgment, based on his experience and careful evaluation of the indi-

(*Text continues on p. 312*)

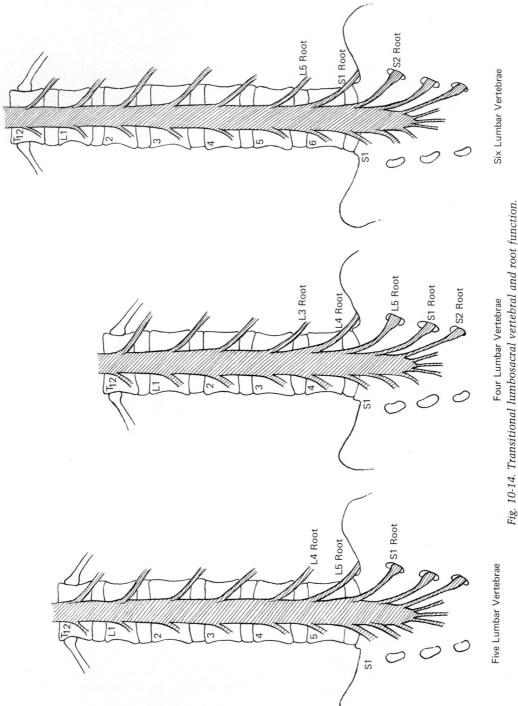

Five Lumbar Vertebrae

Four Lumbar Vertebrae

Six Lumbar Vertebrae

Fig. 10-14. Transitional lumbosacral vertebral and root function.

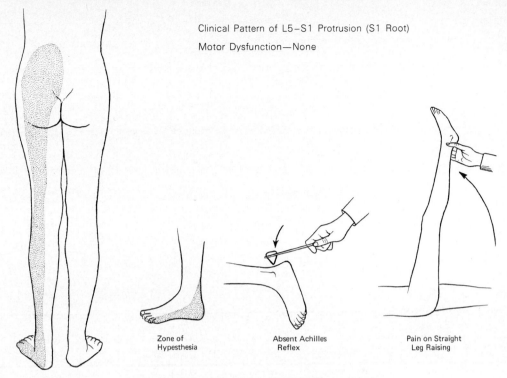

Clinical Pattern of L5–S1 Protrusion (S1 Root)

Motor Dysfunction—None

Area of Pain

Zone of
Hypesthesia

Absent Achilles
Reflex

Pain on Straight
Leg Raising

Fig. 10-15. Clinical pattern of L5–S1 disc protrusion.

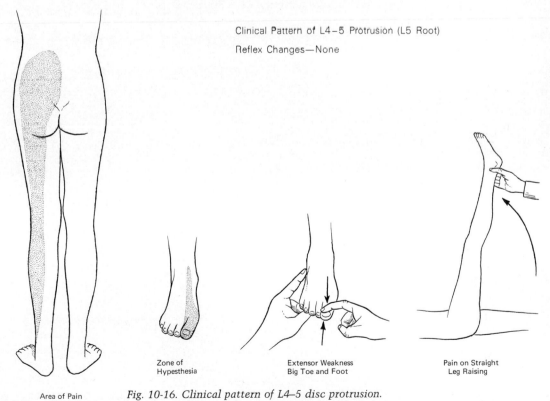

Clinical Pattern of L4–5 Protrusion (L5 Root)

Reflex Changes—None

Area of Pain

Zone of
Hypesthesia

Extensor Weakness
Big Toe and Foot

Pain on Straight
Leg Raising

Fig. 10-16. Clinical pattern of L4–5 disc protrusion.

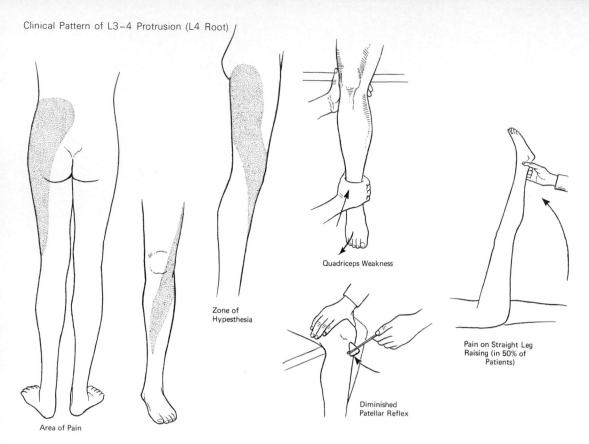

Zone of
Hypesthesia

Quadriceps Weakness

Diminished
Patellar Reflex

Pain on Straight Leg
Raising (in 50% of
Patients)

Area of Pain

Fig. 10-17. Clinical pattern of L3–4 disc protrusion.

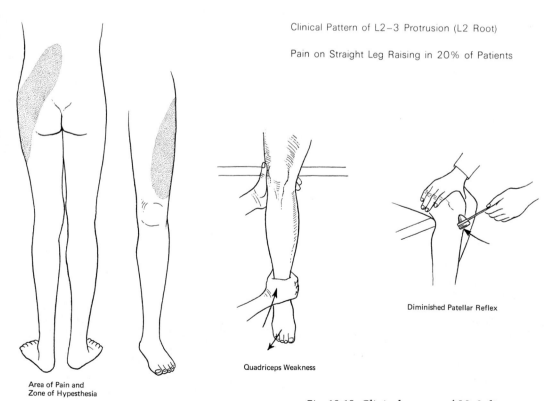

Clinical Pattern of L2–3 Protrusion (L2 Root)

Pain on Straight Leg Raising in 20% of Patients

Diminished Patellar Reflex

Quadriceps Weakness

Area of Pain and
Zone of Hypesthesia

Fig. 10-18. Clinical pattern of L2–3 disc protrusion.

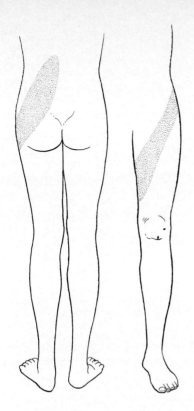

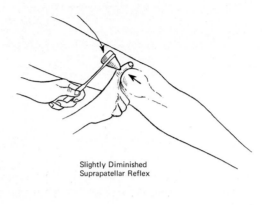

Clinical Pattern of L1–2 Protrusion (L1 Root)

Slightly Weak Quadriceps

No Pain on Straight Leg
Raising

Slightly Diminished
Suprapatellar Reflex

Area of Pain and
Zone of Hypesthesia

Fig. 10-19. Clinical pattern of L1–2 disc protrusion.

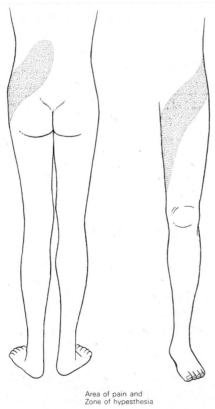

Clinical Pattern of T12

L1 Protrusion (T12 Root)

No Motor Dysfunction

No Reflex Changes

No Motor Dysfunction

No Pain on Straight Leg
Raising

The Clinical Pattern

Area of pain and
Zone of hypesthesia

Fig. 10-20. Clinical pattern of T12–L1 disc protrusion.

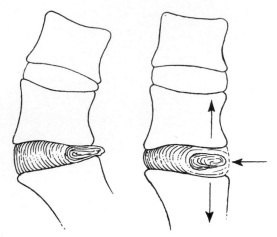

Fig. 10-21. *Positive effect of traction (lumbar flexion) upon protruding fragment of disc.*

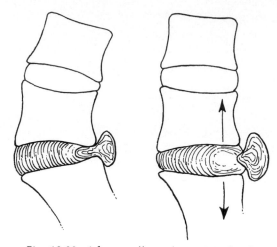

Fig. 10-22. *Adverse effect of traction (lumbar flexion) upon protruding fragment of disc.*

vidual factors, can be relied upon to determine a proper course of treatment (Figs. 10-15 through 10-20).

Conservative Management

Since all of the following methods of treatment which comprise the essentials of the conservative management of lumbar disc disease are presented in more detail in Chapter 6, it is advisable to review these pages.

REST

Almost every patient with lumbar disc disease is helped by rest and worsened by activity. Such a direct cause and effect relationship may not be so readily apparent to the patient, who may be aware of some increase in the stiffness and discomfort of the paraspinal muscles after a period of inactivity, while after walking and performing some light activity will feel more limber. The muscle spasm and pain are not primary symptoms but are secondary effects of the protruding lumbar disc. Goaded by this seemingly paradoxical effect, the patient may intentionally increase the level of physical activities, with the thought of "working out the stiffness in my back." This may all too frequently result in such an acute flare-

up of symptoms as to be completely incapacitating.

TRACTION

Pelvic traction is employed routinely in conjunction with hospital-enforced bed rest (Figs. 10-21 and 10-22). The traction apparatus and the hospital bed are positioned to promote increased lumbar flexion. This spinal position will promote distraction of the posterior elements of the lumbar spine, reducing tensile stress on the annulus fibrosus and widening the intervertebral foraminal apertures at the lower two interspaces Nerve root compression at these levels may be relieved by so altering the position of the lumbar spine. The beneficial effects of traction are probably related to lumbar flexion and bed rest.

PHYSIOTHERAPY

Heat and gentle massage are often helpful in relieving muscle pain and spasm. However, it must be recognized that the muscle symptoms are secondary to protrusion of an intervertebral disc producing annular distension and root pressure (Fig. 10-23). Moving the patient, especially during a period of acute symptoms, may aggravate this primary condition. If transporting the patient to a department of physiotherapy, or any of the physiotherapeutic measures employed, are pain producing, they should be stopped.

TRIGGER POINTS

If a specific, localized area of the lumbar region is persistently painful, Xylocaine infiltration of the site is advocated by some. This may be helpful in providing relief of localized muscle discomfort, but it will probably not affect the overall outcome of conservative management.

The risk of worsening a preexisting neurological deficit must be considered when selecting any mode of therapy (Fig. 10-24). A clear lumbar disc syndrome with radicular symptoms and neurological findings implicating a specific nerve root is not likely to

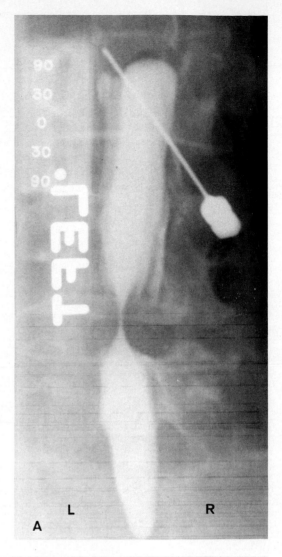

Fig. 10-23. This 48-year-old man was hospitalized with long-standing low back and right sciatic pain. He had typical signs of L5 nerve root compression, with weakness of the right great toe extensor and hypesthesia over the dorsum of the right foot within the L5 dermatome. Conservative treatment consisting of bed rest and pelvic traction was instituted. After 2 days of traction, he noted left sciatic pain in addition to the original right sciatica. Myelography demonstrated a large bilateral filling defect at the L4–5 interspace. At surgery, the disc was completely extruded on the right side and markedly protruded on the left. Prolonged lumbar flexion was probably a factor in aggravating the protrusion on the left side.

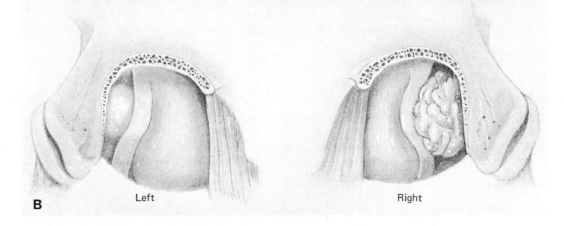

B   Left   Right

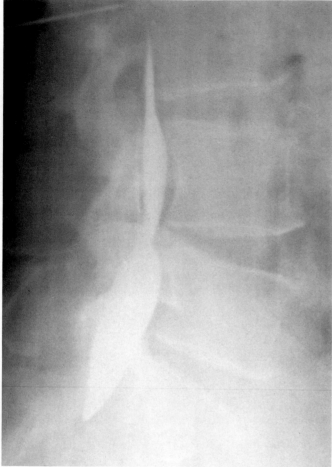

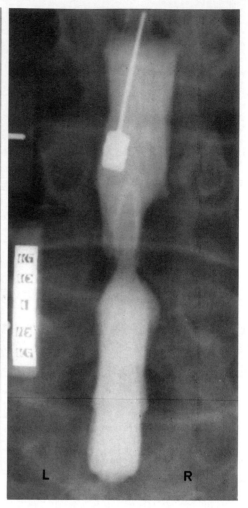

L   R

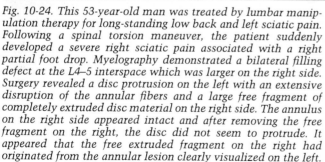

Fig. 10-24. This 53-year-old man was treated by lumbar manipulation therapy for long-standing low back and left sciatic pain.
Following a spinal torsion maneuver, the patient suddenly
developed a severe right sciatic pain associated with a right
partial foot drop. Myelography demonstrated a bilateral filling
defect at the L4–5 interspace which was larger on the right side.
Surgery revealed a disc protrusion on the left with an extensive
disruption of the annular fibers and a large free fragment of
completely extruded disc material on the right side. The annulus
on the right side appeared intact and after removing the free
fragment on the right, the disc did not seem to protrude. It
appeared that the free extruded fragment on the right had
originated from the annular lesion clearly visualized on the left.

benefit from spinal manipulation. Occasionally an adverse effect will follow, such as a
partial foot drop or increase in the severity
and persistence of pain.

If the pain predominantly involves the low
back area with a diffuse myotomal extension
into the buttock and upper thigh, the diagnosis is open to question and manipulation
may be helpful.

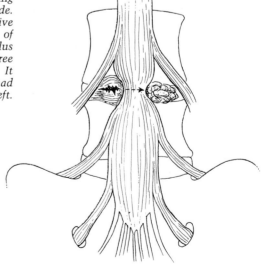

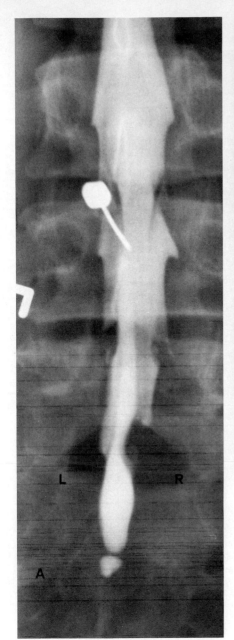

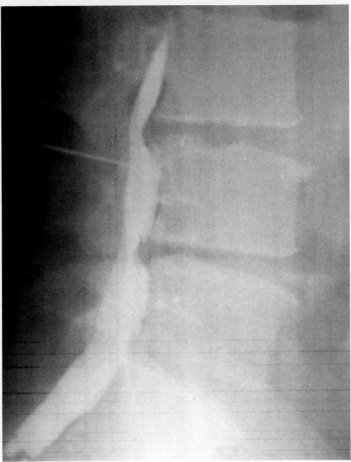

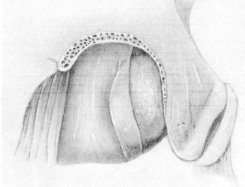

B

Fig. 10-25. **(A)** *This 35-year-old man had no significant low back dysfunction until a fall 6 months prior to admission was followed by severe, intractable low back and right sciatic pain. His signs and symptoms were typical of S1 root compression with an absent right Achilles reflex and numbness along the lateral aspect of the right foot. Myelography demonstrated intervertebral disc protrusions at the L3–4, L4–5, and L5–S1 interspaces. The protruding disc at the L5–S1 level was excised via a right interlaminar approach with no attempt to visualize or decompress the presumably nonsymptom-producing lesions visualized myelographically. The patient has done well since surgery.*

*It must be recognized that this patient will probably be predisposed to low back dysfunction in the future. He has changed his work at my request to a job which is not physically demanding. I do not believe that "prophylactic" disc excision is an acceptable concept and think this patient is best served by confining his surgery to the symptom-producing lesion. **(B)** Large disc protrusion L5–S1.*

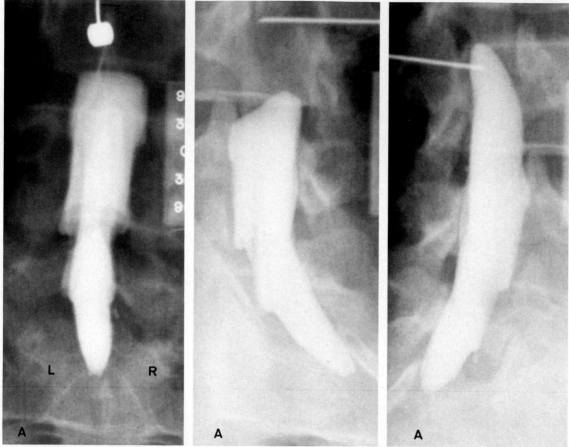

*Fig. 10-26. (**A** and **B**) This 38-year-old woman presented with long-standing low back and right sciatic pain, compatible with L5 root compression from an intervertebral disc protrusion at the L4–5 level. The myelogram was originally interpreted by the roentgenography department as nonrevealing. Careful review and correlation of the films with the clinical picture indicated a significant elevation and curling in of the root sleeve at the L4–5 level on the right, in association with a small defect at that level discovered on the oblique views. Surgery revealed a large, laterally placed disc protrusion at the L4–5 level. (**C** and **D**) This 34-year-old man presented with a 6-month history of low back and right sciatic pain typical of an L4–5 intervertebral disc protrusion. A myelogram performed June 25, 1970, was interpreted as nonrevealing. He was discharged from the hospital and treated conservatively with inadequate improvement. Because of persistent pain, he was rehospitalized and repeat myelography was performed on April 10, 1972. A large filling defect was then seen at the L4–5 level. Surgery revealed a protruding intervertebral disc at the L4–5 level with partial extrusion of disc fragments. A retrospective viewing of the original films reveals significant root asymmetry which was probably due to a protruding disc. The large defect seen on the second myelogram was likely caused by the extruded free fragment. It must be noted that despite the striking change on myelography, the patient's symptoms remained the same from the time of onset.*

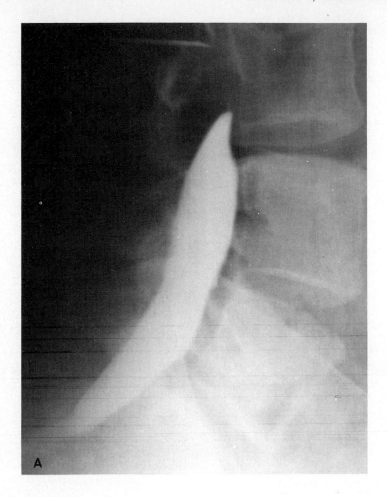

MEDICATION

The dosage and potency of medication should be commensurate with the intensity of symptoms. The patient should be maintained in reasonable comfort. Avoid doling out inadequate amounts of analgesic drugs.

Anti-inflammatory agents are often helpful in the presence of radicular symptoms.

OCCUPATIONAL CHANGES

A number of patients with lumbar disc disease, who are employed in jobs involving

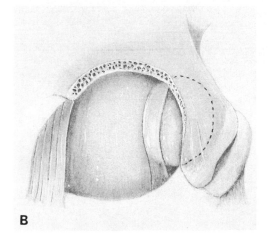

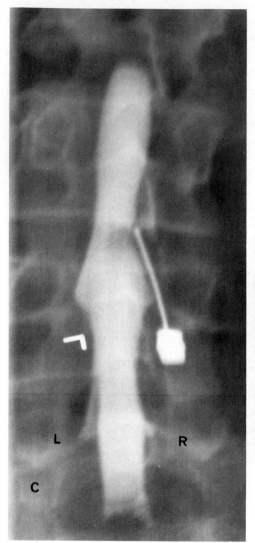

June 25, 1970

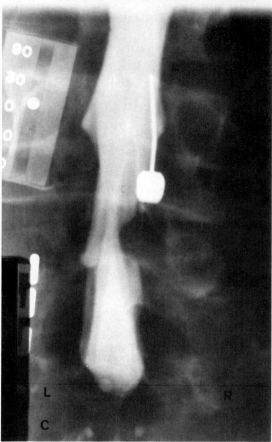

April 10, 1972

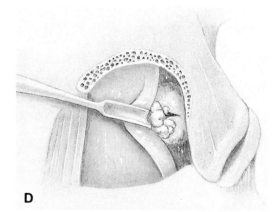

D

heavy labor, manifest a direct and apparent cause-and-effect relationship between their work and the recurrence of symptoms. Every effort must be made to direct and help the patient to obtain working conditions compatible with his disease. To perform lumbar disc surgery on such a patient and then allow him to return to the same work environment may be a disservice to the patient and may reflect poorly upon the surgeon (Fig. 10-25).

ACTIVITIES OF DAILY LIVING

Every routine daily activity that places stress upon the lumbar spine should be thoroughly reviewed with the patient, in order to provide an appreciation of the body mechanics involved in standing, walking, sitting, driving, lifting, and sleeping.

LOW BACK SUPPORTS AND SHOE LIFTS

Following a 10-day period of bed rest, if there is significant relief of symptoms, it is usually necessary to fit the patient with a low back support. This support should be considered a temporary aid to allow progressive mobilization and should not be worn more than 90 days. During this time a corrective exercise and rehabilitation program should be instituted so that this appliance may eventually be discarded. (See Chap. 6, Low Back Supports and Braces.)

If one leg is significantly shorter than the other, a shoe lift in the short leg may be helpful.

Inadequate Response to Conservative Management

INTRACTABLE SYMPTOMS

Despite the intensive employment of all conservative means of treatment, some patients' pain will perversely remain unyielding. This lack of response is not common and is a clinical indication of severity and irreversibility of the disc protrusion.

If after 6 to 8 weeks, such a refractory situation prevails, further definition of the problem may require a Technetium bone scan and a complete medical evaluation by an internist. If the medical workup and bone scan are not helpful, an epidural injection employing a combination of Depo-Medrol and Xylocaine is in order. (The injection technique is discussed in Chap. 13.) This steroid instillation may be helpful in reducing inflammatory reaction and edema of the nerve root, the sinuvertebral nerve, and the posterior longitudinal ligament. It can be performed on either an inpatient or outpatient basis and may need to be repeated on one or two occasions. Before fully assessing the results of epidural steroids, an interval of 4 to 6 weeks should elapse.

A patient who manifests intractable and incapacitating sciatica for 10 to 12 weeks may be considered a potential surgical candidate. If the persisting sciatica is associated either with neurological findings implicating a specific nerve root, or with a positive straight leg raising test, myelography is in order. If the myelogram corroborates the clinical picture, surgery is recommended.

When the lumbar myelogram is normal, lumbar epidural venography may be helpful, especially in revealing the presence of a laterally placed disc herniation which could not be demonstrated by opacification of the medially positioned dural sac.

If the venogram is not helpful, computerized axial tomography of the lumbar spine should be performed. This special study may reveal nerve root impingement from bony encroachment within the extreme lateral angle of the spinal canal or within the intervertebral foramen where both myelography or venography would be nonrevealing.

PERSISTING MOTOR SIGNS

When a course of conservative treatment is given to patients who exhibit motor weakness as a component of their radicular symptoms, they will often note, after several weeks, improvement in their pain but little or no change in motor dysfunction. This inequality in rapidity of response to treatment between pain and motor symptoms is usually seen.

The diminution of pain may be considered an indication to persist with conservative management, in the expectation of deriving an eventual motor improvement.

Delay of surgery, in the face of motor weakness, may be considered ill-advised and dilatory by some, but review of my records bears me out in demonstrating a significant number of such patients with motor weakness who responded favorably to conservative management.

Dr. Anders Hakelius from the Karolinska Institute in Sweden wrote a classic monograph entitled Prognosis in Sciatica, in which he reviewed the long-term prognosis of a large series of patients with herniated lumbar disc syndromes. He compared the follow-up statistics of surgically treated with non-surgically treated individuals, assessing a variety of clinical signs and symptoms. He confirmed that the improvement of motor weakness was not significantly different in those treated surgically than in those treated nonsurgically. So, if sciatic pain subsides and the foot drop persists, a decision to operate in the hopes of improving the motor deficit is probably ill advised.

INTERMITTENT SYMPTOMS

Many patients will note symptomatic improvement from bed rest and traction and while remaining in bed are quite comfortable, requiring no analgesic medication. However, with assumption of a weight-bearing position, recurrence of pain immediately follows. Under these circumstances, bed rest and traction are continued for several additional days, after which very gradual and progressive mobilization is attempted. Before further mobilization is ordered, it may be helpful to have the patient fitted with a low back support, which should be worn prior to weight-bearing efforts. If, despite these measures, weight bearing is not tol-

erated, after 6 to 8 weeks myelography is in order.

SUBJECTIVE RESPONSE

Variations that exist from patient to patient, in response to conservative treatment of lumbar disc disease, are conspicuous to all physicians. One patient may not be happy with an end result that another will gladly accept. These differences relate to individual temperament, mode of living, and the underlying disposition to accept and live with some degree of discomfort.

A patient who leads a more sedentary existence may more readily accept some residual dysfunction than one who by inclination or necessity is physically active. The patient who is forced to earn a living by means of physical labor may not be able to tolerate lumbar disc symptoms of moderate intensity, nor will the sports-minded office worker, who is a devoted golfer or tennis player, be happy with the limitations imposed by such disease.

A decision regarding proper management of these controvertible problems must be based on the experience and judgment of the physician.

Decision Making in Lumbar Disc Surgery

The results of disc surgery relate to a number of factors, unquestionably the most important being patient selectivity (Fig. 10-26). This was corroborated by a clinical review carried out at our clinic in 1977.

Ninety-four patients with failed low back syndromes were referred for consultation to the Crozer-Chester Medical Center Low Back Pain Clinic during the period from July to December, 1976. A detailed history and a physical examination were performed on all patients. Some patients brought complete medical records and roentgenogram studies; others had incomplete records and roentgenogram studies. All such data were carefully reviewed when available. A total of 179 lumbar spine operative procedures had been performed on these patients by 46 surgeons.

Frequency of Surgery in 94 Patients Studied

Patients (No.)	Operative procedures (No.)
41	1
33	2
12	3
5	4
2	5
1	6

Careful review of this relatively small series was carried out in an effort to determine if some common factor or factors could be identified which might be of etiologic significance in the production of the failed low back syndrome. A critical assessment of this material demonstrated that the single most striking factor influencing the outcome of surgery is poor patient selection prior to the initial operative procedure.

As is true with any retrospective study, the benefit of hindsight may create a bias, particularly when attempting to assess a skill as subjective as clinical judgment. With this caveat in mind, the author nevertheless holds to his opinion that the original surgery was not indicated in 76 of the 94 cases (81%) that were reviewed.

It is necessary for the spine surgeon to be able to recognize who is likely to benefit from surgery, and possibly even more important, to identify the patient who is apt to do poorly after surgery. The most that we can reasonably expect, even if the finest surgeon operates on a patient who does not need surgery, is the creation of only minimal iatrogenic dysfunction superimposed on the oroginal problem. Under less optimal circumstances, limitless complications may result.

LUMBAR DISC SURGERY PREDICTIVE SCORE PAD

It must be recognized that any surgical judgment that is primarily based on such a subjective symptom as pain can have as many variables as there are surgeons. All medical judgments relating to therapy are made by assigning positive and negative relative values to various aspects of the clinical picture, with the final decision made by balancing out these relative values. A numerical value system is not commonly used, but such a system may allow us to communicate more easily about this complex problem.

A review of the various clinical factors which play a role in surgical decision making was carried out in 200 postsurgical patients who had a good result and was compared with 96 postsurgical patients who had a poor result. This clinical review was employed as a base on which to list the major positive and negative factors involved in preoperative selection and to assign these factors positive and negative numerical values. Employment of such a system provides a "predictive number" indicating the likely outcome of surgery. In an effort to make the system usable by almost all physicians who are involved in lumbar disc surgery, only the criteria which have broad acceptance and are generally employed were included. Studies which have less widespread use such as electromyogram, discogram, lumbar venogram, CAT scan, and special psychological studies have been purposely excluded.

POSITIVE SCORE CARD FACTORS (Fig. 10-27A)

Factor 1. The key word is incapacitating. If pain is not severe enough to hamper activities of daily living, the patient is often likely to be unsatisfied with the results of surgery.

Factor 2. Excision of a herniated lumbar disc will usually relieve nerve root pain. If sciatica is not the major symptom, and surgery provides relief of sciatica but no improvement of the back pain, the unhappy patient may well ignore the disappearance of the minor sciatica and concentrate on the persisting predominant back pain.

Positive Points	POSITIVE FACTORS	NEGATIVE FACTORS	Negative Points
5	1. Low back pain and sciatic pain severe enough to be incapacitating.	1. **Back pain primarily**	15
		2. **Gross obesity**	10
15	2. Sciatica is more severe than back pain.	3. **Nonorganic signs and symptoms—** entire leg numb; simultaneous weakness of flexion and extension of toes; extension of pain into areas not explainable by an organic lesion.	10
5	3. Weight-bearing (sitting or standing) aggravates the pain; bed rest (in some position) eases the pain.	4. **Poor psychological background—** attempted suicide, unrealistically high expectations from surgery; previous admissions for nonorganic symptoms, hyperventilation, unexplainable chest pains and abdominal pains, intractable incisional pain; alcoholic; not happy with job; physical demands of present occupation excessive; hostility to environment, employer, spouse; much time off from work for medical reasons (man out of work 6 months, woman out of work 16 months).	15
25	4. Neurological examination demonstrates a single root syndrome indicating a specific interspace.		
25	5. Myelographic defect corroborates the neurological examination.		
10 / 20	6. Positive straight leg raising test. Crossed straight leg raising test.	5. **Secondary pain—**work connected accident; vehicular accident; medico-legal adversary situation; near retirement age, eligible for disability pension if symptoms persist.	20
10	7. Patient's realistic self-appraisal of future life style.	6. **History of previous law suits** for medico-legal problems.	10

Positive Total **Negative Total**

Subtract negative total from positive total ☐ for predictive number

SCORING

75 & over .... good
65 - 75 .... fair
55 - 65 .... marginal
below 55 .... poor

Bernard E. Finneson, M.D.
Low Back Pain Clinic
Crozer-Chester Medical Center
Upland, Chester, Pa. 19013

A

Fig. 10-27. (A) Lumbar disc surgery predictive score card. This questionnaire is of predictive value when limited to candidates for excision of a herniated lumbar disc who have not previously undergone lumbar spine surgery. It is not designed to encompass candidates for other types of lumbar spine surgery, such as decompressive laminectomy or fusion. (B) Form letter requesting self-evaluation of the results of lumbar disc surgery. (Figure (A) on facing page.)

Dear (patient's name):

I am writing to obtain your assessment of the lumbar disc surgery I performed on (date).

To facilitate your response I have enclosed a self-addressed postcard. Please check the number (on the postcard) which most closely describes your present condition.

1. If after the surgery your pain was improved and you were able to function well, please check #1.

2. If your pain was improved but you were not able to function without occasional medication and occasional time off from your activities, please check #2.

3. If after surgery your pain was improved but you still have considerable discomfort that requires frequent medication and time off from your activities, please check #3.

4. If after surgery you are either unimproved or worse, please check #4.

I have provided a space on the postcard (COMMENTS) for any additional information you may wish to include.

Thank you in advance for your help.

B

Bernard E. Finneson, M.D.

Factor 3. Body position should affect a lumbar disc syndrome if it is indeed a mechanical problem. Sciatic syndromes that are unaffected by changes in body position are often nonmechanical in nature and will not be alleviated by mechanical removal of pressure.

Factor 4. Self-explanatory (see score card).

Factor 5. It is important that the myelographic defect corroborates the neurologic examination. We must keep in mind the various reports that indicate percentages varying from 25% to 35% of abnormal lumbar myelographs in (low back) symptom-free patients.

Factor 6. The straight leg raising test is a good predictive factor. The crossed straight leg raising test (the nonpainful leg is raised producing aggravation of pain rediating into the painful leg) is twice as effective.

Factor 7. This is an important factor that may easily be ignored by the surgeon. The only way to appreciate the patient's postoperative expectations is to spend some time listening to the patient.

NEGATIVE SCORE CARD FACTORS

Factor 1. This is the reverse of positive factor 2.

Factor 2. Although initially grossly obese people seem to do about the same as those with a more normal habitus, after 1 or 2 years the recurrence rate is somewhat higher.

Factor 3. Simultaneous weakness of great toe flexion and extension cannot be explained by pressure on a single root, and unless some neurologic explanation can be offered for this finding, it should be considered nonorganic.

Factor 4. This is a "mixed bag," but any of these factors should cause the surgeon to be cautious. The alcoholic, for example, may have demonstrated a very steady work history in the past and may never have been hospitalized previously. However, it should be recognized that alcoholic people arise every morning and set about their tasks only with great effort and difficulty. Any break in their routine may produce a behavior reversal.

Factors 5 and 6. Self-explanatory (see score card).

SCORE CARD ANALYSIS

As a logical second step to determine the validity of the predictive number, a retrospective "score card analysis" of patients who had previously undergone lumbar disc surgery was undertaken.

The charts of 596 patients who had undergone lumbar disc surgery at the Crozer-Chester Medical Center between the years 1962 and 1974 were reviewed, and each patient was scored using the lumbar disc surgery predictive score card. After the predictive number had been assigned, mailings were sent to each of the 596 patients (Fig. 10-27B).

For purposes of adapting the patient's mailed self-assessment to the score card, the responses were graded as follows: (1) good; (2) fair; (3) marginal; and (4) poor. Grades 1, 2, and 3 were all improved; grade 4 was either unimproved or worse. Both grades 1 and 2 are considered satisfactory results.

From the 596 mailings there were 303 responses, 23 of which were not considered suitable for inclusion in the study. Several responses which were considered unsuitable were those in which the patient had died and a numerical assessment was submitted by the spouse. The rest were patients who did not understand the instructions and

checked more than one block. One hundred forty-three mailings (24%) were returned marked "addressee unknown." Four hundred forty-six (75%) were accounted for. No answer was received nor was the envelope returned from 150 (25%).

RESULTS OF ANALYSIS

The 280 patients submitting suitable responses indicated self-assessment of their lumbar disc surgery as follows:

Result	Number	Percent	
Good	222	79.3	87.1 satisfactory
Fair	22	7.8	96.0 improved
Marginal	25	8.9	
Poor	11	4.0	
Total	280	100	

The time interval between surgery and score card evaluation of the 280 patients varied from 3 to 16 years with a mean follow-up duration of 8.4 years.

The predictive numbers of each result category were averaged and are as follows:

Result	Average predictive number
Good	75.8
Fair	66.3
Marginal	62.9
Poor	62.3

A comparison of the average predictive number with the scoring box at the bottom of the score card is as follows:

Scoring	Result	Average predictive number
>75	Good	75.8
65–75	Fair	66.3
55–65	Marginal	62.9
<55	Poor	62.3

The average predictive numbers of the good and fair categories fall within the suggested parameters, but the marginal and poor categories demonstrate no significant difference. It is further apparent that the numerical differences between the various categories are not great. The average predictive number for the good category is just above the permissable score of 75. The fair, marginal, and poor categories are numerically so close to each other that one would hesitate to accept these figures as being statistically meaningful.

Since the score card appeared to be of meager benefit in assessing the long-term, follow-up patient, we analyzed the 83 patients (of the basic 280 patient sampling) who had undergone surgery in 1973, 1974, and 1975 with a mean follow-up duration of 3.8 years.

Result	Number	Percent
Good	64	77.2
Fair	10	12.0
Marginal	7	8.4
Poor	2	2.4
Total	83	100

The predictive numbers of each result category were averaged and are as follows:

Result	Average predictive number
Good	78.1
Fair	67.7
Marginal	62.
Poor	55.

A comparison of the average predictive number with the scoring box at the bottom of the score card is as follows:

Scoring	Result	Average predictive number
>75	Good	78.1
65–75	Fair	67.7
55–65	Marginal	62
<55	Poor	55

In comparison with the basic 280-patient sampling, the average predictive numbers of the 83 patients with a mean follow-up duration of 3.8 years fall more clearly within the anticipated parameters of the score card. The numerical differences between the various categories are reasonably disparate and can probably be classified as statistically significant.

Interpretation of Results. The intent in pursuing this project was to determine the relationship between patient selection and the outcome of lumbar disc surgery. Because of the dynamic status of the lumbar spine with the passage of time, patient selectivity seems to be less critical after the first 5 years. For example, a diseased lumbar disc joint which is a source of pain may eventually, as a result of degenerative changes, become relatively nonmobile and pain free. Conversely, a symptom-free lumbar disc joint may, over the course of several years, develop degenerative disc disease which could be painful. The progressive hypertrophic osteoarthritic degenerative changes which may be associated with reduced pain in some instances and increased pain on others can occur at the surgically treated intervertebral disc level and at adjacent levels. These additional variables associated with the long-term, follow-up, lumbar disc surgery patient tend to decrease the significance of the predictive number. For the first 5 years, however, the outcome of lumbar disc surgery seems to be directly related to patient selectivity.

The score card may be utilized as a satisfactory system for presurgical patient selection.

PREDICTIVE FACTORS

The four most important factors in determining a satisfactory outcome for surgery are:

1. Sciatic pain more severe than the back pain.
2. An abnormal myelogram that correlates with the clinical picture.
3. Positive Leségue sign.
4. Neurologic deficit.

The crossed Leségue sign is probably the most specific test for lumbar disc herniation.

If all four of the above are present, technically adequate surgery is likely to produce a satisfactory result. If one of them is absent, the surgeon should be very satisfied with the accuracy of the other three factors. Surgery considered with only one or two of these positive is likely to be associated with a high incidence of less then satisfactory results. With these factors in mind, there are four indications for surgery:

1. Intractable pain.
2. Progressively worsening neurologic deficit.
3. Intractable recurrence of pain.
4. Cauda equina syndrome.

With the exception of the cauda equina syndrome, each of these indications is relative and will depend on how well the patient tolerates the symptoms, on the extent of the neurologic deficit, and on the psychologic and sociologic background of the patient.

CONTRAINDICATIONS FOR SURGERY

1. A first episode of low back and sciatic pain, without an adequate trial of conservative management.
2. Intermittent low back pain associated with occasional pains of equivocal nature, extending into one or the other lower extremity, and an equivocal myelogram.
3. A prolonged history of intermittent low back pain and an equivocal myelogram.
4. Low back and intermittent sciatic pain with a myelogram demonstrating a lesion on the "wrong" or pain-free side. I have seen several patients in whom disc surgery was performed with these criteria, and the two surgeons who elected to proceed on the basis of this information were divided in choosing the side of surgery. The one who operated upon the painful side used as his justification myelographic evidence of disc dysfunction at a specific interspace; since the pain was on the opposite side, he decided it would be best to decompress the root on the side of the pain rather than on the side of the myelographic defect. The surgeon who elected to operate on the side of the myelographic defect rather than on the side of the pain felt that the disc protrusion might cause a shift of the cauda equina enclosed within its dural sac, pressing the opposite root against the lamina and producing radicular symptoms.

5. Improvement of the patient. In the presence of significant motor weakness, if some slight improvement occurs after surgery is scheduled, it may be justifiable to proceed. If pain is the primary symptom, however, improvement is an indication to cancel surgery. I adhere to this principle and have cancelled many scheduled cases on the day of surgery upon being told that the patient no longer had pain or that the pain was markedly improved. Pain surgery performed during an interval of improvement may result in patient dissatisfaction, despite an adequate postoperative result. The patient may be less willing to accept residual symptoms, even of a relatively minor nature, and is more apt to question in retrospect how pressing and indispensable the need was for surgery. If, in the face of improvement, the patient is discharged and subsequently readmitted for surgery with an exacerbation of pain, occasional residual symptoms may present less of a problem and be tolerated more kindly. When contemplating lumbar disc surgery, the indications must be clear to the patient as well as to the surgeon.

Exploratory Lumbar Disc Surgery

Five years ago, the patient who presented with persisting sciatica and a normal myelogram, and who failed to respond to conservative treatment efforts, was often considered a suitable candidate for exploratory lumbar disc surgery. Usually the L5–S1 and L4–5 levels were explored on the symptomatic side. Although some patients were undoubtedly benefited by this approach, a significant group either were not improved or were worse after surgery. At this time, with the additional diagnostic help provided by lumbar epidural venography and computerized axial tomography of the lumbar spine, we are able to assess those intraspinal areas which may previously have been hidden from us. Given these new diagnostic tools, I can't conceive of a suitable indication for a blind exploration based purely on the persistence of pain. The likelihood of finding a surgically treatable lesion if a myelogram, venogram, and CAT scan are all normal is so poor that the era of exploratory lumbar disc surgery is best considered brought to a close.

Surgery

Historical Development

Fifty years ago, an occasional laminectomy was performed for lumbar disc disease and the extruded disc fragments were identified as "chondromata." There was some question regarding the exact nature of these lesions, although some surgeons did recognize them as consisting of displaced intervertebral disc material. The surgical technique utilized in the removal of such lesions invariably involved an extensive bilateral laminectomy. This was usually followed by opening the dura in the midline, separating the nerve roots to either side and by means of a narrow probe, and palpating the anterior spinal canal until the underlying protrusion was identified. The anterior dura was then incised over the most eminent portion of the hump, and through this anterior dural opening, the protruding portion of the disc was exposed and removed.

The entire concept of ruptured intervertebral discs changed after the classic paper of Mixter and Barr. They conclusively and unequivocally demonstrated the origin of these lesions, laid to rest any lingering doubts that they were neoplasms, and documented their etiology as protrusions of the nucleus of an intervertebral disc. They em-

phasized the indications for surgical treatment of this condition. Shortly after the appearance of this paper, surgical technique for protruding lumbar intervertebral discs underwent an important change, with the dura left intact and the protruding disc removed extradurally, although the widespread bilateral laminectomy was continued. Further evolution of surgical refinements followed, including the hemilaminectomy which leaves the spinous process and lamina intact on the pain-free side. Twenty-five or 30 years ago it became common practice to carry out lumbar disc surgery in most cases by means of the unilateral interlaminar approach.

In the past 6 or 7 years, the combined use of a fiberoptic headlight and 2½- to 4½-magnifying-power operating telescopes was accepted by increasing numbers of disc surgeons. The fiberoptic lighting was helpful, not only in providing dependable illumination to the depths of the incision, but in eliminating the technical necessity for the rather long laminectomy incision which extends over three interspaces (though the actual disc surgery was confined to an interlaminar space measuring approximately one half inch). The lengthy skin and muscle incision was required to allow the standard overhead O.R. lighting to illuminate the apex or depth of the operative field. With the brighter beam of light made available with fiberoptic techniques, a much smaller incision is possible (Fig. 10-28). The magnification provided by the operating telescopes aids greatly in assuring delicate handling of tissue and helps prevent nerve root damage. Increasing the magnification to 25 × with the use of an operating microscope has led to development of a specific technique involving a distinct departure from prior surgical concepts. In an effort to minimize reherniations and adhesions, a much more limited removal of disc material is performed. This technique avoids laminectomy, curettement of the disc space, removal of epidural fat, or scalpel incision of the annulus fibrosis and instead employs a blunt probe to perforate this structure.

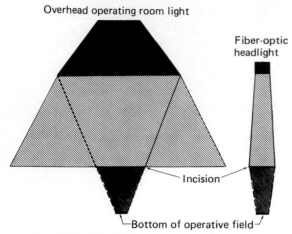

Fig. 10-28. *The brighter, more intense beam of fiberoptic light provides illumination through a small incision. Standard overhead OR lighting requires an incision approximately three times larger to illuminate the depth of the operative field.*

With advances in knowledge and equipment, continued changes can be anticipated.

Choice of Operative Procedure

Once the decision is made that surgery is indicated, the surgeon must determine which operative procedure is most suitable for the patient's particular low back dysfunction.

Is a disc herniation producing a clear single root syndrome? If so, interlaminar disc excision is the procedure of choice.

Is it primarily a stenotic lumbar spinal canal syndrome associated with sciatica produced by foraminal impingement and secondary to a bony spur? Attempting to treat this condition with an interlaminar disc excision is often technically difficult and is likely to have a disappointing clinical result. The operation of choice for a stenotic lumbar spinal canal is decompressive laminectomy and foraminotomy at the appropriate level.

If the symptoms are unilateral and the myelographic defect is bilateral, should surgery be confined to the side of the pain, or should a bilateral interlaminar disc excision be performed? This is often a gray area and may be open to controversy. As a basic principle, I prefer performing the minimal amount of surgery that can adequately relieve symptoms rather than attempting prophylactic surgery of symptoms that have not yet developed. Whichever decision is made in this situation can be wrong. Following a bilateral interlaminar operation, the patient may wake up with postoperative pain in the previously painless leg. Surgery can be confined to the painful side, and in the near or distant future, pain may develop on the nonoperated side.

Should disc excision be followed by a fusion? We do not routinely perform a com-

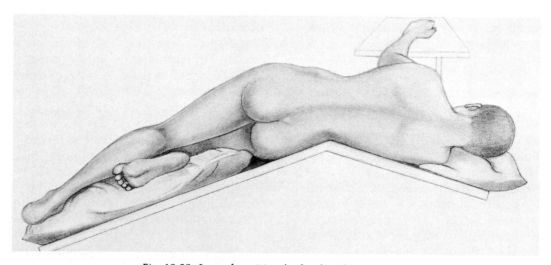

Fig. 10-29. *Lateral position for lumbar disc surgery.*

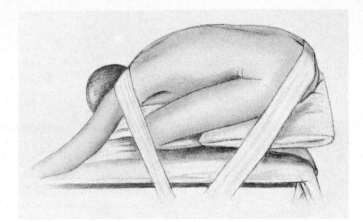

Fig. 10-30. Knee-to-chest position for lumbar disc surgery.

bined disc excision and spinal fusion, but reserve this combined procedure for the unusual situation.

Double-check Side of Lesion

Performing an operative procedure on the "wrong side" is not a common mishap, but it can occur when surgery is performed on any structure that is paired. Patients who have undergone herniorrhapies, hip surgery, cataract surgery, or carpal tunnel decompressions have occasionally awakened from anesthesia and been surprised to find the surgical dressing and the incisional discom-

fort at an unanticipated site. Because the patient undergoing lumbar disc surgery is in the prone position with his "sides reversed," this error may occur with greater frequency than is likely to happen in the supine position. The best way to preclude this blunder is for the surgeon to remain alert to such a possibility and to establish a preventive behavior pattern.

When reviewing spine x-ray films, I make a point of placing the films on the view box as though the patient was in the prone position, with the left marker on my left side. Radiologists, who are trained to visualize films as though the patient is in the

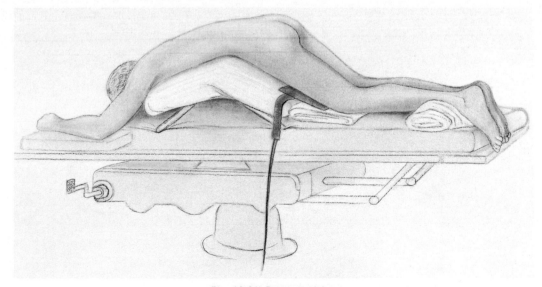

Fig. 10-31. Prone position.

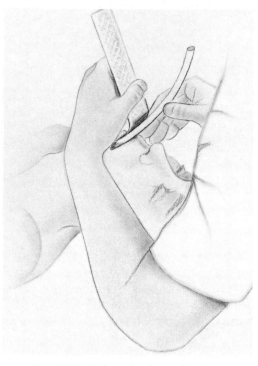

Fig. 10-32. Endotracheal anesthesia.

anatomical position may look with mild disfavor at this heresy. However, it is not the radiologist who will be sued for operating on the wrong side. This practice reinforces a mental image of the spine patient in the prone position.

Another helpful aid to lateralization is the small tatoo that is routinely made at the completion of the myelogram. This permanent mark is radiologically localized at the level of the lesion and placed laterally on the side of the pain.

Prior to induction of anesthesia, the patient is always asked to indicate the painful leg. Of course, the painful side is noted on the chart and the myelograms are also appropriately labeled.

Anesthesia

Many surgeons prefer the use of spinal anesthesia, employing a hypobaric solution; epidural anesthesia also has some advocates.

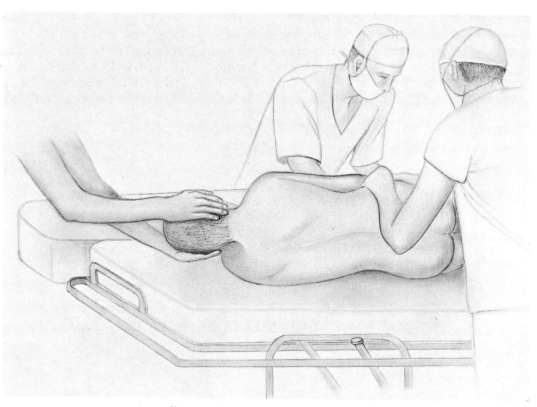

Fig. 10-33. Rolling intubated patient from litter to operating table.

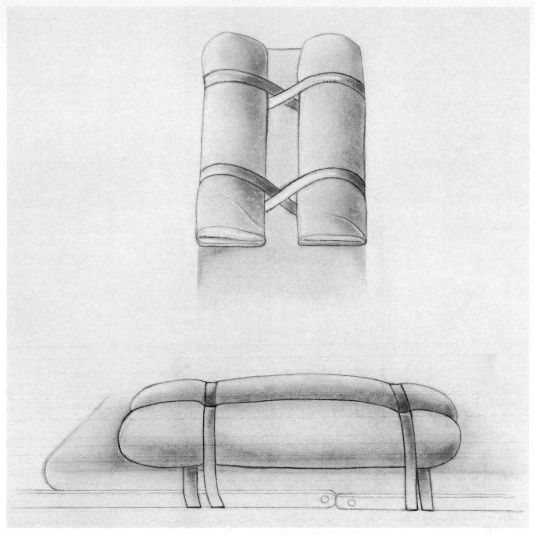

Fig. 10-34. Blanket rolls taped in place.

Intravenous Pentothal supplemented with halothane, nitrous oxide, and oxygen and given through an endotracheal tube is the anesthesia of personal choice and probably utilized by the majority of clinics for lumbar disc surgery.

Position

A variety of positions have been used for operating upon patients with protruded lumbar discs.

For the unilateral disc excision, many people prefer the lateral position (Fig. 10-29). This is the position of choice from the point of view of anesthesia, because it does not hamper respiratory excursions as much as the prone position. The principal surgical advantage is that it allows the abdomen to be relatively free, reducing pressure on the great veins and, in turn, reducing epidural venous distention and bleeding. This position does not allow blood to pool within the depths of the wound, and it promotes posterior lumbar flexion. Another technical advantage is that the surgeon can spread laterally the uppermost interlaminar space by positioning the patient on the table so that the involved disc space is above the flexion break and then flexing the table.

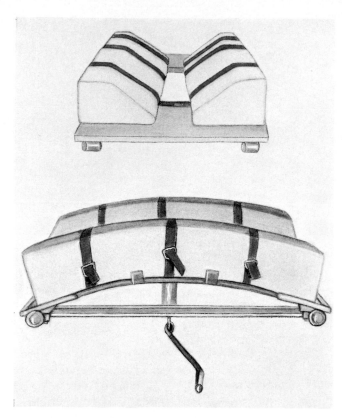

Fig. 10-35. Prone position frame.

The disadvantage of this position is some increased difficulty on the part of the assistant in holding the root retractor or in performing other necessary functions. Those who are not familiar with this position may find it technically more difficult to carry out the paraspinal muscle dissection and interlaminar exposure.

A knee-chest position is utilized by some surgeons, with the purpose of avoiding any pressure whatsoever on the abdomen and so decreasing epidural bleeding. (Fig. 10-30). One minor disadvantage of this position is the number of people required to place the patient in a satisfactory position. A more objectionable disadvantage is the frequent postoperative discomfort the patient suffers from stretching the hamstring muscles and from pressure lateral to the knee which results from this position under the total relaxation of general anesthesia. The dangers of the acute hip and knee flexion associated with this position, exerting a tourniquet effect to the muscles of the lower extremities, must also be considered. Some surgeons are of the opinion that the resulting damage to muscles in the leg triggers the release of myoglobin. The myoglobin in turn can overload the kidneys, while at the same time the degradation products of the muscle globulin seem to be renotoxic. An instructive case of renal failure, following a 4-hour spinal fusion performed in the knee-chest position, was described by Drs. Keim and Drs. Weinstein.[12]

In the early and mid1950s, a number of physicians advocated the sitting position, indicating that this position resulted in freer respiration and was associated with less epidural bleeding. Relatively few clinics continue to utilize the sitting position.

Most lumbar disc surgeons prefer the prone position, in which the patient is intubated on a litter. After the endotracheal tube has been taped securely in place, the patient is rolled onto the operating table,

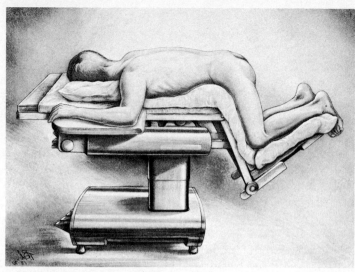

Fig. 10-36. Modified prone position.

which has previously been prepared either with blanket rolls or a "prone position frame" (Figs. 10-31 through 10-36).

A modification of the prone position is obtained by a 90 degree flexion of the hips and knees, with no effort to flex the lumbar spine itself. The hip flexion affords satisfactory flexion of the lumbar spine comparable to the other positions, and it may be associated with somewhat less abdominal pressure. To achieve this position, a minor adjustment of the operating table is accomplished by removal of the adjustable headrest and fitting it to the footrest so that it will provide adequate support for the legs.

The thin patient with a flat belly will do well with either the prone position frame or blanket rolls. Such a position, however, is poorly tolerated by the obese individual, since neither the frame nor the blanket rolls will adequately accommodate a large, protuberant abdomen. Abdominal compression is apt to increase lumbar epidural venous distention, and the resulting hemorrhage will be an impediment to satisfactory visualization. In the presence of copious epidural bleeding, the surgeon may have difficulty concentrating on the prime objective of disc excision and adequate nerve root decompression, since his major efforts will be required to control the hemorrhage. Such an irritating environment may lead to a mishap and is not conducive to the calm and deliberate atmosphere so helpful to safe and smooth surgery.

Several positions have evolved in which the abdomen is completely free and unencumbered. Usually some sort of operating table attachment is required to secure and immobilize the hips and thighs. This support is usually assembled by a friendly hospital maintenance machinist or a handy surgeon.

Dr. Mario Troncelliti, the chief of anesthesia at the Pennsylvania Hospital in Philadelphia, has designed a satisfactory position which enjoys rather widespread use. This is primarily because that institution is graced by two outstanding physicians, Dr. Frederick Simeone and Dr. Richard Rothman, a neu-

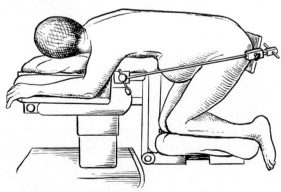

Fig. 10-37. Troncelliti position which avoids compression of a protuberant abdomen.

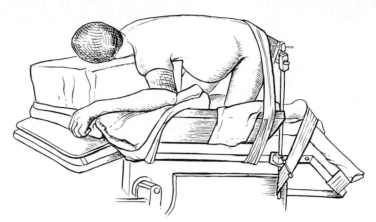

Fig. 10-38. *Modification of Troncelliti position.*

rosurgeon and an orthopedic surgeon, who are extremely generous with their time and efforts in training residents and fellows. In addition to the medical wisdom imparted by these great teachers, the young surgeons depart from training with the Troncelliti position (Figs. 10-37 and 10-38). This is a modification of the previously described modified prone position. The hips and posterior thighs are moved caudally until only the anterior chest is resting on the table and the abdomen is free. The buttocks and posterior thighs are then supported by the operating table attachment.

Surface Landmarks

After the patient is draped, the iliac crests and other bony landmarks providing approximate relationships to spinal level are obscured (Fig. 10-36). For this reason, a surface guide to interspace identification is necessary prior to draping. My preference is the cutaneous tatoo which is made at the level of the disc protrusion using fluoroscopic guidance after completion of the myelogram. If this is not part of the surgeons routine, other aids can be employed.

If a myelogram has been recently done,

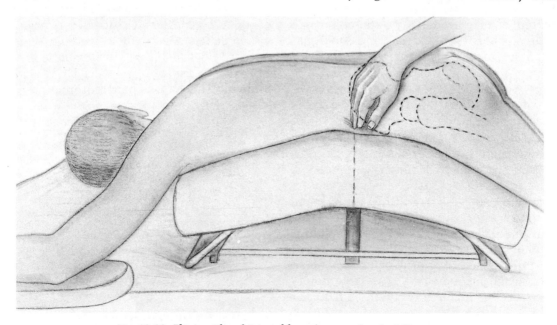

Fig. 10-39. *Flexion "break" in table or frame at level of iliac crest.*

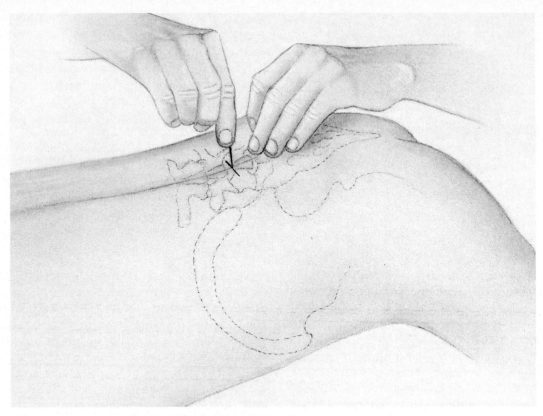

Fig. 10-40. The skin is scratched at the involved interspinous space.

the lumbar puncture mark on the skin is used as a landmark for spinal level. For example, if the lumbar puncture needle is seen on the myelogram films to be at the L3–4 interspace, this will serve as an excellent surface guide for identification of the underlying vertebrae (Fig. 10-39). If a myelogram has not been recently carried out, the first interspace at or immediately below the iliac crest can be considered L3–4; using this as a starting site, one may count down to the involved interspace, scratching a "crosshatch" in the skin at that level with a sterile hypodermic needle subsequent to cleansing the skin with an alcohol sponge (Fig. 10-40 and 10-41).

When utilizing surface guides, the elasticity of the skin must be recognized, particularly in obese patients. This elasticity may permit a surface marking to shift the extent of an interspace, with the distortion from the use of retractors and alterations in the degree of lumbar flexion during surgery.

Preparing the Skin and Draping

A variety of solutions and methods for preparing the skin surface prior to surgery are currently available. After the skin is prepared, sterile drapes can be applied in a variety of ways according to individual choice.

The draping technique I prefer is to place an adhesive transparent plastic covering sheet over the skin initially (Fig. 10-42). A sterile sheet is placed above and below the previously made cutaneous landmark, which will be utilized as a point of reference in draping; a rectangularly perforated sheet is placed overall; and the sheets are then pushed up and down an appropriate distance

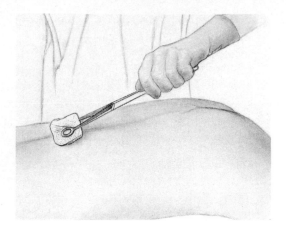

Fig. 10-41. Skin preparation.

usual expectations, the Bovie was not required or used for any portion of the operation. At completion of surgery, upon removal of the drapes, I was dismayed to see a deep cutaneous cautery burn at the site of a towel clip. Since that occurrence, I utilize a plastic Bovie holder. This should prevent such a mishap either from malfunctioning of the apparatus or from the inadvertent activation of the current which may occur when a foot switch is used and the assistant inadvertently steps on the pedal.

Incisions

For many years my routine incision extended over approximately three spinous processes as an aid to interspace localization and to improved illumination, with the ends of the incision permitting overhead lighting to funnel in. I considered the short incision an ego trip on the part of the surgeon. Further experience changed my opinion, and I presently believe that the short incision is beneficial to the patient's postoperative recovery (Fig. 10-44).

There is no question that the patients feel immeasurably better in the immediate postoperative interval with the short-incision operation, compared with a large-incision operation. Of greater importance is the fact that the long incision, which extends over several spinous processes, produces a band of scar extending from the skin and attaching to the spinous processes and laminae along the length of this incision. This scar tissue

and secured at four corners, using towel clips penetrating through the skin and adhesive plastic drape (Fig. 10-43). The placement of the adhesive plastic drape initially and subsequent placement of the plain sheets and lap sheet are done to insure that no contamination will occur by moving a drape back and forth from a "nonprepped" area to the "prepped" area of proposed surgery.

For many years, I routinely attached the Bovie cord to the towel clip on the assistant's side and slipped the suction tubing through the handles of the towel clip on my side. Two years ago, a defective short-circuiting Bovie cord was placed upon the draped operating field in contact with a towel clip and without our knowledge was actively discharging electrical current. The malfunction was discovered prior to the onset of surgery and a substitute cord provided. Surgery proceeded without problems and, contrary to

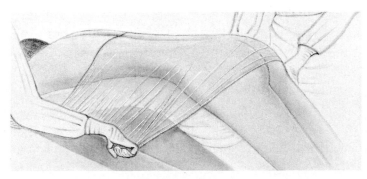

Fig. 10-42. Adhesive plastic skin covering sheet.

is not as supple as nonscarred muscle and fascia. The lack of elasticity and suppleness is not conducive to a nicely disturbed lumbar curvature after wound healing occurs, and this nonsupple lumbar spine probably makes the patient more vulnerable to recurrent low back dysfunction in the future.

When making a small incision, precise localization of the involved interspace is crucial. With the small incision, fiberoptic lighting and magnification are a necessity. The fiberoptic lighting and operating telescopes, or the operating microscope, are a great advantage. For many years I carried out lumbar disc surgery without magnification or special lighting; I tended to label those individuals using such appliances as gadgeteers. However, I presently use a Malis fiberoptic headlight and 4½ power operating telescopes, and, less frequently, the operating microscope. These instruments aid greatly in assuring delicate handling of tissue and in helping to prevent nerve root damage. I consider them an integral and essential aid to surgery.

There is a variety of methods to control skin bleeding, including Michel clips, Ko-lodney clamps, and mosquitoes. Weitlaner self-retaining retractors, which place the skin under tension, will stop most of the minor skin bleeding; the several remaining subcutaneous vessels are easily controlled by cautery (Fig. 10-45). Blood vessel cauterization should not be performed with a hemostat, since it invariably results in considerable tissue destruction. When carried out near the surface of the skin, hemostat cauterization may result in a full thickness skin burn, and the resulting skin slough or necrosis may eventuate into a wound infection. To properly control skin bleeding with a cautery, an assistant should use fine-toothed forceps to evert the skin edge, while the surgeon employs a sucker to locate the bleeding vessel and uses fine-tipped Cushing forceps to cauterize only the vessel, taking care to avoid cautery spread to surrounding tissue.

A second knife ("clean knife") is used to incise through fat to the fascia. If the patient is extremely obese, the Weitlaner retractors may have to be reset more deeply. Additional bleeding is controlled with the use of the cautery. Do not be obsessive about sweeping

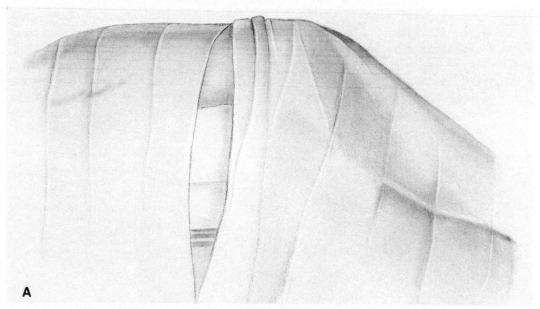

A

Fig. 10-43. **(A)** *Sheets above and below crosshatch, which is used as a reference point in draping.* **(B)** *Draped and clipped surgical area. (Figure continues on p. 338.)*

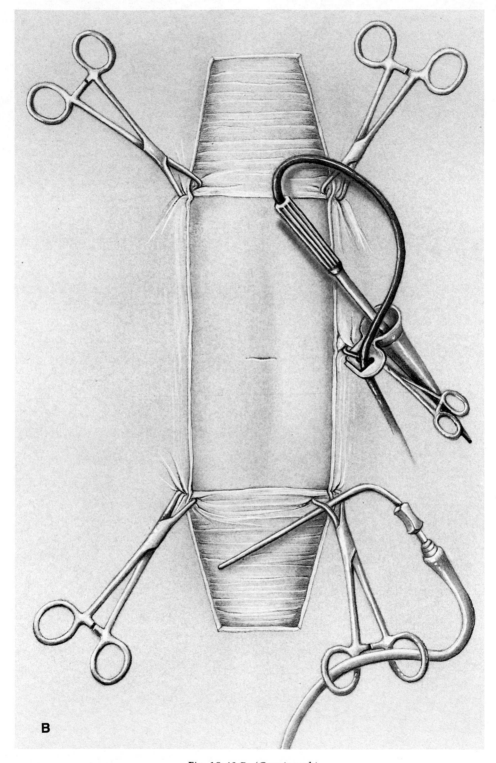

Fig. 10-43 B. *(Continued.)*

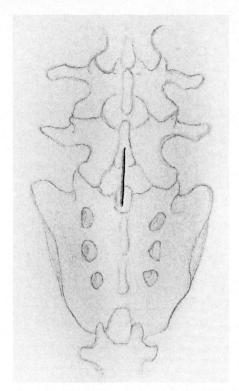

Fig. 10-44. Short incision (compare Fig. 10-45A).

the fat cleanly away from the fascia. Remember you are carrying out a surgical procedure, not an anatomical exposure. This step can only serve to increase the blood loss and, even more serious, to create a false space which may fill with blood in the postoperative period.

Subperiosteal Dissection

The subperiosteal muscle can be dissected by a variety of methods (Fig. 10-46). I prefer to use a periosteal elevator pressed against the edge of the spinous process and to cut directly against the lateral edge of the spine. In this manner I preserve the posterior spinous ligament or supraspinal ligament, a strong fibrous cord that extends without interruption along the tips of the spinous processes from C7 to the median sacral crest and that is continuous with the interspinal ligaments. I believe it is valuable to preserve

this structure and so to avoid unnecessary weakening of the spinal supporting ligaments. To prevent excessive scarring, I use a scalpel rather than a cutting cautery to incise the fascia. The muscles are best stripped from the spinous processes and lamina, using the bimanual 2 periosteal method. One periosteal elevator is used to retract the muscle mass laterally, while the other performs a careful subperiosteal dissection. Peel the periosteum as cleanly as possible from the spinous process and lamina without penetrating muscle which, if torn, may be a source of troublesome bleeding.

After the subperiosteal dissection has been accomplished under direct vision, a sponge extended to its full length is used to strip the bone of any remaining fragments of muscle and fascia. As bone is cleaned with the sponge, allow it to accumulate within the incision to act as a tamponade and prevent muscle bleeding. Any bleeding occurring from the cut edge of the fascia is controlled with cautery. The subperiosteal muscle dissection is carried out laterally to expose the articulation between the superior and inferior articular processes.

After all surface bleeding has been controlled, remove sponges and localize the desired interspace by the time-honored method of palpating the sacrum and then counting up from it (Fig. 10-47). Check this localization with plain spine x-ray films to be sure that the patient does not have a lumbarized first sacral segment or sacralized fifth lumbar segment. Then correlate skeletal localization with the myelographic defect.

If the sacrum cannot be adequately palpated, or if for some other reason you are not totally satisfied with anatomical level identification, stop at this point and obtain definite interspace confirmation with a lateral lumbar spine roentgenogram.

One topic not likely to be profusely discussed in the medical literature is the frequency of interspace misidentification at surgery. I occasionally find such an error in a referred patient and am aware of two occasions when I myself made such a mis-

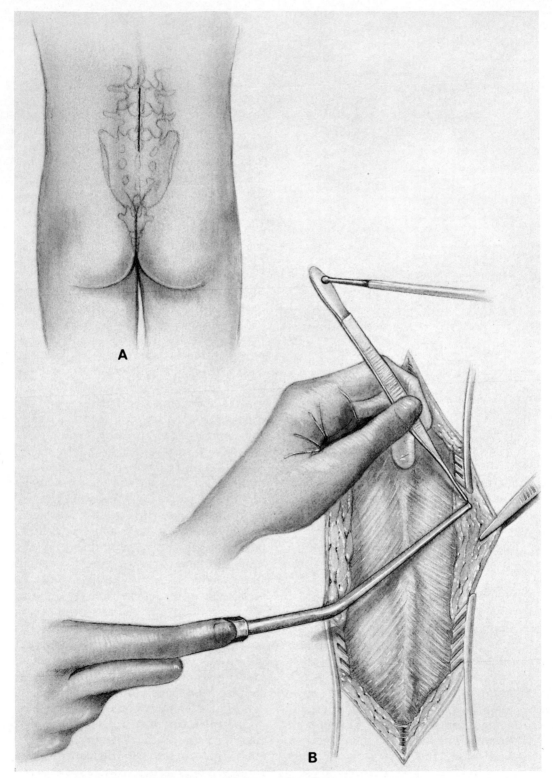

Fig. 10-45. *Superficial vessels in the skin are cauterized.*

take. Both of my mishaps occurred in the 1950s, when I was less aware of my fallability and much too decisive to slow up my surgery for an "unnecessary x-ray film." This error is most likely to occur in either grossly obese patients or patients whose partial lumbarization of the first sacral segment dorsal elements confuses the surgeon.

When in doubt, it is important to obtain a roentgenogram, not only for the surgeon's peace of mind but also so that he can be absolutely certain that the interspace he is working on is the proper one. When pathology is not apparent, at first inspection, such knowledge may provide additional incentive for a most thorough and meticulous interspace exploration and decompression, in-

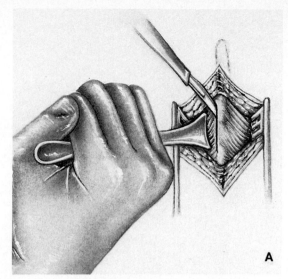

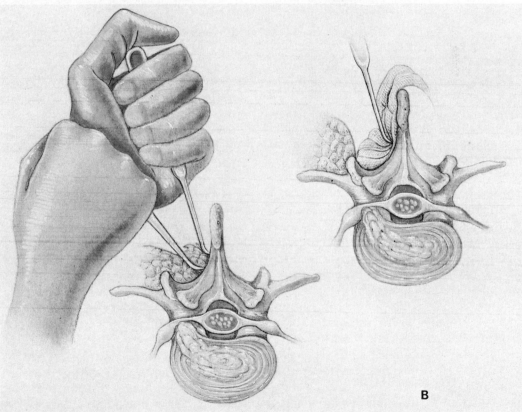

Fig. 10-46. Subperiosteal dissection technique using short incision.

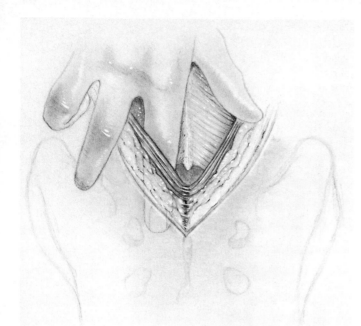

Fig. 10-47. Interspace localization, using
the sacrum as the point of reference.

cluding a generous foraminal decompression.

Once you are completely satisfied that proper localization has been established, place the hemilaminectomy retractors in position (Fig. 10-48). A variety of hemilaminectomy retractors is available, the simplest being the Taylor spinal retractor which consists of a right-angled metal ribbon with a slightly hooked tip, that can be inserted laterally and cephalad to the articular facet. The great advantage of this retractor is its simplicity and lack of any moving parts; the disadvantage is that it has to be either hand-held by the assistant or tied to the base of the operating table or to the foot of the operator. Also, it has the unhappy propensity of occasionally slipping out of place, invariably during the worst possible moment of the procedure.

Most surgeons prefer a self-retaining hem-

ilaminectomy retractor based on the many modifications of the Hoen hemilaminectomy retractor.

When positioning the hemilaminectomy retractors, use the shortest blades possible to achieve adequate exposure, so that the flange of the blades will rest flush with the skin surface. If the flange projects above the skin, it increases the depth through which the surgeon must work. The spinous process blade of the retractor should fit between the spinous interspaces, with the hook or hooks embedded into the interspinous ligaments. The muscle blade should rise above the hump of the articular facet (Fig. 10-49). An occasional error is to impinge the tip of the muscle blade against the facet; this causes the exposure to be needlessly narrow. By placing the paraspinal muscles under tension, the retractors will stop most muscle bleeding. After the retractors are in place

Fig. 10-48. **(A)** Taylor hemilaminectomy retractor; **(B)** Hoen hemilaminectomy retractor. A single-pronged, hooked blade is available for the short incision. **(C)** If the hemilaminectomy retractor blades are longer than necessary, the depth through which the surgeon must work is increased.

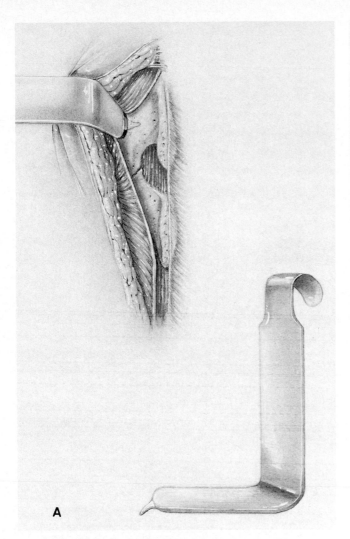

A

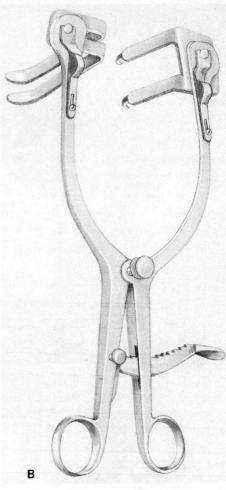

B

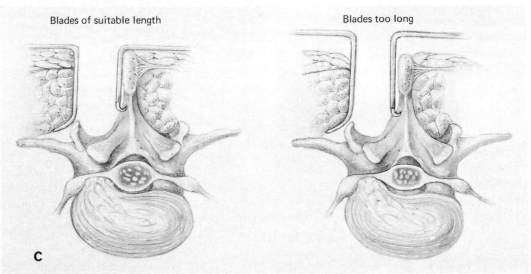

Blades of suitable length   Blades too long

C

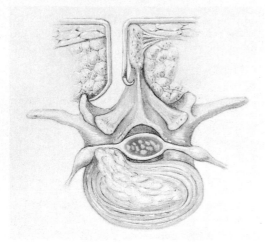

Fig. 10-49. Avoid impinging tip of muscle blade against articular facet.

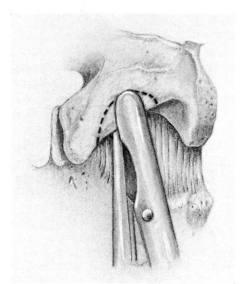

Fig. 10-50. The overhanging edge of the superior lamina is rongeured.

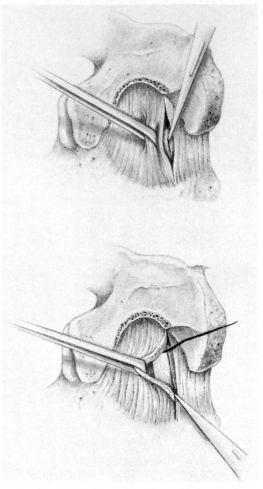

Fig. 10-51. The yellow ligament is cut.

and the exposure is deemed satisfactory, any remaining muscle bleeding is controlled with the use of the cautery.

It must be emphasized that the rest of the surgery takes place in that small keyhole of interlaminar space, and any skin, fascia, or muscle bleeding will funnel directly into the work area. If the assistant has to provide suction to remove the blood, either his head is in the way, obstructing the surgeon's vision or he is poking the suction tip into the wound blindly, which also has its disadvantages. The other alternative is for the surgeon to hold the suction in one hand and operate with the other; this also is not really satisfactory. Therefore, control of bleeding at this stage is a must for smooth, safe surgery.

Developing the Interspace

The laminae vary greatly in width, in angulation, and in position relative to each other, so that occasionally the interlaminar space is sufficiently wide to permit exposure and removal of a protruding intervertebral disc without removal of any, or very much, bone. This widened interlaminar space is

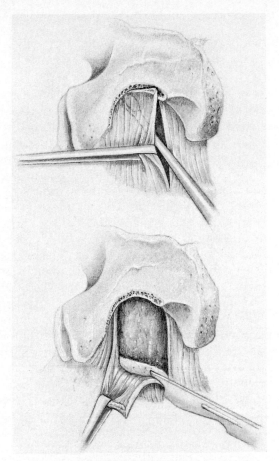

Fig. 10-52. *The yellow ligament is curetted.*

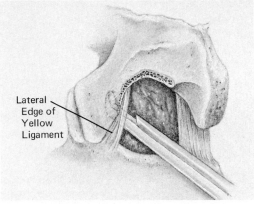

Fig. 10-53. *In widening the interspace, do not mistake the rolled up lateral edge of yellow ligament for the root.*

Lateral Edge of Yellow Ligament

seen most commonly between the L5–S1 levels and much less frequently above that interspace.

The more strenuous bone work of the operation is followed by the relatively delicate soft tissue interspace dissection involving yellow ligament, nerve root, and dura. This strenuous manual work tends to create a hand tremor which is distressingly obvious when performing surgery with magnification techniques such as an operating telescope or microscope. In the hope of reducing a postexertion tremor while manipulating the nerve root and other soft tissues within the interspace, I use air-powered rongeurs for much of the bone work.

When dealing with an interspace of normal dimensions, any rongeur, including duck-billed, Leksell, or Kerrison, can be used to remove the overhanging, inferior edge of the superior vertebrae (Fig. 10-50). If working on the L5–S1 interspace, this would be the inferior edge of the L5 lamina. Some surgeons prefer rongeuring away half of the superior lamina which exposes the superior border of the yellow ligament. This can then be grasped with an Allis tissue forceps and the remainder of the ligament can be excised by sharp dissection with a scalpel. I prefer to remove only one-third of the superior lamina so that the edge of the yellow ligament is not exposed. Bone wax is used to control all bone bleeding from the rongeured edge of the lamina. After the one-third overhang of the superior lamina has been removed, an ample area of the ligamentum flavum is exposed to view. A No. 11 blade on a long handle is used to make a shallow incision in the ligamentum flavum along the fiber. The edge of the incision is grasped with an Allis forceps and tugged laterally in order to spread the incision, allowing the No. 11 blade to incise the entire thickness of the yellow ligament down to the epidural fat (Fig. 10-51 and 10-52). After introducing a small, moistened cotton patty beneath the ligamentum flavum to separate it from the dura, this incision is extended from superior lamina to inferior lamina, taking care to insert merely the tip of the blade beneath the ligament to avoid accidentally cutting into the dura. A second Allis is used to get a firmer grasp on the full thickness of yellow ligament. A curette is introduced below the yellow ligament against the inferior surface of the superior vertebra, permitting a flap of yellow ligament to be curretted laterally with the remainder attached to the dorsal surface of the inferior lamina. This attachment can then safely be excised with scalpel or scissors (Fig. 10-53).

EPIDURAL FAT AND NERVE ROOT DAMAGE

Once the yellow ligament has been excised, the epidural fat can be clearly visualized. Treatment of the epidural fat has recently developed into a conjectural issue. It is now generally agreed that preservation of an epidural layer of fat, especially around the nerve root, will be helpful in preventing encasement of the root within the dense epidural scar tissue that forms following an interspace exploration. For this reason, surgeons attempt to carry out disc excision without disturbing the epidural fat. However, this fatty layer almost always obscures the dura and nerve root. In a laudable effort to prevent future damage of the root by scar tissue, the surgeon may create immediate and possibly persisting injury to the root because of his inability to visualize this structure adequately during surgery.

Frequently, a flap of epidural fat can be retracted so that good visualization of the root and dura is obtained. After completion of the procedure, the epidural fat can be tucked back into position around the root. However, if satisfactory root identification and visualization is not possible with preservation of the fat, excise it. A surgeon is not able to protect a structure that he cannot visualize, and I am aware of two recent postoperative nerve root injuries which two separate surgeons attributed to their desire to preserve the epidural fat. When the epidural fat has been removed, a small stamp of subcutaneous fat can be placed over the dura and root as a free fat graft. Subsequent dissections and explorations have demon-strated a reasonably high incidence of persisting and effective fatty tissue.

Let us remind ourselves that the goal of surgery is adequate decompression of the root, while assuring gentle, safe handling of the root. At this stage of surgery root damage may occur in two ways. One occasional error is to mistake the lateral reflection of the yellow ligament immediately over the root for the root itself. Sometimes after excision of the medial portional this structure the lateral portion rolls up into a band-like, cylindrical appearance which may be quite deceptive. If this band is retracted medially, the underlying root may be mistakenly identified as a bulging disc, which is then attacked with vigor. Another error may occur when we are extending the interlaminar exposure laterally and trimming the lateral reflection of yellow ligament and bone. This portion of the exposure must be performed under good visualization, being careful to hug the inferior bony and ligamentour surface with the jaws of the Schlesinger punch. If the tip of this rongeur is inserted too deeply, it may grasp a bit of the root along with the edge of the yellow ligament and bone. As the surgeon tugs on the instrument, a fairly long, glistening piece of tissue, resembling spaghetti, comes out, followed by bloody spinal fluid. These errors are classifiable as surgical tragedies and can usually be avoided by proper hemostasis, good visualization, and a cautious pace at this point in the operation.

A thin edge of bone is removed from the superior edge of the inferior lamina using a laminectomy punch that is not angled downward. The 40-degree-angled jaw is helpful in working on the superior lamina and laterally, but may produce a dural tear at the inferior lamina (Fig. 10-54).

A slight fold of dura may bulge and be pinched and torn in the jaws of the bone-biting instrument. Most of the fibers in the dura are longitudinal (running up and down); if the instrument catches a fiber and the operator pulls without adequate visualization, to quote George Ehni "the dura will rip open like a seam." Just a small bite of bone can easily cause an inch-long tear in the dura. If the dura is opened, a small hole is usually easier to close than a large one. Therefore dissection should proceed cautiously on the inferior lamina. Do not take a bite of bone with the rongeur and rip it out. Close the instrument carefully and ease the bone out very slowly, so that if the dura is tugged even slightly, the surgeon will be able to visualize the dural tenting and can then release the instrument and inspect the area carefully before proceeding further. This type of complication always occurs before an adequate exposure has been obtained. Cerebrospinal fluid may fill the wound suddenly, becoming tinged with blood, so that it is impossible to see the damaged area. There is a tendency to try to close this opening immediately, but this is a mistake. It is also a mistake to try to visualize the damage by putting a sucker directly into the wound, because the roots may float out of the dural rent with the escaping spinal fluid, catch on the tip of the sucker, and sometimes be severely damaged. Instead of direct suction, insert a cottonoid into the opening, and suck only on the cottonoid until the structures can be seen. Then place a square of Gelfoam over the dural opening, place a cottonoid on top of the Gelfoam square, and tilt the table head down so that spinal fluid pressure will decrease in the lumbar region. If the table is flexed, it should be flattened. Then proceed as though the dura had not been opened. After the disc has been excised and the root decompressed, full attention can be given to the torn dura. Before closing the dural tear, it is necessary to expose both sides and both ends of the tear. Dural closure must be watertight, using 4–0 or 5–0 suture material.

In carrying out a lateral bony exposure, a partial or complete removal of a facet may be necessary for exposure of the lateral margin of the nerve root. The procedure does not appear to result in postoperative weakness or pain when performed unilaterally (Fig. 10-55). Bilateral facet removal and disc excision at that level may produce both spinal instability and pain.

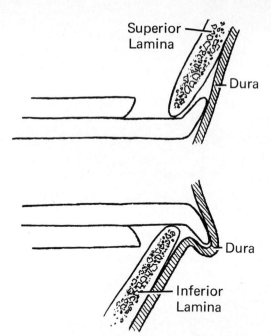

Fig. 10-54. *The laminectomy punch is helpful when working on the superior lamina, but is not suited for the slope of the inferior lamina. The adherent dura is more easily damaged at the edge of the inferior lamina.*

An adequate intervertebral lateral exposure may be of value for three reasons:

1. It facilitates satisfactory disc excision with less danger of overstretching the nerve root and dural sac as these structures are retracted medically. With an adequate lateral exposure, much less root retraction is necessary to afford good access to the disc.

2. With a satisfactory lateral exposure, a partial foraminotomy is accomplished, providing more space for the involved root, which almost always manifests some degree of edema and swelling. Such reduction of root compression is associated with decreased postoperative pain.[15]

3. Years after surgery, hypertrophic osteoarthritic spurring, in association with post-operative epidural scarring, will be less likely to lead to root compression symptoms in the presence of a generous lateral exposure and foraminotomy.

Following adequate bony removal, the epidural fat is completely exposed to view. If the nerve root is obscured by the fat, use

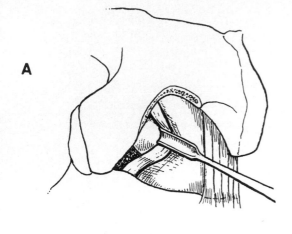

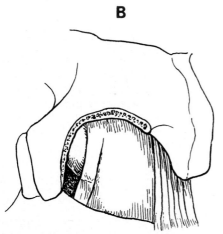

Fig. 10-55. (A) Overstretched root and dural sac with an inadequate lateral bony exposure. (B) Very little root retraction is necessary with adequate lateral bony exposure.

two Cushing forceps to separate the fat from the underlying dura and nerve root. In an effort to preserve the fat, peel it laterally so it forms a retractable flap which can be tucked back into place around the root after disc excision. Only after exposure of the nerve root can blood vessels within the epidural fat be safely cauterized without danger of damage to the root by the cautery current (Fig. 10-56). The Malis bipolar coagulator, using bipolar forceps, allows current flow to go only from one forcep tip to the other. This isolated current, which is associated with much less heat production, reduces the likelihood of inadvertent nerve root irritation or damage by cautery.

Interlaminar Surgery

Although the interlaminar space is rather small, the minute anatomy of this area does vary considerably. It is always amazing to me to see how much can be hidden in this tiny space. An orderly and systematic approach to this area is paramount to successful disc surgery.

Inspection

The field should be dry at this stage. If bleeding remains a problem, decreasing lumbar flexion to a flatter prone position may alleviate abdominal pressure and so reduce engorgement of Batson's lumbar venous plexus. If this change in position is effective in controlling epidural venous bleeding, proceed with surgery in the flatter position.

Is the root elevated or is it flat? Does the root appear swollen or hyperemic; or is it of the same color as the rest of the dura (Fig. 10-57)?

In patients who have had long-standing symptoms, adhesions between the nerve root and the posterior longitudinal ligament are occasionally quite dense (Fig. 10-58). Very careful dissection of the root and the dura may be necessary to allow free retraction and exposure of the protruding disc.

ROOT TENSION

Using a narrow blunt elevator, it should be possible to retract medially without resistance a root that is under no pressure. As a rule, the typical protruding disc will be quite apparent with retraction of the root medially. This manifests itself by slight elevation of the root, and by increased pressure on medial retraction. It is at this stage of the procedure that considerable care must be taken to avoid stretching a compromised root. When the disc protrusion is extensive, it is best not to retract the root too vigorously

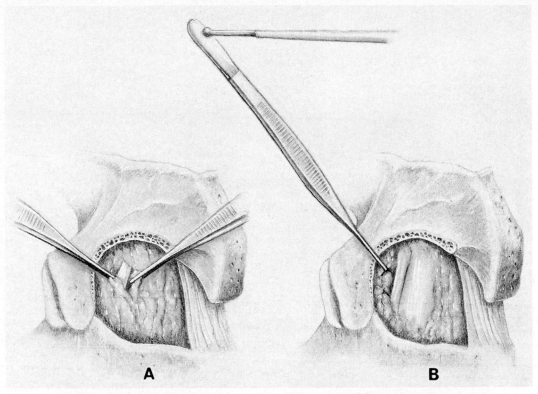

Fig. 10-56. **(A)** *Separate epidural fat to expose dura and root* **(B)** *Avoid cauterization of blood vessels within the epidural fat unless nerve root is completely exposed. Cauterization is best carried out when nerve root is visualized and is out of cautery range.*

over it to avoid excessive root stretch. When the root is under too much pressure to be retracted medially with ease, do not retract the root but work lateral to it to decompress it (Fig. 10-59).

If extruded disc fragments are free within the canal, they can usually be manipulated laterally, grasped with the pituitary forceps, and gently removed. If the disc is not extruded but is bulging so much that the nerve cannot easily be moved medially, work lateral to the disc, introduce the pituitary forceps into the intervertebral disc space, and remove disc fragments piecemeal until the root can be more easily retracted over the partially decompressed annular shell (Fig. 10-60).

The major error at this point comes under the heading of "grandstanding." There is a temptation to demonstrate the pathology to any and all present in the operating room. The root is retracted medially and maintained in an overstretched position while residents, interns, nurses, and visitors are invited to inspect the protruding disc. This is not the time to entertain "the troops," and a herniated disc is not very spectacular looking in any event. Retraction of such a swollen, inflamed nerve is best kept to a minimum to avoid adding to the irreversible damage already caused by the disc protrusion.

Sometimes a disc protrusion is a bit more medial, and the nerve root does not appear elevated or under pressure (Fig. 10-61). However, on attempting to retract the nerve root medially, an obstruction is encountered. The surgeon must then take care to lift the root and dura to determine whether a medially protruding disc is present.

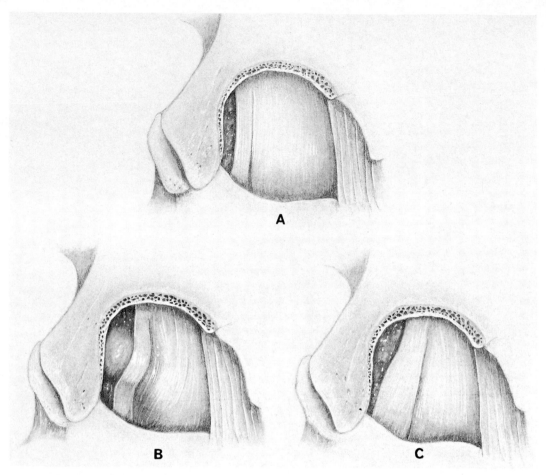

Fig. 10-57. *The root may appear elevated or swollen indicating compression.* **(A)** *Normal.* **(B)** *Elevated.* **(C)** *Swollen.*

Intervertebral Disc Excision

Once the disc has been partially excised, there is little difficulty in retracting the root medially. A nerve root retractor can then be used to expose the disc space more completely. A No. 11 blade is used to make a rectangular slab-shaped window through the annulus, and through this opening an adequate subtotal excision of disc contents is performed (Figs. 10-62 and 10-63). This window extends from the most medial exposure of the annulus to the lateral limits of the bony exposure and comprises the entire width of the intervertebral disc, bounded by the bodies of the superior and inferior vertebrae. I use pituitary forceps of various sizes

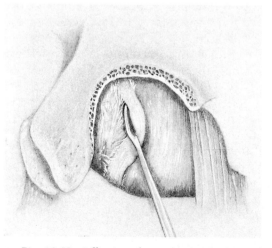

Fig. 10-58. *Adhesions between nerve root and annulus in a patient with long-standing symptoms.*

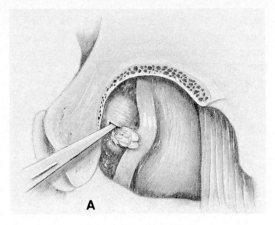

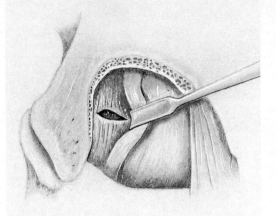

Fig. 10-60. After this partial excision has been accomplished, further root retraction is more easily accomplished over the shell of the protruded disc.

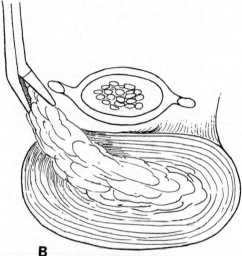

Fig. 10-59. If good exposure of the disc protrusion can be accomplished only by over-stretching the root, attempt only a lateral partial exposure and disc excision.

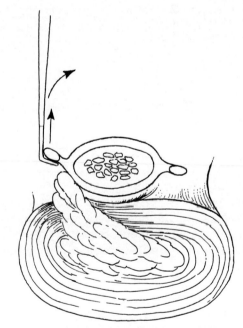

Fig. 10-61. An easily overlooked, medially protruding disc. Exposure requires elevation of the root before medial retraction.

and shapes, as well as a curette, to free up loose fragments of disc material. Excision of a rectangular slab of annulus may prevent the remaining shell of annulus from buckling as the disc space narrows. This buckling is to be prevented because it may fibrose and provide a source of root compression a year or two postoperatively. It is generally accepted that some reduction of the intervertebral space will occur, yet when Foltz and associates checked postoperative patients a year after surgery, no significant thinning was noted.[5] Possibly a year is too short a time for intervertebral narrowing to be visualized, but after a longer interval the change might be more apparent. This seems likely in view of the fact that patients with long-standing disc disease who have not had surgery will often demonstrate interspace narrowing.

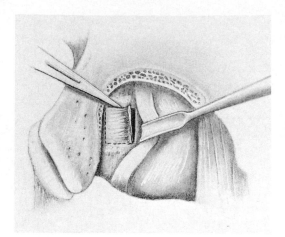

Fig. 10-62. Incision of rectangular window through the annulus fibrosus.

Forceps

A profusion of intervertebral disc rongeur forceps has been designed and modified by a host of surgeons. The variations of the forceps designed by Cushing (pituitary rongeurs) include: Love-Gruenwald, Spurling, Poppen, Cloward, Hoen, Oldberg, Raaf-Oldberg, Schlesinger, Mount, Selverstone, Spence, Voris, Louis, Takahashi, Wilde, Ferris-Smith, Farnum, and Hartmann-Gruenwald. These modifications involve alterations in shaft length, type of grip, jaw shape, size, and angulation.

My personal preference is the Hoen forceps, because its fenestrated jaws can grasp larger fragments of intervertebral disc material than is possible with solid jaws (Fig. 10-64).

In using intervertebral disc rongeur forceps within the intervertebral space, great care is necessary to avoid instrument penetration through the anterior annulus fibrosus and the anterior longitudinal ligament. Such penetration is precarious and may be associated with laceration of one of the great vessels located anterior to the vertebral bodies and within the prevertebral space (Fig. 10-65). Experienced and competent lumbar disc surgeons have suffered this calamity, and when working deep within the intervertebral space, the surgeon must remain

alert to the possibility of this mishap. Degenerative changes affecting an intervertebral disc are generalized and may cause softening of the anterior annular fibers and anterior longitudinal ligament. These structures, when reasonably firm, will usually offer resistance to instrument penetration; but when softened, the surgeon may unknowingly poke through with disc rongeur forceps. After such inadvertant penetration, the iliac artery may be grasped and torn by the forceps. Various methods have been advocated to avoid this problem, including marking the instruments 1½ inches from the tip as a visual remainder of depth pen-

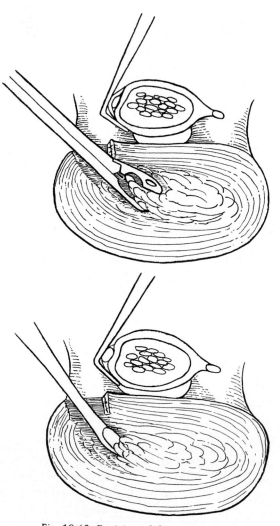

Fig. 10-63. Excision of disc contents.

etration. Good lighting and magnification aid in depth perception and in visualization of the interior of the disc space.

Some years ago, this surgical catastrophe received nationwide publicity when it resulted in the death of a popular Hollywood actor, Jeff Chandler. The residents in those days, mindful of the inherent danger, capriciously referred to the intervertebral space as "Chandler's canal."

Free Disc Fragments

Occasionally the protruded disc is in the "axilla" between the dural sac and the nerve root (Fig. 10-66). A most meticulous dissection of this extruded fragment is necessary, with care in grasping this fragment with an intervertebral disc rongeur forceps to avoid damage to the adjacent laterally displaced nerve root. It is occasionally difficult to recognize a completely free extruded fragment within the axilla. It may resemble epidural fat and in some cases, only the tip of the extruded fragment presents dorsally, with the bulk of it not visible and indenting the inferior portion of the dural sac medially (Figs. 10-67 and 10-68). The surgeon, unaware of this large extrusion, may retract the nerve root and dural sac medially together with the free fragment exposing a bulging or protruding annulus. The disc protrusion will be excised and the interspace evacuated as thoroughly as possible by the usual methods, including curettage and the use of the intervertebral disc forceps. But the offending free fragment, causing root pressure, will inadvertently be left untouched. An indication that such a fragment is present may be the lack of free nerve root mobility. When the nerve root is not free, further inspection is necessary.

A free disc fragment may extrude beneath the posterior spinal ligament. It occasionally will produce a sizable mass capable of producing symptoms that will not be evident to casual inspection. Palpation over the posterior spinal ligament with a thin elevator

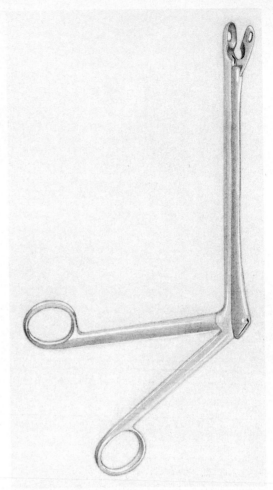

Fig. 10-64. Hoen intervertebral disc rongeur forceps.

will disclose this extrusion, and it can be "milked" laterally, exposing sufficient disc tissue to grasp with the intervertebral disc forceps and remove.

Surgical Judgment

In those patients in whom there is no gross protrusion of the disc, but rather a slightly humped-up annulus, the surgeon must use judgment in deciding whether to excise the high annulus and curette the intervertebral disc space, or to be content with posterior bony decompression of the

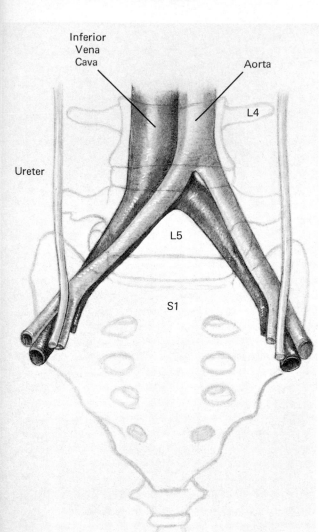

Fig. 10-65. *The major vessels and ureters and their relationship to the anterior lumbar spine.*

nerve root by means of a foraminotomy (Fig. 10-69).

I do not think that any disc should be violated unless it can be seen to be causing nerve root pressure. However, once the disc is violated, thorough disc excision is probably advisable. A bulging annulus does not have to be removed, particularly if the nerve root can be adequately decompressed. The root can easily go over a slight hump, as long as there is no bony counterpressure above it. Sometimes a generous foraminotomy alone is adequate. In equivocal cases, saline injection into the disc, using a 10 ml syringe, may be helpful. If the fulging disc does not take more than 1 or 2 ml of saline without a great deal of pressure, it might be tempting to limit the approach to a decompressive foraminotomy. On the other hand, if the entire 10 ml can be injected into the intervertebral disc space without a great deal of difficulty, such a disc could be considered more pathologic.

NERVE ROOT ANOMALIES

Occasionally the nerve root exiting from the foramen above the surgically exposed interspace will descend medially beneath the facets of the next lower interspace. This minor deviation is not significant unless the surgeon happens to carry out a rather extensively lateral interlaminar exposure. Because the surgeon's attention is focused on the nerve root under his direct vision, he or she may be unaware of an equally vital neural structure which is partially hidden by the lateral reflection of the yellow ligament (Figs. 10-70 and 10-71). Even more rarely, two nerve roots may exit from the same foramen. When the dura and its nerve root is exposed, there is a second root just lateral to the first root. If it is recognized as a nerve root there is no problem, but occasionally the laterally positioned root is mistaken for a bulging disc, and attempts are made to excise it. In doing so the root may be injured beyond repair. There is no substitute for

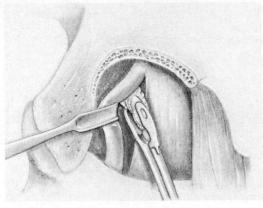

Fig. 10-66. This large free disc fragment between the nerve root and dural sac can easily be overlooked.

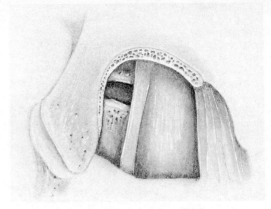

Fig. 10-68. Free nerve root following disc excision and foraminotomy.

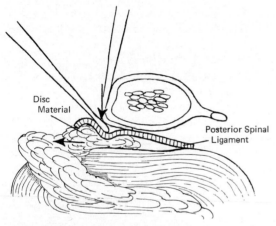

Fig. 10-67. Disc fragments that extrude medially beneath the posterior spinal ligament are easily overlooked and, once identified, not easily removed.

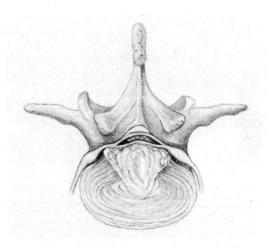

Fig. 10-69. Midline disc protrusion requiring transdural excision.

good lighting and magnification. In addition, the operation should always be done questioningly, since the surgeon is working through a "keyhole," and identification of tissues is extremely important.

After the protruded intervertebral disc has been adequately excised, the operating room table or spinal rest is flattened, so that the originally flexed position is now a relatively straight one. This change in position places the root under less tension, narrows the posterior intervertebral space, and increases the depth between the skin surface and the interlaminar space. The interspace is then reexplored and occasionally several additional fragments of disc material can be removed, with the vertebral bodies closer together. At the termination of the procedure, the nerve root should be under no pressure whatsoever, either anteriorly from the intervertebral disc or from bony constriction within the intervertebral foramina, which should have been partially opened during the original bony dissection.

Bleeding from epidural veins should be carefully controlled before closure of the wound (Fig. 10-72). Removing the lumbar flexion and placing the patient in a flat,

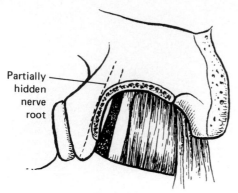

Fig. 10-70. Partially hidden nerve root exiting from foramen above, descending more medially than usual, and passing beneath the facets.

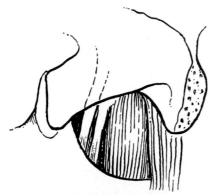

Fig. 10-71. Two roots exiting from the same foramen.

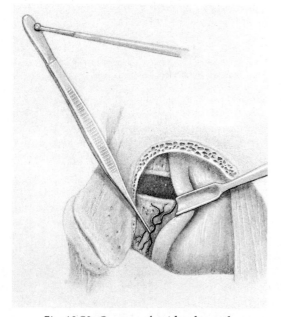

Fig. 10-72. Cautery of epidural vessels.

prone position is helpful in relieving abdominal pressure and reducing lumbar venous engorgement; this change in position alone often controls venous epidural bleeding. Alteration of the table is advisable even if no epidural bleeding is encountered, since it does allow the surgeon to recheck for any retained fragments of disc and changes the minute anatomical relationships of the root and intervertebral space, affording additional inspection. Continued epidural bleeding is controlled with the use of electrocoagulation, and the Malis bipolar coagulation forceps is of great help in preventing spread of the cautery current. Occasionally, a small pledget of Gelfoam is required to control bleeding.

Wound Closure

Suture material of personal preference is 2–0 chromic gut for muscle and fascia, 3–0 plain gut for subcutaneous tissue, and monofilament nylon for skin.

An important, but often overlooked, hemilaminectomy closure technique is elimination of the dead space, which may fill with clot and contribute to postoperative discomfort (Fig. 10-73). This is accomplished with 2–0 chromic suture passed through the interspinous ligament and then into the paraspinal muscles to approximate the paraspinal muscles against the laminae and spinous processes. This hemostatic suture should not be tied so tightly as to cause muscle necrosis.

Vascular and Visceral Injuries During Disc Surgery

Most vascular injuries occur during excision of disc material, when the intervertebral disc forceps produces a laceration of one of the major vessels lying in the prevertebral space such as the aorta, inferior vena cava, or the iliac arteries or veins. Ordinarily, such a catastrophe is signaled by copious bleeding from the intervertebral space immediately after the introduction of an instrument deep

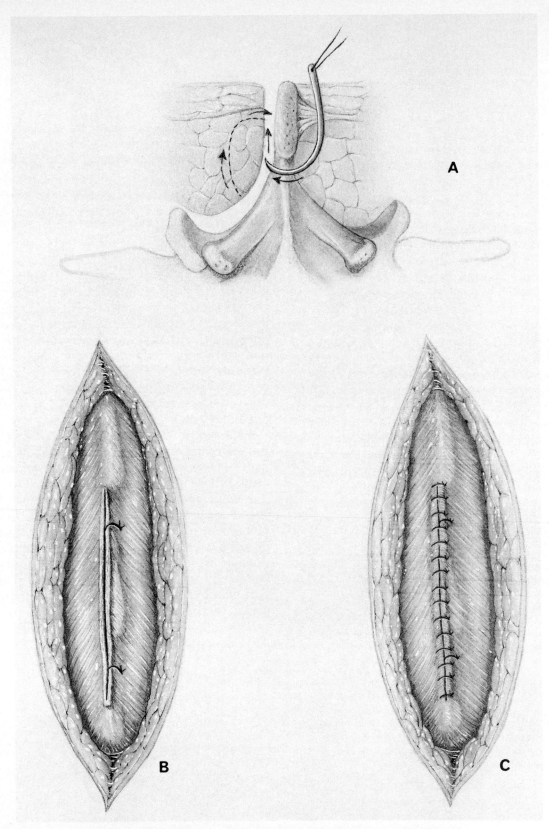

*Fig. 10-73. (**A** and **B**) Muscle closure to eliminate dead space. (**C**) Facial closure.*

within it. Occasionally, no such bleeding is recognized through the intervertebral space, because all bleeding occurs anteriorly; during surgery, the patient will go into shock with sudden hypotension and a rapid, thready pulse.[4] Injury to an artery or a vein may result in the formation of an arteriovenous fistula, which may not be noted for years after the original surgery. Sometimes, the first sign of such an injury is cardiac decompensation.[3,6,11]

As soon as such evidence of vascular injury is recognized, it must be understood that this is a serious surgical emergency which requires immediate action. The anesthesiologist is appraised of the situation and instructed to institute rapid blood transfusion in large volumes. The wound is packed with several large abdominal sponges and closed with a few deep sutures through skin and muscle. The patient is turned to the supine position; and if a general surgeon is available, he should proceed with the laparotomy. If not, the abdominal cavity must be opened by a midrectus incision. Occasionally, no evidence of bleeding is noted in the abdominal cavity, but a large hematoma can be visualized in the retroperitoneal space. The posterior peritoneum is then divided, and the hematoma is evacuated by means of suction. The site of bleeding can then easily be determined, and vascular clamps are applied above and below that region. The lacerated vessel is repaired with vascular suture.

Occasionally, an abdominal viscus such as the ureter, the bladder, and the ileum is perforated.

Operative Report

When dictating the operative report, a detailed description of the significant operative findings is important (Figs. 10-74 and 10-75). Too often, the operative note briefly states that a protruded disc was found and removed. Those subsequently reviewing the case are left to wonder whether there was an extrusion of the nucleus pulposus, a ruptured protruding annulus, a combination of both, or simply a high annulus.

Postoperative Management

Immediately after lumbar disc surgery, postanesthesia care, including monitoring of vital signs and maintenance of an adequate airway, is best managed in the recovery room under direction of the anesthesiologist.

The following postoperative orders are routine:

1. Flat on back 4 hours, then assist patient to turn from side to back to side (alternating sides) every 2 hours. (Traditionally, all spine surgery patients are initially maintained flat and supine in the presumption that this position is associated with decreased venous epidural bleeding and that direct pressure upon the paraspinal muscles will tend to reduce bleeding from this source.)

2. Demerol, 75 milligrams, every 4 hours prn for pain. After the first day, oral medication such as aspirin and codine are employed for pain.

3. Food and fluids by mouth as tolerated.

4. If patient is unable to urinate in the recumbent position, assist patient to sit up or stand while voiding. Insert Foley catheter if these efforts are unsuccessful. (The discomfort of standing on the day of surgery is best endured to avoid the potential complication of a urinary tract infection from the catheter. When a Foley catheter is used, a suitable antibiotic is administered.)

5. First postoperative day:
   a. Dangle legs 5 times
   b. Stand by side of bed once
   c. Assist to bathroom if patient desires

6. Second postoperative day:
   Out of bed in chair. Available in room

7. Third postoperative day:
   Ambulatory

8. One week:
   Sutures out, and discharged wearing nonreinforced lumbosacral support.

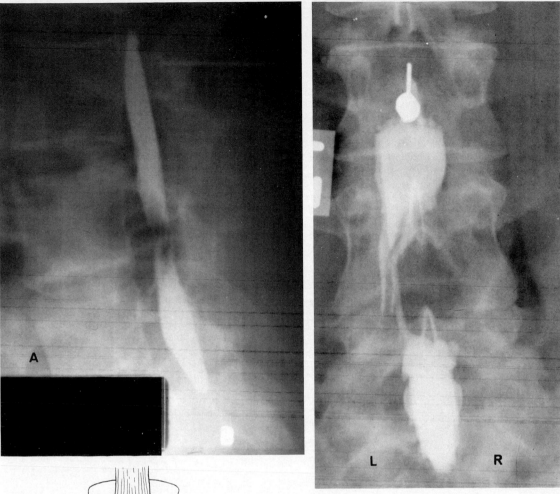

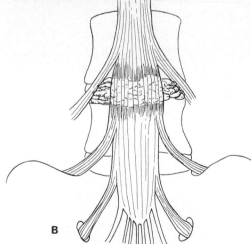

Fig. 10-74. This 39-year-old woman had a history of moderate low back pain and occasional right sciatica for several years. Because of an acute exacerbation of her symptoms, she was hospitalized 2 years previously and responded well to conservative treatment consisting of bed rest and traction. She was relatively pain free until she bent forward over a sink while brushing her teeth and developed a sudden, excruciating low back pain extending into both lower extremities (the right more severe than the left). She was admitted to the hospital with severe weakness of the left foot extensor muscles and slight weakness on the right. Because of inability to void, an indwelling Foley catheter was necessary. **(A)** An emergency myelogram revealed an extensive defect at L4–5 level. **(B)** Surgery performed on same day revealed massive extrusion of the intervertebral disc at the L4–5 level.

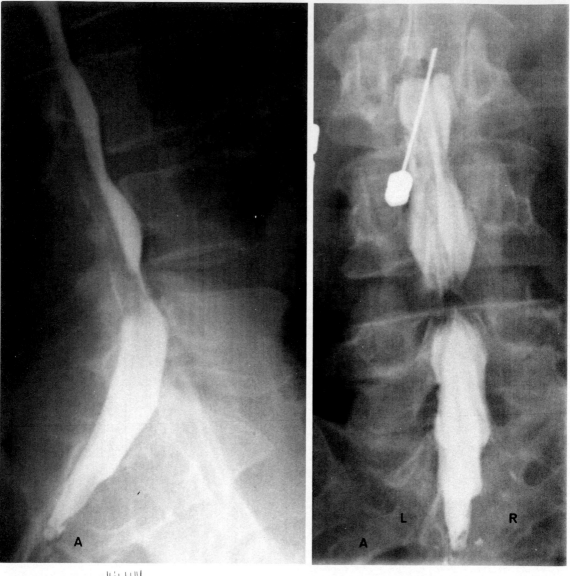

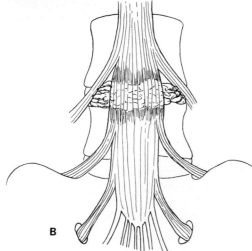

Fig. 10-75. This 67-year-old man presented with a long-standing history of low back pain extending into both posterior thighs. He experienced occasional tingling and numbness but no actual pain below the knees. Myelography revealed a midline intervertebral disc protrusion at the L4–5 interspace with considerable hypertrophy of the ligamentum flavum, producing an annular constriction at the involved level. Because of the dorsal compression from the ligamentum flavum, an L4–5 laminectomy was performed.

(Although the patient is ambulated during the immediate postoperative interval without external support, the increased activities at home are tolerated more kindly with a light canvas support constructed without paravertebral steels.)

9. At home activities gradually and progressively increased:

Ride in car—2 weeks

Drive car—4 weeks

10. Return to work depends largely on the nature of the job:

Clerical and office work—4 to 6 weeks.

Jobs involving heavy physical activities—3 to 4 months

Microlumbar Discectomy

Doctor Robert Williams, a neurosurgeon who practices in Las Vegas, Nevada, has developed a microsurgical technique for lumbar discectomy which differs significantly in several respects from the usual operative approach to lumbar disc disease.

Technique

The surgical microscope is used during the entire surgical procedure from skin incision to skin closure. Doctor Williams employs a one-inch, midline skin incision and performs the usual subperiosteal muscle dissection. When the appropriate interspace is exposed, he prefers to retain the entire lamina and does not remove any portion of it. He uses a scapel to incise the superficial fibers of the ligamentum flavum and makes a final perforation through the deep fibers of this structure with a blunt Penfield #4 dissector to avoid damage to the underlying dura. He uses a small Schlessinger punch to remove the lateral portion of the ligamentum flavum. After he has accomplished this, he identifies the nerve root and retracts it medially with a suction retractor. Upon retracting the root, the annulus fibrosis is visualized under mangification. If the annulus is not ruptured and an extruded disc fragment is not seen, he makes no attempt to incise the intact annulus with a sharp scalpel, instead preferring blunt perforation of the annulus with the Penfield #4 dissector. It is Doctor Williams' presumption that by avoiding an incision through the fibers of this structure he creates a temporary, nonpermanent opening using the blunt Penfield to separate but not cut the annular fibers. Through this limited annular defect, he accomplishs decompression of the herniated disc by taking multiple small bites of intervertebral disc tissue using a special microlumbar discectomy forceps. Care is taken to remove only the disc tissue which can easily be mobilized from the intervertebral disc space, and Doctor Williams specifically avoids curetting the disc space. Following the discectomy, he sometimes observed the annular opening to close partially, in a sphincterlike fashion. He attributes his low recurrence rate to this technique and believes that remaining disc material would be more likely to reherniate if the fibers of the annulus were incised with a scalpel. With this microdiscectomy procedure he reports a 91% satisfactory postsurgical result.

The Four Critical Points

The specific points Doctor Williams emphasizes as being critical to the success of his procedure are:

1. Elimination of laminectomy or facet damage.

2. Preservation of all epidural fat.

3. Blunt perforation of the annulus fibrosis rather than scalpel incision.

4. Preservation of healthy nonherniated intervertebral disc material.

Advantages and Disadvantages of Microlumbar Discectomy

Since Doctor Williams first presented his technique in 1976 at an annual meeting of the Congress of Neurological Surgeons, a

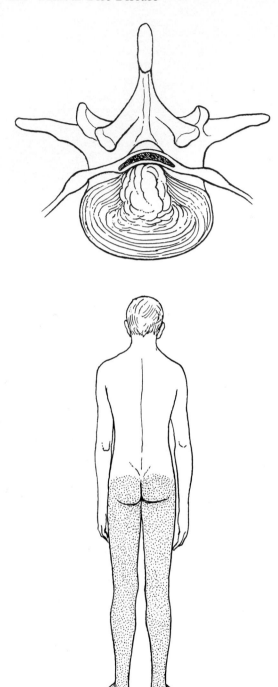

Fig. 10-76. Cauda equina syndrome.

the advantages of excellent lighting and magnification, have gone back to the more traditional approach. The latter includes removal of the inferior ridge of the superior lamina, a foraminotomy to decompress the nerve root, sharp excision of the annulus fibrosis fibers, a generous evacuation of disc tissue, and curettement of the intervertebral disc space (Fig. 10-76). Those physicians who employ the usual surgical approach with an operating microscope are merely using the instrument to provide an excellent light source and magnification. Some discussion may be in order, however, with regard to the points that Doctor Williams raises in carrying out his technique.

1. Avoidance of bony removal presents advantages and disadvantages. Obviously, the less bony removal carried out at a surgically explored interspace, the less weakening of the bony lumbar spine will occur. However, individuals who present with symptoms of lumbar disc disease severe enough to require surgery will usually develop hypertrophic osteoarthritic degenerative changes involving the vertebral surfaces immediately adjacent to the protruding disc. If degenerative change is not seen when the initial disc syndrome presents itself, it tends to occur some years later. With such bony foraminal impingement of the nerve root in addition to the impingement caused by the disc, would not a foraminotomy be of some benefit?

2. A second factor in avoidance of bony removal relates to the minute anatomy of this area. Occasionally the nerve root lies quite medial, and once the lateral portion of the yellow ligament is excised, adequate access to this delicate structure is possible. However, many nerve roots are considerably lateral to this point, and it is only after removing an edge of bone from the lateral margin of the interspace that easy access to the nerve root is possible. Without this lateral exposure excessive stretching or trauma to the nerve root may occur.

3. Preservation of epidural fat is a point that is made by those employing both mi-

number of physicians have adopted the Williams technique. Some continue to follow this specific technique; others, while still using the operating microscope and enjoying crolumbar discectomy and the usual approach; this topic was adequately discussed previously.

4. Blunt perforation of the annular fibers may be a valid concept when we are dealing with a slight bulge of the disc or when annulus fibrosis maintains its full thickness or width. But when the disc is markedly protruding, even if it is not completely extruded, the fibers of the annulus are usually so overly stretched and thinned out that relatively little is gained by attempting to retain this vestigial remnant of a once stout retaining ring.

5. Preservation of healthy nonherniated intervertebral disc material may not be a valid concept. Once a disc becomes damaged enough to require surgery, it is probably no longer healthy. Once we violate this structure surgically, the likelihood of its performing its original biomechanical function does not appear particularly good. Possibly, as generous an excision of the disc as is possible may serve the patient best.

We might speculate that the conservative surgical approach proposed by Doctor Williams may be akin to what is accomplished by injection of Chymopapain or one of the other substances advocated for chemical reduction of disc protrusion. It is quite possible that the procedure that Doctor Willaims recommends is in effect a surgical chemonucleosis.

Let me conclude by stating that I respect and admire Doctor Williams and welcome his innovative technique to the arena of clinical assessment. Further experience and time will provide answers to many of our questions.

Cause of Operative Failure

The most common cause of surgical failure is an error in judgment with regard to the indication for initial surgery. I recently reviewed 94 postsurgical patients with failed low back syndromes; most of them had undergone multiple spinal operative procedures. In this series, the original surgery was not indicated in 76 of the 94 cases (81%) assessed.

If the preoperative symptoms persist after surgery, various questions should be considered. Was the lesion really a symptom-producing, markedly protruding disc, or merely a slightly protruding disc in association with a stenotic lumbar canal? Was a neoplasm overlooked? Were the symptoms primarily due to a lumbosacral strain associated with some slight irritation of the nerve root? Careful analysis may reveal that surgery was not in order, or that a significantly altered surgical procedure was indicated.

Inadequate surgery is the second-ranking cause of operative failure. Was the proper interspace explored? Was a fragment of extruded disc within the axilla between the root and the dural sac overlooked? Did the surgeon fail to identify either clinically or by myelography a second protruding disc? Was evacuation of the disc space inadequate with considerable disc material remaining to cause persisting root pressure?

A most significant cause of persisting pain or even worsening pain following surgery is nerve root damage. This can occur because of excessive medial retraction and stretching of the root, or because of direct root trauma during the removal of intervertebral disc material, with the root being contused, pinched, or sometimes even badly torn. Damage to the nerve root from spread of the cautery current may also be the cause of persisting symptoms.

COMMON CAUSES OF POSTOPERATIVE PAIN

1. Surgery not indicated initially
2. Radiculitis secondary to nerve root trauma at time of surgery
3. Radiculitis secondary to postoperative scarring (intradural or extradural)
4. Persisting nerve root pressure from inadequate disc excision or an overlooked second disc protrusion (less frequently encountered than the other three causes)

Results of Initial Surgery

The results of initial surgery of 1000 cases operated upon by me are classified, on the basis of pain relief and ability to perform physical activity, as satisfactory or unsatisfactory.

Included in the satisfactory classification are those who were advised to change from their physically demanding jobs to occupations that were less physically taxing, and housewives who were placed on restrictions in their daily activities but who were able to continue on this restricted basis in relative comfort.

Included in the unsatisfactory classification are patients who considered surgery "worthwhile" because it reduced the severity of pain, but who were unable to work in relative comfort.

	Satisfactory	Unsatisfactory
Patients	928	72
Percent	93	7
	Secondary Gain	No Secondary Gain
Patients	38 of 343	34 of 657
Percent	11	5

Cauda Equina Syndrome

A cauda equina syndrome secondary to a massive extrusion of an intervertebral disc is relatively rare, and I have personally been involved with the treatment of only six acute cases in 30 years of surgical experience (Fig. 10-76). I am not including the several patients seen each year who have undergone surgery and seek consultation to determine if further treatment is likely to benefit their neurological residuals. Doctor W. B. Jennett reviewed 25 cases of cauda equina compression in 1956, and this remains the largest series in the literature.

Three Stages. The development of the cauda equina syndrome may be divided into three stages:

1. Long-standing intermittent backache
2. Sciatic radiation, often unilateral

3. Sudden onset of pain and weakness in both lower extremities with sphincter disturbance

The third, "final" stage may occur following a strenuous physical action, a cough, a sudden body movement, a spinal manipulation, or it may occur during sleep and first be noted by the patient upon awakening in the morning. Either the first or second stage may not be elicited in the history, and it is remotely possible for the patient not to have experienced either stage 1 nor 2 and to develop stage 3 as their first lumbar spine symptom.

Paradoxical Improvement. Occasionally, a patient who is complaining bitterly of unilateral sciatica will appreciate partial relief of pain after the onset of motor weakness of both lower extremities. This paradoxical improvement of pain, caused by nerve root anesthesia secondary to the increased intraspinal pressure, may lull the physician into delaying myelography and surgery.

SIGNS AND SYMPTOMS

There may be impaired motor function in both lower extremities as well as widespread hypesthesia, extending from the buttocks down to the feet, in association with both bowel and bladder sphincter impairment. Such a condition is considered an emergency, and an expeditious myelogram is in order, to confirm the clinical impression of cauda equina syndrome. This will reveal a complete block at the involved level. Prompt surgical intervention and decompression of this lesion is called for, and delay of treatment in such instances is inadvisable and may add to the permanence of neurological deficit. In situations of such severe compression of the nerve roots, permanent changes may occur, no matter how quickly decompression is performed; delay will probably add to the deficit.

PROGNOSIS OF CAUDA EQUINA SYNDROMES

Most cauda equina syndromes resulting from a massive disc extrusion have residual neurological dysfunction. This may be in the form of motor weakness, sensory changes, sphincter impairment, and persisting pain. It is generally accepted that the delay of speedy decompressive surgery is the most important factor related to the prognosis. For this reason, the cauda equina syndrome is considered a surgical emergency and once the diagnosis is made, an emergency myelogram followed by prompt surgery is generally recommended. My own experience indicates that the promptness with which surgery is carried out may not necessarily be the major factor determining whether neurological residuals will persist following treatment. I would like to present two cases which may illustrate this alternative point of view.

Case 1. F.D. This patient, whom I followed during that portion of my residency spent in a VA hospital, was a 38-year-old chaplain who was permanently assigned to and quartered on the grounds of the hospital. He had a chronic low back pain history and on two previous occasions was hospitalized for severe low back and right sciatic pain. During each of these brief hospitalizations, he received bed rest and traction which eased but did not totally alleviate the pain and enabled him to carry on with his duties as a hospital chaplain. When his low back symptoms worsened, he would seek relief with a Knight spinal brace and oral analgesic medication. On August 2, 1950, while bending forward to pick up a light object, he coughed, and at that moment he experienced an excruciating pain in the back, immediately followed by severe radiating pain and weakness in both lower extremities. Within ½ hour of this episode, which occurred on the hospital grounds, he was seen by the chief of the neurosurgical service. Within 1 hour of the onset of symptoms a myelogram was per-

formed which revealed a complete block at the L4–5 level. The patient was brought to the operating room 2½ hours after the onset of his cauda equina syndrome. A decompressive laminectomy of L4 and L5 was performed, and an enormous fragment of disc material lying free within the spinal canal was removed, after which some additional large disc fragments that were partially extruded from the interspace were removed (Fig. 10-77). The large size of these extruded and partially extruded fragments indicated that the major portion of the intervertebral disc had extruded. All remaining accessible fragments of intervertebral disc material were removed, and the wound was closed in the usual fashion. There was significant improvement in the low·back and sciatic pain postoperatively, but the motor weakness of the right lower extremity persisted. He resumed his duties at the hospital 4 months after surgery but required a Foley catheter for an 8-month interval after surgery. After the Foley was removed, he continued to have urinary sphincter impairment which persisted until the time of his retirement from the VA hospital 4½ years postsurgery. He also had persisting rectal sphincter impairment and required rectal suppositories or enemas for bowel evacuation at regular intervals. He continued to wear a right foot drop brace when he retired as hospital chaplain.

Case 2. C.D. This 41-year-old woman tripped and fell on April 17, 1975, She bruised both knees in the fall, but it was not until the next day that she developed severe back pain. Because of the persistence and severity of her low back pain she was hospitalized at the Sacred Heart Hospital in Chester, Pennsylvania, in May, 1975. She was treated with bed rest and pelvic traction and was discharged with a low back support. Low back pain persisted intermittently, and in August of 1975 she developed numbness "from my waist down" in association with both rectal and urinary sphincter impairment. She was readmitted to the Sacred Heart Hospital

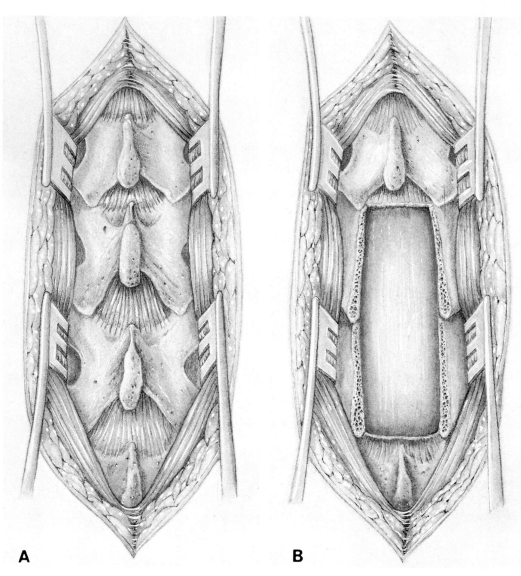

A **B**

Fig. 10-77. (A) Bony exposure. (B) Laminectomy of L4 and L5.

where a myelogram revealed a complete block at the L5–S1 level. Surgery was recommended, but the patient did not wish to have surgery and was discharged. Because of urinary incontinence, she was admitted to the Crozer-Chester Medical Center a month later. A second myelogram was performed which again revealed a complete block at the L5–S1 level. Surgery was recommended but the patient declined. She was discharged from the hospital in June, 1975, with low back pain, a feeling of numbness from the waist down, pain and weakness in both lower extremities, and both urinary and rectal sphincter impairment necessitating the wearing of a diaper. She was first seen by me September 29, 1977. Her complaints included a sensation of numbness from the waist down. The urinary and rectal sphincter impairment was as severe as earlier. She had pain and weakness of both lower extremities and low back pain. She remained incapacitated by these symptoms and had been unable to work as a teacher's aid since the onset of the cauda equina syndrome April 17, 1975. Examination revealed the patient to be obese. Mobility of the lumbar spine was decreased, particularly in flexion, with severe paraspinal muscle spasm in the lumbar region. Sensory examination revealed saddle anesthesia with numbness extending into both lower extremities within the sacral and lower lumbar segments. Straight leg raising was limited to 60 degrees bilaterally, with increased discomfort on the left at that angulation. Both Achilles reflexes were absent. There was weakness of flexion and extension of both feet. Rectal examination revealed lack of tone and the anocutaneous reflex was absent bilaterally. Light touch and vibratory sensation in the feet and appreciation of joint passive motion was retained. She was hospitalized October 2, 1977, and a third lumbar myelogram, performed by me on October 3, 1977, revealed a complete block at the L5–S1 level, in addition to a smaller midline defect at the L4–5 level. Her 1977 myelogram films were compared with her 1975 films and they were found to be essentially the same. At her request, she was discharged shortly after the myelogram and returned for surgery 2 weeks later. A decompressive laminectomy of L4, L5, and S1 was carried out at surgery. The L5–S1 intervertebral disc space was identified and found to be totally calcified with no soft disc material but a significant bony ridge producing cauda equina pressure. To be perfectly sure that we were within the interspace, a small dental chisel was hammered into the calcified disc space and a cross-table lateral film was taken to assure proper anatomical localization. A bilateral foraminotomy was performed at the L5–S1 level. The patient was last seen on followup visit October 5, 1978, just short of a full year after her surgery. At that time she felt well, and her original severe pain in the low back and both lower extremities was no longer present. The numbness and weakness in both lower extremities were completely gone. Diapers for rectal and urinary incontinence

were no longer required but she continued to have urinary frequency and because of this emptied her bladder on a regular basis so that she would not develop incontinence. She does not require a catheter. She has been back to work at her original job as a teacher's aid since April, 1978, and is carrying on quite well. Examination on her last visit revealed some slight hypesthesia to pinprick over the sacrum and perineum. Rectal tone was markedly improved. Both Achilles reflexes remained absent. Motor strength of both feet improved markedly. Straight leg raising was performed to 80 degrees bilaterally.

A NEW LOOK AT PROGNOSIS

These two case reports would, at first glance, tend to fly in the face of standard teaching. The first case is a hospital-based individual who, after developing an acute cauda equina syndrome, was immediately taken in hand, given a prompt myelogram followed by expertly performed decompressive surgery, all within several hours. This patient was left with serious and permanent neurological residuals. On the other hand, the second patient, with an extraordinary delay of more than 2 years, had a much more satisfactory outcome to surgery with fewer and much less severe neurological residuals. This would suggest that even more important than the speed of treatment is the rapidity and force of the original trauma to the nerve roots. A severe and massive retropulsion of an intervertebral disc will probably so severely traumatize the nerve roots, or produce such permanent changes to the vascular supply of the cauda equina, that a serious residual will persist no matter how promptly the pressure is surgically relieved. The second patient, who was extremely obese and had a very acute lumbosacral angle with calcification of the disc, probably had a less acutely developing lesion which produced comparatively less trauma to the cauda equina and provided greater potential for reversibility. Despite the inordinate delay in treatment, she had a quite satisfactory result.

This particular issue is addressed here because of the medicolegal implications. Occasionally, when a less than satisfactory result occurs following surgery, legal action may be taken against the surgeon with the presumption that if more expeditious surgical management had been carried out, the end result would have been better. These illustrative cases may indicate that such conclusions are conjectural.

SURGICAL TECHNIQUE FOR MASSIVE DISC PROTRUSION AND CAUDA EQUINA SYNDROME

When dealing with a cauda equina syndrome, it is best to carry out a most generous and complete laminectomy, for several reasons. A more complete bilateral removal of the protruded disc can be accomplished with generous exposure. Further, the considerable edema and swelling of the nerve roots evoked by such a lesion. A major bony decompression is likely to result in a more prompt and complete neurological recovery than would be the case if there remained bony compression overlying the site of cauda equina insult.

After the laminectomy has been performed, the disc can be removed by means of a bilateral extradural approach. To avoid undue retraction of the nerve roots and dural sac over the large midline protrusion, a very generous foraminotomy and lateral decompression performed on the most symptomatic side is helpful (Fig. 10-78). This enables the surgeon to approach the disc laterally without overstretching the root. If a portion of the extruded fragment can be visualized, it should be grasped with a thin disc removal forceps. The extruded fragment should not be forcefully tugged but slowly and gently delivered, avoiding excessive trauma to the overlying dura and root. Sometimes the extruded fragment is midline in location and an unusually wide dural sac tented over this protrusion prevents visualization of even a small edge of the protrusion without excessive retraction. Under such circumstances, following a generous fora-

minotomy, enter and gradually decompress the lateral portion of the intervertebral disc using various sized pituitary forceps and curettes. After this has been done, the root can more easily be retracted over the shell of remaining disc and the extruded fragment visualized.

TRANSDURAL EXCISION OF MIDLINE DISC EXTRUSION

In the first edition of this monograph, the technique of exploring a midline disc protrusion by means of a transdural approach was discussed. This procedure was advocated by some surgeons as a means of avoiding undue retraction of the nerve roots and dural sac. It involved a laminectomy and dural opening, packing the nerve roots to either side with cotton patties, and exposing the anterior dura. The midline disc is removed through an anterior dural incision.

This is an ill-conceived approach, and I recommend that it not be performed. The disadvantages and potential hazards of opening the dura to remove an epidural lesion far outweigh any potential advantages.

Repeat Operative Procedure

Indications for Repeat Surgery

Reoperation on an intervertebral disc space that has undergone previous surgery is technically more difficult to perform than a primary procedure. The normal tissue planes are usually obliterated by dense fibrous tissue extending from the skin down to the bony elements of the spine.

Of greater importance, both with regard to symptom production and operative difficulty, is the scar tissue enveloping the dural sac and nerve root. The patient who has persisting pain following lumbar disc surgery presents a problem to the physician involving all of the factors that were weighed in the decision to operate initially, and geometrically expanded additional variables related to the previous surgery. Rarely are decisions involving this type of patient easily made.

THE FOUR QUESTIONS

Four questions must be answered to evaluate the clinical problem of repeat surgery properly. The questions are naturally progressive. Each succeeding question is based on a positive answer to the preceding question. A negative response to any of the first three questions eliminates the need to proceed with further consideration of additional surgery.

1. Was the original surgery indicated? Often, this is the most difficult question to answer. If the initial surgery was performed by another physician, a valid reconstruction of the original signs and symptoms may be based on the patient's deficient recollections. When the evaluating physician performed the initial surgery, it should be recalled that objectivity is not likely to be the most conspicuous human characteristic. It certainly "goes against the grain" for a surgeon to conclude that an operation he previously performed was not indicated.

If the physician comes to the conclusion that the initial surgery was not indicated, it is not likely that a "repeat performance" would serve a useful purpose. Only if, in retrospect, the original surgery was deemed warranted, can he proceed with the next logical question.

2. What went wrong? Was the original surgery the procedure of choice? Was it adequately or inadequately performed? Do the postoperative films indicate that the correct side and correct interspace were subjected to exploration, or was a "site error" committed? Did irreversible nerve root damage occur from the original surgery, and is this the cause of persisting symptoms? Does the patient manifest symptoms of a mechanically unstable spine, and should a spinal fusion have been performed at the time of the original surgery? Should a spinal

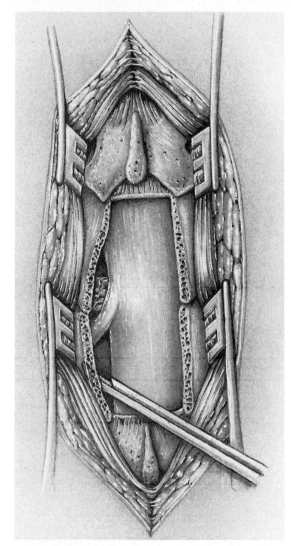

Fig. 10-78. A very generous foraminatory and lateral decompression performed on the most symptomatic side enables the surgeon to approach the disc laterally and avoid undue retraction of the nerve root and dural sac over the large midline protrusion.

fusion be done now? If the answers to these questions enable one to explain the failure of the original surgery, we may proceed to the third question.

3. Is the patient's present dysfunction severe enough to warrant a repeat operation, in the knowledge that the repeat procedure is associated with a higher percentage of failure? An affirmative answer brings us to the last question.

4. What is the indicated surgical procedure? Repeat interlaminar exploration? Complete laminectomy? Fusion?

OPTIMISTS AND PESSIMISTS

The large number of lumbar discectomies performed in this country seems to indicate a wide streak of optimism within the personalities of spine surgeons. At the same time, those of us who tend to see large numbers of surgical failures become increasingly pessimistic and skeptical about the relative value of surgery. Each week I see five or six new patients who remain incapacitated after lumbar disc surgery. Of this group, I may perform repeat surgery on one or two each year, approximating a selection ratio of 1 in 200 patients. Many patients whom I have tried to discourage from having further surgery will eventually find their way to a physician willing to try again. Followup reports or reassessment almost invariably strengthens my conservative point of view.

Patient Selection

It is axiomatic that all surgery should be limited to those who can reasonably be expected to benefit. Since the beneficial results of repeat lumbar spine surgery are relatively meagre compared to the anticipated yield from first surgeries, a very critical patient selection system is in order.

SIX NEGATIVE FACTORS

The following six factors are generally acknowledged as creating negative or unfavorable influence on the prognosis of repeat spine surgery.

1. If the original surgery was not clearly indicated, nothing is to be gained by further surgery. In a recent series of 94 surgical failures which I carefully reviewed and reported, 76 patients (81%) were found to be in this category.

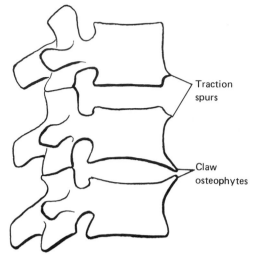

Fig. 10-79. *The "traction spur" described by Doctor Ian MacNab is an excellent radiological indication of excessive lumbar mobility.*

Labels on figure: Traction spurs; Claw osteophytes

2. The postoperative patient who demonstrates myelographic evidence of either adhesive arachnoiditis or perineural and peridural scarring as the principal abnormality offers a poor prognosis for repeat surgery.

3. A history of psychological instability, alcoholism, or drug dependence is often associated with a poor long-term result. This may be construed as an unfair blanket indictment. Certainly, an alcoholic or a patient with a significant emotional dysfunction may also be burdened with an organic lesion within the lumbar spine. Withholding surgical correction of this lesion might be considered as reprehensible as failing to treat a fractured arm because the patient is a neurotic. Theoretically, this is sound reasoning, but in practice such a nondescriminating course of action will lead to an intimidating incidence of unfortunate results. It may be helpful to remind ourselves that a recurrent disc is usually far more complex than a fractured arm.

4. Patients who are involved in a work-connected secondary gain situation or who have ongoing litigation relating to their clinical problems are not likely to do as well as those free of such negative factors.

5. A history of no improvement after surgery or a relatively short interval of relief

(of less than a year after the initial operation) indicates a poor prognosis for repeat spinal surgery. This rule does not hold if it can be determined that the original surgery was performed inadequately, on the wrong side, or within the wrong interspace.

6. The number of previous operations is a significant prognostic factor. A patient who has had one prior operative procedure and who demonstrates a specific indication for repeat surgery may have a reasonably favorable prognosis. The patient with two previous spinal operations is more likely to be made worse rather than better by repeat surgery, and the prognosis becomes increasingly worse with additional operations.

FOUR POSITIVE FACTORS

Pain of itself is not considered a specific indication for repeat lumbar spine surgery. However, persistent and incapacitating pain is implicitly included with any of the following four entities in order for repeat surgery to be warranted. They are listed in prognostic order, with the first, spinal stenosis, having the best prognosis, and the last, pseudoarthrosis, the worst.

1. Spinal Stenosis. This condition may occur either as a complication arising from previously performed surgery or as an entity that was present prior to the original surgery. Occasionally after a midline fusion, overgrowth of the fusion mass may result in cauda equina compression. This is much less common than the patient who had a preexisting one level lumbar stenosis prior to surgery. Because the presurgical symptoms primarily involved a single root syndrome, a limited surgical approach would initially have been employed. Most commonly this would take the form of a partial disc excision and foraminotomy. Sometimes such an approach is adequate, but occasionally the postoperative development of peridural scar tissue verging on the preexisting spinal stenosis will create recurrent symptoms. A decompressive laminectomy could be helpful.

2. Lumbar Spine Instability. Sometimes, following a lumbar discectomy, the patient's sciatic pain is relieved but is replaced by severe back pain. This new back pain is worsened by weight bearing and movement and is eased by bed rest and immobility. Carefully studied lateral lumbar spine films in flexion and extension will often demonstrate an abnormally mobile interspace. If the films are obtained during a severe exacerbation of pain, the patient may be too uncomfortable to flex and extend the lumbar spine through a sufficiently extensive range to make an x-ray film diagnosis of instability. The "traction spur" described by Doctor Ian MacNab is an alternative roentgenographical indication of excessive lumbar mobility (Fig. 10-79). This spur is easily differentiated from the more commonly seen degenerative osteophyte which develops at the edge of the vertebral body and which curves toward its matching osteophyte at the edge of the opposing vertebral body. In contrast, the traction spur arises approximately 1 mm away from the discal edge of the vertebral body and projects horizontally, instead of curving toward the opposing vertebra. The spur is produced when greater than normal mobility places a traction strain upon the outermost fibers of the annulus fibrosis. It is because these outermost annular fibers attach to the vertebral body beyond the epiphyseal ring that the spur develops just short of the vertebral discal border.

3. Lumbar Disc Reherniation. Lumbar disc reherniation is subject to a wide spectrum of definitions and individual interpretations. What one physician might choose to label as a lumbar disc reherniation, a second might identify as persistence of a lesion that was inadequately excised. The additional element of postoperative perineural and peridural scar tissue provides additional opportunities for shading of opinion.

The usual clinical picture is exemplified by the patient with a single root syndrome

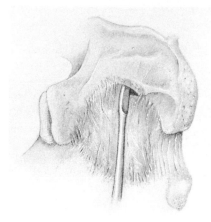

Fig. 10-80. Dissecting adherent dura from undersurface of the superior lamina.

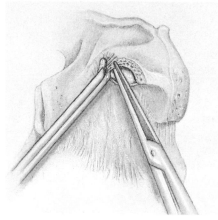

Fig. 10-81. Avoid tugging on epidural scar tissue.

who had a lumbar discectomy followed by improvement. Because of recurrent symptoms, a second myelogram is performed which reveals a filling defect that is essentially similar to the myelogram prior to the first operation.

Before deciding on a surgical approach to this problem, a very careful evaluation of the lumbar spine films is important. If the original surgery included a lateral decompression and generous foraminotomy at the level of the filling defect, the prognosis with additional surgery is not likely to be good. Conversely, if the spine films demonstrate that the original surgery was limited to an interlaminar discectomy and a lateral bony decompression, and a foraminotomy may be performed during the second procedure, the prognosis for improvement after surgery may be fairly good.

The basis for such a prognostic disparity is the likelihood that nerve root symptoms may arise from impingement within the lateral recess or the intervertebral foramen. Removal of these bony strictures will permit a nerve root to pass asymptomaticaly over a bony spur, a residual disc protrusion, or epidural scar tissue. If the spine roentgenograms indicate that all possible lateral and foraminal bony encroachment was removed during the original surgery, the existence of an intractable nerve root irritation syndrome

which will not benefit from further surgery is more likely.

4. Pseudoarthrosis. This is listed as one of the 4 indications for repeat spine surgery, but it has the worst prognosis of the group. Repair of a pseudoarthrosis is not easy; when the secondary procedure is unsuccessful, a worsening of symptoms often occurs. Even when a successful repair of an unstable fusion is accomplished, the improvement from this surgery is often very disappointing. Before deciding to carry out surgery on this condition, the physician should fully explore all alternatives to surgery.

Technical Considerations in Repeat Spinal Surgery

The scarred paraspinal muscle is removed from the spinous processes and laminae in the same manner as in the primary procedure. However, the surgeon now must be much more careful to avoid injury to the dural sac and nerve roots by an instrument that may inadvertently slip between the widened interlaminar space at the site of the previous operative procedure. Scar tissue will be tightly adherent to the dura, and great care must be taken to avoid tearing the dura and arachnoid when sweeping the muscles laterally over the previously explored interspace (Fig. 10-80; see also Fig. 10-54). Once the muscle dissection has been satis-

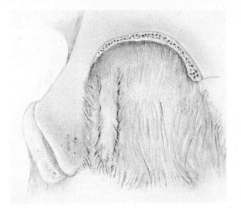

Fig. 10-82. *The nerve root, surrounded by scar tissue, is more easily damaged at the edge of the inferior lamina.*

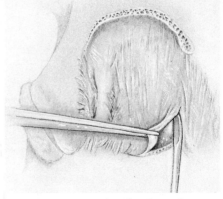

Fig. 10-83. *Dissection of epidural scar from upper edge of inferior lamina. This dissection is continued medially until the superior lamina is reduced. The root is best exposed from the superior lamina downward.*

factorily accomplished, a new plane of cleavage must be established to allow adequate dissection of the dura and nerve root. The easiest way to start this dissection is to insert a thin elevator between the scar and the undersurface of the remaining lamina above. After a small area beneath the superior lamina has been freed, a 40°-angled, small jawed laminectomy punch rongeur is introduced to bite a small rim of bone and expose a zone of dura that has not previously been dissected. Once this first bite has been accomplished, the dura-scar dissection is carried a bit more laterally, allowing a second bite. This is continued cautiously until a thin rim of superior lamina has been completely removed. This dissection is best not hurried, and care is taken to avoid tugging on scar tissue which is adherent to the underlying dura and which may tear the dura and arachnoid (Fig. 10-81). After this plane of cleavage has been carried laterally to the facet, it may be possible to separate the remaining dura from the overlying scar tissue.

If the scar tissue is too dense and adherent despite the bony removal, it may be necessary to interrupt the dissection at the superior lamina and resume a similar dissection at the inferior lamina. This may be more technically difficult, since the superior edge of the inferior lamina dips downward and is angled more anteriorly. The down-

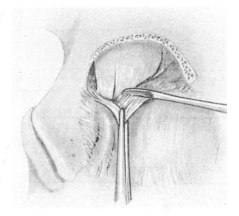

Fig. 10-84. *Exposure of root encased in scar is best started at point of exit from dural sac rather than from a site where the root is free.*

ward slope, in association with epidural scarring, creates a potential hazard of tearing the dura, which is increased by use of the 40°-angled jaw laminectomy punch. The danger to the root at this site is great. While dissection beneath the superior lamina exposes the origin of the nerve root as it separates from the dural sac, inferior lamina dissection exposes the free nerve root completely detached from the dura, making identification of the scar-encased root more difficult and giving rise to possible root damage (Figs. 10-82 through 10-84). In the presence of dense, adherent scar tissue, do not attempt to carry out the dissection laterally at the

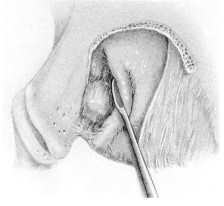

Fig. 10-85. Retracting the nerve root.

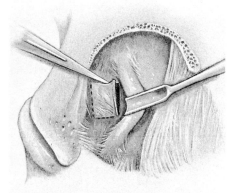

Fig. 10-86. Slab-shaped incision into recurrent disc.

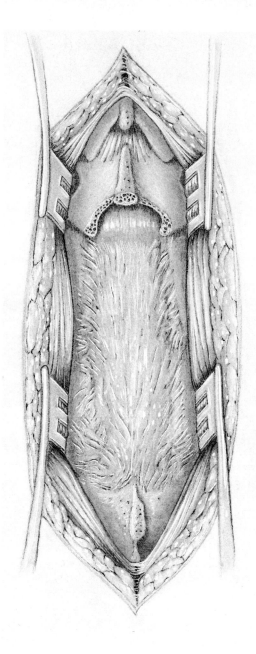

Fig. 10-87. Reexploration of complete laminectomy. The inferior edge of the L3 lamina has been excised to expose unscarred dura.

inferior lamina. The reason for developing the dura inferiorly is to provide an additional plane of cleavage between dura and scar tissue. In many cases, this will allow the scar tissue to be more easily peeled away from the dura, so that the dissection can once more be carried out at the superior lamina. Use of the 40°-angled, small jawed laminectomy punch rongeur will achieve a more lateral bony exposure. Each time a bite of bone is taken, which carries with it scar tissue adherent to the underlying dura and root, refrain from tugging on the scar; instead use a Metzenbaum scissors to cut the bone fragment free. With careful dissection, the dura and root can eventually be adequately exposed and freed of most of the scar tissue. In some cases, it is necessary to perform a hemilaminectomy to develop a satisfactory scar-dural cleavage plane. Only after the dura and root are well identified can these structures be safely retracted medially, exposing the underlying intervertebral space (Fig. 10-85).

Previously explored intervertebral discs,

in addition to recurrent annular protrusions, often manifest a significant mass of fibrous scar tissue, which in combination are capable of producing nerve root compression. At one time it was believed that painful root compression could occur solely from the development of epidural scar tissue. I have not observed this and am of the opinion that in addition to scar tissue, some degree of disc protrusion or bony encroachment within the lateral recess or intervertebral foramen is necessary before root compression symptoms will develop. Such abnormal intervertebral discs should be reexplored, using a long-handled No. 11 blade to make a generous slab-shaped incision within the annulus. This facilitates radical evacuation of old degenerated disc material, debris, and cartilaginous plates (Fig. 10-86). Following previous surgery it is advisable to carry out a much wider, bony decompression, either a hemilaminectomy, or, if the myelogram reveals considerable compression resulting from scar tissue, a complete bilateral wide laminectomy.

Some years ago, in the face of myelographic evidence of adhesive arachnoiditis, it was considered advisable to open the dura and free up or "comb out" the nerve roots. This is often associated with increased nerve root pain and is seldom, if ever, helpful. Also, it may result in further scarring and potential root damage.

In some cases where the articular facets have been partially entered into by previous surgery, the articular capsules are stretched and dysfunctional. Resection of such abnormal capsules and facets may be symptom alleviating.

Reexploration Following Complete Laminectomy

In some instances it will be necessary to reexplore following a complete laminectomy (Figs. 10-87 and 10-88). This presents much more difficulty, because the scar tissue is intimately associated with a considerable area of dura, adding greatly to the possibility

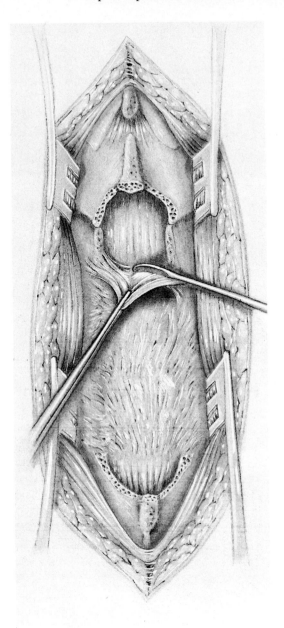

Fig. 10-88. This illustrates trouble in the making. Excision of scar tissue adherent to the dura wastes precious anesthesia time and is a good way to tear the dura.

of a dural tear. In such a situation, the first step is a bilateral, subperiosteal dissection of the intact vertebrae immediately above and below the laminectomy opening. After this has been accomplished, it is possible to approximate the depth of the dural sac be-

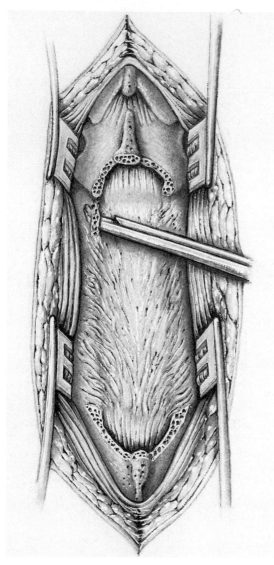

Fig. 10-89. *After establishing a plane of cleavage between the dura and scar tissue by removing a thin edge of lamina superiorly, avoid the midline scar adherent to the dura, and continue to develop the dissection laterally with an angled Schlesinger punch.*

tween these two points. Working from intact bone and using meticulous dissection, the overlying scar tissue can be dissected free from the dura. Additional bony removal, at least a thin margin of untouched bone above and below the previous laminectomy, is most helpful in developing a plane of cleavage between the dura and the adherent scar tissue.

Probably the most common reason for repeat surgery on a previously performed bilateral laminectomy is persisting nerve root pressure symptoms. These symptoms are presumably due to an inadequate lateral recess decompression during the original procedure. Under such circumstances, a complete dissection of the midline scar tissue adherent to the dura is not indicated. The outer, denser layer of scar contiguous with the paraspinal muscles is easily dissected and should be excised. The underlying, thin layer of scar tissue that intimately adheres to the dura is best left undisturbed. Removal of this layer not only dissipates precious time and energy but may be dangerous. It is at this point in the procedure that the obsessive surgeon who attempts to remove all scar tissue and restore the dura to its original smooth blue appearance may create a dural tear. Once torn, this nonelastic, scarred dura may not lend itself to a satisfactory watertight closure and could give rise to concerns about CSF fistula and meningitis. After establishing a plane of cleavage between the dura and scar tissue by removing a thin margin of previously untouched lamina superiorly, continue to develop this dissection laterally (Fig. 10-89). Use an angled Schlesinger punch to unroof the lateral recess and perform foraminotomies.

Results of Repeat Procedures

Of 146 patients requiring repeat spinal surgery, 31 manifested symptoms on the side opposite the original complaint; 8 manifested symptoms on the same side but developed disc disease at a different interspace from the original lesion; 107 manifested dysfuction related to the site of previous surgery. Of these 107, 14 were considered lumbar instability, with back pain absent and radicular symptoms, and had fusions with no interspace reexploration; 61 had interspace reexploration followed by fusion; and 32 had interspace reexploration not followed by fusion.

Of the 107 patients with dysfuction related to the site of previous surgery, 79 (74%) had satisfactory results, 28 (26%) unsatisfactory results. Of the 31 with dysfunction on the side opposite the original complaint, 27 (87%) were satisfactory, and 4 (13%) were unsatisfactory.

References

1. Andrew J: Sacralization: Aetilogical factor in lumbar intervertebral disc lesions, and cause of misleading focal signs. Br J Surg: 42:304, 1954
2. Barr JS, Mixter WJ: Posterior protrusion of the lumbar intervertebral discs. J Bone Jt Surg 23:444–456, 1941
3. Finneson BE: A lumbar disc surgery predictive score card. Spine 3(2):186–188, 1978
4. Finneson BE, Cooper VR: A lumbar disc surgery predictive score card. Spine 4(2), 1979
5. Foltz EL, Ward AA Jr, Knopp M: Intervertebral fusion following lumbar disk excision. J Neurosurg 13:469, 1956
6. Fortune C: Arterio-venous fistula of left common iliac artery and vein. Med J Aust 43:660, 1956
7. Freeman DG: Major vascular complications of lumbar disc surgery. Western J Surg 60:175, 1961
8. Geiger LE: Fusion of vertebrae following resection of intervertebral disc. J Neurosurg 18:79, 1961
9. Glass BA, Ilgenfritz HC: Arteriovenous fistula secondary to operation for ruptured intervertebral disc. Ann Surg 14:122, 1954
10. Goldner JL, McCollum DE, Urbaniak JR: Anterior Disc Excision and Interbody Spine Fusion for Chronic Low Back Pain. American Academy of Orthopedic Surgeons, Symposium on the Spine. St. Louis, CV Mosby, 1969
11. Hakelius A: Prognosis in sciatica. Acta Orthop Scand, (Suppl) 129, 1970
12. Harman P: Anterior extraperitoneal disc excision and vertebral body fusion. Clin Orthop, 18:169, 1961
13. Hasner E, Jacobsen HH, Schalimtzek M, Snorrason E: Lumbosacral transitional vertebrae. A clinical and roentgenological study of 400 cases of low back pain. Acta Radiol 39:225, 1953
14. Hoover NW: Indications for fusion at time of removal of intervertebral disc. J Bone Joint Surg, 50A:189–193, 1968
15. Horton RE: Arteriovenous fistula following operation for prolapsed intervertebral disk. Br J Surg 49:77, 1961
16. Jennett WB: A study of 25 cases of compression of the cauda equina by prolapsed intervertebral disc. J Neurol Neurosurg Psychiat 19:109–116, 1956
17. Keim HA, Weinstein JD: Acute renal failure—a complication of spine fusion in the tuck position. J Bone Joint Surg 52A1248, 1970
18. Knighton RS, Hitselberger WE: A study of patients ten to seventeen years following operation for herniated nucleus pulposus. West J Surg 72: 134–138, 1964
19. Love JG: Removal of protruded intervertebral disks without laminectomy. Proc Mayo Clin 14:800, 1939, 15:4, 1940
20. MacNab L: Negative laminectomy, J Bone Jt Surg 50A:838, 1968
21. Mixter WJ, Barr JS: Rupture of the Intervertebral Disc Without Involvement of the Spinal Canal. New England Surgical Society, Boston, Sept 30, 1933
22. Moore CA, Cohen A: Combined arterial, venous, and ureteral injury complicating lumbar disk surgery. Amer J Surg 115:574, 1968
23. Rolander D: Motion of the lumbar spine with special reference to the stabilizing effect of posterior fusion. Acta Orthop Scand (Suppl) 90, 1966
24. Shenkin HA, Haft H: Foraminotomy in the surgical treatment of herniated lumbar disks, Surgery 60:274, 1966
25. Spangfort EV: The lumbar disc herniation; A computer-aided analysis of 2,504 operations. Acta Ortho Scand (Suppl) 142, March 1972
26. Speed L: Spondylolisthesis: Treatment by anterior bone graft. Arch Surg, 37:175, 1938
27. Stewart DY: The anterior disc excision and interbody fusion approach to the problem of degenerative disc disease of the lower lumbar spinal segments. New York, J Med, 61:3252, 1961
28. White JC: Results in surgical treatment of herniated lumbar intervertebral discs. Clin Neurosurg 13:42–54, 1966

Lumbar Spine Fusion 11

Mark D. Brown

Fusion of a lumbar intervertebral joint is indicated when the spine cannot protect the neural elements, support the body, or allow normal motion. If disc space narrowing results in nerve entrapment, one method of treatment is to restore the disc intervertebral space height and fuse the spine. Abnormal motion as the result of a degenerated disc, which may result in recurrent painful disability from repeated ligament sprains, can be managed by spinal fusion. Destruction of a vertebral body by malignant tumors usually requires bone replacement and fusion for support.

Spine fusion can be defined as the permanent internal fixation of part or all of the intervertebral joint(s). An intervertebral joint is composed of two adjacent vertebrae and their posterior bony elements connected by an intervertebral disc, ligaments, and two facet joint capsules.

Materials Used in Spine Fusion

The materials used for arthrodesis of these joints (Fig. 11-1) include autogenous (one's own) bone or allogeneic (banked) bone, with or without internal fixation. Internal fixation is used alone without bone in patients who have destructive lesions as the result of malignancy. Materials utilized for internal fixation include rods, hooks, wire, metallic

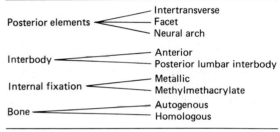

Fig. 11-1. Techniques in spinal fusion.

mesh, plates, bolts, screws, and cement (methylmethacrylate).

Arthrodesis for Malignancy Involving the Spine

Since loosening is an inevitable occurrence at the junction between the internal fixation devices and living bone, internal fixation by itself should be used only in patients with a limited life expectancy. However, an accurate estimate of life expectancy of patients with malignancies is becoming more difficult because of the recent advances in their medical management. It is not uncommon to see patients with metastatic diseases surviving much longer than would have formerly been expected. In these patients, failure of fixation will invariably occur with time. However, the use of wire, mesh, and cement for internal fixation can provide excellent long term fixation (Fig. 11-2).

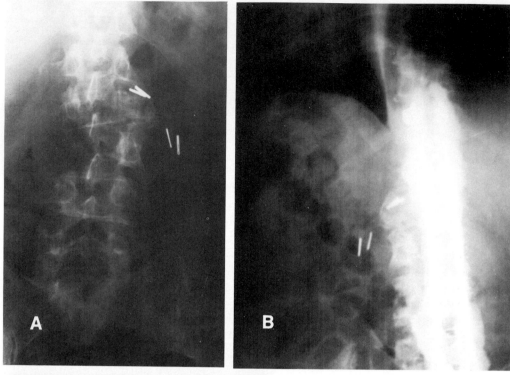

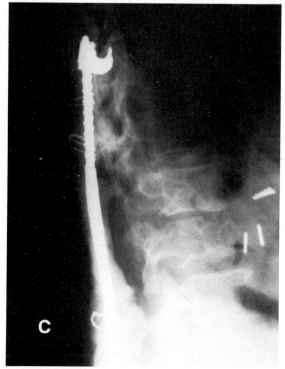

Fig. 11-2. **(A)** An anteroposterior roentgenogram demonstrates bone loss of the L3 vertebral body and pedicle secondary to metastatic hypernephroma. Internal fixation with two destraction rods, wires, and methylmethacrylate (**B** and **C**) gave enough fixation to allow the patient to ambulate without support and free of pain.

Bone Grafts

I advocate the use of bone grafts with or without supplemental fixation in all but the most unusual cases. Once union of the grafts with the spine has occurred and the graft has been replaced with viable new bone by the process of **creeping substitution,** the fusion should last a lifetime.

Autogenous Bone Graft

The most rapid fusion occurs with the patient's own bone. The optimum grafts for rapid fusion are cortico-cancellous, matchstick grafts measuring approximately 5 mm in diameter. These grafts, when placed in the region of a good blood supply (*i.e.,* across the transverse processes under the paraspinal muscles), usually incorporate quickly, act as a scaffolding for new bone, and induce osteogenesis from the surrounding mesenchymal tissue in the wound hematoma. We obtain a 95% fusion rate at the lumbosacral level and an 85% fusion rate between L4, L5, and the sacrum using autogenous posterolateral bone grafts placed across the transverse processes and the lateral surfaces of the superior facets.

INTERTRANSVERSE FUSION

The intertransverse lateral fusion technique, using autogenous grafts from the ileum, has evolved as the standard technique for spinal fusion by the posterior approach for the following reasons. The operation can be done through a traditional midline posterior incision used for decompression of the spinal canal and spinal foramen. Bony overgrowth leading to spinal stenosis, and spondylolisthesis aquisita (potential complications with posterior fusions) do not occur following this procedure. The lateral intertransverse fusion offers a good biomechanical support for resistance to torsional forces which are detrimental to the abnormal intervertebral joint. The thought that compression alone is the most important force to overcome in the abnormal joint is no longer true. We are now aware that torsion may be the more important motion to avoid for the degenerated intervertebral joint.

Banked Bone Graft

With the advent of modern tissue banking techniques, banked bone is readily available to the spinal surgeon. In our hands, banked bone has proven to be useful for arthrodesis of the lumbar spine under certain circumstances. Infectious processes and vertebral body destruction secondary to primary or metastatic tumor (Fig. 11-3) require anterior stabilization and replacement of the lost bone. We have found banked bone to be a logical source of graft material both to fill the gap and at the same time to provide a stable biomechanical construct. Tubular cortical bone allografts from the midshaft of the femur or tibia are remarkably strong, and they are easy to contour and fit with a

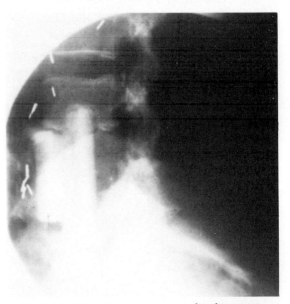

Fig. 11-3. *Lateral roentgenogram lumbar spine shows cortical tubular banked bone graft used to replace the L4 vertebra previously destroyed by metastatic carcinoma. The patient was ambulated without support in the immediate postoperative period.*

high-speed air burr (Fig. 11-4) I supplement these grafts by packing the medullary cavity with autogenous cancellous bone chips from a rib or anterior iliac crest, and by placing autogenous bone fragments around the graft to enhance the fusion of the graft to the spine. We look upon the banked grafts as bioresorbable spacers that induce new bone formation. They are excellent for replacing one or more destroyed vertebral bodies, and they provide immediate support to the spine.

A case illustrating this method of fusion technique is shown in (Fig. 11-5). The case is presented to show that cortical banked bone grafts can be used even in the presence of osteomyelitis, if the graft bed has been adequately debrided and the patient has received specific systemic antibiotic therapy. This patient suffered from severe lumbar spinal stenosis, hematogenous osteomyelitis with marked vertebral bone loss, and disc destruction. She was paraplegic, secondary to an epidural abscess. The diagnosis, *Proteus mirabilis* disc space infection, was made by closed Craig needle biopsy. Following specific antibiotic therapy, an anterior debridement of the epidural space, necrotic vertebral bodies, and intervertebral disc was performed, followed by an application of a cortical tubular banked bone graft. A stable biomechanical construct was obtained at the operating room table, and the patient was mobilized rapidly postoperative. She could not tolerate an external support. Her paraplegia resolved and bowel and bladder function returned. She was eventually rehabilitated and could walk without support. A year and a half following the initial salvage surgery, she underwent elective posterior decompression for spinal stenosis. Following the posterior decompression, an intertransverse spinal fusion with autogenous iliac bone graft was performed to supplement the previous anterior fusion. It was anticipated that following bilateral foraminotomies at three levels to decompress the spinal stenosis, the anterior graft would be subjected to abnormal torsional strain, and that the lateral fusion would prevent this from happening. The patient's satisfactory clinical result has proved this approach to be correct 2 years postoperatively.

Interbody Fusion Techniques

Since 80% of the weight-bearing function of the intervertebral joint occurs at the intervertebral disc, an interbody fusion would theoretically produce good clinical results. Cloward's long-term results in patients with solid interbody fusions, reviewed by two independent observers, would bear this out. Several other centers throughout the world where clinical data regarding his technique is being compiled would seem to substantiate his results. Dr. Cloward's posterior lumbar interbody spinal fusion technique has the advantage that during a single operation, one can decompress the spinal canal and foramen, remove the nucleus pulposus,

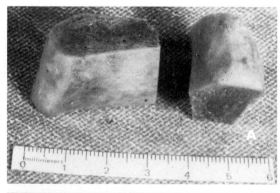

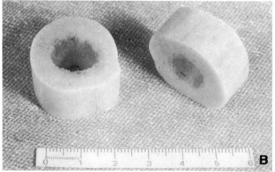

Fig. 11-4. Wedge grafts (A) from iliac crest utilized for interbody fusions. Tubular cortical banked bone grafts (B) for vertebral body replacement.

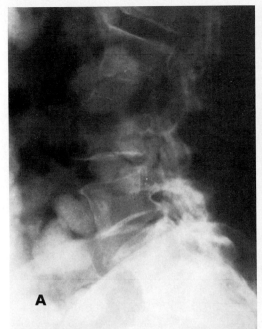
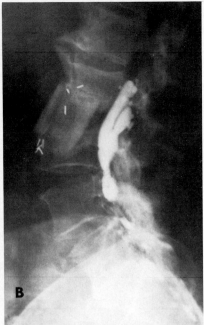
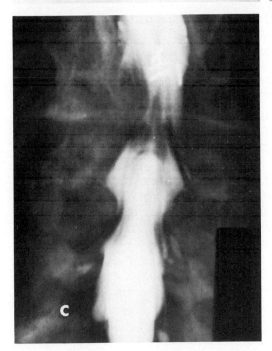

Fig. 11-5. Hematogenous disc space infection with osteomy-
olitis of the L2 and L3 vertebral bodies **(A).** One year postoperative interbody fusion with cortical tubular banked graft
(B). An AP roentgenogram of a myelogram **(C)** shows spinal
stenosis of the L3–4 intervertebral joint which was relieved
by posterior decompression and lateral spinal fusion.

restore the intervertebral space height, and
establish immediate mechanical stability.
The patients exhibit surprisingly little postoperative pain, and if the graft fuses and is
replaced by new bone before collapse or
rejection intervenes, they can anticipate an
excellent long-term relief of low back pain
and radicular pain (Fig. 11-6).

The major theoretical disadvantages of
interbody grafting techniques are biological.
The graft must be able to support the interspace and yet must allow bone induction

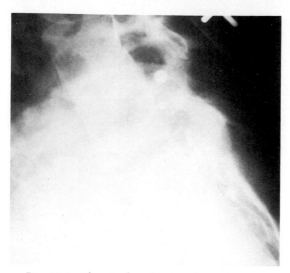

Fig. 11-6. Chronic low back pain and severe sciatic list for 1 year following an L4 disc excision in a 17-yr-old female were cured by this successful posterior interbody lumbar fusion. Patient is now a flight attendant.

and scaffolding for creeping substitution. To fulfill these two requirements, one must use a large amount of cortical cancellous bone graft at each interspace.

Both posterior and anterior interbody techniques require a large amount of cortical cancellous bone graft. One lumbar disc space requires four rectangular grafts averaging 2.5 cm in length, 1.2 cm in height, and 1.5 cm in width (see Fig. 11-4). It is frequently difficult to obtain this volume of bone from the patient's own iliac crest and, therefore, most surgeons performing this operation have turned to banked bone. Banked bone grafts perform satisfactorily under compression as compared to autogenous grafts, but the bone is still subject to low-grade immunological rejection. The fusion rate averages 85% at one level and 70% at more than one level.

It is imperative that all the nucleus pulposus of the disc space be removed. If residual nucleus pulposus fibrocartilage remains, it will proliferate into new fibrocartilage and actually erode the bone graft.

The posterior interbody fusion has the disadvantage of being technically difficult and requires long operative time even in the hands of experienced spinal surgeons. The complications of this technique are pseudoarthrosis of the bone graft, infection, constricting peridural scar, graft migration, nerve root trauma, and the possibility of great vessel damage.

There are no studies comparing rates of success with autogenous versus banked bone in lumbar interbody fusions performed by the same technique and surgeon. I have not decided whether Cloward's technique with banked bone will withstand the test of time. I am impressed with the quality of the clinical result obtained when the fusion does occur. The problem that concerns me is how to salvage those cases which do not show healing.

Anterior Lumbar Interbody Fusion

The other approach to interbody fusion is anterior, by either the retroperitoneal or transperitoneal route. Theoretical advantages and disadvantages of these methods are for the most part the same as those described for the posterior interbody lumbar technique. Dr. Leonard Goldner has long-term experience with the anterior interbody technique. He applied this technique to salvage spine cases where it is impossible to perform additional surgery from the posterior approach because of numerous previous scars or previous posterior infection. The advantage of this procedure is that one does not have to work in an area of previous spinal surgery and thus one eliminates the tedious and time-consuming dissection of epidural and perineural cicatrix. The anterior approach also avoids further nerve root trauma and scarring.

The major disadvantages of the anterior interbody technique are the lack of familiarity with the anterior approach by most spinal surgeons, the time that it requires per interspace, the large volume of bone need, and the pseudoarthrosis rate (*i.e.*, 28% for a two-level anterior fusion compared to 12% at two levels by the posterior lateral technique, according to Dr. Goldner). There is a reported incidence of thromboembolic disease of 5% to 8%, probably secondary to retraction of the iliac vessels. Although there have been reports of retrograde ejaculation, a better understanding of the anatomy of the presacral sympathetic plexus, which can be avoided by not dissecting the anterior surface of the sacrum, help us to prevent this complication. Solid interbody fusions by the anterior approach lead to a good quality of clinical result for the patient, according to the long-term experience of Dr. Goldner.

Fusion for Degenerative Disease of the Intervertebral Joint

The majority of patients for whom we consider spinal fusions suffer from the consequences of degenerative disc disease and osteoarthritis of the facet joints. The spinal surgeon must have a thorough understanding of the pathophysiology and pathologic anatomy of the degenerated intervertebral joint, in order to develop proficiency in determining which patients should undergo intervertebral joint arthrodesis.

Disc degeneration results in the loss of the hydraulic ballbearing properties of the nucleus pulposus. Disc narrowing results in subluxation of the facets with a consequence of secondary degenerative osteoarthritis of the joints. The nucleus pulposus normally distributes the load on the disc so that the fibers of the annulus fibrosis function under tension. In a degenerated disc the annulus fibrosis is subjected to direct compression loads. The fibrocytes in the annulus fibrosus begin producing fibrocartilaginous matrix, and the annulus fibrosus takes on the appearance of the nucleus pulposus. With even slight narrowing of the disc height, the angles of insertion of the collagen fibers of the annulus fibrosis are changed. The peripheral annulus fibrosus fibers thus become susceptible to rupture even under normal physiologic torsional loads. Even moderately degenerated discs can withstand compression loads to a greater degree than adjacent vertebral bodies before failure, but they cannot withstand resistance to torsion. Radial tears

in the annulus fibrosus with migration of the nucleus pulposus eventually may lead to disc prolapse or disc protrusion as a result of torsion on a degenerated disc. The eventual consequences of disc degeneration and facet joint osteoarthritis are narrowing of the vertebral foramen, the lateral recesses, and the spinal canal itself.

Degeneration of the annulus fibrosus, the longitudinal ligaments, and the facet joint capsules may lead to stiffening of the joint through normal healing processes. However, the degenerative process may be overwhelmed by recurrent injury. If the degenerative changes progress to the point where the healing potential is exhausted, there may result a mechanically unstable intervertebral joint.

Only rarely (Fig. 11-7) do we see the degenerative process lead to complete resorption of the nucleus pulposus (see the nitrogen gas shadow in its place) and attrition of the annulus fibrosus and longitudinal ligaments to such a degree that one vertebrae slips forward onto another. Although this patient had some disabling intermittent attacks of mechanical back pain (*i.e.*, moderate activity, low back sprain, back pain requiring rest for four or five days), she had no evidence of nerve root compromise (note the large neural foramen).

One must view each individual patient in light of knowledge of the pathophysiology described above in considering the indication for spine fusion and the methods and materials to be utilized. In considering the list of relative indications for spinal fusion for degenerative disc disease, keep in mind that we are not fusing spines but treating patients with symptoms. The patient in whom roentgenograms are shown in (Fig. 11-7) had a history compatible with mechanical back pain. On physical exam, she exhibited the classical extension lag, that is, pain and a jog of motion on extending from a standing flexed position. We considered a posterolateral spinal fusion on her because extensive degenerative changes in the vertebral bodies from abnormal weight bearing would preclude good bone stock for an in-

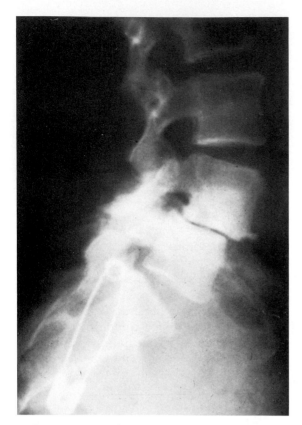

Fig. 11-7. Lateral roentgenogram lumbar spine. Severe degenerative disc disease with gas shadow in place of nucleus pulposus, pseudospondylolisthesis, and marked sclorosis of vertebral bodies. The patient had no radicular symptoms, but classic mechanical low back pain.

rehabilitation, a solid spinal fusion will not alter the eventual outcome. The patient must know the nature, benefit, and risks of the procedure and the alternatives of care and must participate in the decision for any reconstructive surgery.

Normal control of torsion strain in the lumbar spine depends upon the integrity of the facet joints. If the facet joints are surgically removed, I feel a lateral fusion is indicated to resist torsion at that level which already has a susceptible degenerated disc (Fig. 11-8). The exceptions to this rule are patients over the age of 60 in whom degenerative changes have resulted in a very stiff, functionally fused joint or in whom very little activity is anticipated postoperatively.

I have found that it is difficult to determine

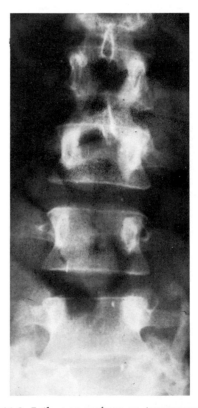

Fig. 11-8. Failure to perform an intertransverse fusion at the time of extensive posterior decompression shown in this anteroposterior roentgenogram will lead to mechanical symptoms at those interspaces that are already suseptible because of disc degeneration. These are difficult cases to salvage.

terbody fusion. We felt a successful lateral fusion would eliminate torsional strain on the abnormal intervertebral joint and thus eliminate repeated ligamentous sprains.

The patient was still in her 40s, poorly trained, on welfare, and had no motivation for rehabilitation. She refused surgery, although her history, physical findings, and roentgenograms were compatible with mechanical insufficiency, secondary to severe degenerative changes. We continue to follow her and will fuse the segment if she agrees. It is important to realize that the majority of patients on whom we are called upon to perform arthrodesis for degenerative disc disease will be asked to undergo elective reconstructive surgery. If they are not psychologically or physiologically capable of

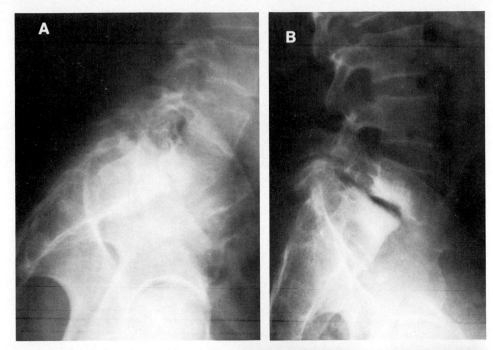

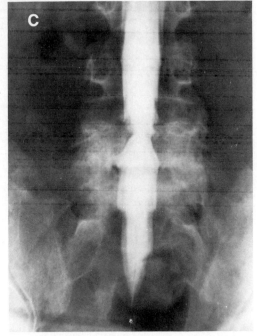

Fig. 11-9. Lateral in flexion **(A)** *and extension* **(B)** *standing roentgenograms demonstrate segmental instability secondary to spondylolisthesis and advanced disc degeneration.* **(C)** *Anteroposterior view of the myelogram shows spinal canal stenosis. A wide decompression and spinal fusion gave the patient relief.*

which degenerative joints will be stiff and which will be loose prior to surgery. We have not had much success in most patients with preoperative stress films to determine which joints are loose. We, therefore, advocate the maneuver of rocking the vertebral bodies one on another with two Kocher clamps on adjacent spinous processes at the time of surgery. If the joint is floppy and a unilateral or bilateral foraminotomy is indicated, then I perform an intertransverse lateral fusion. The patient's whose roentgenograms are presented in (Fig. 11-9) is a 63-year-old diabetic laborer who supported

Facetectomy (unilateral, bilateral)
Severe disc degeneration (gas shadow)
Positive stress films
Extension lag
Chronic mechanical low back pain
Repeat disc excision same level
Central disc prolapse L4-5
Wide disc space
Bilateral disc displacement
High demand activity (sports, laborer etc.)
Relative youth
Loose joint at surgery

Fig. 11-10. Reasons for arthrodesis of lumbar intervertebral joints for degenerative diseases.

his family of seven until a year prior to the time he sought medical help. He had severe pseudo-intermittent claudication and bilateral L5 radiculopathy. The plain x-ray films showed severe disc degeneration (gas shadow) at the L5 interspace associated with a 50% spondylolisthesis. The patient was weaned from cigarettes and pain medica-

tions and was asked to donate three units of blood over a 3-week period prior to planned surgery.

At surgery, the dura was adherent to the overlying degenerated ligamentum flavum between the L4 and L5 lamina. A portion of the inferior half of the L5 pedicles and the posterior lateral corners of the L5 vertebral bodies were removed to decompress the L5 roots on both sides. The annulus fibrosus was not compromised. Bilateral foraminotomies were necessary for complete decompression of the L5 spinal nerves. A bilateral intertransverse autograft with cortical cancellous iliac crest bone was performed. The patient had an excellent clinical result, with relief of intermittent claudication and radiculopathy and no back pain. No homologous blood was necessary. Even though this patient was over 60, we felt an

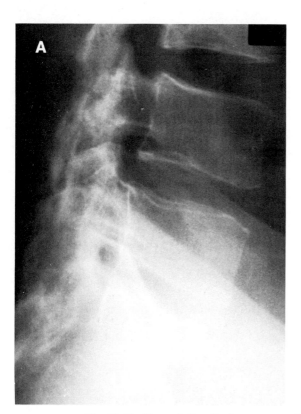 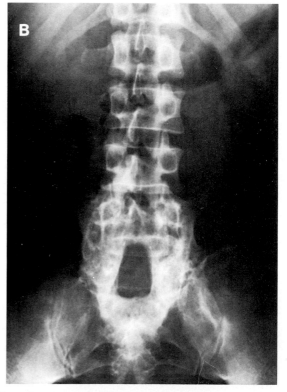

Fig. 11-11. Central disc displacement and lateral recess encroachment on L5 and S1 nerve roots bilateral in a 30-yr-old hospital orderly. Lateral (A) and AP (B) roentgenograms 4 years postoperative and 3½ years after returning to full employment shows a complete laminectomy at L5 with a solid lateral intertransverse fusion.

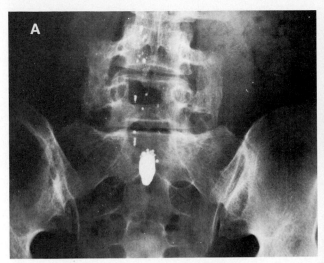

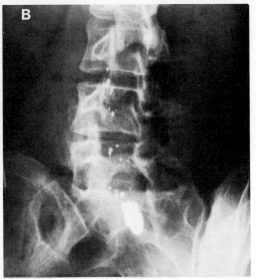

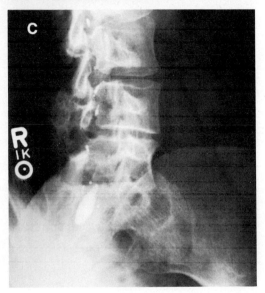

Fig. 11-12. Postoperative roentogenograms of a 30-yr-old housewife with recurrent list and mechanical low back pain for 2 years following an L4 laminotomy and disc excision. Symptoms completely cured by an intertransverse lateral fusion. Note the inferior facet of L4 on the left had previously been excised.

intertransverse fusion was necessary, because a bilateral foraminotomy was required for neural decompression at an interspace where the disc was so degenerated that a gas shadow was present. This extensive surgery in an elderly individual can be successfully performed if one prepares the patient physiologically. We feel that the demands that this patient had placed on the spine in the past and would place on his back in the future also dictated a spinal fusion.

Predicting the Necessity for Spinal Fusion

For degenerative disc disease and osteoarthritis of the intervertebral joint, we list a number of features which would make us lean towards fusion at the time of surgery (Fig. 11-10). For example, a 30-year-old hospital orderly and father of five children had been suffering attacks of low back pain for

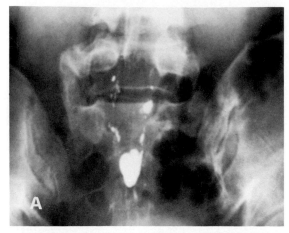

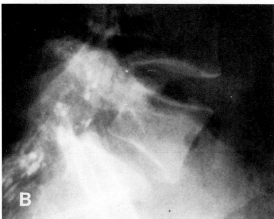

Fig. 11-13. Anteroposterior (A) and lateral (B) roentgenograms demonstrate bilateral foraminotomy and intertransverse lateral fusion successfully used to treat a young man with back pain and leg pain. He had 25% spondylolisthesis, disc prolapse, and bilateral L5 radiculopathy.

5 years. He developed acute bilateral radiculopathy in association with disc displacement at L4–5 and L5–S1. A complete laminectomy and disc excision at L4 and L5 was followed by an intertransverse lateral fusion. The roentgenograms shown in (Fig. 11-11) were taken 4 years following surgery and 3½ years following return to full duty. We predicted the necessity for spinal fusion in this patient at the time of his initial surgery, because he had six of the twelve criteria listed in Figure 11-10.

A solid intertransverse fusion at the L4–5 level completely cured the chronic mechanical back pain syndrome in this 30-year-old woman who underwent a previous laminotomy and disc excision at the L4 level (Fig. 11-12).

Spondylolisthesis

A neural arch defect with forward slipping of one vertebrae on the other, usually at the L5 level, occurs in approximately 5% of the North American population. The defect in itself does not necessarily mean the patient will have symptoms. However, the patient noted in (Fig. 11-13) was a young truck driver with an L5 radiculopathy. At the time of neural arch decompression and foraminotomy for adequate decompression of the L5 nerve root, an intertransverse lateral fusion was performed. The patient went back to lifting heavy objects and driving a large tractor trailer. He is completely asymptomatic. Although he was young, he had had a history of chronic intermittent back pain for approximately 10 years.

Occasionally, a patient under the age of 20 will develop mechanical low back pain symptoms associated with spondylolisthesis. An example (Fig. 11-14) of a patient without nerve root involvement is shown to demonstrate the efficacy of fusion alone in these cases. This young man was able to play sports in high school following the fusion.

Trauma

A list of indications for spinal fusion is given in (Fig. 11-15). Two examples are shown. The first patient (Fig. 11-16) required internal fixation and fusion because of the extent of posterior decompression. The fixation allowed for immediate mobilization and rehabilitation. The second patient (Fig. 11-17) presented with a nonunion of a fusion through the lamina, pars, and pedicle of L2 on the right. He had mechanical back pain and L2 radiculopathy. A decompression of

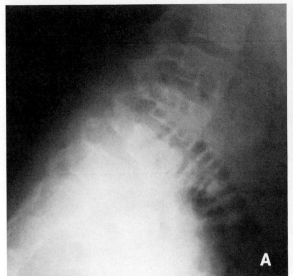

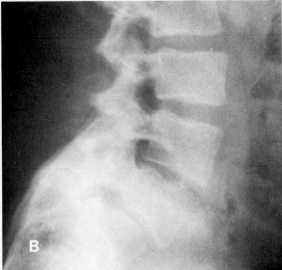

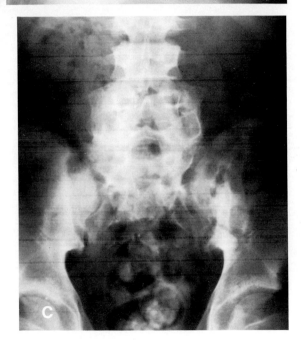

Fig. 11-14. *Lateral roentgenograms of a 14-yr-old boy standing, in flexion with 20 pounds held* **(A)**. *Note 40% spondylolisthesis compared to a lateral x-ray film without stress* **(B)**. *Lateral* **(B)** *and AP* **(C)** *roentgenograms of solid fusion 2 years postoperative. The patient had mechanical low back pain, no neurologic deficits, and a negative myelogram prior to surgery.*

the L2 and L3 nerve roots and lateral fusion alleviated his symptoms.

A prospective controlled study, using a standard surgical technique for degenerative disc disease and osteoarthritis of the intervertebral joint in the lumbar spine with and without fusion, has not been done. This study is required before spinal surgeons can

---

Unstable fracture and/or dislocation

Traumatic spondylolisthesis

Vertebral fracture involving lower lumbar discs

Surgical decompression

Fig. 11-15. *Indications for spinal fusion for trauma victims.*

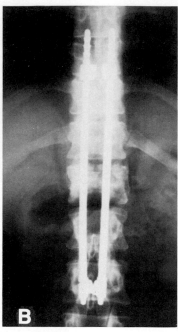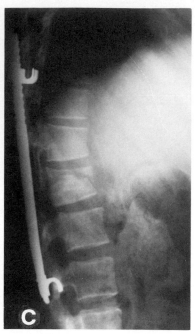

Fig. 11-16. Unstable fracture of the L1 vertebral body and posterior elements with associated paraplegia (A) managed by decompression and internal fixation with two distraction rods to allow early rehabilitation by allowing patient in chair 1 week postinjury (B and C).

make definitive statements regarding the indications for spinal fusion at the time of neural decompression. At the present state of the art, the indications for spinal fusion require experience and judgement based upon a thorough history, physical examination, and correlation of laboratory studies.

A great deal of preplanning and technical skill is required for a successful outcome in this type of elective reconstructive surgery. The aim should always be towards rehabilitation of the patient. The indications and techniques of lumbar spine fusion remain a challenge to the spinal surgeon.

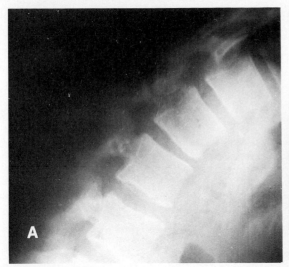

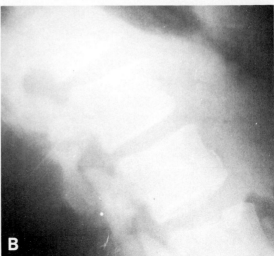

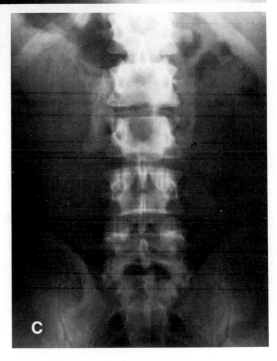

*Fig. 11-17. Nonunion of L2 neural arch fracture noted in lateral flexion (**A**) and extension (**B**) roentgenograms. The patient suffered from chronic right L2 radiculopathy and mechanical back pain for 1 year. He was successfully treated by decompression of the nerve and lateral fusion (**C**).*

The Cloward Technique 12

Ralph B. Cloward

Removal of Disc

The surgical technique for removal of ruptured lumbar intervertebral discs has changed very little since it was introduced by Mixter and Barr in 1934.[11] Protrusion of the nucleus pulposus or rupture and intraspinal herniation of fragments of the annulus fibrosus occurs most often in a posterolateral position causing unilateral nerve root compression. A unilateral operation, either a hemilaminectomy or an interlaminar approach, is employed to remove the lesion from the spinal canal.

The technique of the interlaminar operation used by most neurosurgeons (Spurling,[14] Semmes,[13] Raaf[12]) consists of a vertical midline skin incision, unilateral stripping of lumbosacral fascia and muscles, and exposure of spines and lamina on the side of the lesion. Part of the ligamentum flavum is removed, a notch is made in one or both margins of the laminae with a rongeur or Kerrison punch, and an oval opening into the spinal canal, usually about 1.0 to 1.5 cm in diameter directly over or medial to the nerve root, is created. A narrow blade is inserted, and the nerve root is forcibly retracted medially to expose the intervertebral disc. Bleeding from epidural veins in this area is often troublesome and must be controlled before the disc lesion can be visualized, located, and removed.

The technical difficulties and surgical failures encountered with this operation can be partially attributed to an inadequate exposure of the spinal canal. The small opening precludes extensive exploration above, below, and medial to the nerve root which is necessary to locate and remove multiple and elusive disc fragments. Forceful manual retraction of the nerve root is required to arrest bleeding and to visualize and remove the disc fragments. This may account for postoperative pain and neurological deficits. Yct it is not unusual to hear surgeons boast of "taking out a disc in 20 minutes without even removing any bone."

A different surgical technique is described for removal of a ruptured lumbar intervertebral disc. By making an ample interlaminar opening into the spinal canal, the problems of exposure of the lesion, control of hemorrhage, and damage to the nerve roots are mostly eliminated and actual overall operative time is reduced. This technique has been used by the author for over 36 years.[2]

The operation utilizes a transverse skin incision and a wide bilateral stripping and retraction of fascia and muscles. The ligamentum flavum is not removed, but detached and reflected medially in a flap. Bone is removed only from the margins of the lamina and the articular facets. A complete laminectomy is never done except for spondylolisthesis, when the separate neural arch is disarticulated and removed.[7] Using a "vertebra spreader," an interlaminar exposure is developed two to

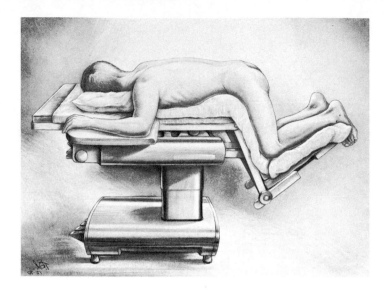

Fig. 12-1. Position on operating table. Pad under iliac crests. Abdomen free.

three times larger than that obtained by the "standard" technique. The advantages are obvious.

Operative Technique

Position and Anesthesia

The patient is placed in the kneeling position over the lower end of the operating table. A vertically placed sponge rubber roll beneath each ilium prevents pressure on the abdomen (Fig. 12-1). General endotracheal anesthesia is used. After antiseptic preparation of the skin, ½% Marcaine with adrenalin and Wydase* is infiltrated intracutaneously in the line of the incision; 50 cc of this solution injected bilaterally into the paravertebral lumbar muscles will prevent muscle bleeding and diminish postoperative pain.

Skin Incision

An 8-cm transverse skin incision is made over the lesion (Fig. 12-2). Bleeding from skin is arrested by fixing a towel to the skin with multiple small towel clips or skin clips placed 1 cm apart. Skin bleeders are never cauterized. The skin and subcutaneous fat is undermined and retracted vertically with an Adson retractor (Fig. 12-3).

*Trademark of Wyeth Co.

Fascia and Muscles

A midline incision of the desired length is made with a scalpel through lumbosacral fascia and muscle attachments to the tip of the spinous processes. Using two large, sharp periosteal elevators, the muscles are stripped subperiosteally laterally beyond the capsule of the articular facets. The blades of the self-retaining laminectomy retractor are inserted on each side. The new retractor handle with a ratchet opening is attached and spread, giving a wide bilateral exposure of the entire lamina (Fig. 12-4). About 1 cm of the adjacent margins of the spinous processes and the interspinous ligament is removed with a rongeur, and the raw bone surfaces are waxed.

Ligamentum Flavum and Laminae

On the side of the lesion a narrow, full curved sharp periosteal elevator is worked deep beneath the upper laminae to release the attachments of the ligamentum flavum from its lower margin and anterior surface (Fig. 12-5). Using a chisel 6 mm wide, the lower one-third of this lamina (about ½ to 1 cm) is removed from the base of the spinous process laterally to include the lower one-third of the superior articular facet (Fig. 12-6). A slightly curved osteotome is used to remove the anterior half of this lamina, that is, the surface of the lamina facing the spinal

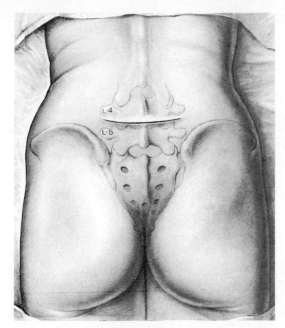

Fig. 12-2. Transverse skin incision.

sufficient to permit insertion of the tips of the new vertebra spreader beneath the margins of the lamina. By turning the thumb screw of the spreader, the physician widens the interlaminar opening, putting the ligamentum flavum on a stretch. The upper fibers of the ligament still attached to the lamina are carefully divided with a No. 11 scalpel blade as far lateral as possible (Fig. 12-7). Then the ligament attachments to the lower lamina are cut, being careful not to puncture or incise the dura or epidural veins which lie immediately beneath (Fig. 12-8). A small, grooved director or a patty beneath the ligament may be used here. The incision is continued laterally along the laminar edge and then superiorly along the medial margin of the inferior facet until it meets the lateral cut of the upper incision. A heavy silk retention suture is passed through the lateral edge of the ligament, and the flap of ligament is reflected medially and secured to the laminectomy retractor on the opposite side (Fig. 12-9). One cm of the margin of the lower lamina is removed with the narrow chisel from the base of the spinous process to the facet. This bone is usually thin compared to the upper lamina, so chiseling is done carefully and with a prying action, and the bone is removed with a heavy disc

canal. This is chiseled off to the upper pedicle and laterally as far as possible. The AP diameter of the spinal canal is thus enlarged, permitting greater exposure and visualization of the upper nerve root. The bone edges are waxed. On the opposite side of the spine, the ligament is partially detached from each laminar margin with the narrow elevator,

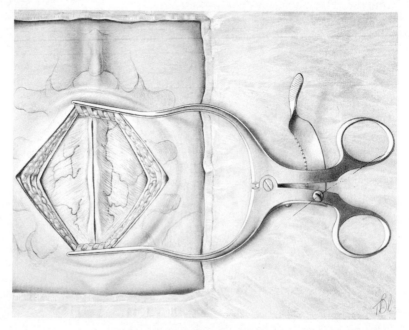

Fig. 12-3. Midline incision lumbosacral fascia.

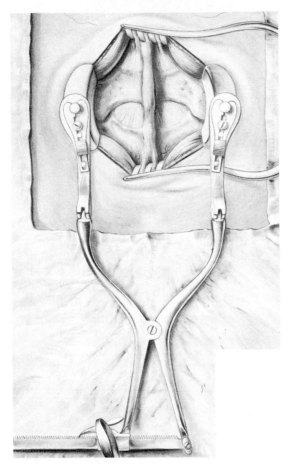

Fig. 12-4. Cloward lumbar lamina retractor.

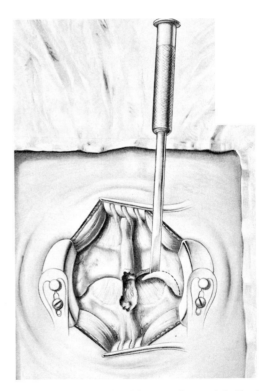

Fig. 12-5. Cloward sharp periosteal elevator, curved (8″).

Fig. 12-6. Removal of lower edge and half of lower facet.

rongeur. The chisel is next placed in a vertical position about 3 mm lateral to the medial margin of the lower facet cutting this overhanging edge (Fig. 12-10). A second vertical cut is made in the facet parallel and lateral to the first, then a third lateral to it. If the facet is unusually large, each cut is 3 mm wide. The lateral bone slices are first removed by grasping with a disc rongeur. On removing the medial margin, bleeding may occur from the epidural veins. This is arrested with Gelfoam* and thrombin. Bone bleeding is waxed.

Removal of the medial half of the inferior facet will expose 1 cm or more of the spinal canal lateral to the nerve root. This area is full of epidural fat and veins. These are separated from the lateral margin of the nerve root and dural sac, and the latter is

* Trademark of Upjohn

gently retracted medially with a flexible retractor blade held manually or by a self-retaining retractor.[1] The veins and fat are grasped with tissue forceps and obliterated with the electrocoagulator, using the cutting current at a low setting (Fig. 12-11). A broad self-retaining retractor blade with a "shoe" tip is placed under the nerve root and dural

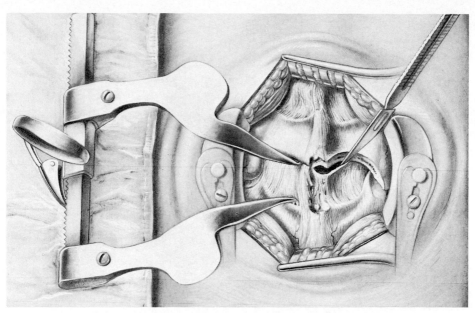

Fig. 12-7. Cloward lumbar lamina spreader.

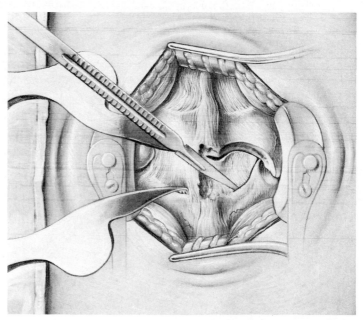

Fig. 12-8. Fibers of ligamentum flavum are carefully divided with a No. 11 scalpel blade as far lateral as possible.

sac, gently retracted to the midline, and secured in this position to the clamp on the laminectomy retractor (Fig. 12-12). This eliminates strong manual retraction of the nerve root and possible trauma to it, yet gives a wide exposure of the spinal canal. All vessels lateral and anterior to the dura are methodically cauterized under direct vision with little or not blood loss. The charred tissue is clipped with scissors and removed with a disc rongeur. Venous bleeding under the upper lamina beyond the surgeon's vision is "packed off" with Gelfoam and thrombin and a string-patty. Bone bleeding from the posterior surface of the vertebral body is burned with the cutting current. With the anterior wall of the spinal canal completely dry and widely exposed, the op-

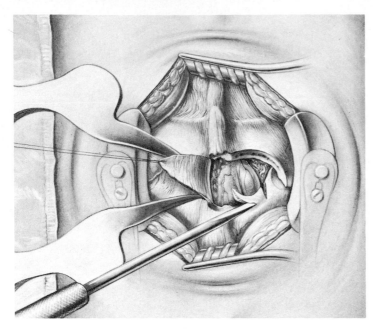

Fig. 12-9. Removal of edge of lower lamina.

erative attack on the intervertebral disc is more easily and effectively accomplished.

Disc Removal

From this point on, the surgical treatment of the disc lesion will differ with the surgeon's discretion. Three operative procedures used are as follows: (a) only the mass of disc which protrudes or has sequestrated in the spinal canal is removed (Fig. 12-13); (b) the posterior fibers of the annulus fibrosus are incised and the interior of the disc is curreted, usually removing remnants of the nucleus pulposus and any loose fragments of the annulus; or (c) an interbody fusion is

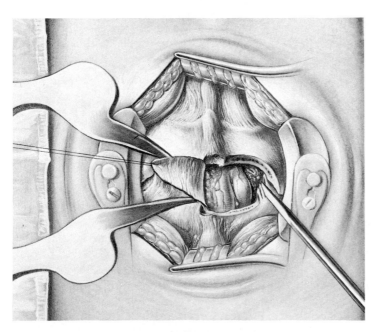

Fig. 12-10. Removal of medial ⅔ of upper facet.

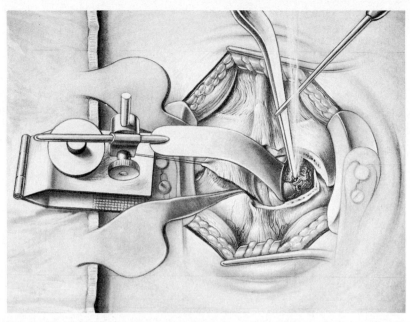

Fig. 12-11. (Left) Cloward nerve root retractor, self-retaining with two malleable blades, 5/16 in and ½ in wide (blade length 4"; blade and shaft length 8¼"). This instrument can be attached to any laminectomy retractor. The blade is engaged beneath the nerve root, retracted medially to the desired position, and held in place by the turn of the wheel. (Center) Cloward flexible nerve root retractor (8½"). (Right) D'Errico dressing forceps, bayonet shape (8¾").

done by removing the entire disc, including the cartilage plates and the cortex of the adjacent vertebral bodies and inserting four large blocks of bone into the intervertebral space. The latter technique is used by the author. (See Posterior Lumbar Interbody Fusion, this chapter.) Interrupted No. 0 synthetic absorbable sutures (Vicryl or Dexon)* are used to close the lumbar muscles and fascia and No. 00 in the subcutaneous layer. This skin is closed with Steri-tapes*. A Jackson-Pratt drain is always used.

Discussion

The reasons for radical departure in operative technique from that almost universally used requires further explanation.

*Trademarks.

Transverse Skin Incision

This was first used by the author in the late, 1940s for lumbar disc surgery, when bone from the interbody fusion was removed from the patient's ilium.[2] Both operations were done through a single transverse incision. A wider lateral exposure is made possible with a transverse skin incision. When the incision is made parallel to the normal skin lines, it heals better with less scar.

Ligamentum Flavum

Almost all "disc" surgeons remove this ligament. The defect resulting from its removal fills with dense scar tissue which may encompass and possibly compress the dural sac and nerve roots. If the entire ligament is preserved by separating its attachments from the lamina and reflecting it in a flap, a larger opening into the spinal canal is obtained and

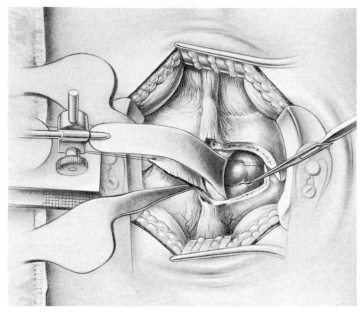

Fig. 12-12. Posterior disc fibers cut with #11 blade scalpel.

the replaced flap protects the dura and prevents scarring (Fig. 12-14).

Use of Chisel and Hammer

Spinal rongeurs, including the Leksell and the Kerrison, have been the standard instruments used by neurosurgeons for laminec-

tomy or laminotomy. The operative technique described here recommends the use of narrow, sharp chisels and hammer. The rongeurs may be used to remove part of the laminar edge, but the hard bone of the facet must be removed with a chisel or air drill. When the surgeon becomes accustomed to the use of the hammer and chisel technique

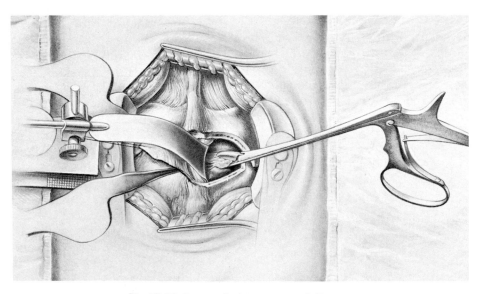

Fig. 12-13. Removal of sequestrated disc.

to contour the interlaminar exposure as well as the bed for the intervertebral grafts for interbody fusion, he will find that it can be more effective than using rongeurs or other instruments.

Articular Facets

It is the recommendation of most orthopedic surgeons to leave the articular facets of the lumbar spine intact in lumbar disc surgery. Removal of all or any part of these vertebral elements is not advised for two reasons: (a) they are considered major elements in the articulation of the vertebral joint; and (b) they must be preserved as an essential bony surface to be used in posterior spinal fusion operations (Hibbs, Albee). The reluctance to remove a part of the articular facets is one reason for failure to obtain an adequate lateral exposure in the spinal canal for effective surgery. In the author's experience, the advantages from removing a part of the articular facets far outweigh the disadvantages.

Disc Removal

Once the ruptured and symptomatic lumbar disc is diagnosed and exposed at operation, its removal may be "simple" or "radical." Either the intraspinal mass is simply removed (Fig. 12-10) or, in addition, the intervertebral space is opened and a portion of its contents evacuated. The reasons given to justify the latter procedure are based on a false assumption that the persistent low back pain which frequently follows the simple disc removal is caused by disc substance remaining in the intervertebral space. Patients are often subjected to repeat operations for removal of "more of the disc." The same theory is used to explain the recent use of proteolytic enzymes to "remove the disc" chemically.[9]

The author's experience has shown that the persistent disabling pain following rupture and loss of the supporting function of the intervertebral disc is caused by move-

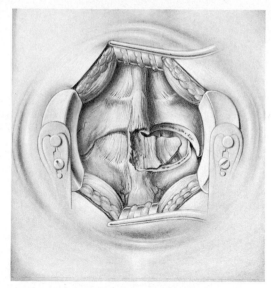

Fig. 12-14. The replaced flap of ligamentum flavum protects the dura and prevents scarring.

ment of the abnormal painful joint, as well as from retained disc substance.[7] This pain can most effectively be cured by total disc removal followed by interbody fusion. This arrests joint movement and relieves the back pain.

Postoperative Cortisone

Intrathecal cortisone was used after lumbar disc operations for 13 years. When the medication Meticortelone was discontinued by the manufacturers, I changed to intramuscular steroids (Decadron) for the first 3 days postoperative. This aids in relieving post operative pain and temperature. Whether it prevents the formation of postoperative adhesions is questionable.

Posterior Lumbar Interbody Fusion (PLIF)

In the treatment of lesions of the lumbar intervertebral disc, the question of whether the patient should or should not be treated by a spinal fusion operation always arises.

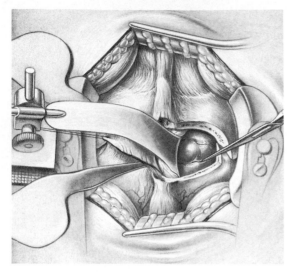

Fig. 12-15. A No. 11 blade is used to cut out the posterior half of the disc.

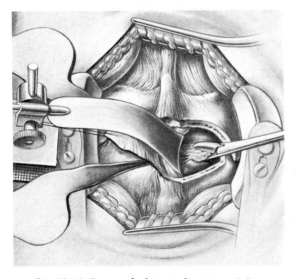

Fig. 12-16. Removal of incised portion of disc.

There is no unanimity of thought among neurosurgeons and orthopedic surgeons, and one of the founding fathers of lumbar disc surgery, when asked this question, replied: "If an operative procedure can be devised which will give satisfactory fusion as well as satisfactory removal and without lengthening the convalescent period, then I will concur with the idea of a fusion as part of the original operation."[8] These criteria laid down by Dr. Mixter are fully met by the operation of posterior lumbar interbody fusion.

This operation was originated by the author and has been used for 36 years in the treatment of over 2000 patients with lumbar disc disease.[2,5,11] A complete cure rate of approximately 96% has been accomplished. The operative technique of PLIF is not difficult for the average disc surgeon to learn. However, there are three necessary prerequisites for the success of this operation.

1. The surgeon must be motivated to spend the necessary time at the operating table to properly perform and complete the operation.

2. The surgeon must have available and be properly trained to use the special instruments designed for and required to do this operation.

3. The surgeon should have a bone bank with adequate supply of good quality bone to use as bone grafts.[6]

If these criteria are met, most lumbar disc operations will be gratifyingly successful.

Disc Removal

Exposure of the anterior wall of the spinal canal and the posterior surface of the intervertebral disc by an interlaminar approach has been described. Special instruments are used to prepare a wide exposure of spinal canal, both to retract the nerve root and dural sac and to eradicate epidural vessels in preparation for removal of the disc.

A long scalpel handle with No. 11 Bard Parker blade is used to cut out the posterior half of the disc. A vertical incision is made in the disc in the midline beneath the retracted dura and nerve root. Then horizontal incisions are made following the margins of the adjacent vertebral bodies, extending as far lateral as possible, usually beyond the pedicle of the lower vertebra (Fig. 12-15). The incised disc is withdrawn with a large disc rongeur, giving an opening into the

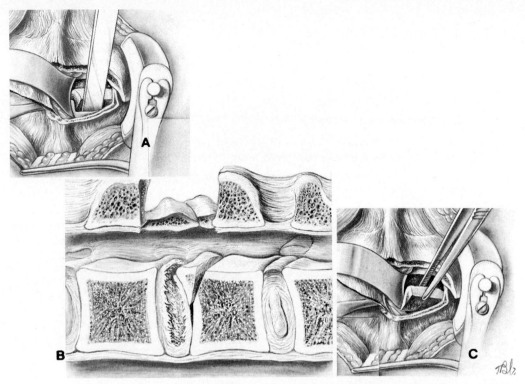

Fig. 12-17. Removal of bony ledge of posterior superior margin at the lower vertebral body.

intervertebral space through which the remainder of the disc is removed (Fig. 12-16).

The bony ledge or "shelf" of the posterior superior margin of the lower vertebral body which overhangs the interspace is removed (Fig. 12-17). This bone margin is first cut vertically in the midline beneath the dural sac with a 7 mm osteotome (Fig. 12-18A). Then the second cut is made as far lateral as possible, usually into the base of the pedicle (Fig. 12-18B). A wide osteotome (10 mm) connects these two cuts with a transverse one about 3 to 5 mm behind the margin of the vertebra (Fig. 12-17A). The osteotome is hammered straight down, passing through bone and cartilage and into the intervertebral space (Fig. 12-17B). Removal of this wedge of bone gives a wide opening into the interspace (Fig. 12-17C). A strip of Gelfoam soaked in thrombin is packed over the bleeding surface of the vertebral body. This im-

mediately arrests bone bleeding which may be brisk. The cartilaginous plate remaining on this vertebral body and on the entire plate of the upper one is stripped free with a long curved thin osteotome used as a manual elevator. Half of the interspace is thus cleaned of all soft tissue down to the anterior longitudinal ligament using a large disc rongeur, an English rongeur, and a ring currette.

The cortical surfaces of the vertebral bodies are methodically removed using an 8 mm curved or straight osteotome and hammer (Fig. 12-19A). The cartilage plates may be removed with the bone. Repeated curls are made using a prying action until the vertebral bodies are completely decorticated (Fig. 12-19B). The cortex removal is extended medially beneath the dural sac and laterally to or beyond the vertebral pedicle. This will prepare a wide space for larger and more bone grafts.

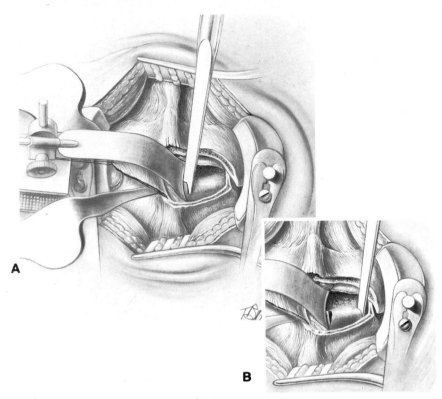

Fig. 12-18. Medial and lateral vertical cuts into bony ledge of posterior superior margin of the lower vertebral body.

Bone Grafts

If bone is to be obtained from the patient, it is advisable to remove the grafts the day before the spinal fusion. The best donor site is the left posterior ilium. With the patient in the prone position, a transverse skin incision is made parallel to and below the iliac crest from the posterior superior iliac spine to the cluneal nerves. These large sensory enrves, which cross the ilium from above downward about 6 to 8 cm lateral to the midline, should be carefully dissected out and protected from injury to prevent painful postoperative neuromata from developing at the donor site.

The gluteal muscles are stripped subperiosteally from the posterior surface of the ilium and retracted, using one long and one short self-retaining retractor blade. With a wide, thin-blade, straight osteotome, five parallel vertical cuts are made about 1½ cm apart, starting at the iliac crest and driving downward approximately 3 cm (Fig. 12-20A). These cuts are connected at their base by a transverse cut made with a wide-curved osteotome driven inward to the inner table of the ilium. The three medial bone plugs thus outlined are removed by chiseling from above downward with a wide-curved osteotome, getting as thick a graft as possible, but leaving the inner table of the ilium intact (Fig. 12-20B). The fourth graft, most lateral, is removed, full thickness of the ilium. Thus, three grafts will have cortex on one side and one will have double cortex. The raw exposed bony surface of the ilium is covered with bone wax to arrest all bleeding. The wound is closed in layers with a rubber tissue drain in place. The bone grafts are placed in a sterile jar containing streptomycin solution, sealed, and kept in a deep freeze until used.

The bone grafts preferred for this operation are obtained from the bone bank.[1,2]

These grafts or "plugs" were previously

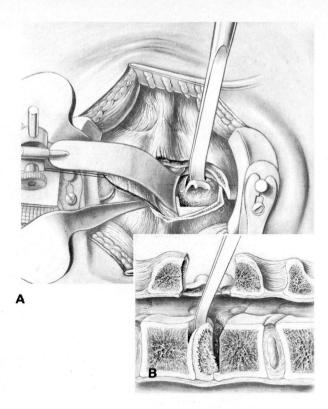

Fig. 12-19. Removal of cortical surfaces of the vertebral bodies.

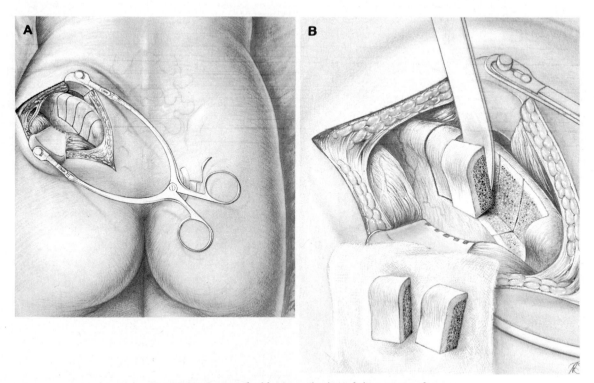

Fig. 12-20. Removal of bone grafts from left posterior ilium.

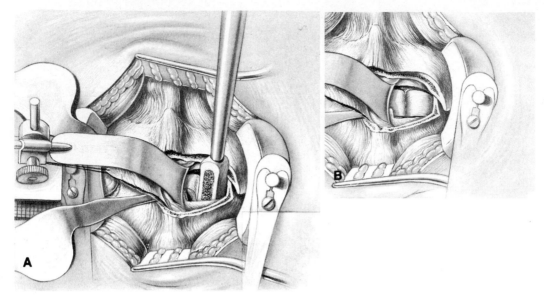

Fig. 12-21. Impacting second "plug" into interspace.

prepared from the ilium of a fresh cadaver removed under sterile conditions, cultured, and preserved by freezing. This bone bank method has been recently replaced with a new technique. Under unsterile conditions the iliac bones are removed from the cadaver and cut into various size grafts with an amputation saw. After soaking the grafts in tap water or a weak solution of hydrogen peroxide, all soft tissue elements including blood, fat, marrow, and so on, are completely removed by thorough washing with a jet stream of tap water. The grafts are then dried, double packaged in appropriate paper, and sterilized, with other hospital equipment, in the ehtylene oxide gas chamber. After adequate aeration, the packages of bone are stored at room temperature. The sterile grafts are received at the operating table, washed, and placed in a solution of neomycin until used.

BONE GRAFTING

A gauge is dropped into the prepared intervertebral space to measure its depth. A vertebra spanner, of various widths, is used to measure the vertical diameter of the disc space. Using these two measurements, the bone graft is trimmed with the air drill and ronguer to the exact width and 3 mm shorter than the measured depth, so the grafts can be recessed below the anterior wall of the spinal canal. Several turns are made on the thumb screw of the interlaminar spreader to widen the intervertebral space for insertion of the large bone graft. The graft is grasped with a tooth forceps, and its lower end is inserted into the center of the prepared disc space. Bone graft impactors are available in various sizes and shapes depending on the contour and the consistency of bone on the upper end of the bone graft. If the graft has cortex on the end, an oval or round impactor with a sharp pin is used (Fig. 12-21A). This prevents it from slipping as the graft is driven into the interspace. If the graft has no cortex on its upper end, the impactor with a broad base and lip is used to prevent the graft from breaking or crumbling with hard pounding (Fig. 12-22A). An attempt is made to drive the bone graft in a perpendicular direction so that its cancellous surface will be parallel to the vertical walls of the interspace (Fig. 12-22B). If the thickness of the bone graft is much less than the width of the prepared hemi-interspace, a "puka" chisel may be placed on one or both sides of the graft for

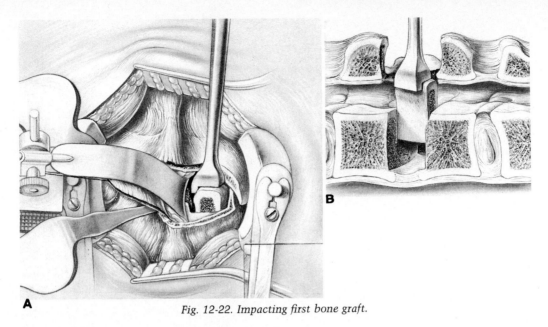

Fig. 12-22. *Impacting first bone graft.*

vertical support to prevent the graft from twisting or rotating.

The next step is to move the first bone graft medially to enlarge the opening lateral to it for insertion of the second or third graft. This is accomplished by using the two puka chisels. These instruments have heavy, flat, dull blades with holes perforating the handle. They are inserted or driven vertically into the interspace lateral to the bone graft. The T-shaped handle is inserted into a hole of the medial chisel to create a prying, twisting action against the lateral chisel. This will "walk" the bone graft toward the midline (Fig. 12-23).

The second plug is trimmed to fit the opening, prepared, and impacted into the interspace (Fig. 12-21B). If this graft does not fill the space, the puka chisels are again used to crowd this graft medially and prepare a space for a third graft. Bleeding from epidural veins may result from jarring the spine when the grafts are impacted. This is arrested with Gelfoam and packing. Bleeding from the cancellous bone of the vertebral bodies is arrested by the compression force of the bone grafts. The bone margin of the vertebral bodies not covered by the bone graft is waxed.

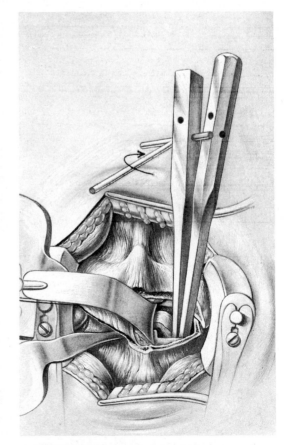

Fig. 12-23. *Use of the two "puka" chisels to move the first bone graft medially.*

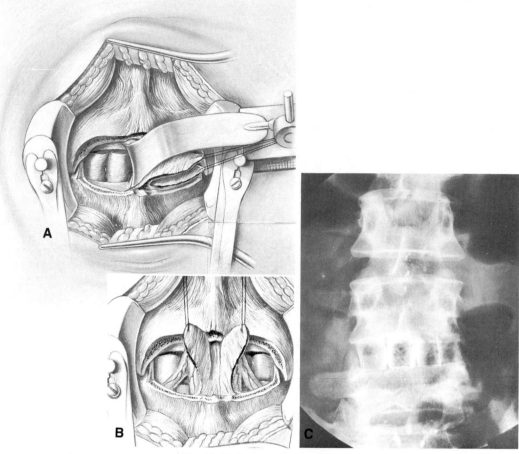

Fig. 12-24. Bone grafts in place.

The self-retaining retractor blade is removed from the nerve root and dural sac, and these structures are permitted to return to their normal position. The space lateral to the nerve root is filled with a large strip of Gelfoam, and the flap of ligamentum flavum is replaced over the dura and nerve root. This half of the wound is then packed off with a gauze sponge.

On the opposite side of the spine, a similar operative procedure is carried out. The vertebra spreader is not required to increase the width of the intervertebral space, since this has been accomplished by the inserted bone grafts. However, the spreader may be used to widen the interlaminar space. The inter-vertebral space on this side is prepared in the same manner, removing disc, cartilage, and cortical end-plates. The first bone graft is moved forcibly toward the midline until it is in close proximity to the medial graft inserted from the other side (Fig. 12-24A). After the final graft is impacted, the instruments and all sponges and Gelfoam are removed from the spinal canal (Fig. 12-24B).

The two flaps of ligamentum flavum are elevated, and the nerve roots and dural sac are gently compressed to the midline with a bayonet forcep to allow inspection of the entire grafted area (Fig. 12-25). This is done to assure that all grafts are equally recessed

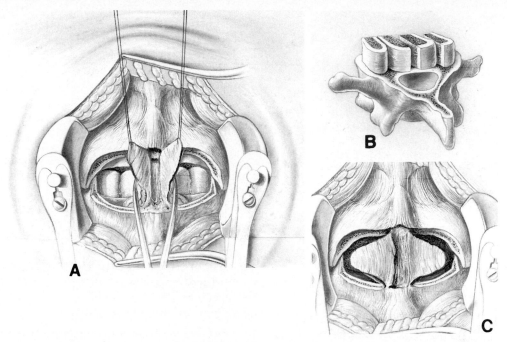

Fig. 12-25. **(A)** *Inspection of grafts.* **(B)** *Bone grafts in place.* **(C)** *Flaps of the ligamentum flavum are replaced over dural sac and nerve roots.*

and that there is ample space between the anterior surface of the nerve roots and dural sac and bone grafts.

Wound Closure

Flaps of the ligamentum flavum are replaced over the dural sac and nerve roots (Fig. 12-25C). The open space lateral to the roots is filled with a strip of thrombin-soaked Gelfoam. A long strip of gauze is packed over the lamina and interlaminar space and the blades of the self-retaining laminectomy retractor are removed. An Addison retractor is placed in the lumbar fascia and retracted.

The large paravertebral muscles which bulge into the field are closed with No. 0 Vicryl or Dexon sutures, using a large full curved cutting needle which is passed around the muscle belly on each side (Fig. 12-26). The deep gauze sponge is removed and a wide (10 mm) Jackson-Pratt drain is placed transversely to reach both sides of the interlaminar exposure. The muscle sutures are tied loosely to approximate this layer. The lumbosacral fascia is closed tightly with No. 0 interrupted Vicryl sutures. The round tube of the Jackson-Pratt drain exits through the upper end of the fascia incision and is sutured snugly. A small stab wound is made 3 to 4 cm above the transverse skin incision, a curved hemostat thrust through the subcutaneous tissue, and the tube grabbed and pulled through the small incision. The suction-reservoir bulb of the Jackson-Pratt drain is attached. The subcutaneous layer is sutured with a No. 00 or No. 000 Vicryl suture. The stitch is placed as close as possible to the under side of the dermis and inverted with a knot down, giving an excellent skin closure. No needles are passed through the skin. Steritapes close the skin line. A thin gauze dressing is applied over the wound and the drain sealed with 3M tape.

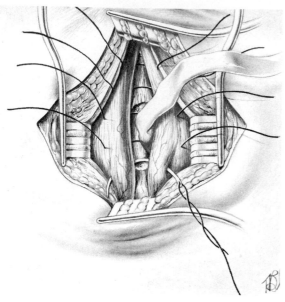

Fig. 12-26. Closure with Jackson-Pratt drain inserted down to the lamina before the muscle sutures are tied.

Postoperative Care

The patient is placed supine in bed, taken to recovery, and before he recovers from the anesthetic, his bladder is emptied by a single catheterization. This practice has eliminated the need for further catheterization. The patient receives intramuscular steroid drugs (Decadron 4mm) for the first 3 postoperative days, decreasing the dosage interval daily from 4, to 6, to 8 hours. Morphine is administered for pain, but it is not frequently required. The Jackson-Pratt drain is permitted to aspirate blood and serum from the wound until less than 10 cc is obtained in an 8-hour period. This usually requires 2 to 3 days. The patient is permitted to sit on the side of the bed or stand to void the same day of his operation. The following day he may walk to the toilet and ambulate as desired thereafter. With this regimen, hospitalization has been reduced to 5 to 7 days. Postoperative roentgenograms of the lumbosacral spine are obtained prior to discharge (Fig. 12-24C). No corsets, braces, belts or casts are used. The patient is encouraged to bend and stretch his back muscles after the

10th post operative day. By gradually increasing the exercises, the patient is assured a flexible painless back when healing is complete. Follow-up roentgenograms will demonstrate fusion of the bone grafts in 3 to 5 months (Fig. 12-27).

Discussion

Fusion of the vertebral bodies by the posterior approach through the spinal canal (PLIF) is a superior method of fusion for the lumbar spine. It has many advantages over other types of spinal fusion currently in use either by the anterior or posterior approach.

1. PLIF permits visualization and removal of disc fragments protruding into or invading the spinal canal, causing compression of the nerve root or the cauda equina.

2. Posterior marginal osteophytes and displaced or enlarged facets of spinal stenosis are completely removed. These are frequently associated with nerve root compression and adhesions.

3. Ankylosis of the vertebra is more rapid than other types of spinal fusion.

a. The bone grafts are placed at right angles to the weight-bearing axis of the spine.

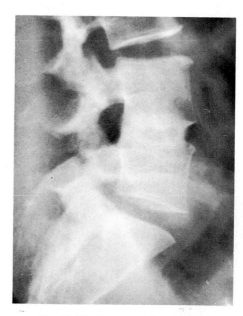

Fig. 12-27. Post operative x-ray.

b. The vertebral joint is mechanically fixed at operation, eliminating the need for external support or braces.

c. Compression of the bone grafts against the raw surface of the vertebral bodies is conducive to early vascularization and rapid fusion.

4. Morbidity of the operation is lower, and limited exposure of the spine preserves muscle and ligament attachments. Steroid drugs, Marcaine, and the Jackson-Pratt drain permit a temperature-free and more painless postoperative course.

5. Recovery is rapid. The patient walks on the first or second postoperative day and leaves the hospital in less than a week.

6. The percentage of complete cures without disability is higher owing to the following factors:

a. Infrequency of nerve root and cauda equina scarring, which may cause persistent postoperative pain;

b. Minimal stiffness of lumbar muscles due to fibrosis and shortening which frequently follows long periods of immobilization;

c. Low rate of pseudoarthrosis (less than 5%)

References

1. Cloward RB: Creation and operation of a bone bank. J Neurosurg 23:682–688, 1970

2. Cloward RB: The degenerated lumbar discs. Treatment by vertebral body fusion. J of ICS 22:375–386, Oct 1954

3. Cloward RB: Gas sterilized cadaver bone grafts for spine fusion operations. A simplified bone bank. Spine 5:4–10, 1980

4. Cloward RB: The Jackson-Pratt drain in anterior cervical spinal operations. Surg Neurol 7:205–208, 1977

5. Cloward RB: Lesions of the intervertebral discs and their treatment by interbody fusion methods. (The painful disc) Clin Orthop 27:51–77, 1963

6. Cloward RB: A self-retaining spinal dura retractor. J Neurosurg 9:230–232, 1952

7. Cloward RB: The treatment of ruptured lumbar intervertebral discs by vertebral body fusion. I. Indications, operative techniques and after care. J Neurosurg 10:154–165, 1953

8. Cloward RB: Vertebral body fusion for ruptured lumbar discs. Roentgenographic study. Ann Surg 90:969–976, 1955

9. Flor LT: Clinical use of chymopapain in lumbar and dorsal disc lesion. An end-result study. Clin Orthop 67:81–87, Nov-Dec 1969

10. Mixter WJ: Symposium on intervertebral discs and sciatic pain. (Discussion) J Bone Joint Surg 29:468, 1947

11. Mixter WJ, Barr JS: Rupture of the intervertebral disk with involvement of the spinal canal. New Eng J Med 211:210, 1934

12. Raaf J: Removal of protruded lumbar intervertebral discs. J Neurosurg 32:604, 1970

13. Semmes RE: Ruptured lumbar intervertebral discs: Their recognition and surgical relief. Clin Neurosurg 8:78–92, 1960

14. Spurling RG: Lesions of the lumbar intervertebral disc. Charles C Thomas, Springfield, Ill. 95–99, 1953

Analgesic blocks using a combination of local anesthetic and corticosteroids are often helpful in managing the patient with severe low back and sciatic pain. Fifteen years ago the subarachnoid instillation of corticosteroids was commonly used as a method of treating low back and sciatic pain. If a patient with a lumbar disc syndrome had a normal myelogram, 40 or 80 ml of methyl prednisolone acetate suspension was often introduced into the subarachnoid space prior to withdrawal of the lumbar puncture needle used for the myelogram. This often resulted in a remission of symptoms for a variable, sometimes quite prolonged, duration. In the past 10 years, we have become increasingly aware of the possible occurrence of adhesive arachnoiditis many years after subarachnoid instillation of almost any substance including local anesthetics, pantopaque, and corticosteroids. To avoid such an undesired inflammatory reaction of the delicate pia and arachnoid membranes, epidural injections were advocated with the presumption that the dura would provide an adequate natural barrier to the instilled medicines. The lumbar epidural block and the caudal block are both epidural injections.

Mechanism of Effect

The exact mechanism of action of epidural corticosteroids is uncertain. It is presumed that the potent anti-inflammatory effect may modify the reaction to either pressure or tension of various neural elements within the spine. The patients who are most likely to benefit from these injections are those who manifest a significant degree of radicular pain, while patients with primarily low back pain seem to have minimal or no improvement in their symptoms. This might imply that nerve root edema and inflammation, secondary to the pressure or tension of a disc protrusion or bony spur, may be reduced by corticosteroids. The duration of effect may be related to the nerve root tension to edema ratio. If the predominant element is tension with minimal root edema, a short-term benefit can be anticipated. If root inflammation edema is predominant, a prolonged beneficial effect may occur.

PATIENT SELECTION

1. Lumbar disc syndrome and a normal myelogram.
2. Lumbar disc syndrome with medical contraindication to surgery.
3. Patient with low back and radicular pain with multiple myelographic defects and the absence of hard neurological signs implicating a specific nerve root.
4. Diagnostic problem with lower extremity discomfort which may be due to nerve root irritation, hip dysfunction, or vascular

415

disease. A lack of response to an epidural block in the face of such an uncertain situation may indicate that the non-spine entities deserve further consideration.

Lumbar Epidural Block

The lumbar epidural block, a form of peripheral nerve block, is accomplished by introducing the anesthetic agent into the peridural or the epidural space. Although the anesthetic drug is deposited into the extradural space, the site of drug action is more peripheral, since in most instances the drug solution must spread out into the intervertebral foramina before the spinal nerve sheath is sufficiently permeated.

SITE OF INJECTION

When this technique is used for patients who have never previously had surgery, the injection is carried out in the low lumbar region as close as possible to the site of suspected dysfunction. However, many of these blocks are performed on patients who have had previous low back surgery and continue to manifest symptoms. With these patients it is well to carry out the block away from the site of the original incision for two reasons.

1. If the needle is inserted into the dense scar, it will not be possible to recognize the various tissue levels which the bevel of the needle is penetrating. This may lead to an inadvertent puncture of the dura.

2. Because the dura is usually quite adherent to the overlying laminae following surgery, an adequate epidural space is eradicated, making it impossible to carry out an injection successfully at that site. Since most lumbar laminectomy scars extend over the sacrum, the postoperative peridural injection is best performed at either the L1–2 or L2–3 levels.

POSITION

The lateral recumbent position is preferred (Fig. 13-1). When performing a lumbar puncture the sitting position is advantageous because it creates increased hydrostatic pressure within the caudal sac, making it easier for the spinal needle to penetrate the distended dura and arachnoid cleanly. Since our objectives here, however, are to avoid penetrating the dura and to place the bevel of the needle in the extradural space, it is advantageous to have as little distention of the caudal sac as possible. For this reason the lateral recumbent position is advantageous. Since the injected medication will

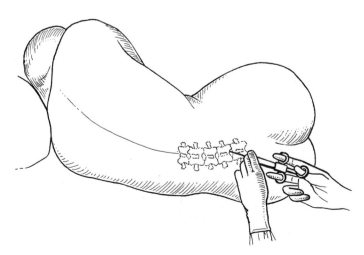

Fig. 13-1. Technique for introducing needle into epidural space.

spread to some extent on the basis of gravity flow, the patient is instructed to lie on the painful side so that the involved nerve roots will be lowermost and be affected by the medication to the greatest extent. It is important that the patient be well flexed with the thighs upon the abdomen, because it is felt that flexion increases the "negative pressure" within the peridural space and allows easier identification when the needle bevel reaches this level.

TECHNIQUE

A 25-gauge hypodermic needle is used to make a local anesthesia wheal over the desired interspace, and a 20-gauge, short, beveled spinal needle is introduced between the spinous processes. After penetrating the interspinous ligament, the stylet is removed and the needle connected to a 10-cc, "three-ringed" syringe that is half filled with air. Using gentle pressure on the plunger of the syringe, the needle is slowly advanced toward the extradural space (Fig. 13-2). The entrance of the bevel of the needle into this space is signaled by a sudden absence of any resistance to injection of the air; as a result, the syringe is usually emptied into the peridural space. This air injection often causes discomfort or paresthesia in the low back.

It is necessary to observe the hub of the needle carefully for a minute or two to be sure that no CSF drainage is present as a result of partial penetration of the dura. Gentle aspiration of the needle is now attempted, with great care being taken not to dislodge or move the needle in any way. If spinal fluid is obtained, the block is terminated, since dural puncture is a contraindication to epidural block. If blood is aspirated, the stylet is reinserted, and after a 3- to 5-minute wait for coagulation to occur, aspiration is reattempted. If the second aspiration is negative, the block may be done, but at frequent intervals aspiration with the injecting syringe is carried out. After the satisfactory position of the needle has been established, 6 cc of 1% Xylocaine, specifically prepared for spinal anesthesia without fixatives, is injected. The needle is left in place and the stylet inserted. A mixture of 75 to 100 mg of prednisolone acetate suspension is prepared with normal saline to a total volume of 8 cc. After several minutes, some degree of anesthesia is appreciated as a result of the Xylocaine injection, and the patient's discomfort is reduced. The prednisolone acetate suspension mixture is then injected and the needle is withdrawn. Some physicians feel that in addition to the effects of the medication there is a possible neurolysis effect by mechanically breaking up adhesions.

Following the injection, the patient is placed in a hospital bed with the head slightly elevated and the knees flexed. After approximately ½ hour, he is allowed to leave in a wheelchair and can be driven home but must rest in bed for at least 2 hours. If a patient has no one to drive him home, he must remain in the hospital for 2 or 3 hours.

The two major complications of epidural

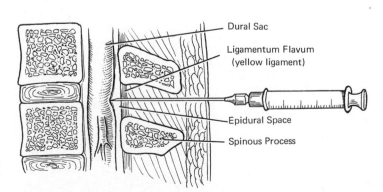

Fig. 13-2. The "potential" epidural space is in part created by needle pressure upon the nondistended dura.

block are inadvertent injection of the local anesthesia either into the subarachnoid space or into a blood vessel. If a subarachnoid injection has occurred, the patient is given a spinal anesthesia and requires the usual precautions and supportive measures necessary with this form of anesthesia. Oxygen, vasopressor drugs, and intravenous fluids may be in order. If ascent of anesthesia level causes impaired respiration, intubation and mechanical ventilation may be necessary. If these measures are instituted in time, the spinal anesthetic effect will eventually recede, spontaneous respirations will resume, and the blood pressure will improve.

Following inadvertent injection of the local anesthetic into a blood vessel, it is quite likely that no untoward reaction will ensue. The two possible complications include seizures or cardiovascular collapse. If seizures occur, routine anticonvulsant measures include an airway both for aeration and for prevention of tongue maceration, avoidance of extremity damage from tonic and clonic movements, oxygen, and anticonvulsant drugs. Cardiovascular collapse requires oxygen, intravenous fluids, vasopressors, and vagolytic drugs such as Atropine to treat bradycardia. Some are of the opinion that more effective pain relief is obtained with the epidural block. Occasionally, for technical reasons such as extensive scarring, or the personal preference of the injector, the caudal block is used.

Caudal Block

The caudal block is a form of peridural analgesia or anesthesia performed by injecting the solution into the caudal or sacral canal through the sacral hiatus. Because the injection is into the sacral canal, the normal anatomy of the sacrum and the sacral canal and the anomalies of this structure should be known. Many of these anamolies present unfavorable conditions both for needle insertion and for the satisfactory dispersion of the injected solution.

SACRAL CANAL

The sacral canal is merely the sacral prolongation of the vertebral canal (Fig. 13–3). Viewed laterally, its longitudinal axis is curved like the sacrum with anterior concavity. The anterior floor of the canal is formed by the fused vertebral bodies and the overlying posterior longitudinal ligament. The lateral boundaries are formed by the sacral pedicles and the intervertebral foramina. The posterior roof is formed by the fused laminae. Occasionally, as a result of the transverse ridges found between the fused sacral vertebrae, the anterior floor is so irregular as to prevent the needle from advancing cephalad during caudal injection.

A continuation of the caudal sac extends from the lumbar region into the upper segments of the sacral canal. Generally, the terminal end of the caudal sac extends no further than S2. This is far from an absolute rule, however, as is apparent to those who review lumbar myelograms which demonstrate the considerable variability of the end of the dural sac in relationship to the sacrum. This anatomical variability is of considerable technical importance in the performance of a caudal block, which is based on installation of solution into the peridural space but not into the subarachnoid space (Figs.

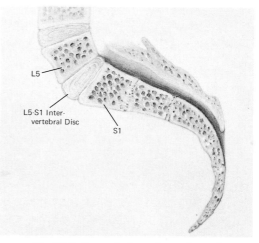

L5

L5-S1 Inter-
vertebral Disc

S1

Fig. 13-3. Lateral view of sacral canal.

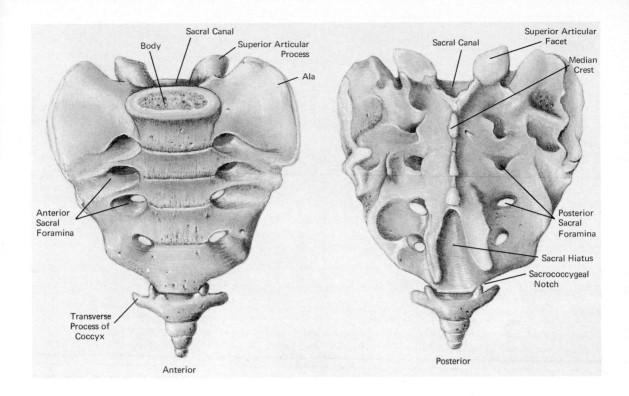

Fig. 13-4. Anterior and posterior views of sacrum.

13-4 and 13-5). The length of the sacral canal varies from 7 to 9 cm and the distance between the apex of the sacral hiatus and the end of the dural sac exhibits even greater variation (from 2 to 7 cm with an average of 4.5 cm). When performing a caudal block on patients who have had previous myelography, it is most helpful to review the films, since this will give a clear indication of the exact termination of the caudal sac in relationship to the sacral canal.

When the caudal sac terminates, it ends in a dural strand called the filum terminale, which passes through the sacral canal and fuses to the periosteum of the dorsal surface of the coccyx. The sacral nerve roots are surrounded by sleeve-like extensions from the caudal sac. These dural prolongations are variable in their extent, in some cases reaching below the caudal end of the dura. This anatomical variation, usually revealed by the myelogram, is also of practical im-

portance in considering a caudal block. In addition to nerve roots and their enveloping membranes, the sacral canal contains blood vessels, fat, loose areolar tissue, and lymphatics. The blood vessels are primarily veins and are most prevalent along the anterior lateral aspect of the canal, like the lumbar epidural vessels.

SACRAL HIATUS

The caudal portion of the sacral canal terminates as an inverted U-shaped or V-shaped opening on the dorsum of the sacrum called the sacral hiatus (Fig. 13-6). Its formation is due to a fusion failure of the last one or two (4th and 5th) sacral laminae. It is about 5 cm above the tip of the coccyx and is usually a centimeter or two above the upper limit of the gluteal crease. Two bony prominences on either side of the sacral

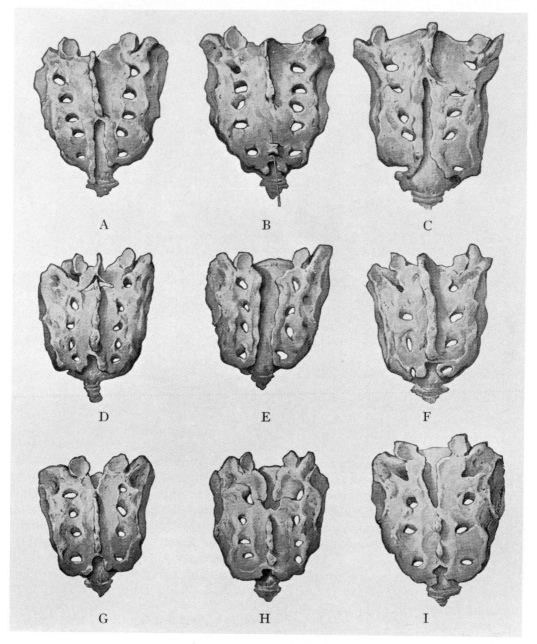

Fig. 13-5. Common anomalies of the sacrum: **(A)** Deformity of lateral borders of hiatus with upward extension. **(B)** Fairly normal hiatus but with an additional foramen in a sacral spinous process through which the needle has been inserted. **(C)** Hiatus extending upward to the level of the body of the first sacral vertebra. **(D)** Deformity of the sacrum resulting from injury. **(E)** Open sacral canal. **(F)** Flattened anteroposterior diameter of canal. **(G, H, I)** Failure of fusion of lamina of the first sacral vertebra. (Courtesy M Williamson)

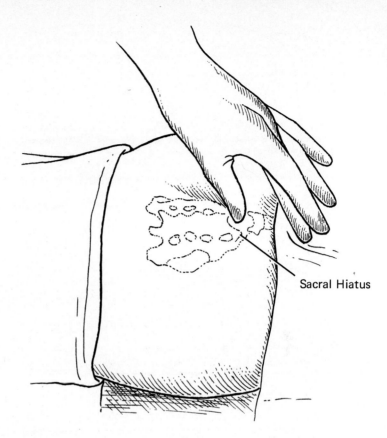

Sacral Hiatus

Fig. 13-6. Locating the sacral hiatus.

hiatus are valuable as landmarks when performing a caudal block. These are referred to as the sacral cornua. Completely covering the sacral hiatus is the posterior sacrococcygeal ligament, which actually forms the caudal end of the vertebral canal. Superficial to this ligament lie the subcutaneous tissues and skin.

TECHNIQUE

The patient is placed in the prone position with two pillows beneath the pubis to make the power portion of the sacrum more prominent. The sacral hiatus is palpated by running the finger up and down from the midline of the sacrum down to the gluteal crease and palpating a slight depression just below the inverted U-shaped opening. Further identification is obtained by palpating the lateral walls of this hiatus, the so-called sacral cornua. Another confirmation of position is to palpate the tip of the coccyx and then proceed cephalad approximately 5 cm again ending at the slight depression just above the gluteal crease.

Little difficulty is encountered in identification of the sacral hiatus in thin patients, but if a patient is obese, difficulties may arise. Occasionally, the knee-chest position in obese patients is helpful.

After establishing the location of the sacral hiatus, the hair overlying this site is shaved and the area cleansed with antiseptic solution and draped with a sterile towel. A local anesthetic skin wheal is made over the sacral hiatus with a 25-gauge hypodermic needle. The needle is introduced deeper to infiltrate the subcutaneous tissues and the sacrococcygeal ligament (Fig. 13-7). The 25-gauge needle is temporarily allowed to remain in place as a landmark. A 19-gauge lumbar puncture needle with stylet in place, maintained perpendicular to the skin, is then introduced directly through the center of the

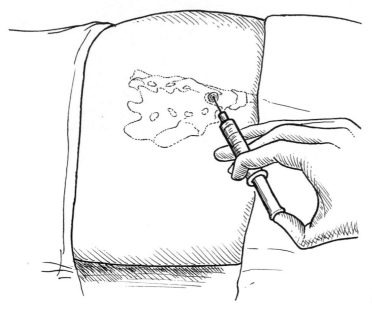

Fig. 13-7. Local anesthetic wheal over sacral hiatus.

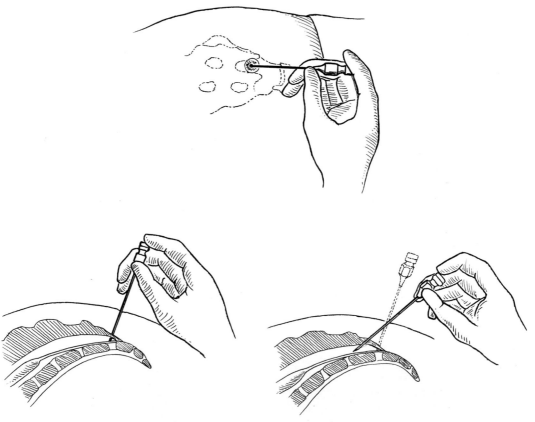

Fig. 13-8. Spinal needle placement.

sacral hiatus, through the skin and subcutaneous tissues (Fig. 13-8). As the needle penetrates the sacrococcygeal ligament, it is met with firm resistance which suddenly subsides. The bevel of the needle will then encounter bony resistance, indicating that it has impinged upon the body of the S4 vertebra. At this point, the needle is withdrawn slightly and the shaft is depressed and is then advanced 2 or 3 cm, bringing the bevel to the level of S3. Because of a high transverse ridge between the last two sacral vertebrae, the needle is occasionally obstructed before it can be adequately introduced into the sacral canal. If this occurs, the shaft and hub of the needle are depressed further, causing the bevel to move upward so that, hopefully, it will be able to glide over this bony ridge. In some instances, either the sacral canal is so small or the obstructing ridge is so great that the needle cannot be further advanced. If such is the case, an attempt can be made to inject the solution without further needle advancement.

At this point it is most important to be sure that the needle is neither in the subarachnoid space nor in a blood vessel. Careful aspiration of the needle is done at least three or four times and before each aspiration ½ cc of air is injected through the needle to be sure that it is not obstructed by fat or areolar tissue. If spinal fluid is obtained, the block is terminated, since dural puncture is a contraindication to caudal block. If blood is aspirated, the needle is moved back by ½ cm, the stylet is reinserted, and after a 3- to 5-minute wait for coagulation to occur, aspiration is reattempted.

After the physician is satisfied that the needle is neither in a blood vessel nor in the subarachnoid space, 8 cc of 1% Xylocaine without fixative, specifically prepared for spinal anesthesia, is initially injected (Fig. 13-9). The needle is left in place with the stylet inserted. During this injection, it is good to place the hand over the sacrum to be sure that a subcutaneous injection is not being made directly over the sacrum. Occasionally, marked resistance to injection is encountered, usually indicating that the point of the needle has become embedded in the periosteum. In such a case, a slight withdrawal of the needle is usually helpful. After injection of the anesthetic solution, the patient may note reduction of discomfort in 5 or 10 minutes. One hundred milligrams of prednisolone acetate suspension is diluted to 12 cc, making a total of 20 cc of medication injected.

The level achieved by a caudal block primarily depends upon the volume of solution used. Other factors are speed of injection and the position of the patient. The more rapid the injection, the higher the level. A patient in head down position may obtain anesthesia or analgesia reaching one or two segments higher.

Some anesthesiologists feel that in addition to relieving pain, a measure of therapeutic effect may be achieved in the use of

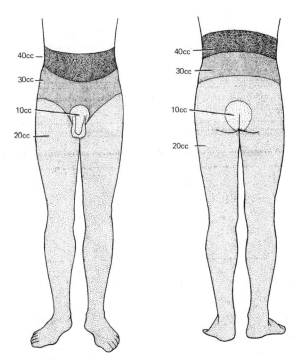

Fig. 13-9. Amounts of anesthetic solution necessary for various levels of anesthesia.

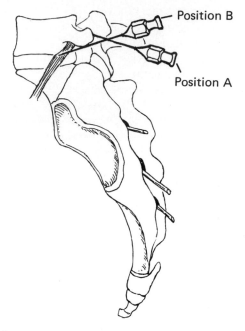

Fig. 13-10. Cross-section of paravertebral block.

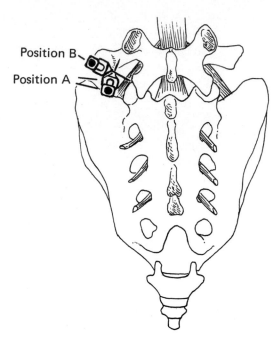

Fig. 13-11. Spinal needle placement for para-vertebral block.

the caudal block by mechanically relieving "nerve root adhesions" within the spinal and sacral canal.

COMPLICATIONS

The major complication of caudal block is inadvertent injection of the local anesthesia either into the subarachnoid space or into a blood vessel. If this occurs, the patient should be provided with supportive measures. Oxygen, vasopressor drugs, and intravenous fluids may be in order.

If the inadvertent injection was intravascular, it may be associated with convulsions (which must be treated by intravenous anticonvulsant medication) or with cardio-respiratory collapse (which is treated by vasopressor drugs, intubation, artificial respiration, and general supportive management). Another complication of caudal block may be hypotension due to paralysis of the sympathetic vasoconstrictors. This complication usually occurs only if the block is quite extensive. It is prevented by vasopressor medication prior to the injection.

Paravertebral Block

INDICATIONS

The paravertebral block can be applied as a diagnostic aid in determining whether a specific root is the source of pain (Fig. 13-10). When a dorsal rhizotomy is contemplated for surgical relief of pain, it can be employed in the form of a short-term presurgical therapeutic trial. Since the L5 and S1 nerve roots are the two most commonly invovled roots, the technique of injecting these nerves will be discussed.

TECHNIQUE

The patient is positioned on the x-ray table in a prone position with either two pillows or a large foam rubber sponge beneath the abdomen to achieve some degree of lumbar flexion. What is estimated as the L5–S1 interspace is identified using roentgenographic guidance. A 25-gauge hypodermic needle is used to place a local anesthesia skin wheal 4 cm lateral to the L5 spinous

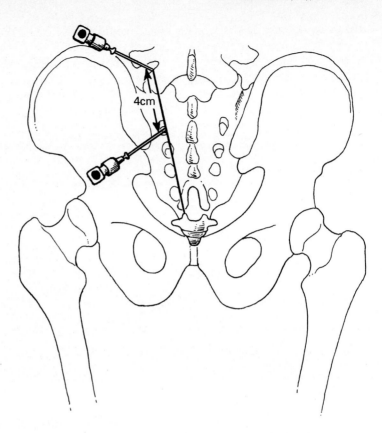

4cm

Fig. 13-12. Localization of first sacral foramen.

process, and again roentgenographic guidance is used to check the accurate position of this hypodermic needle (Fig. 13-11). An 8-cm, 22-gauge, needle with a depth marker is introduced in a direction perpendicular to the skin and advanced until its point impinges upon the L5 lumbar vertebra transverse process, a depth between 4 to 6 cm. The depth guide on the needle is then placed 3 cm from the skin. The needle is withdrawn until its point is in the subcutaneous tissue and then redirected slightly more medially and caudally so that it will pass inferior to the transverse process toward the intervertebral foramen and the exiting L5 nerve root. The needle is advanced very slowly and as soon as paresthesia is produced by the needle striking the L5 nerve root, its progress is immediately stopped. At this point, the needle is aspirated for either spinal fluid or blood. If the aspiration is negative, 3 to 5 cc of 1% Xylocaine is injected into the nerve

root. Do not inject the anesthetic solution until a recheck x-ray film is taken.

After performing the paravertebral L5 root block, we now prepare to do the transsacral (paravertebral sacral) block. The sacral hiatus and cornua are identified, and a line is drawn between the sacral cornu on the side of the block and the previously inserted L5 root block needle. The first posterior sacral foramen is located approximately 4 cm caudad from this needle on the previously drawn line (Fig. 13-12). The 8-cm, 22-gauge, needle is introduced through the wheal in a slightly medial direction so that the roof of the sacrum is contacted. After this bony impingement has occurred, the depth marker is placed 1.5 cm from the skin. The needle is slightly withdrawn and reinserted in a more perpendicular fashion. As the needle contacts the first sacral foramen, penetration of the ligament covering the foramen will produce a slight sensation of resistance which immediately disappears. The needle is advanced until paresthesia is experienced by the patient or until the depth marker is flush with the skin. If no paresthesia is appreciated, and a roentgenographic check indicates the needle within the S1 foramen, 5 cc of 1% Xylocaine can be injected.

Complications of the paravertebral block are smiliar to those discussed under caudal block, but generally of a lesser magnitude.

Stenotic Lumbar Spinal Canal Syndrome 14

Stenotic Lumbar Spinal Canal

In the past 10 years the concept of the "stenotic lumbar canal" has received increasing emphasis. Among the physicians most responsible for directing our attention to this syndrome is George Ehni of Baylor University College of Medicine in Houston, Texas. He has redefined this clinical entity with specific signs and symptoms separating the stenotic lumbar spinal canal from other conditions affecting the lumbar spine. His important five-part article was originally presented as part of a panel discussion he chaired on "syndromes of the small lumbar spinal canal" at a meeting of the Southern Neurosurgical Society, New Orleans, Louisiana on February 17, 1968.[7] The increasing use of computerized axial tomography to visualize the cross-sectional configuration of the spinal canal and measure its dimensions, has added to our understanding of this condition.

HISTORICAL DATA

In a case report published in 1900, by Bernard Sachs and J. Fraenkel, two New York City neurologists, a patient was described with lumbosacral pain who walked in a stooped forward position.[17] A laminectomy was carried out and apparently was helpful in relieving some of the symptoms. At the time of surgery Dr. Arpad Gerster, the surgeon, noted unusual heaviness of the laminae and thickness of the periosteum but found no evidence of mass or infection. This early case report was followed by others of a similar nature in which laminectomy was found to be helpful. The explanation in most cases indicated hypertrophic osteoarthritic changes in addition to hypertrophy of the yellow ligament, causing compression of the nerve roots of the cauda equina. Included in these early papers was one written by Charles Elsberg.[8] In his paper, which was a review of 60 laminectomies for various spinal dysfunctions, he mentioned several patients with "symptoms very much like those of tumor of the cauda equina, although nothing is found at the operation that can be relieved by surgical means. All of the patients improved very much after the operation, and the result can only be ascribed to the laminectomy." Throughout the subsequent years, this entity has been called to our attention by a number of authors in various ways. In 1947, M. A. Sarpyener discussed "congenital stricture of the spinal canal."[18] H. Verbiest of Utrecht, Holland, who recognized the importance of the stenotic canal long before anyone else, has written on this subject from 1949 to the present.[25,26,27] J. A. Epstein, another pioneer and innovator in this field, and his associates, have written several papers describing nerve root compression caused by narrowing of the lumbar spinal canal.[9,10] From 1965 on, increasing numbers of papers have been written discussing this entity.

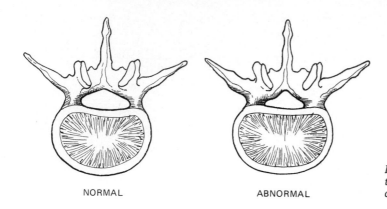

NORMAL   ABNORMAL

Fig. 14-1. Anatomic differences between the normal and stenotic lumbar spinal canal.

Cervical Versus Lumbar Spinal Canal Stenosis

Two decades prior to recognition of the stenotic spinal canal syndrome, encroachment upon the cervical spine resulting from a stenotic cervical spinal canal had been generally accepted as a recognizable clinical entity (Fig. 14-1). A number of patients whose neurological symptoms initially led to a diagnosis of multiple sclerosis, amyotrophic lateral sclerosis, or other neurological degenerative disease, were found to have spondylotic encroachment upon the cervical cord, documented by cervical myelography.

Roentgenological interest in the size of the lumbar spinal canal paralleled the lack of clinical involvement in this area. This discrepancy is now corrected. New awareness of the stenotic lumbar spinal canal syndrome has given impetus to special roentgenographic techniques specifically created to measure this space.

ANATOMICAL CHARACTERISTICS

Putting aside changes of the vertebrae resulting from degenertion and other factors which would decrease the dimensions of the spinal canal, a clinically significant individual variation in both the size and configuration of the canal exists. Using specially designed calipers, Dr. Henk Verbiest measured the diameters of the spinal canal at surgery. He considers an AP diameter of less than 12 mm likely to be symptom producing.

Of equal importance to the AP measurement is the configuration of the spinal canal. The following four anatomical characteristics are associated with constrictive lateral recesses and constriction of the intervertebral (neural) foramina.

1. Short and thick pedicles
2. Short and thick laminae
3. More acute angle between the right and left halves of the laminae
4. Enlarged, bulbous articular facets

ROENTGENOGRAPHIC CHARACTERISTICS

Clinically, the AP dimension is most important with the so-called shallow canal. In many cases the side-to-side diameters of the canal are also limited, but this is usually not delineated by a diminution in the interpedicular measurements. These usually remain normal, and are seldom helpful in determining the size of a spinal canal.

Measurements on conventionally made lateral lumbar roentgenograms are usually done using the Epstein (and associates) technique. The AP diameter is measured from the posterior margin of the lumbar intervertebral foramen to the posterior surface of the vertebral body. This measurement can be used from L1 to L4 but not at the L5–S1 level, because the oblique orientation of the foramen at that level causes it to appear deceptively smaller and would produce an inaccurate measurement. Dr. Epstein considers any measurement below 13 mm to represent an abnormally shallow lumbar canal (Fig. 14-2).

LUMBAR MOBILITY

In patients with a stenotic lumbar canal, any changes which further decrease the space within this canal are more likely to produce symptoms than would be the case in a normal-sized spinal canal. Movements of the lumbar spine will cause minor changes of the structures within the canal. When the spinal canal is of normal size and configuration, these changes are of no clinical significance. However, in the case of a small lumbar spinal canal, such changes may be symptom producing.

Flexion of the lumbar spine produces the following changes.

1. Decrease in intraspinal protrusion of lumbar intervertebral disc
2. Slight increase in the length of the anterior wall of the spinal canal
3. Significant increase in length of the posterior wall of the spinal canal
4. Stretching and decreased bulge of the yellow ligaments within the spinal canal
5. Stretching and decreased cross-sectional area of nerve roots

The overall effect of spinal flexion is to produce a general increase in spinal canal volume and decreased nerve root bulk.

Extension of the lumbar spine produces these changes.

1. Bulging of intervertebral discs into the spinal canal
2. Slight decrease of anterior canal length
3. Moderate decrease of posterior canal length
4. Enfolding and protrusion of yellow ligaments into the spinal canal
5. Relaxation and increase in cross-sectional diameter of nerve roots

It can be seen that spinal extension produces an overall decrease in the volume of the lumbar spinal canal and increased nerve root bulk.

CLINICAL CHARACTERISTICS

It must be recognized that coexistence of the stenotic lumbar spinal canal with either the herniated lumbar disc or lumbar spondylosis is extremely common. It is also clear that a congenitally stenotic lumbar spinal canal that is present from birth is not usually associated with symptoms in early life, but tends to develop after the age of 35 or 40 years. This implies the occurrence of secondary changes causing further encroachment and eventually leading to the production of symptoms. These changes include subperiosteal thickening over the vertebral body and the laminal arch, and thickening of the capsular ligaments and the ligamentum flavum.

The stenotic lumbar spinal canal syndrome has certain of the following clinical characteristics which allow us to distinguish from spondylosis or lumbar disc disease in a canal of normal size.

1. Patients often have multiple root involvements with a greatly increased frequency of bilateral leg pain. In lumbar disc disease it is usually possible to identify a "single root lesion" with the examination pointing to one specific root. In the stenotic lumbar spinal canal syndrome, two and sometimes three roots on the same or both sides may be involved.

2. The position of maximal comfort differs considerably in this syndrome from a typical herniated lumbar disc picture. Most lumbar disc patients are improved with bed rest and are reasonably comfortable when lying flat. But in the small lumbar spinal canal syndrome, often the only position of comfort is with the hospital bed angulated in such a fashion that the patient's head is elevated from 40 degrees to 60 degrees and the hips and knees are flexed allowing lumbar flexion to occur. In many instances the patient may be completely relaxed after 24

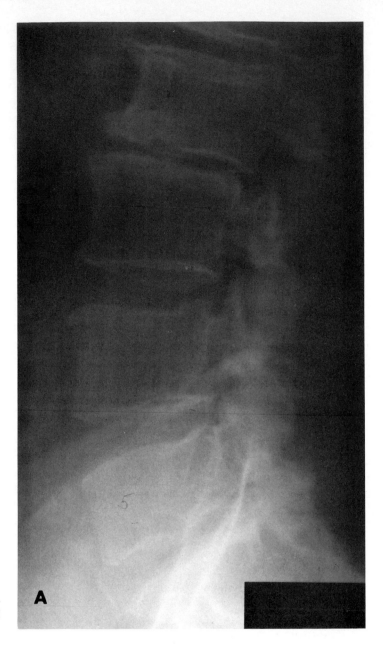

Fig. 14-2. Compare this stenotic lumbar spinal canal (A) with normal sized spinal canal (B).

to 48 hours of this position and be in no discomfort whatsoever. If the bed is then flattened out, so that the position of lumbar flexion is changed to a slight lumbar lordosis, the pain may immediately and promptly recur to almost its original severity. This is a fairly reliable clinical sign that we are dealing with a stenotic spinal canal.

3. The patient often is unable to walk with comfort unless he bends forward, producing a reversal and flexion of the normal lordotic curve.

4. On examination it is noted that straight leg raising is often much less painful than might be expected, despite the fact that the patient may have pain radiating down one or both legs. Forward bending, which ordinarily causes considerable discomfort in

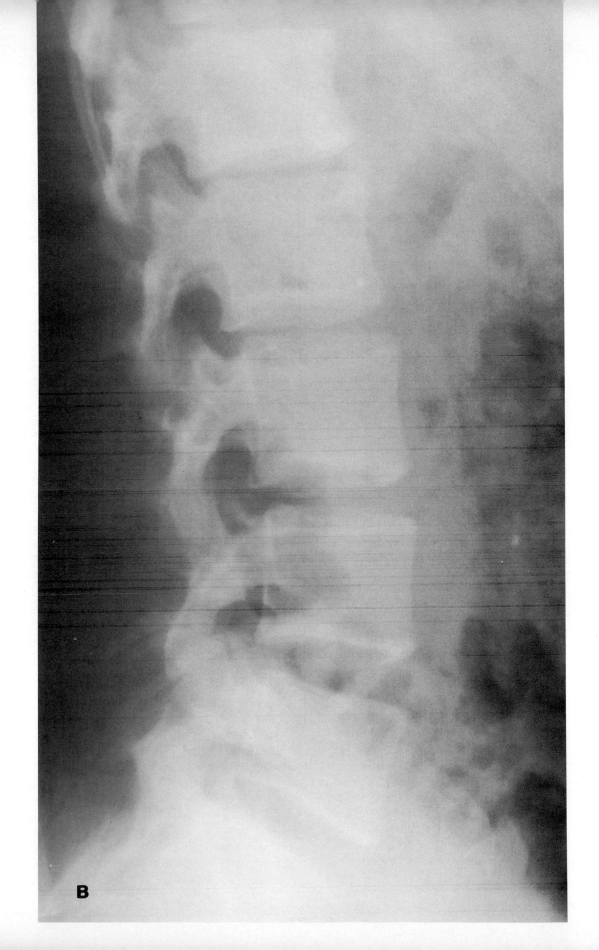

B

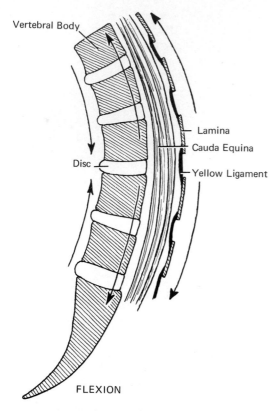

Fig. 14-3. Increased spinal canal volume and decreased nerve root (cauda equina) bulk with flexion.

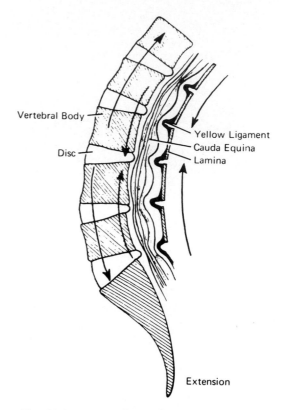

Fig. 14-4. Decreased spinal canal volume and increased nerve root bulk with extension.

lumbar disc disease, is not at all painful and may actually ease the pain (Figs. 14-3 and 14-4).

PLAIN ROENTGENOGRAPHIC CHANGES

1. Flattening of the lumbar lordotic curve.
2. Slight spondylolisthesis of L4 on L5 without a pars defect.
3. Increased density of facets.
4. Hypertrophic osteoarthritic spurs and interspace narrowing. (This finding must be given increased clinical significance. In a normal-sized spinal canal a considerable amount of arthrosis may be well tolerated, but with the preexistence of a stenotic canal such changes may cause symptoms. In this regard one must look for facet enlargement, heaviness of laminae and spondylolisthesis. Narrowing or vertebral malalignment at the L5–S1 interspace in association with a stenotic lumbar canal is less likely to be symptom-producing than even a slight L4–5 spondylolisthesis. This is because there is a great deal of space between the neural elements and the bone at the L5–S1 level; considerable hypertrophic spurring can exist at that site without compromising the nerve roots. However, at the L4–5 level the roots are normally more snugly enclosed within their bony boundaries, so that a minimal "offset" may be symptom producing.)
5. An AP spinal canal diameter of less than 13 mm (from the posterior margin of the intervertebral foramen to the posterior surface of the vertebral body.

MYELOGRAPHY

The myelogram is frequently misinterpreted in stenotic lumbar spinal canal syndrome (Fig. 14-5). Because the roots are compressed against each other and not freely floating, as is the case when the spinal canal is of normal size, introduction of the myelographic spinal puncture needle is often painful and may be associated with slow CSF flow. The myelographer may feel that technical deficiencies on his part are producing both the pain and the sluggish passage of Pantopaque. In many cases the interpretation of the myelogram is erroneous and may be mislabeled as a subdural injection or adhesive arachnoiditis. It is most disturbing for me to review old myelograms that I had either originally interpreted as "technically inadequate" or diagnosed as adhesive arachnoiditis, when actually they were diagnostic of a stenotic lumbar spinal canal. The symptoms in retrospect fit this syndrome quite well. One must always consider a needle that is properly placed and in the midline but is pain producing, as being in a pathologic process.

Lumbar Spondylosis and the Stenotic Lumbar Spinal Canal

Lumbar spondylosis is a condition in which there is a progressive degeneration of the intervertebral disc leading to changes of the adjacent vertebrae and ligaments. Although it is also called hypertrophic arthritis, osteoarthritis, and lumbar spondylitis, the term spondylosis is considered preferable, since the condition is a degenerative rather than an inflammatory one. For the past 20 years this term was utilized primarily in relation to the cervical spine and was generally accepted as meaning a generalized deterioration of the cervical intervertebral disc and its associated ligamentous and osseous structures. Cervical spondylosis implies an accumulation of degenerative changes in the cervical spine resulting in narrowing of the vertebral canal. It is associated with cervical cord compression, nerve root compression, and, in many cases, vertebral artery compression resulting in a vertebrobasilar ischemia.

The term lumbar spondylosis invites the clinician to recognize that degenerative changes can occur in the lumbar spine as well as in the cervical spine, and that these changes will also produce diminution and narrowing of the spinal canal, creating specific clinical symptoms.

Lumbar spondylosis has been confused with other disorders capable of producing low back and sciatic pain such as disc herniation, lumbosacral strain, adhesive arachnoiditis, neoplasm, and functional backache. Some of the unsatisfactory responses and disappointments resulting from treatment can be avoided if this entity is recognized and appropriately treated.

It is important to distinguish between the relatively benign and often inconsequential symptoms of lumbar spondylosis in the normal canal and the severe encroachment produced by a similar degree of spondylosis in a stenotic canal. The latter may result in multilevel interferences with cauda equina function requiring surgical decompression of several levels.

Lumbar Disc Dynasty

The chief hindrance to recognition of the importance of lumbar spondylosis is the domination of lumbar disc disease. Beginning in the mid1930s, the term lumbar disc disease assumed considerable popularity and was utilized to explain low back pain with radiation into one or both lower extremities. As the neurosurgeons and orthopedic surgeons who practiced lumbar disc surgery became technically proficient, a large group of successfuly treated patients gave increased authority to this entity. This led to a sort of mental despotism, so that any lumbar sciatic pain syndrome was essentially considered a "disc problem." A patient was identified as a herniated lumbar disc suspect, and efforts in investigation and management were directed toward that specific entity. If the usual course of conservative management did not alleviate the pain, a myelogram would be performed to "verify

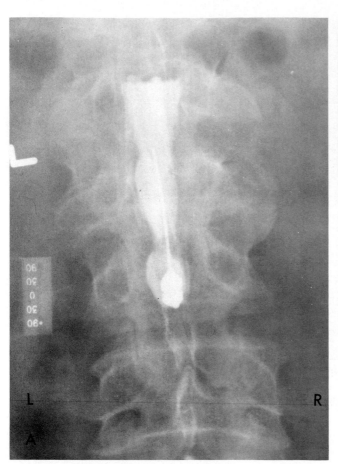 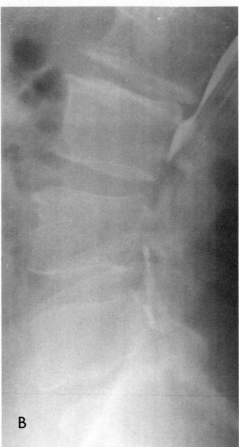

*Fig. 14-5. (**A** and **B**) Myelographic demonstration of stenotic lumbar spinal canal. Six cc of Pantopaque was injected through the lumbar puncture needle, inserted at the L1–2 interspace; free flow of dye column cranially. Block is at midportion of L3. (**C** and **D**) Three cc of Pantopaque was injected through the second lumbar puncture needle injected at L5–S1 interspace; the dye column is blocked at the L4–5 level. The lateral view reveals no evidence of disc herniation at L1–2, L2–3, L4–5, L5–S1. L3–4 is not adequately visualized.*

the existence of a herniated lumbar disc." When such a lesion was disclosed by myelography, interlaminar excision of the symptom-producing fragment of extruded disc was often followed by an excellent clinical improvement. However, a number of myelograms reveal some constriction of the dural sac with a slightly protruding intervertebral disc in the lower lumbar region. On the basis of persisting symptoms and an equivocal myelogram, many of these patients are subjected to interlaminar explorations, in the course of which a firm, slightly protruding intervertebral disc is violated and excised. Occasionally, because no significant disc

protrusion is visualized at surgery, a "negative exploration" results. Included in this sizable group of patients are many cases of lumbar spondylosis in association with a stenotic lumbar spinal canal. As a result of such inappropriate management, they do not fare well.

Pathology of Lumbar Spondylosis

Whenever we attempt to understand what produces degenerative changes within an anatomical structure, we must have an appreciation of its primary functions. Although

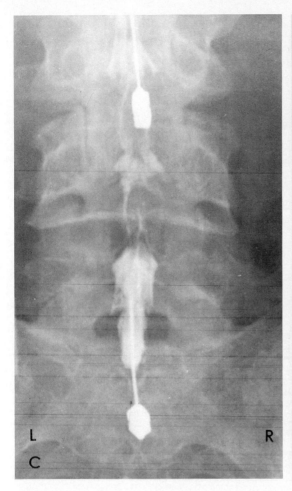

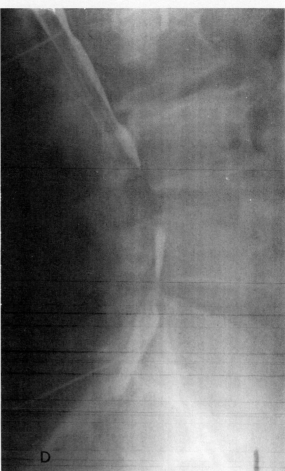

we are using the term lumbar spondylosis to emphasize the similarities involving degenerative changes of the cervical and lumbar spines, the significant differences in function between these two areas must be recognized. The **cervical spine** is structured primarily for mobility and secondarily for weight bearing; the **lumbar spine** is structured primarily for weight bearing with mobility being of secondary importance. These differences would imply that degenerative changes involving the lumbar spine arise primarily from the stresses of weight bearing and to a lesser extent from mobility, whereas the opposite is true in the cervical region.

Spondylitic changes of the lumbar spine involve narrowing of the intervertebral disc spaces, "lipping," and osteophyte formation around the margins of contiguous vertebral bodies, which may occur anteriorly or laterally but also often posteriorly. In addition, hypertrophic changes involving the posterior intervertebral joints are present affecting the joint capsules and ligaments, which become swollen. This is usually seen as a multilevel process, symmetrical bilaterally, with hypertrophy of the laminae, facets, and usually the yellow ligaments.

Progressive Development of Lumbar Spondylosis[3]

DEGENERATION OF THE NUCLEUS PULPOSUS

Exactly why degeneration occurs in some persons and not in others is an issue that is not completely settled. It is generally felt

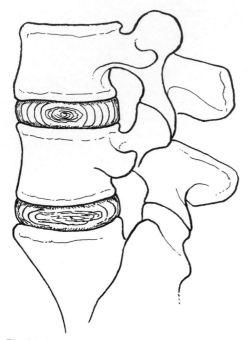

Fig. 14-6. Degeneration of the nucleus pulposus.
Illustrations 14-6 to 14-10 demonstrate the progressive stages of lumbar spondylosis at the
L5–S1 level; the L4–5 level is depicted as normal
for purposes of contrast. It should be emphasized
that lumbar spondylosis is a generally occurring
clinical condition and is not usually limited to
a single interspace.

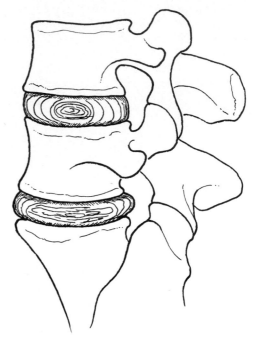

Fig. 14-7. Degeneration of the annulus fibrosus.

that the intrinsic tissue strength of the nucleus pulposus, the stress of weight bearing,
and the deteriorative changes of aging are
the determining factors. The nucleus pulposus softens, disintegrates and eventually
becomes fragmented (Figs. 14-6 through 14-
10).

DEGENERATION OF THE ANNULUS FIBROSUS

As the nucleus pulposus degenerates, it
can no longer function as a semi-incom-
pressible fulcrum for intervertebral movement and is unable to distribute pressure
equally over the annulus and vertebral end-
plates. This degeneration subjects the annulus to increased compression which, because of the normal lumbar lordosis, falls
mainly in its posterior portion. As noted
above, it is weight bearing or compression

which is a major factor in producing degenerative changes. The abnormal and constant
pressure often leads to fissuring of the posterior portion of the annulus fibrosus, the
fissures usually occurring within a relatively
small area and often unilaterally.[14] The most
common site of annular fissure is at the site
where it is least reinforced by the posterior
longitudinal ligament. At this stage in the
degenerative process the nucleus pulposus
develops a degree of fibrosis somewhat in
excess of the normal state of fibrosis seen in
the normal aging process. It is also at this
phase of degeneration that a divarication
occurs and one of two separate and distinct
entities (disc herniation or spondylosis) will
develop.

HERNIATION OF THE NUCLEUS PULPOSUS

In less than 20% of patients with weakening or tearing of the fibers of the annulus
fibrosis, a large fragment of disc material
will completely extrude through the opening
in the annulus, producing a mass effect large

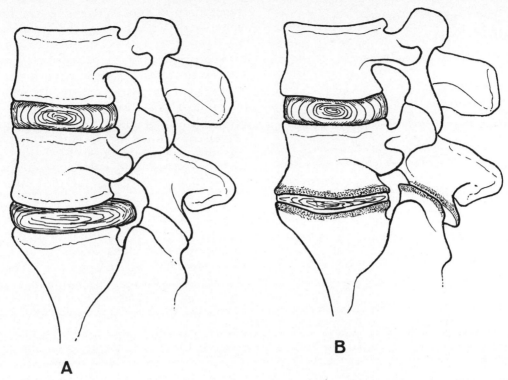

Fig. 14-8. (A) Herniation of the nucleus pulposus. (B) Spondylosis.

enough to cause nerve root compression. In such an instance, the symptoms are those of a herniated lumbar disc.

SPONDYLOSIS

In most cases, despite the stress placed on the annulus fibrosus, no complete rupture occurs. The annulus becomes softer and weaker, but never completely loses its integrity, so that it contains the disc contents within its bounds. If such a situation occurs, the disc becomes anatomically fixed but functionally impaired, and no actual nuclear tissue displacement has occurred to cause nerve root compression. In some instances, a minimal disruption of the annular fibers occurs with weakening and a slight protrusion. Although there is some increased bulge of the intervertebral disc into the spinal canal, it is relatively minimal, and fibrosis susbsequently occurs with the eventual disc protrusion becoming quite fibrous and stable in its consistency and mobility.

FIBROSIS

Fibrosis is associated with decreased tissue bulk and loss of sponginess and elasticity. The tissue of the annulus fibrosus shrinks and becomes increasingly fibrous. Decreased elasticity will produce sclerotic changes in the vertebral bodies, with sclerotic bone replacing the cartilaginous end-plates, and new bone formation around the periphery of the contiguous vertebral surfaces. The intervertebral space narrows as a result of increased fibrosis and loss of tissue mass within the intervertebral disc. The posterior diarthrodial joints become involved as a result of the loss of the normal nuclear fulcrum for movement. This involvement, in combination with a decrease in the intervertebral space, alters the planes of the articular surfaces of the diarthrodial joints

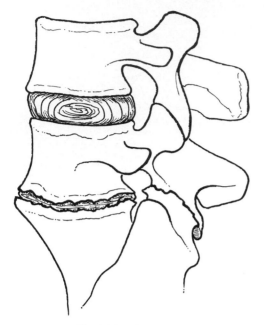

Fig. 14-9. Fibrosis.

so that they are no longer congruous and subjects the joints to abnormal stresses and strains. Such stresses are productive of degenerative arthritis, including narrowing of the posterior diarthrodial joint spaces, subchondral sclerosis, peripheral new bone formation, and periarticular fibrosis.

COMPLETE FIBROUS ANKYLOSIS OF THE INTERVERTEBRAL JOINT

In rare cases, if the ankylosis becomes completely stable with no movement whatsoever, the patient's low back symptoms may improve. However, such changes take many years and in most instances involve more than one interspace, each of which is undergoing degenerative changes at a different stage. When improvement occurs, it is very gradual and over a time span of many years.

Roentgenographic Changes

Lumbar spondylosis is roentgenographically apparent. Plain x-ray films of the lumbar spine reveal changes which are usually generalized throughout most of the lumbar spine and almost invariably involve the L3–4, L4–5, and L5–S1 interspaces. It is rare to see one interspace grossly affected and the rest not involved. Osteophyte formations often occur anteriorly or laterally, but they may occur posteriorly. In addition, hypertrophic changes involving the posterior intervertebral joints are present; they involve the joint capsules and ligaments which become hypertrophied with facet enlargement and heaviness of laminae.

Extensive roentgenographic evidence of lumbar spondylosis may be seen as an incidental finding in a patient who gives no history of significant low back or sciatic discomfort. In association with a stenotic lumbar spinal canal, such findings are of clinical importance.

The myelogram may reveal invaginated yellow ligaments and moderate multilevel bulging of discs which, in a constricted spinal canal, are capable of producing pressure on the cauda equina from all sides.

Lumbar Spondylosis with Spinal Canal of Normal Dimensions

Most patients with lumbar spondylosis are older than those with primary lumbar disc lesions. A chief symptom is low back pain, often described as aching, which usually is both generalized and specific and involves certain areas of point tenderness. Activity, as a rule, worsens the discomfort; rest eases it. However, since prolonged immobility is often associated with stiffness and aching discomfort, the patient may become uncomfortable while resting in bed and require a limited duration walk for relief. A compromise device such as a rocking chair allows the patient to rest while avoiding painful immobility. The pain experienced with lumbar spondylosis differs from that of lumbar disc disease in that it produces a more unrelenting discomfort with relatively low peaks of pain, never quite as severe or as crippling as lumbar disc disease and without its pain-free remissions. Sciatic pain is rare and when present is less acute or specific and more generalized, involving one or both lower extremities and more than one root within the distribution of the pain.

EXAMINATION

Examination of the low back reveals moderate paraspinal muscle spasm in the lumbar region with some limitation of mobility of the lumbar spine in most movements. Extension is usually a bit more restricted than flexion. There is invariably some flattening of the normal lumbar lordosis. Usually moderate paraspinal muscle spasm is elicited. As a rule, straight leg raising is not as painful as with lumbar disc disease. Occasional sensory, motor, and reflex changes are elicited, but they are not frequent nor are they as specific as those seen in lumbar disc disease. The mechanism of nerve root symptoms is twofold. Lipping of the posterior portions of the vertebral bodies may cause root compression identical to the soft disc protrusion. In addition, the posterior intervertebral joint involvement, including the joint capsules and ligaments, develops hypertrophy of these structures in the area of the intervertebral foramina productive of nerve root compression and irritation. The clinical picture created by nerve root compression within the foramen differs in some respects from the more frequently encountered root syndrome resulting from lumbar disc protrusions.

Foraminal Root Compression Syndrome

Anatomically, the size of the foramina decreases progressively in the lumbar region from L1 to L5, and the size of the nerve root increases a bit from above downward, so that the lower lumbar roots are most likely to be effected by hypertrophic changes. The lumbar roots depart from the dural sac ap-

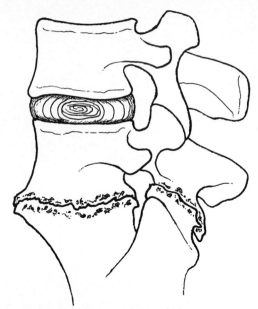

Fig. 14-10. Complete fibrous ankylosis of the intervertebral joint.

proximately 2 cm above the point of exit through the intervertebral foramen. The L4 nerve root exits from the L4–5 intervertebral foramen, the L5 root from the L5–S1 foramen, and the S1 root from the first sacral foramen. This is often a source of confusion, since the level of root involvement with disc protrusion is one segment lower. A disc protrusion at the L5–S1 level will result in an S1 root syndrome, while foraminal root compression at the L5–S1 level will produce an L5 root syndrome. The discrepancy in root levels is due to the different areas of root compression (Fig. 14-11). A disc protrusion usually impinges the nerve root within the spinal canal approximately ½ cm before it separates from the dural sac. The foraminal syndrome impinges the root as it is exiting from the spinal canal 2½ cm (the height of a lumbar vertebra) below the site of disc protrusion.

MECHANISM OF FORAMINAL ROOT COMPRESSION

1. Disc degeneration and intervertebral disc space narrowing

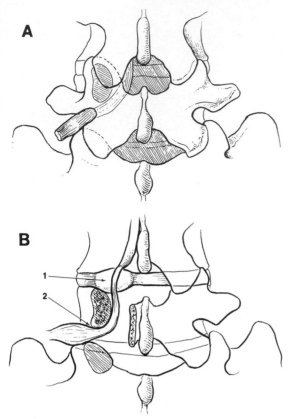

Fig. 14-11. **(A)** *Course of exiting L5 nerve root.* **(B)** *Different sites of L5 root compression with:* **(1)** *disc herniation,* **(2)** *stenotic spinal canal.*

2. Hypertrophic osteoarthritic involvement of the posterior lumbar joint

3. Degenerative spondylolisthesis associated with pathologic mobility of the involved segment

4. Posterior joint telescoping and reduction of the foraminal aperture

5. Fibrosis and thickening of the foraminal reflection of the yellow ligament producing further foraminal encroachment

6. Root impingement between the pedicle of the cephalad vertebra and the superior facet of the caudal vertebra

DISTINCTIVE CLINICAL CHARACTERISTICS

1. Straight leg raising often not particularly painful

2. Lateral flexion, lumbar torsion, and lumbar extension possibly painful

3. Radicular pain more diffuse and spotty as compared with lumbar disc protrusion

4. Hard neurological findings such as reflex or motor changes less frequent in comparison with lumbar disc protrusion

Lumbar Spondylosis with Stenotic Lumbar Spinal Canal

HISTORY

The patient has a long history of intermittent low back pain, often related to specific positions and activities. He frequently is unable to sleep in a prone position, which would tend to increase the lumbar lordosis, and finds it necessary to sleep on his side with hips and knees flexed in the fetal position, assuring substantial lumbar flexion. Since prolonged car driving is often associated with considerable discomfort, he may achieve more comfort in moving the car seat as far forward as possible, requiring increased flexion of the hips and knees and providing increased lumbar lordosis. In addition to low back pain, nerve root symptoms often occur which may be monoradicular, less commonly involving compression of several roots or even the entire cauda equina. Occasionally, pain is only a minor complaint, some patients present with predominantly motor weakness.

A history of neurological deficit, produced during anesthesia while in a position of lumbar hyperextension, is occasionally elicited. Normally, patients with lumbar spondylosis in association with a stenotic lumbar spinal canal manifest protective pain mechanisms which will restrict excessive lumbar extension. Under anesthesia, these protective mechanisms are lost, making it possible to obtain extreme extension with the potential of cauda equina compression.

A number of case reports in the literature attest to serious neurological dysfunction involving the cauda equina following extension of the lumbar spine, with or without anesthesia. One of the earliest reports documenting such a phenomenon was by Goldthwaite in 1911, whose 39-year-old patient with hypertrophic arthritis of the lumbar spine complained of low back pain for 7 years. Right-sided sacroiliac joint displacement had been diagnosed and "replaced" under anesthesia. However, intermittent pain persisted until one day, upon getting out of a hot tub, the patient was unable to assume an erect posture, and remained in a stooped forward position and complained of intense bilateral leg pains. He received another sacroiliac joint "adjustment" under ether anesthesia which did not relieve his pain. A decision was made to encase the patient in a body cast and he was placed supine on an orthopedic frame for cast application. Just as his lumbar spine was extended, he complained for a moment of intense pain, after which he relaxed. Moments later his legs where found to be numb. His neurological status progressed rapidly to sphincter incontinence and complete motor and sensory paralysis of the lower extremities. This neurological picture was reversible, and function returned to a considerable extent when he was placed on his side in bed, but when placed in the supine position he worsened. Following an interval of supine recumbency, he developed persisting motor, sensory, and sphincter paralysis associated with "explosive" cutting pains in the legs, feet, and rectum. This state continued for 6 weeks until a lumbar laminectomy was performed by Dr. Harvey Cushing who found nothing other than narrowing of the bony canal at the lumbosacral level. Gradual improvement reportedly followed the surgery. In a 5-year period Dr. George Ehni encountered six instances of cauda equina palsy following anesthesia, with the patient in increased lumbar extension. A number of additional episodes of sphincter dysfunction and motor and sensory disturbances in the lower extremities have followed anesthesia (for abdominal, pelvic, or chest surgery) and have been reported mainly as presumed complications of spinal anesthesia. The various explanations, including root trauma from the lumbar puncture needle, neurolytic effects or occult actions of the anesthetic agent, inadvertent introduction of chemical contaminants, and infection, are some of the factors mentioned. In retrospect, a certain number of these problems may have resulted from acute compression of the cauda equina by hyperextension of the lumbar spine while the patient was under anesthesia.

Occasionally, a history of intermittent claudication, similar in certain respects to the vascular occlusive syndrome produced by painful contraction of anoxic muscle, is due to spondylitic changes affecting the cauda equina. Both types of intermittent claudication produce signs and symptoms that appear after the patient has walked a predictable distance, and they disappear when he has rested. There are certain differentiating characteristics that will enable the clinician to establish a proper diagnosis (Fig. 14-12).

The pain of anoxic muscle contractions characteristically occurs in the calves, and is the principal symptom associated with arterial insufficiency. Pain in cauda equina claudication may be absent but when present it has distinctly paresthetic qualities described as numbness, coldness, or burning. The location of the pain is in the lumbosacral or sciatic distribution.

Sensory deficits in arterial insufficiency are rare and when seen are peripheral, involving toes and feet. In cauda equina claudication numbness and paresthesia begin in the lumbar region and buttocks may remain confined to these areas, but often descend ein the distribution of the lower lumbar and sacral dermatomes. Or they may begin in the feet and ascend to the buttocks. Such a sensory "march" is common. Motor deficits are rare in arterial insufficiency, although during muscle anoxia the calf muscles often cramp and become tight. In cauda equina claudication, sensory symptoms precede motor dysfunction causing the patient to stop walking. If, however, he continues walking beyond the appearance of discomfort or paresthesias, the legs may become weak to the point of collapse.

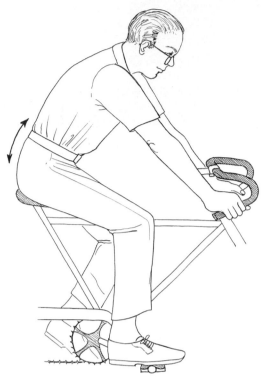

Fig. 14-12. The stationary exercise bicycle, available in most departments of physical medicine, is most helpful in differentiating vascular from cauda equina claudication. The patient with cauda equina claudication can pedal "endlessly" in a lumbar flexed position, but the vascular occulsive patient will develop painful muscle ischemia in a short time.

EXAMINATION

The physical examination in lumbar spondylosis with a stenotic lumbar spinal canal is often surprisingly unrevealing, despite intermittent cauda equina compression symptoms that are often severe. If a patient is examined immediately after such an episode, sensory deficits and loss of reflexes may be noted that will subside as the patient's symptoms disappear.

The diagnosis is tentatively made by careful history and physical examination, and measurements of the lumbar spine films, and confirmed by computerized axial tomography of the lumbar spine and myelography.

TREATMENT

The symptoms of lumbar spondylosis in the presence of a spinal canal of normal dimensions are almost always nonsurgical.

A combination of medications and exercise, as well as alteration in the mode of daily living, is usually adequate. A low back support is rarely necessary. (See Conservative Treatment, Chap. 6.)

The treatment of spondylosis in the presence of a stenotic spinal canal is a generous decompressive laminectomy and facetectomy.

Impacted Spinous Processes

An unusual source of osteoligamentous spinal pain is occasionally encountered when long-standing increased lumbar lordosis produces impaction or "kissing" of two of the spinous processes of the lumbar spine. This can occur at any lumbar level, and the site of impaction is generally the site of maximal pain (Fig. 14-13).

The exact cause of the pain is uncertain. There is speculation that a traumatic neuritis occurs of a branch of the posterior primary division of the spinal nerve which supplies the interspinous ligament and the surrounding soft tissues.[28]

Digital pressure between the spinous processes with the patient standing elicits pain; such tenderness is increased in hyperextension and decreased during flexion. Occasionally, a small cystlike mass can be palpated during hyperextension that disappears on flexion. The pain is frequently related to position, with lumbar flexion often affording relief.

Roentgenographically, lateral films of the lumbar spine will reveal a weight-bearing pseudoarthrosis between two lumbar spinous processes with contact sclerosis and sometimes visible "crumbling" at the point of contact.

If the pain is due to this condition, infiltration of the involved interspinous ligament with 1 or 2 cc of 1% lidocaine will alleviate the pain. If relief is obtained with the local anesthetic, the needle should be allowed to remain in place and then be utilized for a methylprednisolone acetate injection (Fig. 14-14). This may provide temporary improvement, but an exercise and postural correction program must be instituted for satisfactory long-term management of the lumbar lordosis associated with disc degeneration and segmental instability.

Achondroplasia and the Stenotic Lumbar Spinal Canal

The achondroplastic dwarf has been recognized as a distinct physical entity for centuries. There are many historic drawings and documents describing the typical physiognomy: large head, prominent forehead, extremely short arms and legs. Achondroplasia is a disease of unknown etiology which relates to a dysfunction involving endochrondral ossification. The condition is familial and occurs not only in humans but, by selective breeding, can be developed in animals. The dachshund and bassett hound, French bulldog, and the Pekingese are examples of achondroplastic dwarf forms created in dogs through selective breeding.

Abnormalities of the Spine

Many physicians are under the impression that from a neurological point of view achondroplasia is consistent with a normal life. However, abnormalities of the spine are a regular occurrence in this condition. In addition to the well-recognized increased lumbar lordosis, there are also changes produced in the individual vertebrae as well. There is a decrease in the height of the individual vertebral bodies, and it is this that accounts for the relative shortness of the entire spine. The pedicles are extremely short, particularly in the thoracic and lumbar region,

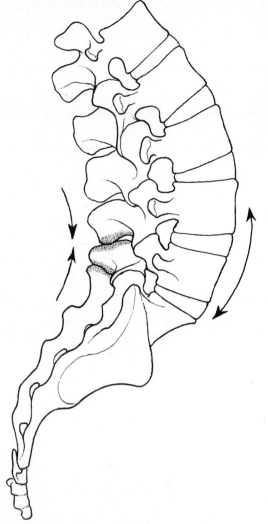

Fig. 14-13. *Impacted spinous processes.*

resulting from premature synostosis of the ossification centers of the vertebral body with those of the laminae; the laminae are almost in contact with the dorsum of the vertebral bodies. This results in a diminution of the AP diameter of the spinal canal. In addition to the AP diameter, there are changes in the transverse diameters of the lumbar vertebral bodies. Normally, the transverse diameters of the lumbar vertebrae increase slightly caudally, so that L5 is the widest of the lumbar vertebrae. In achondroplastic dwarfism there is a progressive terminal lumbar stenosis which is exactly opposite to that seen in the normal state. The vertebral canal is not only narrowed in the AP diameter but tapers progressively downward, narrowing also in the transverse diameter in the lower lumbar region.[5] The spinal cord, cauda equina, and conus medullaris are normal in width, so these changes in the size and configuration of the bony spine subject the neural elements to constriction.

SPINAL DEGENERATIVE CHANGES

It is rare for neurological changes in the thoracic or lumbar region to occur in childhood or early adulthood. However, since the spinal cord, cauda equina, and conus medullaris are normal in width, these elements fit very snugly into the small bony canal. Any encroachment on the lumen of the spinal canal or the intervertebral foramina has a constricting effect upon the cord and the spinal nerve roots.

The dorsolumbar segment of the achondroplastic spine is often unstable and may develop a dorsal kyphosis with large osteoarthritic spurs, as well as changes involving the articular processes. By the time an achondroplastic dwarf becomes an adult, his spinal canal is further compromised by marginal hypertrophic osteoarthritic spurring of the vertebral bodies and occasionally by protrusion of intervertebral discs.[6]

Signs and Symptoms

Degenerative changes of the lower lumbar region will cause low back pain and lower extremity paresthesia, particularly on standing. Motor dysfunction in the lower extremities, such as foot drop, may occur. If the compression is in the thoracolumbar region, a spastic paraparesis may develop with bladder and bowel disturbances. Usually such changes occur after the age of 40. Both the conus medullaris and the cauda equina also may be severely constricted after the age of 40, when osteoarthritic spurs and degenerative changes in the intervertebral discs develop. All of these encroach further upon the very snug spinal canal.[28]

Achondroplastic Dogs

The changes that are seen in human achondroplastic dwarfs are also seen in breeds of dogs that are typically achondroplastic. These dogs show an increased incidence of disc degeneration and will occasionally develop paraplegia with remissions and exacerbations. The highest incidence of disc protrusion in dogs is at the thoracolumbar interspace (the nineteenth interspace). The analogy between these occurrences and human achondroplasia is striking.[14]

Myelogram

As in all stenotic lumbar spinal canal syndromes, attempts at performing a lumbar puncture are often unsuccessful. Even though the puncture has been performed properly and the Pantopaque has been successfully deposited in the subarachnoid space, the space is often so narrow that free flow of the contrast material is not possible. The Pantopaque often puddles at each of the concavities of the bodies of the lumbar vertebrae, resulting in an erroneous interpretation of the myelogram as technically unsatisfactory and a subdural or extradural injection. Because of this, it may be necessary to introduce the Pantopaque from above, either by a cisternal puncture or through the lateral approach between C1 and C2.

The following case report is of interest for two reasons. In addition to describing the fairly typical history of a stenotic lumbar spinal canal syndrome presented by an achondroplastic dwarf, it provides a somewhat different concept regarding aggravation of preexisting stenotic lumbar canal symp-

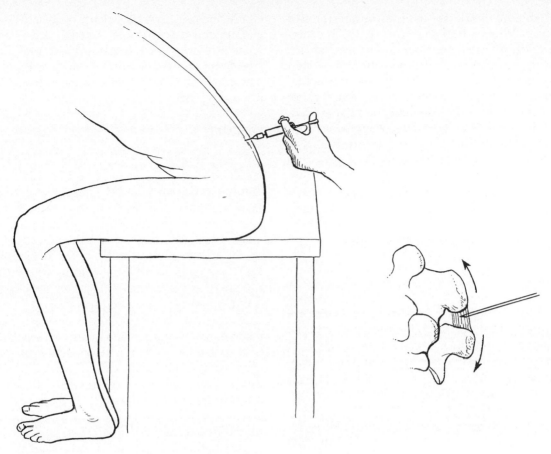

Fig. 14-14. Injection of interspinous ligament.

toms following myelography. It is generally believed that the worsening of symptoms is due to the technical difficulty of injecting Pantopaque into a diminished subarachnoid space, which is often smaller in dimension than the bevel of the lumbar puncture (LP) needle. Because of less than satisfactory flow of CSF through the LP needle, insertions at multiple levels are often attempted, each insertion being associated with pain or discomfort. Such direct nerve root trauma is undoubtedly responsible for some postmyelogram worsening of symptoms. In this case, however, the physician who originally managed the patient recognized the potential hazards of performing a lumbar puncture and took the precaution of injecting the Pantopaque by means of a cisternal puncture.

W.W. A 52-year-old achondroplastic dwarf had intermittent low back symptoms occasionally associated with right hip discomfort for 4 or 5 years. In 1972, he developed incapacitating cervical symptoms involving pain and motor weakness of the left upper extremity. A cervical myelogram was performed in July, 1972, by means of a cisternal tap and was followed by a decompressive cervical laminectomy which was beneficial in relieving the cervical symptoms. The Pantopaque, when allowed to flow into the lumbar area, revealed partial blocks at L1–2, L2–3, L3–4, and L4–5 levels. Immediately after the myelogram, the patient developed increased pain in the low back and both lower extremities which was intractable and incapacitating. He remained incapacitated because of his low back symptoms and was unable to work as an entertainer for 2–4 years. When I first saw him in 1975, examination revealed considerable muscle spasm in the lumbar area with poor lumbar mobility, normal reflexes, hypesthesia of much of the left lower extremity, normal motor power, and normal straight leg raising.

On April 28, 1975, a decompressive laminectomy of L1 to L5 was performed. Immediate improvement of the low back and bilateral leg pain followed. Although he continues to have intermittent low back symptoms, these are controlled with mild analgesic medication and exercises. He is able to pursue his career as an entertainer.

Treatment

The treatment of this condition is decompressive laminectomy. In some patients the changes found at surgery are so severe that despite adequate decompression, no clinical improvement will occur. In the face of such severe cauda equina constriction, favorable results will be derived from surgery only in the early stages of compression. A laminectomy should not only be wide but also extensive, involving at least two laminae above the site of the block and two below. In many cases a laminectomy of the entire lumbar spine and the first one or two thoracic laminae is necessary. If there is a protruded intervertebral disc, this should be excised at the time of the laminectomy.[1]

Paget's Disease of the Lumbar Spine (Osteitis Deformans)

Sir James Paget, the English Surgeon who first described this disease as a clinical entity in 1877, believed the bony changes were related to an inflammatory process. Because the chief clinical manifestation was the deforming nature of bony changes, he called the disease "osteitis deformans."[16] This condition, particularly in its milder forms, is fairly common, affecting approximately 3% of all persons over 40 years of age. It is a generalized disease, but it often affects the spine and may particularly involve the lumbar region producing lumbar and sciatic pain. The cause and mechanism of Paget's disease are unknown.

Pathology

The changes of Paget's disease are the result of a combination of both destructive and reparative processes. These changes are slowly progressive, starting in a solitary site and gradually extending to involve larger areas and more bones. The bones most commonly involved are the tibia, femur, pelvis, vertebrae, and skull. Aside from the skull, the greatest incidence is in bones subject to the most weight-bearing stress.

During the early and most active phase, resorption exceeds deposition. Deossification first occurs along the cortical surfaces, causing the bone to weaken and distort under pressure. Such distortion produces microfractures (infractions) of the cortex. Cortical demineralization is widely disseminated in patchy areas.

The osteolytic phase is followed by an osteosclerotic phase in which, in an attempt to repair the spongelike, weakened, and deformed bone, the balance swings in favor of deposition. Osteoblastic proliferation within the remaining cortex produces some bony replacement.

In response to the bony distortion and resulting cortical infractions, the periosteum lays down new bone to strengthen the weakened bone. This periosteal osteogenesis is additive, causing widening of the bone as a whole without decreasing the medullary volume. This added bone is very primitive. The involved areas of bone are extremely vascular and may even exhibit arteriovenous shunts.

MICROSCOPIC CHANGES

In normal bone, the outermost layer of the osteon (haversian canal with its lamellae) takes the hematoxylin stain more readily than surrounding tissue. When cut in cross-section, the result is a heavy blue line, called "the cement line," demarcating one osteon from its neighbor.

In Paget's disease, portions of osteons are irregularly eroded and to these areas of erosion, osteoblasts reparatively apply new osteoid in an erratic fashion. When cut in cross-section, an irregular mosaic pattern is seen. This typical mosaic pattern of alternating mature and immature bone, which was first described by Schmorl, is characteristic of fully developed Paget's disease.[19]

ROENTGENOGRAPHIC CHANGES

In general the roentgenographic changes reflect osteolysis and excessive repair, either alone or in combination, resulting in areas of radiolucency and opacity. Initially during the osteolytic phase, there is a demineralizing process which causes skeletal radiolucency, deformity, and a coarsening and prominence of the larger trabeculae in the line of weight bearing. The coarse trabeculations in affected vertebral bodies tend to be horizontal and to accentuate the margins of the body. Compression fractures are not uncommon; they result in narrowing of the vertebral body anteriorly. As the disease progresses, areas of density appear which may eventually overshadow the surrounding normal bone, resulting occasionally in almost homogenous opacity of a vertebral body.

Oblique views may reveal narrowing of the intervertebral foramina, resulting from bony thickening of the foraminal boundaries. Convex masses of partially calcified osteoid tissue frequently project beyond the vertebral bodies and displace the paraspinal shadow. These changes are seen best in the thoracic area.

MYELOGRAM

The myelogram reveals multilevel vertebral encorachment with narrowing of the subarachnoid space. There is usually bilateral and often anterior compression. Occasionally, the body of the vertebra is so distorted that the resulting deformity produces a marked angulation and dorsal displacement of the Pantopaque column, best seen on the cross-table lateral view. In some instances, this dorsal displacement is extensive enough to produce a complete block. The intervertebral discs remain intact, and the deformity is almost always centered over the midportion of the vertebral body rather than the disc.

Signs and Symptoms

Frequently, Paget's disease is limited to a solitary bone (monostatic osteitis deformans), is noted as an incidental x-ray film finding, and may remain asymptomatic throughout life. Those cases that are symptomatic usually are polyostatic (affecting numerous bones).

The characteristic clinical picture of mature Paget's disease is striking. Collapse of the anterior portions of the vertebral bodies causes a typical kyphosis of the thoracic spine which thrusts the head forward and downward. The femurs bend outward, producing bowing and accentuating the deformity by an outward and forward bowing of the tibias. The stature is shortened by these lower extremity curvatures. Softening of the sacrum and the iliac bones, in association with a coxa vara from softening of the femoral necks, results in a waddling gait. In severe cases, the ribs and sternum are involved, causing lateral flattening and increased anteroposterior diameter of the thorax. This thoracic deformity, together with the kyphosis, interferes with normal respiratory excursions and is often associated with dyspnea. The forward curvature of the spine causes the abdomen to protrude. The calvarium is much enlarged.

Despite the rather unique and grotesque characteristics of this disease, the onset is so insidious that both the patient and associates who observe him at close intervals do not usually become aware of the changes until the condition is far advanced. The patient may first be aware of this condition when his hat seems too small. As a rule, the gradually increasing disabilities and deformities are attributed to old age, and may be overlooked by family and physicians alike.

Periosteal bone formation may impinge upon the foramina of emerging cranial and spinal nerves and interfere with motor and sensory nerve function; it may also produce pain. Cardiac output is considerably elevated, and the impaired respiratory excursions may add to the increased workload of the heart. Cardiovascular disease is the most common cause of death in advanced generalized Paget's disease.

LABORATORY FINDINGS

The serum alkaline phosphate is always markedly elevated when the disease is disseminated but may be within normal limits when the disease is localized. Serum calcium is rarely elevated and serum phosphorus levels remain normal. Anemia is uncommon, despite considerable fibrosis in medullary hematopoietic areas.

Diagnosis

Patients suffering from Paget's disease involving the lumbar spine complain of pain in the low back area, the pain varying in intensity and character from a dull soreness to a most intense paroxysm. Some degree of pain is invariably present and, although activities such as heavy lifting, stooping, and bending tend to aggravate the pain somewhat, rest will not relieve the pain. In many cases, periods of prolonged immobility are associated with increased pain described as "severe stiffness of my back." The pain is frequently worse at night, preventing sleep. Unilateral or bilateral nerve root irritation is occasionally present. The root symptoms are presumed secondary to narrowing of the intervertebral foramina from subperiosteal deposition of bone. Although the back pain is usually constant, the nerve root pain is

generally intermittent, frequently related to activity and often eased with rest.

The localized periostitis over the anterior tibial areas produces exquisite pain which is aggravated by pressure over the affected bone. Severe and persisting cramps in both lower extremities are common. The anterortibial pain and calf cramps occasionally may be mistaken for root compression symptoms.

I have treated two cases of spinal cord compression secondary to Paget's disease of the spine, both of which involved the thoracic cord. Although osteitis deformans involves the lumbar spine more frequently than the dorsal spine, when cord compression occurs as the result of this condition it almost always develops in the dorsal region.[15,20] The probable explanation for this predilection is that the smallest cross-sectional area of the spinal canal is in the thoracic region. Therefore, any thickening of the bony vertebral ring would be more apt to manifest itself at this level.[2]

Cauda equina compression resulting from Paget's disease of the lumbar spine is quite rare. The only case I have personally encountered with cauda equina compression, involved sarcomatous degeneration of osteitis deformans.[11] It is estimated that 4% of all patients with symptomatic Paget's disease have superimposition of a malignant tumor, either osteosarcoma or fibrosarcoma, which occurs in an area previously affected by Paget's disease.[4,12,13,17,21,22,24]

Treatment

Significant advancements have been made in the treatment of this condition. Calcitonin, the polypeptide hormone of the C cells of the thyroid, has been effective in relieving the pain of active Paget's disease and in decreasing the vascularity of Pagetic bone. The commercially available forms are calcitonin, derived from the ultimobronchial glands of salmon, or synthetically prepared calcitonin. The drug reduces serum calcium by the reduction of osteoblast-mediated bone resorption. Following its use, reversal of paraparesis and paraplegia due to intraspinal compression of neural element from Pagetic bone has been seen to occur.

Calcitonin is administered subcutaneously in an initial dose of 100 M.R.C. units followed by a daily dose of 25 to 200 M.R.C. units. An improvement in bone chemistry is demonstrated with therapy, after which the elevated levels of serum alkaline phosphatase and hydroxyproline in the urine revert toward normal. Side-effects may include flushing, local erythema and tenderness, nausea, and swelling of hand and fingers. Secondary hyperparathyroidism may occur with long-term use.

Diphosphanates or disodium etidronate (EHDP) is effective in improving the clinical and biochemical abnormalities of Paget's disease and can be administered orally. Intermittent courses of 5 mg of EHDP/kg body weight/day for 6 months has the best risk to benefit ratio and is preferable to cintinuous therapy. Higher doses will produce greater biochemical improvement but are associated with increased side-effects.

If the neurological symptoms do not improve following a course of calcitonin or EHDP, theoretically there should be a decrease in the hypervascularity of the involved bone, which should facilitate subsequent surgical intervention. Long bone pain improves to a significantly higher degree than low back pain with these medications.

I have treated seven patients with radiculitis secondary to foraminal compression from Paget's disease. Three did reasonably well with bed rest and a low back support. Two improved with intrathecal instillation of methylprednisolone acetate. Two did not derive adequate relief with conservative measures and required foraminotomies.

With regard to surgical technique, greater than usual care is required in performing a subperiosteal paravertebral muscle dissection when the underlying laminae are involved by Paget's disease. Direct downward pressure with the periosteal elevators may fracture a softened lamina and damage the underlying neural elements.

Following the subperiosteal paravertebral muscle dissection, the lumbar laminae and spinous processes may often appear as a single monolithic sheath of bone. Certainly, the anatomy will be sufficiently distorted to make precise localization uncertain. A cross table "marker film" with an instrument at the site of the presumed involved interspace is often most helpful in localization.

There is an increase in vascular attachments between the paraspinal muscles and diseased lamina. The blood flow through bone affected by osteitis deformans has been measured and found to be increased many times over that of normal bone. This observation is well confirmed by the difficulties in achieving adequate hemostasis during the performance of a laminectomy.

References

1. Alexander E Jr.: Achondroplasia (Significance of the small lumbar spinal canal). J Neurosurg 31:513, 1961
2. Amyes EW, Vogel PN: Osteitis deformans (Paget's disease) of the spine with compression of the spinal cord: Report of three cases and discussion of the surgical problems. Bull Los Angeles Neurol Soc 19:18, 1954
3. Armstrong JR: Lumbar Disc Lesions; Pathogenesis and Treatment of Low Back Pain and Sciatica. Edinburgh E, S Livingstone, Ltd, 1965
4. Bird CE: Sarcoma complicating Paget's disease of the bone: Report of 9 cases, 5 with pathologic verification. Arch Surg 14:1187, 1927
5. Caffey J: Achondroplasia of pelvis and lumbosacral spine. Some roentgenographic features. Am J Roentgenol 80:449, 1958
6. Duvorsin RC, Yahr MD: Compressive spinal cord and root syndromes in achondroplastic dwarfs. Neurology 12:202, 1962
7. Ehni G, Clark K, Wilson CB, Alexander E: Significance of the small lumbar spinal canal (5 parts), J Neurosurg 31:490, 1969
8. Elsberg CA: Experiences in spinal surgery. Observations upon 60 laminectomies for spinal disease. Surg Gynecol Obstet 16:117, 1913
9. Epstein JA: Diagnosis and treatment of painful neurological disorders caused by spondylosis of the lumbar spine. J Neurosurg 17:991, 1960

10. Epstein JA, Epstein BS, Levine L: Nerve root compression associated with narrowing of the lumbar spinal canal. J Neurol Neurosurg Psychiatry 25:165, 1962
11. Finneson, BE, Goluboff B, Shenkin HA: Sarcomatous degeneration of osteitis deformans causing compression of the cauda equina. Neurology 8:82, 1958
12. Geschickter CF, Copeland MM: Tumors of Bone. ed. 3. Philadelphia, JB Lippincott Co., 1949
13. Gruner OC, Scringer F.A.C, Foster LS: A clinical and histological study of a case of Paget's disease of the bones with multiple sarcoma formation. Arch Intern Med 9:641, 1912
14. Hoelein BF: Canine neurology: Diagnosis and Treatment. Philadelphia and London, WB Saunders, 1965
15. Latimer FR, Webster JE, Guardjian ES: Osteitis deformans with spinal cord compression: Report of three cases. J Neurosurg 10:583, 1953
16. Paget J: On a form of chronic inflammation of bones (osteitis deformans). Med Chir Tr 60:37, 1877. Also reprinted in Med Classics 1:29, 1936
17. Sachs B, Fraenkel J: Progressive ankylotic rigidity of the spine. J Nerve Ment Dis 27:1, 1900
18. Sarpyener MA: Spina bifida aperta and congenital stricture of the spinal canal. J Bone Joint Surg 29:817, 1947
19. Schmorl G: Ueber Ostitis Deformans Paget. Arch Path Anat 283:694, 1932
20. Schwarz GA, Reback S: Compression of the spinal cord in osteitis deformans (Paget's disease) of the vertebrae. Am J Roentgenol 42:345, 1939
21. Sear HR: Some notes on diagnosis of bone tumors. Brit Med J 1:49, 1936
22. Sear HR: Osteogenic sarcoma as a complication of osteitis deformans. Brit J Radiol 22:580, 1949
23. Sherman RS, Soong KY: A roentgen study of osteogenic sarcoma developing in Paget's disease. Radiology 63:48, 1954
24. Summey TJ, Pressly CL: Sarcoma complicating Paget's disease of bone. Am J Surg 123:135, 1946
25. Verbiest H: Sur certaines formes rares de compression de la queue de cheval. Hommage a Clovis Vincent. Paris: Maloiue, 161, 1949
26. Verbiest H: A radicular syndrome from developmental narrowing of the lumbar vertebral canal. J Bone Joint Surg 26B:230, 1954
27. Verbiest H: Further experiences on the pathological influence of a development narrowness of the bony lumbar vertebral canal. J Bone Joint Surg 37B:576, 1955
28. Vogl A: The fate of the achondroplastic dwarf (Neurologic complications and achondroplasia). Exp Med Surg 20:108, 1962
29. Williams PC: The Lumbosacral Spine. New York, McGraw-Hill, 1965

Spondylolisthesis and Its Treatment 15

Leon L. Wiltse

Few conditions have fascinated the surgeon as has spondylolisthesis. Literally thousands of articles have been written on the subject, and still scarcely a week goes by without a new one appearing in the world literature. In 1782 Herbinaux, a Belgian obstetrician, noted that there were times when a bony prominence in front of the sacrum caused problems in delivery. He is generally credited with having first described spondylolisthesis, probably the complete type in which the body of L5 is actually lying in front of the sacrum (in other words, "spondyloptosis").[26]

Spondylolisthesis is the slipping of all or part of one vertebra forward on another. The term, coined by Kilian in 1854, is derived from the Greek "spondylos" meaning vertebra, and "olisthesis" meaning to slip.[32] Kilian did not recognize the defect in the pars but believed the lesion to be caused by a slow subluxation of the lumbosacral facets. One year later Robert of Koblenz established the location of the fundamental lesion of the isthmic type to be in the pars interarticularis, but he did not recognize the nature of the defect.[53] Lambi demonstrated the lesion in the pars in 1855.[33] Neugebauer in 1881 made an extensive study of anatomic specimens throughout Europe and was the first to recognize that slip can occur by elongation of the pars without their coming apart.[41] He did confuse the degenerative type with the isthmic type.

The types of this condition are as varied as its causes. The type of most clinical importance in persons under the age of 50 is the one in which the lesion is in the isthmus or pars interarticularis. However, there are several other conditions that permit forward slip of one vertebra on another. This discussion will be limited to the lumbar spine, except to note that the disease does occur in the cervical spine and that a few reports of pars defects in the thoracic spine have been published. However, these are so rare as to be of little importance. The classification of spondylolisthesis is both anatomic and etiologic.

Classification of Spondylolisthesis

The following classification of spondylolisthesis and spondylolysis has been derived from previous ones published by various authors.[36,44,67]

I. Dysplastic (congenital). In this type congenital abnormalities of the upper sacrum or the arch of L5 permit the olisthesis to occur.

II. Isthmic. The lesion is in the pars interarticularis. Three types can be recognized.

A. Lytic: fatigue fracture of the pars

B. Elongated but intact pars

C. Acute fracture of the pars (not to be confused with "traumatic"; see IV)

451

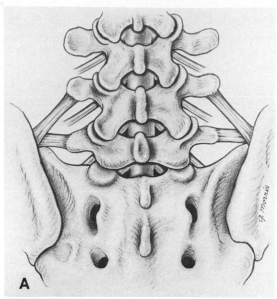

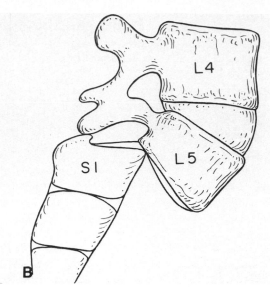

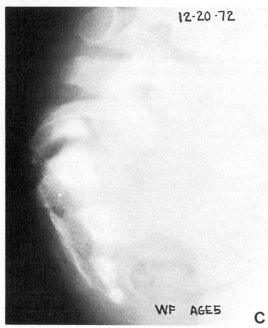

*Fig. 15-1. Dysplasia (congenital spondylolisthesis). **(A)** Congenital spondylolisthesis. Note inadequate superior articular processes of sacrum. **(B)** Lateral drawing of dysplastic spondylolisthesis. **(C)** Lateral radiograph of patient with dysplastic spondylolisthesis. Pars are not really elongated but the deformity of the inferior articular processes of L5 gives that impression. (Wiltse L: Common problems of the lumbar spine: Spondylolisthesis and its treatment. Jr Cont Educ Ortho July, 1979)*

III. Degenerative, due to long-standing intersegmental instability

IV. Post-traumatic, due to fractures in areas of the bony hook other than the pars

V. Pathologic: generalized or localized bone disease

Dysplastic Spondylolisthesis

In this type there is congenital dysplasia of the upper sacrum or the neural arch of L5. Because of this dysplasia, there is insufficient strength to withstand the forward thrust, and the last free lumbar vertebra gradually slips forward on the one below. The pars interarticularis may remain unchanged (Fig. 15-1). If it remains completely unchanged and the ring is intact, slip cannot exceed more than about 35% or there will be too much pressure on the cauda equina.

It is the author's impression that this type is most likely to produce tight hamstrings

(Fig. 15-2). However, usually the pars interarticularis either elongates or comes apart. If it elongates, it is very difficult roentgenographically to distinguish the dysplastic type from Type II, Subtype B. If it separates, it may be impossible to distinguish from Type II, Subtype A; but, if exposed at operation the abnormal relationship and subluxation of the facets will be apparent in the dysplastic type.

Fundamental to this type is that S1 or L5 has congenital changes of such a nature that the joint is incapable of withstanding the forward thrust of the body weight above. The pars interarticularis in these patients is often rather poorly developed to begin with, predisposing it to cracking and separating.

Often there is a wide-open sacrum and the L5 vertebra will show wide spina bifida. In a study by Wynne-Davies and Scott,[72] eleven of twelve patients with a dysplastic lesion had either spina bifida occulta or segmental defects in the lumbosacral area, and often both were present. There are no large series indicating the sex ratio between male and female, but in the Wynne-Davies and Scott series, there were seven males and five females (sex ratio 1.4) in the dysplastic group.[72]

There is a strong genetic element to the dysplastic type of spondylolisthesis. In the dysplastic type one in three relatives will be affected (33%), according to the study by Wynne-Davies and Scott.[72]

Isthmic Spondylolisthesis

The basic lesion in this type is in the pars interarticularis. Secondary changes (*e.g.*, alteration in the shape of the body of L5) may occur, but these are not fundamental to its etiology.[68]

Subtype A, Lytic. Lytic spondylolisthesis is due to separation or dissolution of the pars. It is always a fatigue fracture and is the most common type below age 50.[68] Statistically it is seldom seen in patients below age 5, but it does occasionally occur. The author's youngest patient having an unques-

tioned lesion of the pars was only age 8 months when the lesion was first discovered.[65] This child's father also had the same lesion. Kleiger[6] reported a patient in whom the lesion was first discovered when the child was only age 4 months.

If a group of 100 children of age 5 were to be studied roentgenographically, there probably would not be one with pars defects. However, if the same children were examined toward the end of the first grade (in other words, approaching age 7), the incidence would be around 4.4%, which is just slightly below the national average.[56] Baker performed a study such as this.[4] He was also able to examine the same group roentgenographically when they were approaching adulthood. He found that the incidence had increased 1.4% by the time the group reached age 18. Most of this increase occurred between ages 11 and 16, the time of life when boys and girls are engaging in the very strenuous athletics which produce fatigue fractures (Fig. 15-3).

Just why the age period 5.5 to 7 is the one during which the lesion appears so frequently is not well known. One might postulate that it is because this is the age when children start school and begin to push each other and tumble about, or that for the first time they sit for long periods with a lordotic posture. However, neither seems an adequate explanation.

It is not known whether fracture in the pars is due to flexion or extension stresses. (It is probably due to both plus torsional stresses.) There is considerable controversy concerning this point. It is known that the fracture never occurs in animals below man, and only man has true lordosis.[15,28,58,63] There is a strong hereditary component in the etiology of this type.[5,73] In the study by Wynne-Davies and Scott, 14.9% of the close relatives of patients with isthmic spondylolisthesis had the defect. Table 15-1 is from their article.

Subtype B. Elongation of the pars without separation is fundamentally the same disease as Subtype A. It is secondary to repeated

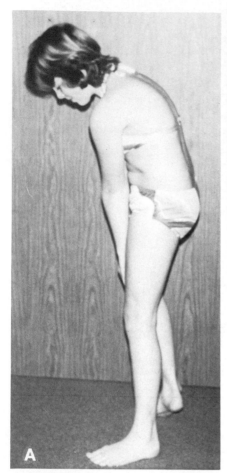

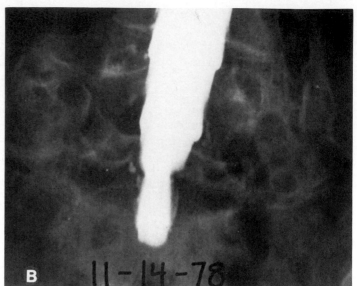

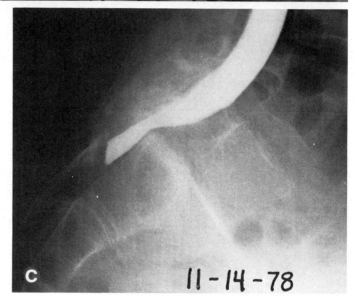

Fig. 15-2. A picture of a child with congenital spondylolisthesis with relatively small amount of slip. **(A)** Extremely tight hamstrings even 8 months post bilateral one-level L5–S1 fusion done through a paraspinal approach. **(B)** AP myelogram taken 6 months post fusion. Note the cauda equina is choked off but not severely so, and far less than many. **(C)** Lateral myelogram 6 months post fusion. (Continued opposite page)

microfractures which allow the pars to heal in a somewhat elongated position as the body of L5 slides forward. The author has x-rayed all available members of five families in which the probands had an elongated but intact pars, while several other members of each of their immediate families had typical spondylolysis or spondylolisthesis with the classic pars defect seen in Subtype A (Fig 15-4).[68]

The pars may remain in continuity as it elongates, or it may thin out and finally separate, leaving stumps with a combined length much greater than that of a normal pars. When this separation occurs, the lesion is reclassified to Type II, Subtype A, since it

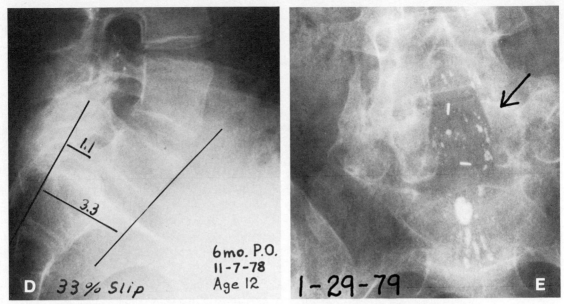

Fig. 15-2 (Continued). **(D)** *Lateral roentgenogram. Note slip is only 33%. The very severe tightness of the hamstrings must be because there is no defect in the pars.* **(E)** *A midline decompression was done and the tight hamstrings began to disappear within a few weeks and now a year later are nearly gone.*

cannot be differentiated from this subtype. The fundamental disease is the same.

Subtype C, Acute Pars Fractures. These are always secondary to severe trauma and are extremely rare.[66] In the author's total experience he has not seen more than three cases. Olisthesis may be present but more frequently there are pars fractures with spondylolysis only.

To sum up, in the types presented so far, there is no doubt that a lumbosacral midline lesion or other segmental defect in the lower lumbar spine is common among individuals with spondylolysis or spondylolisthesis. However, since this is not associated with an increased family incidence of neural tube defects and the two are not etiologically related, it seems probable that there is a genetic element to both the dysplastic and isthmic types of spondylolisthesis.[72] As of this writing, the pattern of inheritance is not known for certain. Haukipuro and colleagues feel that the pattern is definitely due to a dominant gene; so do Amusco and Mankin.[1,24] Wynne-Davies and Scott believe

Table 15-1.   PROPORTIONS OF FIRST-DEGREE RELATIVES WITH SPONDYLOLSIS OR SPONDYLOLISTHESIS

Patients	Parents	Siblings	Children	Total	Percent
12 Dysplastic type	6 of 18	2 of 12	3 of 3	11 of 33	(33.0%)
35 Isthmic	5 of 32	7 of 51	5 of 31	17 of 114	(14.9%)
47 Total	11 of 50	9 of 63	8 of 34	28 of 147	(19.0%)
	(22.0%)	(14.32%)	(23.5%)		

(Wynne-Davies, Scott, JHW: Inheritance and spondylolisthesis, a radiographic family survey. Jr Bone Jt Surg 61B(3), 1979)

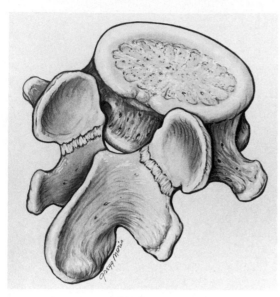

Fig. 15-3. Drawing showing the defect is isthmic spondylolysis, classification IIA. (Ruge D, Wiltse LL: Spondylolisthesis and its treatment: Conservative treatment, fusion with and without reduction. In Spinal Disorders—Diagnosis and Treatment. Lea & Febiger, Philadelphia, 1977.)

it lies between autosomal dominant inheritance with reduced penetrance, and multifactorial inheritance.

From our own studies done in the 1950s, we felt the pattern of inheritance was due to a recessive gene with incomplete penetrance, but in some families the gene involved showed incomplete dominance in that some affected individuals are carriers (heterozygous) for the gene.

Degenerative Spondylolisthesis[30,37,42]

The degenerative lesion is due to long-standing intersegmental instability. There is remodeling of the articular processes at the level of involvement (Fig. 15-5). It is the belief of Farfan that there are multiple small compression fractures of the inferior articular processes of the vertebra that slip forward.[15] Because of this, the bone of the articular processes has a peculiar appearance grossly resembling the bone in Paget's disease. As the slip progresses, the articular processes change direction and become more horizontal. One side virtually always slips down more than the other, and rotation at the level of olisthesis is an integral characteristic.

In the patients who come to the doctor with clinical symptoms, degenerative spondylolisthesis occurs six times as frequently in females as in males, six to nine times more frequently at the L4 interspace than at adjoining levels, and four times more frequently when the L5 is sacralized than when it is not.[54] When the lesion is at L4, the L5 vertebra is more stable and in less lordosis than average. The author has not seen this lesion in any patient under age 40.

Slipping never seems to exceed 33% unless there has been surgical intervention. The predisposing factor is thought to be a straight, stable lumbosacral joint which sits high between the ilia. This arrangement puts increased stress on the joint between L4 and L5, leading to decompensation of the ligaments, hypermobility and degeneration at the articular processes, and multiple microfractures of the inferior articular processes of L4, allowing forward slipping.[54]

Post-traumatic Spondylolisthesis

The post-traumatic type is secondary to an acute injury which fractures some part of the supporting bone other than the pars, and allows forward slip of the upper vertebra on the one below as a secondary phenomenon. This is unlike the acute isthmic fracture in that an isolated pars fracture is not present (Fig. 15-6).

This type of spondylolisthesis is always due to severe trauma. Essential to this type is that the slip occurs gradually. It is not an acute fracture dislocation. This type is fairly rare, I see about one new case a year. Fractures have also been reported in the pedicle of the lumbar vertebrae which permit spondylolisthesis.[48,62]

Pathologic Spondylolisthesis

Because of local or generalized bone disease, the bony hook mechanism (consisting of the pedicle, the pars, the superior and inferior articular processes) fails to hold the forward thrust of the superincumbent body weight, and forward slip of a vertebra onto the one below occurs. It is a rare type and is of little importance. It is included here only for completeness.

Generalized. In this type there are widespread generalized bony changes as in the following examples:

1. Albers-Schoenberg disease. In this condition fractures of the pars are frequent. These sometimes heal and refracture. Spondylolysis occurs and often spondylolisthesis.[50]
2. Arthrogryposis. In a type of arthrogryposis called Kuskokwim disease, several pedicles (but L5 in particular) may be elongated producing spondylolisthesis of L5 on S1 (Fig. 15-7).[49]
3. Paget's disease. Patients have been seen in whom one pair of pedicles has become elongated, allowing the related vertebral body to assume a forward position on the one below.
4. Syphilitic disease. Spondylolisthesis in the lumbar spone secondary to syphilitic gummas of the articular processes has been reported by Karaharjii.[31]

Localized. *Spondylolysis or Spondylolisthesis Adquisita.*[2,23,64] In this type of spondylolisthesis there is a fracture of the pars at the upper end of a lumbar spinal fusion. This is a fatigue fracture, but other factors (*e.g.*, injury to the pars when doing the fusion, or interference with the venous drainage of the area of the pars caused by stripping of the tissue) may contribute to the etiology. So we place this type under "pathologic," but a good argument could be made that it is simply a stress fracture of the pars due to the increased stress resulting from the long lever arm. This type is not seen if a lateral mass fusion is done, and as a result it is now virtually nonexistent.

Treatment of the Various Types of Spondylolisthesis in Children

In children the principal types of spondylolisthesis which will be encountered are the dysplastic and isthmic types. Treatment can usually be conservative. However, if symptoms persist, surgery should be done. Generally speaking, persistent symptoms in a child will require surgery more often than the same symptoms in an adult. The reason is that symptoms appearing so early in life as this mean a great many years of trouble for the child and at an age when he wishes to engage in the more strenuous activities usual for children and young adults. The older a person is when symptoms begin, the more likely that he will be satisfied to cut down his activities and live with his discomfort without resorting to surgery.

Before deciding upon surgery, it is important to allow several months to elapse after the onset of symptoms to see if the symptoms will disappear spontaneously. Also, the back symptoms may be caused by something else (*e.g.*, intervertebral disc disease), the spondylolisthesis or spondylolysis being only an incidental finding.

The pattern of olisthesis is different in different children. In the young athlete with spondylolysis or spondylolisthesis, no more than first-degree slip is the rule. Only rarely do these children have more. I have seen one case, a 13-year-old boy who developed a stress fracture in the pars and slipped to 50% by age 15 (Fig. 15-8). Sagittal rotation such as this has been called "roll" by Newman and Fitzgerald, and "slip angle" by Boxall and associates.[7] Then there is the child, usually between ages 9 and 13 when first seen (but maybe as young as age 5), who has a very high degree of slip. These can be

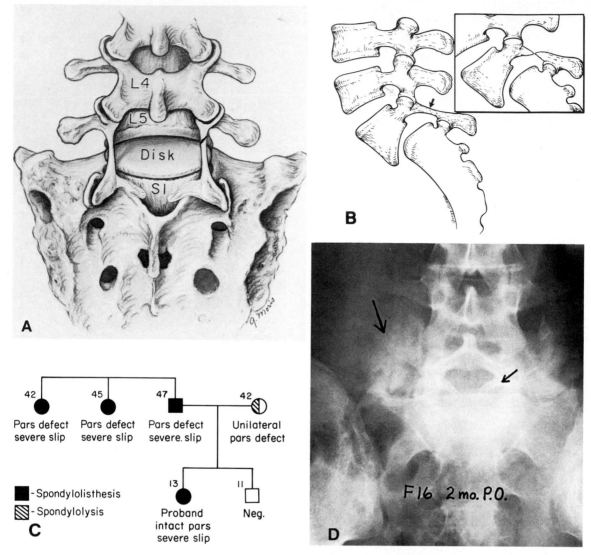

Fig. 15-4. Elongated by intact pars (IIB in classification). **(A)** Drawing made at surgery of elongated but intact pars. On the right, the right pars has cracked through and the left has elongated but remained intact. It might have healed even if the fusion had not been done. **(B)** Lateral drawing of type IIB. The pars may stretch for years and then crack and come apart. (Ruge D, Wiltse LL: Spondylolisthesis and its treatment: Conservative treatment, fusion with and without reduction. In Spinal Disorders—Diagnosis and Treatment. Lea & Febiger, Philadelphia, 1977). **(C)** Family of one of the author's patients with elongated but intact pars. Only the proband had elongated but intact pars. All others had typical type IIA lesions in the pars. (Wiltse LL, Newman PM, Macnab I: Classification of spondylolysis and spondylolisthesis. Clin Orthop 116, 1976). **(D)** AP radiograph post fusion of the drawing in A. (Continued opposite page).

either the dysplastic or the isthmic type. These children usually have the typical spondylolisthesis build: short torso and flat buttocks (Fig. 15-9). This particular shape of the buttocks arises from the fact that the sacrum is vertical rather than at the normal 42 or 43 degrees from the horizontal. These children walk with a peculiar "spastic" gait

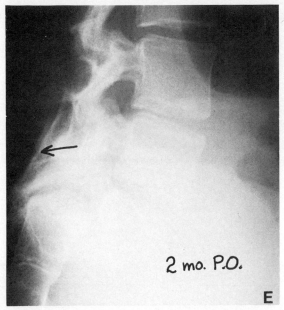

2 mo. P.O.

E

Fig. 15-4. (Continued) *(E) Lateral roentgenograph post fusion of the patient represented in B.*

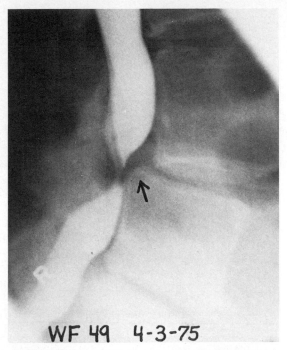

WF 49   4-3-75

Fig. 15-5. Lateral myelogram of a patient with degenerative spondylolisthesis. (Wiltse L: Common problems of the lumbar spine: Spondylolisthesis and its treatment. J Cont Educ Orthop July, 1979)

owing either to stretching or to pressure on the nerves of the cauda equina as the nerves pass over the top of the sacrum. Also the L5 nerve root may be compressed between the proximal stump of the pars or the base of the transverse processes of L5 and the body and ala of S1. These cases with high-grade slip are not common in the general population. Orthopedists see them relatively often, because the problem is so striking that the pediatrician or family physician immediately refers these children to a specialist. These also are the children who are most often symptomatic.

The author has observed patients in whom the L5 nerve roots were compressed to thin ribbons between the distal ends of the proximal stumps of the pars of L5 and the body of the sacrum. Compression can occur to the other components of the cauda equine (*i.e.,* the S1, S2, S3 spinal nerve roots which also innervate the hamstrings), but these nerves are compressed by the lamina of L5 as they pass over the top of the sacrum.[18] Gill has reported a case with high-grade slip where the traction was great enough to pull

one of the sacral nerves apart. A nerve can function normally and still be reduced by compression to 25% of its normal size when the compression occurs slowly, but beyond this some reflex and sensory changes are likely to occur.[14] The hamstrings function well and usually show no electromyographic changes, yet are in enough spasm to contribute to the peculiar gait.

Another reason for this peculiar gait is that the pelvis is held in such an extremely flexed position that the hips have reached the limit of their extension and still are not in a stright line with the trunk. Notice in Figure 15-10 that the sacrum is in a vertical position. A line drawn across the top of the body of S1 would be nearly horizontal instead of 42 or 43 degrees from the horizontal as is normal for an adult. That means that the pelvis is flexed 42 or 43 degrees. Most people are unable to extend their hips to that extent.

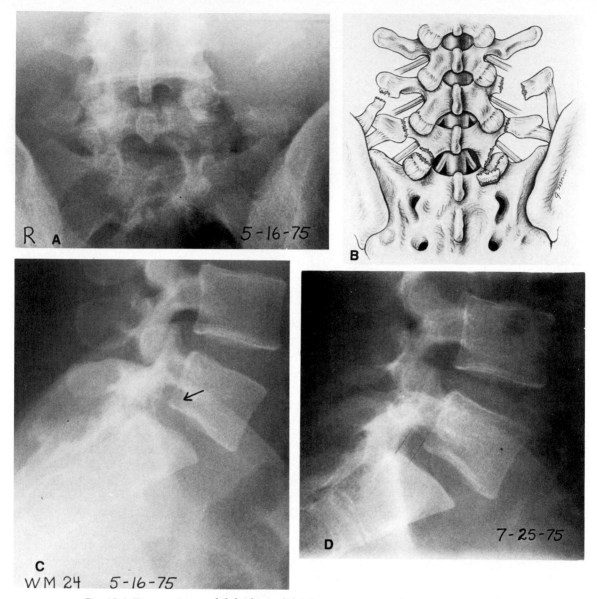

Fig. 15-6. Traumatic spondylolisthesis. *(A) AP roentgenogram of a man age 25 in whom spondylolisthesis (type IV in classification) developed. He had been in a severe auto accident 2 weeks previously. Note fracture of the transverse processes and the articular processes. (B) Drawing of the fracture shown in A. (C) Lateral x-ray film of the same patient taken 14 days post injury. Note minimal slip of L5 on S1. (D) Lateral roentgenogram of patient shown in A, taken 14 days post surgery. Note olisthesis is progressing. (Continued opposite page)*

These children often have functional scoliosis, the so-called "sciatic scoliosis."[52] This is secondary to muscle spasm produced by irritation of the neural elements due to pressure or traction. It may also be due to the fact that the L5 vertebra slips forward asymmetrically causing curvature in the lower lumbar spine. Later this becomes structural scoliosis.

In the author's series there were just about

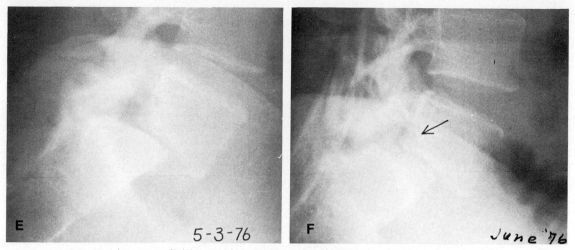

5-3-76

June '76

*Fig. 15-6 (Continued) **(E)** Lateral x-ray film 1 year post injury. Note fairly severe slip. This progressive slip is typical of traumatic spondylolisthesis. **(F)** A bilateral lateral fusion was done through the paraspinal approach, stopping further slip. The patient was allowed up immediately post operation, but a standing spot lateral roentgenogram was taken at frequent intervals to watch for further olisthesis.*

twice as many girls with this high-grade slip as there were boys, an interesting statistic inasmuch as the overall incidence of isthmic defects is just about twice as high in boys as in girls. It may be, however, that these patients with severe hamstring spasm are mostly of the congenital type where the incidence is more nearly the same in the sexes.[72]

In most instances with even high grades of slip, the parents haven't been aware of the child's unusual appearance, and it has often been called to their attention by the school nurse or the gymnasium teacher. The fact that the slipping of these vertebrae is so seldom detected early points to the importance of close observation of children with spondylolisthesis.

When the child with pars defects is first seen, a standing spot lateral roentgenogram of the lumbosacral joint should be taken. If surgery is not resorted to, the same type of x-ray is repeated at 4-month intervals in order to detect further slip. Once all growth has been obtained, no additional slip is likely to occur and no further roentgenograms are necessary.

The risk factors as regards the likelihood of further slip are as follows, to quote Boxall

and associates.[7] When these are present, it behooves the surgeon to watch the child very carefully and to do a fusion if in doubt.

Age: the younger the child, the more risk of further olisthesis. Once growth stops, further slip is unlikely but should be watched for another few years.

Sex: girls have at least four times the likelihood of developing severe slip as do boys.

Presence of spina bifida: this increases the likelihood of further slip.

Wedging of L5: the so-called trapezoidal L5 body is a bad prognostic sign. The percentage of wedging is determined by the method of Laurent and Einola and represents the trapezoidal shape of the body of the olisthetic L5 vertebral body (Fig. 15-11)[34] It is calculated as:

$$\frac{\text{Posterior height of body of L5}}{\text{Anterior height of body of L5}} \times 100$$

$$= \% \text{ of wedging of L5}$$

Erosion of the anterior portion of S1: this has been called the "superior sacral contour" by Boxall and colleagues. If it is severely changed and rounded off starting far posterior, this is a bad prognostic sign.[7]

Diminished anteroposterior dimension of S1: in the series of Boxall and associates, patients with a very high-grade slip (grade V) nearly all

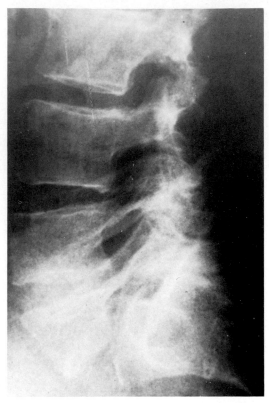

Fig. 15-7. Roentgenogram in Kuskokwim disease. Note elongated pedicle of lower three lumbar vertebrae (Courtesy Dr. Gilbert Wright, Sacramento, CA, 1970)

had significant narrowing of the anterior posterior dimension of the body of S1.[7]

Increased lumbar lordosis: a very high grade of lumbar lordosis (*i.e.*, the angle between the top of L5 and the top of the first level vertebra) goes along with a high grade of slip. It may be questioned if this portends increased olisthesis or is simply a result of increased slip.

Measuring the percent of olisthesis: Figure 15-12 shows our method of measuring the percentage of olisthesis. We prefer to use the widest point of S1. The top of S1 is often rounded, so we choose the widest point. The amount of slip is divided by the width of S1, and this gives us the percent of olisthesis. The lines drawn to measure the percent of slip are at right angles to the line along the back of the body of S1.

Sagittal rotation: this has been called roll and also slip angle.[7,17] As L5 slides forward it rolls or undergoes sagittal rotation (Fig. 15-13).

Superior sacral contour (Fig. 15-14): Boxall and colleagues have divided the top of S1 into four parts according to Meyerding's classification.[7] If the erosion starts half way back, this would be a No. 2 contour; three-fourths of the way back would be a No. 3 contour. The further back the rounding starts, the poorer the prognosis as regards the likelihood of further slip.

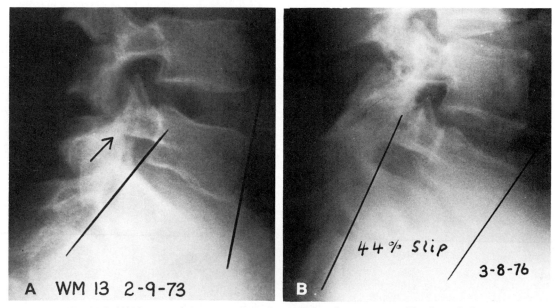

Fig. 15-8. (A) Note crack in pars on lateral x-ray film. This was missed by the radiologist. Note how L5 rolls around the top of the sacrum as it slips forward. (B) Two years later, 44% slip has occurred.

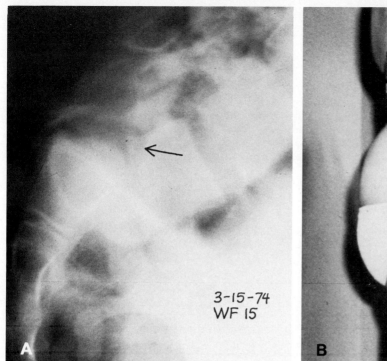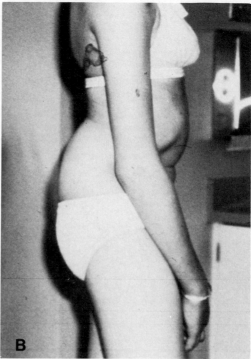

3-15-74
WF 15

Fig. 15-9. **(A)** *Lateral roentgenograph of a girl age 15 with at least 50% slip of L5 on S1.* **(B)** *Lateral photograph of the child whose x-ray film is shown in A. Note flat buttocks and short torso typical of this condition.*

SURGICAL TREATMENT IN THE CHILD

If conservative therapy (consisting of time, routine back care, abdominal strengthening exercises, and perhaps a corset) does not bring about cessation of pain, spinal fusion is indicated. Persistent symptoms in the child require operation in a much higher percentage than in adults. The author also believes that the child should undergo a fusion procedure if the olisthesis is progressing, even a small amount.

A child can often have a surprising amount of olisthesis of L5 and S1 without much change in appearance. Figure 15-15 shows such a child.

Following are the basic differences between the child with spondylolisthesis and the adult, and hence the reasons operation may be more imperative in the child.

1. Further olisthesis may occur in the child but rarely in the adult.

2. Solid arthrodesis is effected more readily in the child than in the adult.

3. The child has a great many years ahead of him and it is too much to expect that he cut down his activities indefinitely.

4. For reasons not entirely clear, the subjective results, that is, relief of pain after operation are very much better in the child than in the adult.

5. The adult can and often is willing to cut down on his activities and live with his pain to avoid surgery.

If symptoms persist for more than 8 months in the child, we do a fusion. In the child who has principally back pain, a one-level fusion through the paraspinal approach without decompression is indicated. If he has severe one-sided leg pain with neurologic

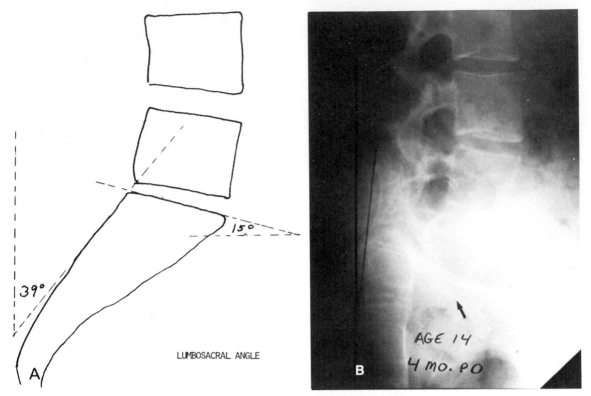

LUMBOSACRAL ANGLE

Fig. 15-10. **(A)** *In measuring the lumbosacral angle (sacral inclination) in spondylolis-thesis, a line is drawn along the back of the body of S1 and this is compared with a vertical line. This may give quite a different figure than a line drawn across the top of the body of S1 as is usually done. We must use the back of the body of S1 because the top of S1 has such a marked change of contour that a satisfactory reference line cannot be drawn. This drawing is from an actual x-ray film of a patient with degenerative disc disease.* **(B)** *The line drawn on the back of S1 shows the lumbosacral angle to be very small, 4°. However, this child has a high grade of lumbar lordosis.* **(C)** *Method of calculating lumbar lordosis. The fronts of the bodies are chosen as points to draw the reference because they are less prone to variation than are the tops of the vertebral bodies.* **(D)** *Note on same lateral as B above that the lumbar lordosis is 47° but the sacral inclination is 4°.*

changes, unilateral decompression is occasionally done. In recent years I have simply fused *in situ* without decompression, even in the child with leg pain and neurologic change. So far, all have returned to neurological normalcy over a period of months. In the rare case where nerve decompression is done, it is the author's practice to preserve as much of the lamina as possible and always to fuse the loose element to the sacrum while leaving the spinous processes in place and the interspinous and supraspinous ligaments intact (see the paraspinal approach in the following pages).

It has not been necessary to keep these patients flat postfusion except for those with very tight hamstrings. In the latter instance, they are kept supine for a few weeks so the hamstrings will settle down. Even in the child with high grade slip who has tight hamstrings, the paraspinal approach is used, leaving the loose element in place. If the olisthesis is progressing rapidly at the time of fusion, we keep the child in bed for 8 to 10 weeks as a precaution against further slip.

In the child with severe bladder or bowel symptoms, decompression is achieved by removing the loose element and removing the laminae of L4 as well as possibly also removing the posterior superior corner of

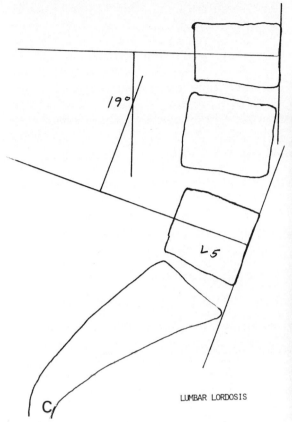

LUMBAR LORDOSIS

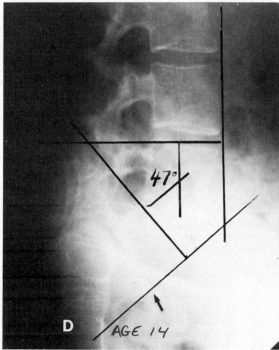

the sacrum. These children must be kept flat for 3 or 4 months post operation to prevent further slip. Fusion would be postponed to a later date. This has been extremely rare in the author's experience. It is likely that some type of metallic internal fixation should be used in addition to fusion.

In the adult with high-grade slip, it is difficult to get a transverse process fusion to "take" if the loose element has been removed and only the transverse processes remain as an area for fusion to the sacral ala. I do not recommend immediate fusion after a Gill operation. This has not been a problem in children, because their bones fuse so readily.

In the child, because the L4 disc is not ordinarily a matter for concern, a one-level fusion is usually performed. In the presence of very high-grade slip, however, it is often difficult to avoid extension of the fusion to

L4. Such an extension does not lower the incidence of success, probably because fusion takes place readily in children.

In the child with non-structural sciatic scoliosis, a one-level fusion suffices unless there is definite pathology at the L4–5 joint. If this is the case, the fusion should be extended to include L4. If there is structural scoliosis, it may need to be treated as a separate entity. However, surprisingly often, after a lumbosacral fusion has become solid, the scoliosis improves or even disappears.[16,27]

If a severe subarachnoid block is suspected, a myelogram may be indicated. Often only a trickle of contrast medium runs through at the level of defect (if Pantopaque is used). Unless there is substantial neurologic change, however, the author's practice is simply to fuse even these lesions in situ. Once the fusion is solid, the nerves appear to accommodate to the cramped quarters,

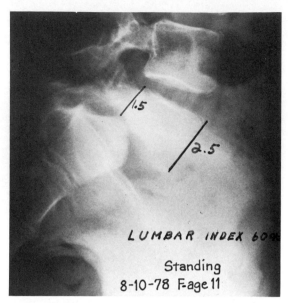

Fig. 15-11. *Wedging of L5. This 11-yr-old white female has a percent of wedging of 60% calculated by the formula seen here:*

$$\frac{\text{Posterior ht of L5 body } 1.5}{\text{Anterior ht of L5 body } 2.5} = 60\%$$

This child has 53% slip at this time. She disappeared from followup (against medical advice) for 8 months and, when seen again, had slipped to 78%. An L5 to S1 fusion was done at that time.

and the tightness of the hamstrings disappears over a period of several months. If necessary, decompression can be done very satisfactorily once a wide fusion has become solid.

The physician should be alert to tethering of the spinal cord due to a tight filum terminale. This has been described in association with spondylolisthesis.[70] The Metrizamide (not Pantopaque) myelogram usually shows a low-lying conus medullaris and tight filum. If this condition is present, surgical release of the tight filum should be done.[70] This is so rare that it is difficult to say just what surgical procedure should be performed. It is the author's impression that it would be best to make a midline approach, do a bilateral laminectomy of L4, L5, and S1, open the dura, and cut the tight filum terminale. A transverse process fusion of L5 to S1 could be done at the same time. This

child should then be kept flat for 2 months, because removing this much bony support will probably permit further olisthesis. Even then, after the child is allowed to stand, upright spot lateral roentgenograms should be taken frequently to watch for further slip. If the slip progresses, 3 more months in the horizontal position is recommended.

Another approach, especially if the degree of slip is not too great (below 33%), would be to release the tight filum and then allow the child to be up and about. He might not need a fusion. If he does, it could be done a few months later through the paraspinal approach and no period of recumbency would be necessary.

To sum up, the indications for surgery in the child are as follows:

1. Symptoms severe enough to interfere with usual activities over a period of 8 months or more
2. Persistent, severely tight hamstrings
3. Progressive olisthesis or sagittal rotation of L5 on S1 (in an L5 spondylolisthesis)

THE PARASPINAL SACROSPINALIS-SPLITTING APPROACH TO THE LUMBAR SPINE

The paraspinal approach to the lumbar spine passes across the sacrospinalis. The sacrospinalis muscle is split about two finger-breadths lateral to the midline.[70] The transverse processes and lateral masses are reached more directly through this approach, and there is no more bleeding here than with other approaches to the lateral parts of the vertebrae.

OPERATIVE TECHNIQUE

The patient is placed on the operating table in either the prone or the kneeling position (Fig. 15-16). A midline skin incision is made but, once through the skin, the skin is retracted so that the fascial incisions can be made (Fig. 15-16A). The incisions are made in the fascia about two finger-breadths lateral to the spinous processes and three-quarters of the way out laterally on the sacrospinalis. These fascial incisions may curve slightly toward the midline at their distal ends (Fig. 15-16B). The index finger can then be used to dissect through the muscle mass down to the sacrum; it is then slid down the back of the sacrum to the articular process of the L5 and S1 vertebrae, as well as to the space between the transverse process of L5 and the sacral ala (Fig. 15-16C).

It should be noted that the muscle fibers do not split cleanly (up at L3 they do), because at this level they run in various directions. They can be separated, however, and any tag ends of loose muscle are simply cut off before the wound is closed. It is wise to do so, as this muscle has been denervated in any case, and only enough muscle for adequate closure need be left.

If a lumbosacral fusion is being done, care must be taken not to dissect too far cephalad, or one will inadvertently expose the L4 vertebra. (There is a natural tendency to do this.) Two Gelpi retractors bent to a right angle at a point 2 inches from their tips are very good instruments for retracting the muscle. These are standard in most operating rooms. One must be sure to choose the orthopedic variety which are extra strong.

The sacrospinalis is split only enough to expose the vertebra to be fused. The top of the sacral ala should be denuded of soft tissue. The posterior surface of the sacrum should not be denuded any more than is necessary for exposure, because bone grafts will mainly be placed in contact with the top of the ala.

The laminae of the vertebrae to be fused are exposed about 1.5 cm medial to the facet joints. The lumbar transverse processes should be denuded of soft tissue completely out to the tips and well around the superior and inferior borders. Especially in the child with high-grade slip, the iliolumbar and intertransverse ligaments are carefully preserved to prevent further slip. The spinal nerves are in front of the transverse processes and intertransverse ligaments. These nerves will not be injured, provided the

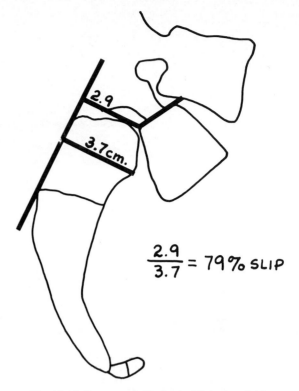

$$\frac{2.9}{3.7} = 79\% \text{ SLIP}$$

Fig. 15-12. Percent of olisthesis. There is a fairly definite point at the superior extremity of the pedicle where it joins the vertebral body. This gives a point on the body of L5 for measurement of the amount of slip. The back of the body of S1 also is a definite reference point.

exposure is not continued anteriorly. If care is taken, there is little danger of damaging a spinal nerve.

The lumbar arteries and veins, which pass just above the bases of the transverse processes and at the angle of the medial point of the sacral ala, often bleed freely and can be difficult to stop with cautery. These bleeding "holes" should be plugged with a piece of Surgicel about 3 cm by 3 cm in size. Vessels coming out of the superior sacral foramina may also bleed rather profusely; these also can be staunched with Surgicel. This material should be removed later. However, no harm comes if a small wad of it is inadvertently left in. If bleeding does not stop, replace the Surgicel with a wad of Gelfoam* and

* Trademark Upjohn.

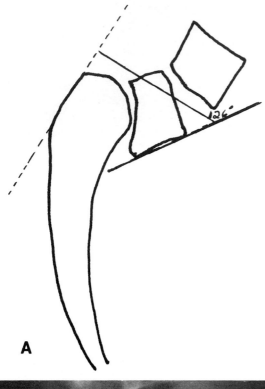

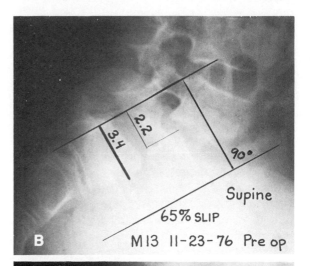

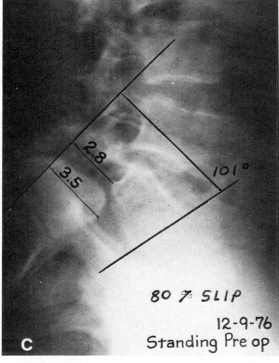

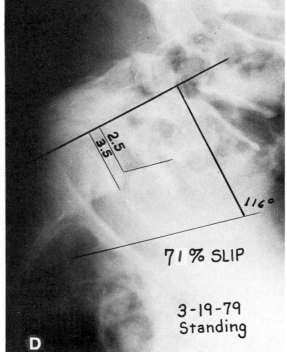

Fig. 15-13. Degree of roll, sagittal rotation of L5. **(A)** We use the angle between a line drawn along the back of S1 and the front of L5. The larger this angle is, the more sagittal rotation L5 has undergone. **(B)** 13-yr-old male. Prone x-ray film on 11/23/76 taken immediately preoperation shows 90° of sagittal rotation of L5 and 65% slip. **(C)** A few days later on 12/9/76 a standing lateral shows 101° of sagittal rotation of L5 and 80% slip. **(D)** Over 2 years later. On 3/19/79 a standing lateral film after an L4 to S1 fusion has become solid shows slight reduction of the slip to 71% but further sagittal rotation to 116° (Continued opposite page)

leave it in. Only bipolar cautery should be used on these vessels which accompany the posterior rami, as damage to the anterior rami theoretically can occur with unipolar cautery. For a detailed description of the vessels in this area, see the article by Macnab and Dall.[38]

Only the lateral surface of the superior articular processes of the topmost vertebra to be included in the fusion should be denuded. Care should be taken not to remove the capsule, or to damage the adjacent joint, nor to expose any part of the vertebra immediately above the fusion area. By observing these precautions, any tendency for the fusion to extend upward will be avoided. Within the fusion area, the lateral surface of the SAP, as well as the pars interarticularis and lamina to a point just medial to the facets, are meticulously denuded of soft tissue. The spinous processes are not exposed, thereby preserving their ligamentous attach-

ments and some of their blood supply. Except in the case of a very loose posterior element or spina bifida, the intervertebral joints within the fusion area are carefully exposed, and the articular cartilage in the posterior two-thirds of each joint is removed.

The graft bed is prepared as in a classic Hibbs fusion. A flap of bone from the top of the ala of the sacrum, based anteriorly, is turned forward and cephalad to form a bridge to the transverse processes of L5 (Fig. 15-16D). Enough iliac graft for both sides can be obtained from one side of the pelvis through the same midline skin incision. (The author's group has never used bone from more than one side.) The inner cortex is left intact. Cancellous bone is impacted between the denuded articular processes, and strips of cancellous iliac and cortical bone are tamped very securely around the transverse processes, with care not to break them. The softer, pure cancellous bone is packed in first because it stays down well against the host bone. Cortical bone has a tendency to spring back from the transverse processes.

The wound is then closed. The muscle itself is sutured loosely with fine chromic catgut suture. The heavy fascia is easy to close and should be securely sutured.

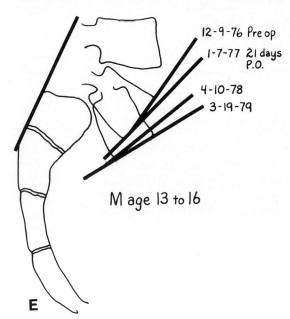

E

*Fig. 15-13 (Continued) **(E)** Drawing showing the sagittal rotation of L5 which took place in this 13-yr-old boy from date of fusion on 12/10/76 until he was finally considered solidly fused on 3/19/79. This case emphasizes the importance of taking a standing preop lateral film. If we had had only the horizontal preop lateral we would have thought that a great deal of slip and roll had occurred between operation and the time the fusion became solid.*

POSTOPERATIVE MANAGEMENT

After fusion is done through the paraspinal approach, the patient is encouraged to get out of bed when he feels able (usually in a few days) and is allowed to walk as much as he likes. It is preferred that he sit in a straight-backed chair and avoid deep over-stuffed sofas for 2 months. A routine of exercises is started 2 or 3 days after operation. All patients are trained to avoid motion of the low back by rolling like a log instead of twisting, and by bending the knees when stooping. Corsets or braces are not used unless the patient prefers to wear one, because no increase in the incidence of fusion has been observed with the use of these devices.

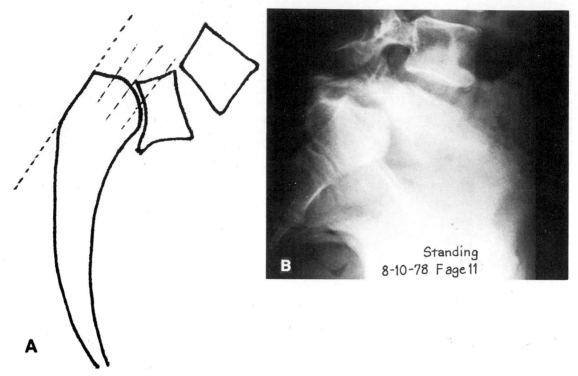

Fig. 15-14. Superior sacral contour. *(A) The further posteriorly the eroding of S1 starts, the poorer the prognosis. In this drawing, the sloping-off of S1 starts between the 1st- and 2nd-degree points. Thus it is between a Grade II and a Grade III contour. (B) This standing lateral film of an 11-yr-old girl shows a marked rounding of the front of the superior surface of the body of S1. This is a poor prognostic sign as regards further slip. This child did develop further slip. Here she had 53% slip (anterior translation) and by the following March had slipped to 78% and so was fused. (She had disappeared from followup.)*

In the approach described here, relatively few of the supporting ligaments are cut and, although minimal increase in slip and roll has occurred in some patients, serious further olisthesis has not developed.

For the past 15 years the author's group has allowed most of these children to get up immediately, no matter how much slip is present, but they are followed carefully with standing spot lateral x-ray films of the lumbosacral joint. It is our practice always to take standing spot lateral roentgenograms of the lumbosacral joint just before operation to use as a baseline. Then, after the child has been up for 3 or 4 days, another standing spot lateral film is taken of L5 and S1; a week later the spot lateral film is repeated. If there is any sign of slip, the child is put to bed until the fusion becomes solid, which occurs in about 3 months. If, as is usual, no further slip or roll occurs, the weekly roentgenograms are continued another 2 weeks and then at monthly intervals. The gonads should be shielded with lead but, because only a single spot standing lateral roentgenogram is taken, the total amount of radiation received during the entire healing phase is still about the same as with one standard low back series.

If the loose posterior element has been removed in a patient with spondylolisthesis, there is likelihood that further slipping will occur. If the annulus has been incised for removal of a ruptured disc at the same level in addition to removal of the loose element, and then if the patient is allowed up before the fusion is solidified, progression of slip is virtually certain.[60] There is evidence that, if

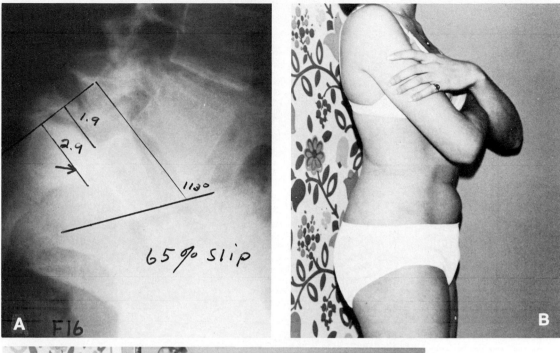

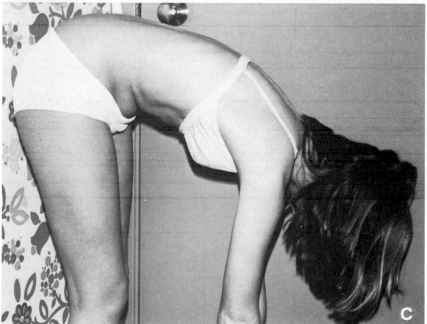

Fig. 15-15. (A) Lateral film shows 65% slip and 113° of sagittal rotation of L5. (B) Standing lateral shows surprisingly little change in body contour. (C) Note very good ability to bend. No tightness of hamstrings.

further slip is going to occur, even keeping the patient down 3 months is not always sufficient to prevent it, as it takes a very long time for the graft to mature.

When decompression of the cauda equina and nerve roots is indicated, it can be accomplished through the paraspinal approach better than through a midline, because this

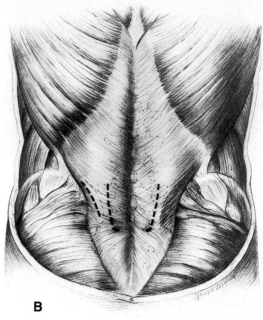

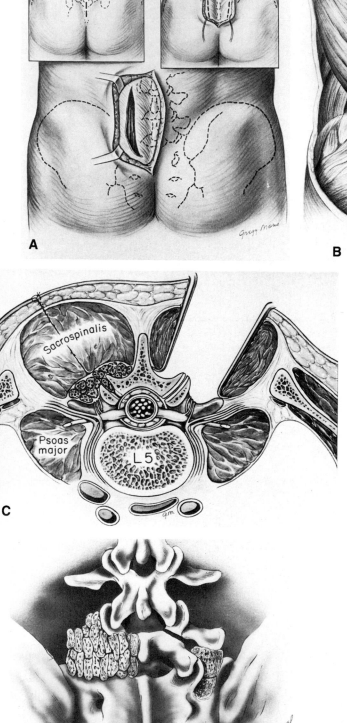

Fig. 15-16. Paraspinal approach for spinal fusion. **(A)** Composite drawing of the paraspinal approach. A midline skin incision is used once through the skin, the incision is pulled over, and the fascia is cut two finger-breadths lateral to the midline. (Wiltse LL, Bateman JG, Hutchinson RH et al: The paraspinalis approach to the lumbar spine. Clin Orthop 91:52, 1973) **(B)** Dotted lines show where the incisions in the fascia are made. The line over the posterior superior iliac spine indicates the line of incision in the fascia if a bone graft is to be taken. One iliac crest will usually supply enough bone for both sides. **(C)** Two Gelpi retractors seem to be the best instruments for retraction of the muscle. Note location of bone grafts after closure of the wound **(left)**. **(D)** Extent of bone graft used by the author. The graft covers the lateral surface of the superior articular process of the first sacral vertebra, and the joint between L5 and S1 is fused. The joint between L4 and L5 is not injured, but the graft extends onto the lateral aspect of the superior articular process of L5. An identical area is fused on the opposite side also. **(Right)** A flap of bone is turned upward from the ala of the sacrum so it bridges the gap between the ala and the transverse process. (Continued opposite page)

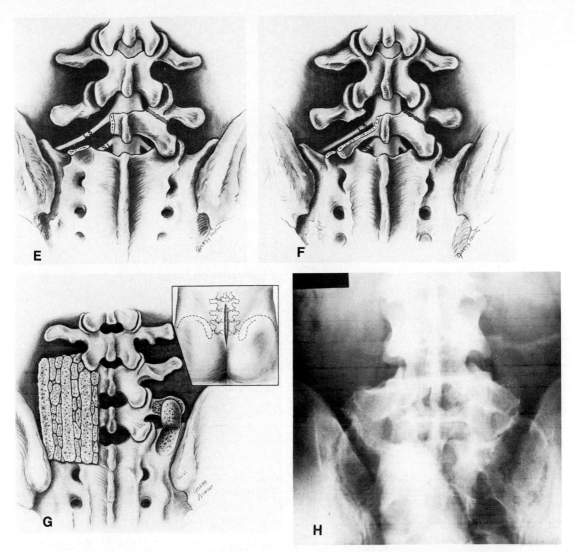

Fig. 15-16 (Continued) **(E)** *Identifying and decompressing the nerve root is more easily done once part of the defective pars interarticularis has been removed. The author ordinarily does not remove this much bone, preferring to remove only that amount shown in B.* **(F)** *It is advantageous to leave part of the lamina as shown here. The remaining portion of the loose lamina is fused to the sacrum and thus rocking of this loose fragment, which may produce pain, is prevented. (Wiltse LL, Bateman JG, Hutchinson RH, et al: Paraspinal sacrospinalis-splitting approach to the lumbar spine. J Bone Joint Surg 50A:920–923, 1968)* **(G)** *Paraspinal fusion, two levels. Bone covers no more than the lateral half of the laminae (Wiltse LL: Common problems of the lumbar spine: Spondylolisthesis and its treatment. J Cont Ed Ortho July, 1979)* **(H)** *Successful fusion done for a spondylolisthesis in a 19-yr-old male with 30% slip. X-ray film taken 3 years post fusion.*

approach is centered almost directly over the region where the nerve root compression occurs (Fig. 15-16F). It is not necessary to do a complete laminectomy. With only a portion of the lamina removed, it is possible to trace the spinal nerve laterally and decompress it completely. If there are bony ossicles or fibrocartilaginous mass associated with spondylolisthesis, they lie in the direct line of approach and can be removed easily. In

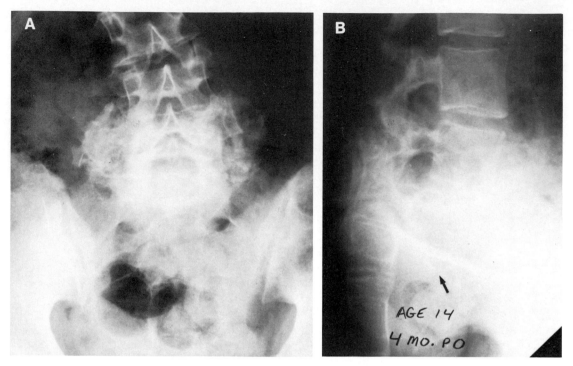

Fig. 15-17. **(A)** *AP roentgenogram of girl age 14 who had a fusion from L4 to S1 through the paraspinal approach. With such a high degree of slip, L4 is often included in the fusion.* **(B)** *Lateral roentgenogram of the same child. Note the vertical sacrum. (Wiltse LL: Common problems of the lumbar spine: Spondylolisthesis and its treatment, J Cont Educ Ortho July, 1979)*

this connection it is worth noting that, except in instances of high-grade slip, it is the L5 nerve that is compressed in the presence of spondylolisthesis of the L5 vertebra. This may give the clinical picture of a ruptured disc at the interspace between L4 and L5, since an L4 disc usually compresses the L5 nerve root. In the rare case when it is believed that the posterior superior border of the sacrum must be removed, a mildline approach is better.

Through a paraspinal approach either a one-level or a multi-level fusion can be done. The anatomy of this approach is somewhat more complicated than that of the midline approach, because one does not have the exposed spinous processes to serve as guides.

The question has arisen: can this approach be used with a very high-grade slip? Figure 15-17 shows a roentgenogram of a child with an extremly high-grade slip who was oper-

ated on through a paraspinal approach. It is noted that this child has almost a vertical sacrum with the body of L5 around in front of S1. In this case, because of the very severe slip, the fusion was extended to L4. However, if one can fuse only L5 conveniently, this is what we would do. There is an advantage in fusing only the pathologic area in the adult, because one-level fusions are more frequently successful than two-level fusions in this age group.

THE MIDLINE APPROACH FOR ARTHRODESIS IN SPONDYLOLISTHESIS

There are occasions in children when one may choose to do a transverse process fusion through the midline after removal of the loose element. This technique has the following disadvantages.

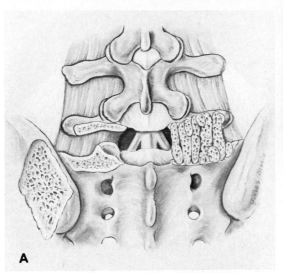
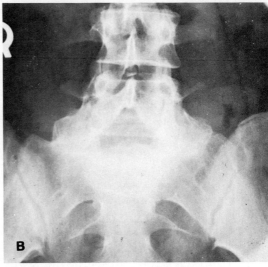

*Fig. 15-18. One-level spinal fusion done through the midline after removal of the loose element according to the technique of Gill. **(A)** Drawing of one-level fusion after loose element has been removed. **(B)** Roentgenogram taken 5 years after a one-level fusion was done following removal of the loose element. (Ruge D, Wiltse LL: Spondylolisthesis and its treatment: Conservative treatment, fusion with and without fusion. In Lumbar Spine Fusion. Lea & Febiger, Philadelphia, 1977)*

1. There is a real danger that a piece of bone graft may fall on a nerve and compress it. Bone may also creep medially onto the dura.

2. Since all midline structures are cut, if there is already high-grade slip, further olisthesis is likely to occur. A long period in bed is necessary as a prevention.

3. Even after the fusion seems to be solid, further slip is likely to occur until the graft is mature.

4. The incidence of failure of fusion was higher in our series than with the paraspinal approach. However, in a recent report by Sherman and associates, the incidence of failure of fusion was found to be no higher after a Gill operation than in cases where the loose element was left in.[60] This may be true in the child but was not true in the adult in our series.

Fusion through the midline is indicated after midline laminectomy has been done as, for example, in the rare case where it is necessary to release a tight filum terminale. The technique has been well described before.[57] Figure 15-18A shows a drawing of the technique. Figure 15-18B shows a roentgenogram of a child who had an L5 to S1 fusion by this technique. We no longer do posterior fusion in adults in conjunction with a Gill operation. If a fusion must be done, it is done anteriorly or at a later date, if done posteriorly.

Treatment of Isthmic Spondylolisthesis in the Adult

The conservative treatment of the adult with lytic spondylolisthesis is much like that for backache from other causes. The same exercises are prescribed, although the author has found them to be less effective in spondylolisthesis than in disc disease. The same type of corset is used with about the same chance of success.

SURGICAL TREATMENT IN THE ADULT

The principal reason for surgical treatment in the adult is for relief of pain, not (as is the occasional misconception) to prevent progression of slip. Slip rarely increases in the adult when there has been no surgical intervention. When it does progress, the increase is small and is not in itself an indication for surgery. Usually, but not always, slip is due to narrowing of the disc space. Occasionally, a high grade of slip which has been present since childhood causes neurologic difficulties in an adult and must be treated surgically.

In patients under age 24, a one-level fusion is usually all that is needed. Whether to extend the fusion to L4 depends on the status of the L4 disc. Thus, it is necessary to ascertain, if possible, the status of the L4 disc. The electromyogram gives valuable information and often confirms the impression gained by the physical examination. The fifth spinal nerve may be involved, owing either to a bulging disc at the L4 space or to the entrapment of the L5 spinal nerve at the L5 pars defect. If myelography shows a definitely bulging disc at the L4 space, the L4 disc should be removed and the fusion extended to include L4. If myelographic findings are normal at L4, further study by discogram using the pain reproduction test is indicated. Posterior bulging noted on the myelogram, if associated with a positive pain reduction test, requires surgical removal of the L4 disc and inclusion of L4 in the fusion. The failings of the discogram and the pain reproduction test as diagnostic tools are well recognized, but the tests do give some valuable information in the specific situation mentioned here.

Recently the author's group has found the CT scan to be very useful in determining the status of the L4 disc. Since the advent of multiplanar tomography (axial, sagittal, and coronal), a great deal of information which was previously unavailable can be obtained. The incidence of successful fusion in the adult using a paraspinal approach in the author's series is about 94% in the adult if limited to one level. This incidence drops to 84% for two-level fusions. Thus there is a distinct advantage in performing a one-level fusion, even at the risk of having to treat the L4 disc later.

REDUCTION OF SEVERE SPONDYLOLISTHESIS

The first reported reduction of a severe spondylolisthesis was by Jenkins in 1936.[29] Using strong longitudinal traction, he achieved reasonable correction which he followed with anterior interbody fusion. A follow-up on Jenkins' patient many years later demonstrated that the bony grafts had resorbed and that all the reduction had been lost.[45] A. M. Hendry in the early 1940s attempted unsuccessfully to reduce severe spondylolisthesis with longitudinal traction applied through flexed hips.[45] Since then, many workers have attempted to reduce severe spondylolisthesis.[21] Persistent problems were the high risk of producing a cauda equina lesion, and the fact that maintaining reduction was difficult, if not impossible.[22,43] More recently, Harrington and Dickson have advocated posterior reduction by instrumentation and fusion.[20] However, in some cases this operation has increased the kyphotic deformity, and the patient has been left with a fixed flexion deformity of the spine. Daymond has used halofemoral traction in nearly 20 patients since 1969 as a preliminary form of correction for severe spondylolisthesis, followed by posterior fusion and internal fixation.[12] DeWald combined this posterior instrumentation with anterior fusion at the lumbosacral level.[13]

Recently, reports on techniques for reduction of severe spondylolisthesis have been made by Bradford and also by McPhee and O'Brien using halofemoral traction.[9,40]

Both Bradford, and McPhee and O'Brien, used halofemoral traction combined with removal of the loose element according to the technique of Gill. An intertransverse fusion is done either from L4 to S1 or L5 to S1. A few days later an anterior approach is made, and an anterior interbody fusion at L5 is done. The patient must remain horizontal for 3 or 4 months, but good reduction and maintenance of position is reported by both groups.

Ascani of Rome has developed a method whereby ordinary femoral pin traction is used for several days.[3] Then the patient is severely hyperextended in a cast while further traction is applied. The lumbar spine is fused through a hole in the back of the cast. Rene Louis of France has developed a method using both anterior and posterior arthodesis and internal fixation with a special four-pointed, star-shaped, plate.[35] Matthias of Germany has developed a plate which attaches to the sacrum and to the pedicles of L4.[39] Both anterior fusion and posterior fusion are done. Snijder and colleagues have developed a method in which, through a posterior approach after a Gill operation, both an anterior interbody and intertransverse fusion are done, and the L5 vertebra is held back in position by a wire through the base of the spinous process of L4. This wire passes out through the skin and is attached to a spring-loaded coil and a modified Milwaukee brace.[61]

Ohki and associates of Japan described a procedure combining the methods of Bradford and O'Brien and also using the transcutaneous traction wire of Snijder.[47] The spring-loaded traction device is fastened to an outrigger on the halofemoral apparatus (Fig. 15-19). There are undoubtedly many more methods or combinations of methods being used throughout the world.

It would seem likely that, as techniques for reduction become simpler and more reliable, it will become standard procedure to reduce the slip in patients with high-grade olisthesis. Whether this becomes the rule will depend on whether future experience shows that the patient's appearance can be improved enough by reduction, as compared with fusion in situ, to warrant the rather formidable procedure.

Perhaps if school children where checked as they are for scoliosis, the high grades of slip could become a thing of the past. An attempt is being made in Long Beach, CA. to do this.

At the present state of the art, it is my opinion that reduction is never necessary if the slip is less than 50%. Actually, many patients with even more than 60% slip show relatively little change in body contour and

do well with fusion *in situ* (Fig. 15-15). It has been stated by Bradford that after reduction, even though the fusion is solid, recurrent slip may occur owing to remodeling of bone if the olisthesis is high grade.[8] This finding has in fact been true in the author's experience and is probably due to the fact that there is such a great tendency for the affected vertebra to slip back to its original position. This, coupled with the fact that it takes many months for a graft to mature, accounts for the phenomenon of gradual redisplacement even after fusion is thought to be solid.

To summarize, I would say that relatively few patients with spondylolisthesis who need fusion need to be reduced. Most can be fused *in situ*. Reduction should be attempted only by the surgeon who has made a very careful study of all available methods and has had a good deal of experience in spine surgery. An orthopedist who only occasionally sets out to reduce spondylolisthesis is likely to have trouble.

REMOVAL OF THE LOOSE ELEMENT ONLY

In 1950 Gill described the operation in which the loose element is removed along with any fibrocartilaginous mass or other bony mass which might be impinging upon the spinal nerve (Fig. 15-20).[19] The important thing in doing a Gill operation is not only to remove the loose element but also to trace the L5 spinal nerve well out into the muscle, removing all constricting scar tissue or bony ossicles. In addition, the proximal stump of the pars should be cut back to the pedicle. Even the base of the transverse process can squeeze the nerve between itself and the sacral ala and in these cases should be partially removed.

Davis and Baily reviewed their experience with the Gill operation done on 39 patients between 1952 and 1967.[11] Results in 83% were rated as satisfactory from a clinical standpoint. Among their patients, those with moderate to severe arthritic changes in the lumbosacral area had the poorest results.

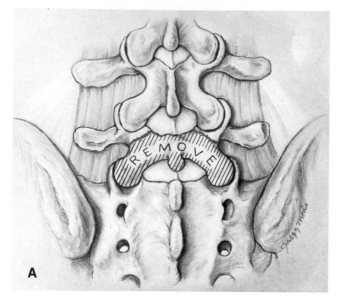

Fig. 15-19. Drawings of the Gill operation. **(A)** Loose element in isthmic spondylolisthesis (type IIA). **(B)** After the loose element is removed, the L5 spinal nerve is channeled and the proximal stump of the pars cut off as on left. **(C)** The dotted line across the proximal stump of the pars indicates where this bone is cut off to remove the pressure on the L5 spinal nerve. Note the L5 nerve is pinched between the stump of the pars of the lateral mass and the superior border of the body of L5. (Wiltse, LL: Common problems of the lumbar spine: Spondylolisthesis and its treatment. J Cont Educ Orthop 7:13–31, 1979)

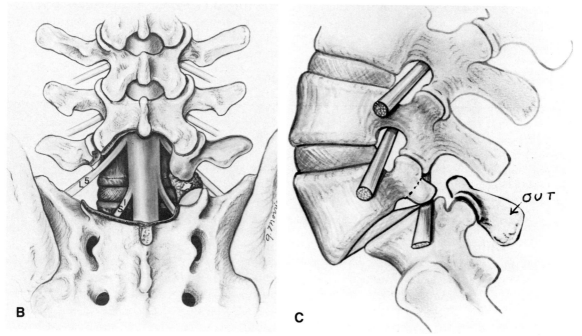

Younger adults who had little or no arthritic changes had the best results. This seems like an inconsistency but it is not. The patient who has a great degree of arthritic change around the level of defect will obtain relief from sciatica by simple removal of the loose element, but the degenerative disc and the severe arthritic changes may continue to cause pain. Also, in these arthritic patients

there is a strong tendency not to decompress far enough laterally. This, in the author's opinion, notwithstanding the findings of Davis and Baily, accounts for the poorer results in the older patient with osteoarthitic change. The author uses the Gill operation alone in the older adult (past age 60) who has considerable osteoarthritic change and disc space narrowing and who has significant

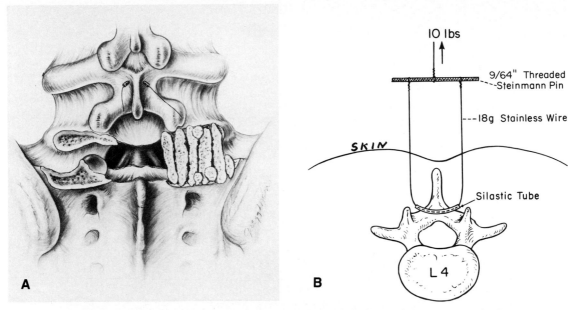

Fig. 15-20. **(A)** *The approach is made posteriorly and the loose element removed. The disc is then completely removed by a technique similar to Cloward's. The olisthesis is reduced and an interbody iliac graft put in place. An intertransverse fusion is then done.* **(B)** *Method of putting in the traction wire. The wire can be pulled out.*

sciatica. I do this because I have found fusion to work so well in the younger patient that I would not want to stop fusing these younger patients. In the older patient, especially with a narrow L5 disc space and osteoarthritic changes, there is enough stability that further slip is not likely to occur when only a Gill operation is done.

INTERBODY FUSION FOR SPONDYLOLISTHESIS OF THE LUMBAR SPINE

During the last 30 years we have used interbody fusion for the treatment of spondylolisthesis only occasionally. Our preference has generally been a posterior intertransverse fusion through the paraspinal approach. We have used interbody fusion only in patients who have had previous attempts at posterior fusion. It is my belief that the incidence of failure of interbody fusion in most surgeons' hands is high in the lumbar spine. However, some techniques yield an adequate success rate (Fig.

15-21A). When Douglas Freebody's technique is employed, the success rate is satisfactory. We have never used this technique except in the presence of very high-grade olisthesis when there have been one or two failures (Fig. 15-21B, C) of posterior surgery and when there is gross instability noted on flexion and extension.

Freebody Technique. A midline incision is made in the lower abdomen and the abdominal contents are moved to one side. A catheter should be placed in the urinary bladder preoperatively to keep it as small as possible. A longitudinal incision is made in the posterior peritoneum overlying the vertebrae to be fused. Before this is done, the tissue overlying the bodies of L4 and L5 to S1 are infiltrated with saline and epinephrine. This maneuver facilitates the identification of structures, permitting the presacral nerve and vessels to be pushed laterally with a "pusher" as they pass over the sacral promontory. Bleeding also is diminished by the epinephrine. Electrocoagulation should never be used here. If the bifurcation of the

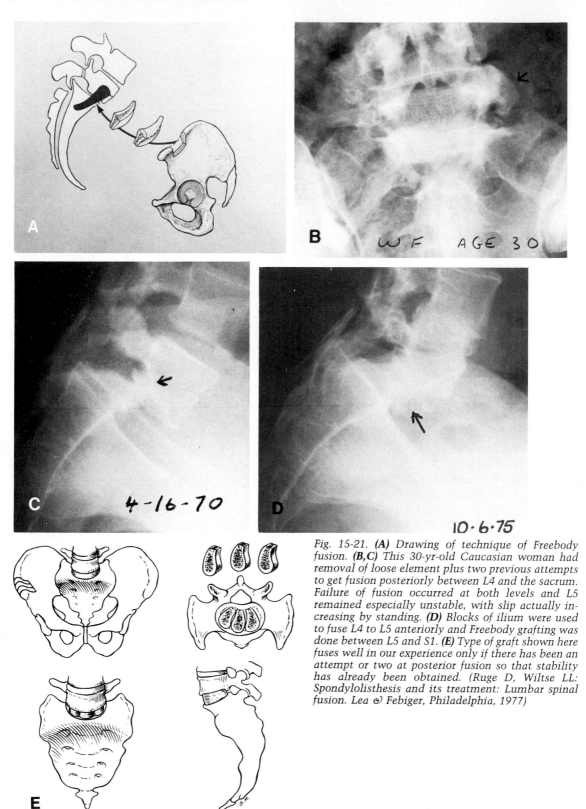

Fig. 15-21. **(A)** *Drawing of technique of Freebody fusion.* **(B,C)** *This 30-yr-old Caucasian woman had removal of loose element plus two previous attempts to get fusion posteriorly between L4 and the sacrum. Failure of fusion occurred at both levels and L5 remained especially unstable, with slip actually increasing by standing.* **(D)** *Blocks of ilium were used to fuse L4 to L5 anteriorly and Freebody grafting was done between L5 and S1.* **(E)** *Type of graft shown here fuses well in our experience only if there has been an attempt or two at posterior fusion so that stability has already been obtained.* (Ruge D, Wiltse LL: *Spondylolisthesis and its treatment: Lumbar spinal fusion.* Lea & Febiger, Philadelphia, 1977)

great vessels is high, the fifth disc can be approached between them. If the bifurcation is low, the vessels can be retracted to the right after ligation of the left lumbar vessels, which pass laterally around the vertebral bodies. The large vessels are carefully pushed over as far as possible to expose the disc, and retractors are driven in place. A flap of annulus based to the right is then freed, and the disc is completely excised. A portion of the end-plates is removed to raw bone.

A trap door is taken out of the front of the body of L5 as seen in Figure 15-21D. Through this trap door, access is gained to the top of S1. With a curette (or if the bone is too hard, a large drill) a hole is made through S1 to about the center of S2, perhaps 4 cm in depth into the sacrum.

An osteoperiosteal flap is then lifted off the crest of the ilium, and a full-thickness bone graft is removed from the top of the iliac crest at its thickest point. This graft is about 2.5 by 6 cm and is about the shape and size of a man's thumb. It is driven into the prepared slot across L5 into S1. The trap door is impacted back into the body of L5. The spaces on either side of the graft which have been occupied by disc tissue are curetted to bleeding bone and tamped full of cancellous bone. The prepared flap of annulus is sutured back into place, and the wound is closed. The patient is kept in a plaster bed for 6 weeks before ambulation is permitted, and then may only walk in a molded plastic jacket which he wears until the fusion appears solid.

Our success rate with the Freebody arthrodesis has been only fair. In several of our cases nonunion resulted, even though the procedure seemed to have been performed well technically and the patient kept immobilized postoperatively as recommended.

It is not necessary to fuse two levels in most patients with spondylolisthesis, but many have already undergone extensive surgery posteriorly and the fourth disc space has been curretted. Under these circumstances, we feel it advisable to stabilize this space also, but at this level we prefer to use multiple blocks of ilium cut from the top of the iliac (Fig. 15-21E). If there is high-grade slip we prefer the transperitoneal approach when we do an anterior fusion between L5 and S1. In such cases it is virtually impossible to perform a satisfactory fusion of the L5–S1 interspace through a retroperitoneal approach.

Left Flank Approach. Abdominal hernia occurs occasionally in the line of incision with both of the above approaches. For this reason, we have adopted a left flank incision similar to that used for nephrectomy or sympathectomy when we intend to fuse the L3 or L4 but not the L5 level. This approach is easily closed and is free of complications. The incision is an oblique one, halfway between the lower rib cage and the iliac crest error. It is usually necessary to extend the incision an inch or two more medially than is required for a sympathectomy. The incision is then carried through the external oblique, internal oblique, and transverse abdominal muscles. The vertical muscle bundles encountered generally have to be divided to obtain adequate exposure. To enter the retroperitoneal space, the posterior peritoneum is gently and bluntly dissected medially, a maneuver that exposes the anterior surface of the psoas muscle. The ureter has to be carefully mobilized so that it is not damaged. Exposure is continued by blunt dissection primarily, but it is a matter of mobilizing the vascular structures proximally and distally enough to expose the appropriate lumbar intervertebral space. Surgical hemoclips are helpful in the control of small bleeders, but one troublesome problem is fragile lumbar veins which can bleed profusely if torn.[10] Another real advantage of this approach is that iliac bone for the fusion can easily be removed without a separate skin incision.

ANOTHER TECHNIQUE FOR INTERBODY FUSION

Using Fibula Only. To fuse just one level we most often use fibular bone (Fig. 15-22). We prefer one level, because enough fibula

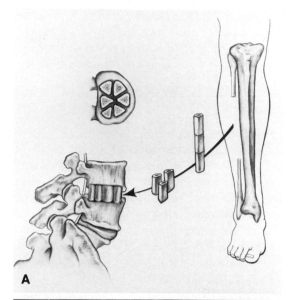

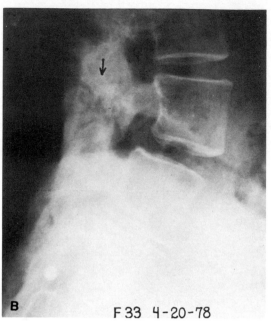

F 33 4-20-78

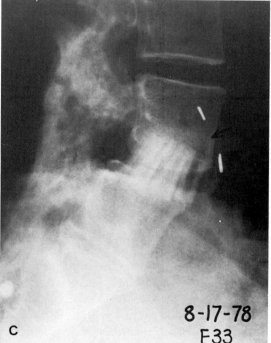

8-17-78
F33

Fig. 15-22. *(A) Fibular grafting procedure. (B) Lateral film shows failure of fusion at L4 after three attempts at posterior fusion. (C) Lateral film 4 months after fibular grafting at L4. The patient has now been followed another year and the grafts are solid. If they tip over post operation, failure of fusion will result. (A & C—Wiltse LL: Problem of the multioperated back patient. AAOS Instructional course lectures, Vol. XXVIII. C.V. Mosby, 1979)*

to fuse two levels is difficult to obtain from one leg. It is not advisable to remove fibula below the junction of its middle and lower thirds, or less than 2 inches from the top. When fibular struts are used, the vertebral end-plates are only partially excised, preserving good hard bone, and the bodies spread severely. The segments of fibula are sawed with a reciprocating saw and impacted into place securely. They are stood on end between the bodies. It is mandatory that these fibular grafts be held in place securely and that they be in a straight up-and-down position between the vertebral bodies. If they tip over, fusion will not occur. Great care must be used in taking out the fibula. We

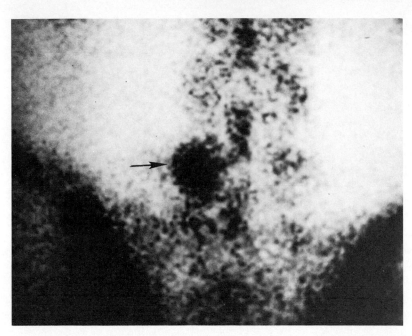

Fig. 15-23. *This is a scan of a 16-yr-old male athlete complaining of back pain. He had been performing extremely competitive high school football. Back pain had been present for 3 weeks. This scan shows only one pars to be "hot."*

use Henry's approach.[25] It is very easy to injure the superficial branch of the peroneal nerve as it passes distally along the front of the shaft of the fibula. Even vigorous retraction can injure this nerve. Use small periosteal strippers and retract carefully.

One should not attempt anterior interbody fusion without special retractors and, if not adept at handling the great vessels, should ask a vascular surgeon to make the approach.

Spondylolisthesis in the Young Athlete

As mentioned previously in this chapter, the incidence of pars defects in 5-year-olds is virtually zero, but at the end of the first grade when the child is approaching age 7, the incidence is about 4.4%. Boys have about twice as many pars defects as girls. This may change as girls enter so-called "male" sports. Between the end of the first grade and adulthood, the overall incidence increases by about 1.4% with boys still having about twice as many defects as girls.

This 1.4% appears to occur largely between the ages of 9 and 15. This is the age of rapid growth and the age at which the young athlete for the first time engages in very competitive sports. When the young athlete comes to the orthopedist with severe back pain, a set of roentgenograms is ordered. If the x-ray film is negative and the pain persists, a bone scan is done. If both the bone scan and the x-ray film are negative, no stress reaction is developing in the pars, and the condition should be treated as an ordinary back strain.

If the x-ray film is negative but the bone scan indicates a stress reaction in the pars interarticularis, then the physician must decide what course to take (Fig. 15-23). If the youngster is permitted to continue with vigorous athletics, he may develop full-blown pars defects. On the other hand, if the young athlete is taken off athletics and put into a corset (largely as a reminder), the stress reaction will usually disappear without going on to defects. If the roentgenogram shows early defects already present and the technetium scan shows the lesions to be "hot," then taking him off athletics and putting him in a corset may arrest the process, and the lesions may heal. If the child persists in vigorous athletics, it is likely that these lesions will not heal (Fig. 15-24).

If the lesion is present and is cold on the bone scan, then the lesion is well established

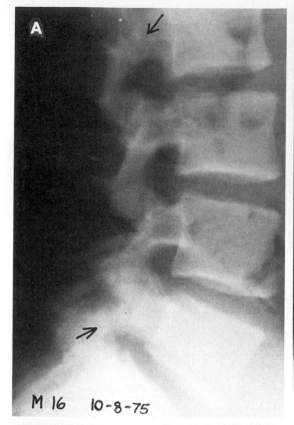

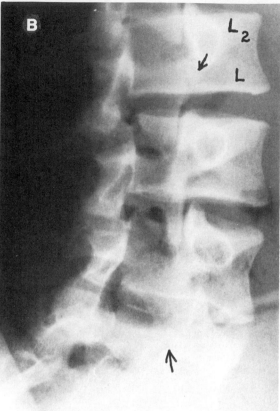

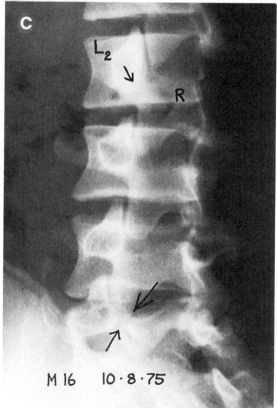

Fig. 15-24. *(A-C)* This young male athlete presented with low back pain and paraspinous muscle spasm. The initial roentgenograms showed bilateral pars interarticularis defects at the L5 level. The early defect of the left L2 pars interarticularis was not appreciated. (Continued opposite page)

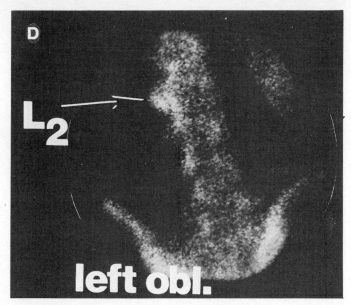

Fig. 15-24. (Continued) **(D)** *The left oblique bone scan showed increased activity in the left L2 posterior elements. The right pars at L2 and the L5 pars defects showed no increased activity (cold) on the scan. (Jackson D, Wiltse LL, Cirincione RJ: Spondylolysis in the female gymnast. Cl Ortho 117, June 1976)*

and will not heal. (A lesion will become "cold" in about a year.) The child should then be treated as if he had an ordinary back sprain. In other words, let him go back to playing as soon as his acute back symptoms subside.

We have seen a few new lesions develop even in college football players. Very rarely will olisthesis occur in college boys. However, at an earlier age (*i.e.*, about 7 and 12), we have seen several develop first-degree spondylolisthesis and one developed 50% slip (see Fig. 15-9). This is the exception.

Since we are dealing with a lesion which is not a terribly serious one and certainly not crippling, taking the youngster off his cherished sport very often is a serious psychological blow and often it is unnecessary.

As for the college football player, if the lesion is already established as it usually is, he can go ahead and play as he wishes since slip will not progress further. He is in no more danger of a serious injury than any other player.

If he can put up with the pain and discomfort, then let him play. He can be treated as for any other backache.[59] Semon and Spengler, in a retrospective study of 506 college football players, showed no increase in time

loss disability in the group with proven spondylolysis, compared with a control group without pars defects.

The question has been asked: what about spinal fusion for these young athletes? In early adolescence, if the child cannot participate in the usual activities for his age group and the pain persists for at least 8 or 9 months, then a one-level spinal fusion should be done. He will have to be off his sports at least 1 year and probably 2, but at this age he can be back in competitive sports by the time he reaches senior high school and college. On the other hand, to fuse a college football player with the idea that he will get back to really competitive football is probably unrealistic.

The same, of course, is true for other very vigorous sports. It is generally better to let the athlete play with his spondylolisthesis if pain permits. If he can't participate in athletics, then take him off the very strenuous sports and, if he can live comfortably doing ordinary activities, this is probably best. On the other hand, if he can't even perform at this level, then a fusion should be done.

The surgeon should be sure he is fusing the correct level, since the nonspondylytic

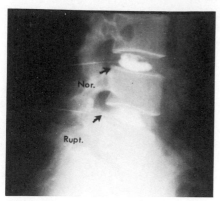

Fig. 15-25. *Discogram. Fusion had been decided upon but the question was, should L4 be included in the fusion? The myelogram was negative. In this case the pain reproduction test was positive at L4 but negative at L3. Fusion was done to include L4. Note also the bulge at L4 noted on the discogram but the relatively normal L3 discogram.*

L4 space can give trouble too. In selecting the correct level, we check with a venogram or myelogram. If the L4 level is negative, we then do a discogram at L4 to see if pain can be reproduced by the saline acceptance test (pain reproduction test). If the discogram is fairly normal and pain is not reproduced on injection, we feel fairly safe in doing a one-level fusion at the L5–S1 level (Fig. 15-25).

Treatment of Degenerative Spondylolisthesis

Degenerative spondylolisthesis results from forward slip of the entire vertebra (Fig. 15-26). The pars remains intact. By far the most frequent site of occurrence is between L4 and L5 with the L3 next in order of frequency.[54]

TREATMENT

Symptomatic therapy is adequate in the vast majority of patients but, when the pain is unrelenting and constant, surgery is most gratifying. Advanced age is not a contraindication.

Pain is the primary indication for surgery. Most patients have little or no neurologic deficit, but a very few have rather severe changes. The myelogram is characteristically dramatically abnormal. Circulatory change in the legs is not part of the syndrome.

The markedly enlarged inferior articular processes of L4 at the level of slip give them the appearance of being closer to the midline than average.[17] The bone has an unusual granular appearance.

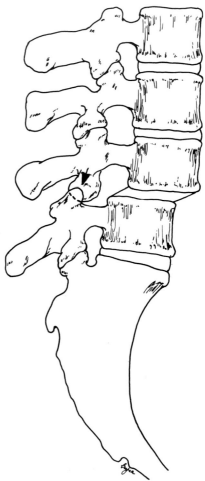

Fig. 15-26. *Lateral drawing. In this diagram of the lumbar spine with degenerative spondylolisthesis, the L5 vertebral body is square and the lumbosacral angle characteristically reduced but much more so than average. There is no pars defect. The whole L4 vertebra has slid forward. (Wiltse LL: Common problems of the lumbar spine: Degenerative spondylolisthesis and spinal stenosis. J Cont Educ Ortho May, 1979)*

The L4 spinal nerve which passes out at the level of slip (when the olisthesis is at L4), is seldom involved (Fig. 15-27).[55] In 48 patients whose histories we reviewed, there was only one instance of slight improvement of the L4 spinal nerve noted on the electromyogram; this occurred in a patient who had undergone a previous chemonucleolysis. The electromyographic changes may have been due to a slight nerve injury by the needle at the time of injection.

It has been the author's custom to decompress as depicted in the series of drawings in Figure 15-28. The lateral 80% of the zygapophyseal joints is preserved at the level of olisthesis.[11] Even so, further olisthesis at this level usually occurs. Occasionally in removing the lamina, the inferior articular process of the vertebra is broken off.[69] To avoid this, a side-cutting burr is used on a high-speed drill. This must be applied with care, however, as it will cut the nerve if allowed to go too deep.

Rosenberg, and Fitzgerald and Newman, have recommended the smaller area of decompression shown in Figure 15-29.[17,55] They reported that removing the distal half of the lamina and spinous process of the affected vertebra and the proximal half of the one below gives sufficient decompression. Two questions naturally arise: is this an adequate decompression, and will it prevent further olisthesis any better than the somewhat longer decompression shown in Figure 15-29?

One thing is certain: if the articular process is inadvertently broken off on both sides in a patient who does not have a very narrow disc space at that level, further olisthesis will nearly always occur. If, in addition, the disc is entered at the level of olisthesis and a generous portion of the posterior longitudinal ligament is cut, further slip may be very severe. Thus, this extensive bone removal should never be done. Even with increase in olisthesis, the L4 nerve is not impinged because it occupies the upper half of the neural canal. Removal of the disc after bony decompression at the level of olisthesis is especially to be condemned.

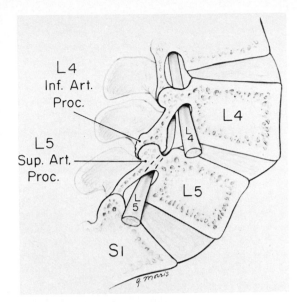

Fig. 15-27. Parasagittal view. Drawing of a parasagittal section through the area of olisthesis in degenerative spondylolisthesis at L4. This drawing was made from a computerized axial tomogram. Note how the inferior articular processes of L4 compress the L5 spinal nerve (not the L4 spinal nerves). (Wiltse LL: Surgery for intervertebral disc disease of the lumbar spine. Clin Orthop 129, 1977)

If the patient is below age 65, the author performs a transverse process fusion at the involved level (Fig. 15-30). This produces stability if arthrodesis is achieved. If the lateral masses and facets have been preserved, the chances for successful arthrodesis are very good. There may be a thickened, scarred blanched dura with an absence of fat at the level of compression.

The question has often been asked whether increased olisthesis, after decompression, causes increased symptoms? One would think so, but there is no real evidence that it does. The claudication and sciatica are usually gone. The residual back pain, if any, is usually tolerable and may be helped by a corset.

The area of actual compression in L4–L5 degenerative spondylolisthesis is between the inferior articular processes of L4 and the upper edge of the body of L5. The amount of bone which must be removed probably

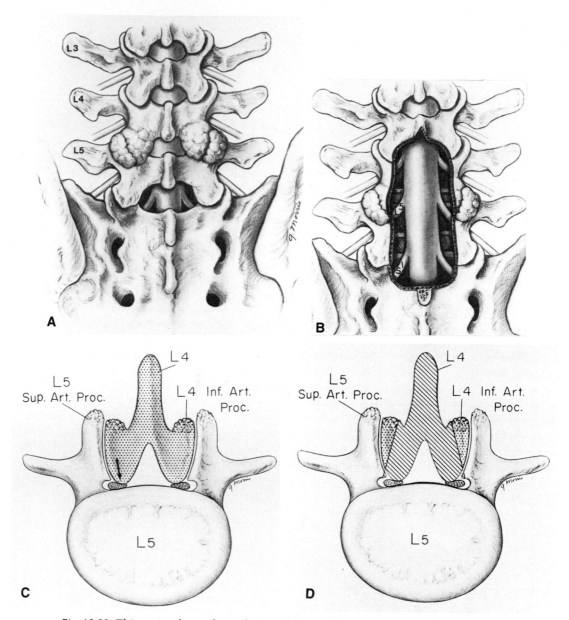

Fig. 15-28. This series shows the author's technique of decompression for degenerative spondylolisthesis at L4. **(A)** Artist's drawing taken from a dried specimen. **(B)** Area of decompression most commonly done by the author. The bone is cut with an air-driver, side-cutting burr to avoid breaking the remnants of articular processes. **(C)** Note how inferior articular processes of L4 compress the L5 nerve between themselves and the upper border of the body of L5. Drawing is from a computerized axial tomogram of degenerative spondylolisthesis at L4. **(D)** The cross-hatched area is removed. Note that the osteotomy is angled laterally so more bone is removed anteriorly. (Continued opposite page)

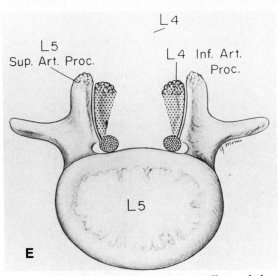

*Fig. 15-28. (Continued) **(E)** The small stippled areas represent remnants of the interior articular processes of L4 as seen in cross-section. One can readily see why the remaining portions of the inferior articular processes of L4 often break during the surgery unless great care is exercised. (Wiltse LL: Surgery for intervertebral disc disease of the lumbar spine, Clin Orthop 129, 1977)*

need not be terribly extensive. The problem is that, once even the smaller amount of bone has been removed, the connection is broken, and further olisthesis may occur. So one may as well do a bilateral laminectomy of both L4 and L5 and thus be absolutely certain of removing all compression. The exception would be if one intended to do an Albee graft between the remaining portions of the spinous processes of L4 and L5 as described by Fitzgerald and Newman.[17] In that case, it would be advantageous to keep the gap as small as possible.

In a study of patients with degenerative spondylolisthesis operated on by the author and reported by Reynolds on June 8, 1978, at the International Society for the Study of the Lumbar Spine in San Francisco, the following findings were reported.[51]

1. The pain was predominantly of the sciatic type in 70% and claudicant in 30%.

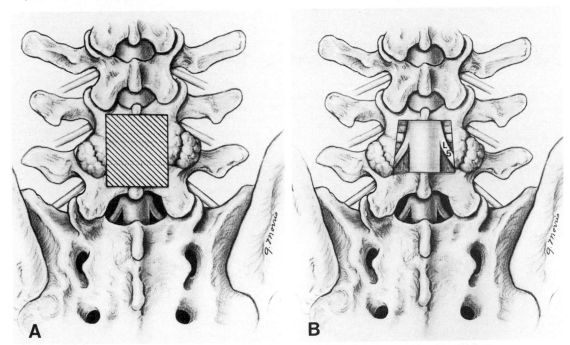

*Fig. 15-29. **(A)** In this drawing of degenerative spondylolisthesis, the cross-hatched area represents the decompression as recommended by Rosenberg, Fitzgerald, and Newman (see text). **(B)** This smaller amount of decompression as shown in the drawing cuts away as much support as does the larger decompression but may be advantageous if an interspinous fusion is to be done as advocated by Fitzgerald and Newman. Interspinous fusion is easier because the remaining portions of the spinous processes of L4 and L5 are closer together. (Wiltse LL: Surgery for intervertebral disc disease, Clin Ortho 129, 1977)*

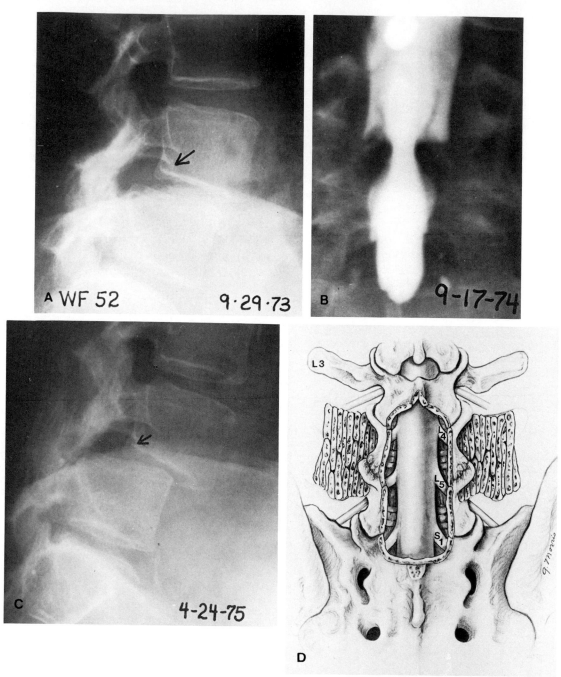

Fig. 15-30. This series of drawings and x-ray film studies is of a woman age 52 who had degenerative spondylolisthesis with bilateral leg pain. She could walk only a block or so without sitting down. (A) Degree of olisthy of L4 on L5 preoperatively. (B) Severe hourglass constriction in the AP myelogram. (C) Postoperative lateral roentgenogram. Note there has been some increased olisthy. This is usual. (D) One-level transverse process fusion was done. This is usually performed in patients under age 65. An L4 to L5 fusion is sufficient as the L5–S1 joint is nearly always stable. (Continued opposite page)

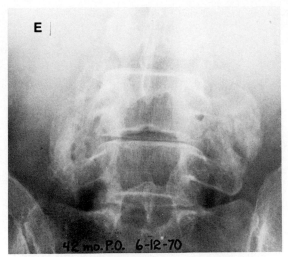

E |

42 mo. P.O. 6-12-70

Fig. 15-30. (Continued) *(E) AP x-ray film taken about 22 months postoperatively. Bending films showed the fusion to be solid. (Wiltse LL, Kirkaldy-Willis WM, McIvor GWD: The treatment of spinal stenosis. Clin Ortho 115, 1976)*

2. The electromyogram was abnormal in 41%. Of this 41%, the nerve below the level of slip was involved.

3. The degree of olisthesis was from 2 to 13 mm with an average of 6.7 mm and a mode of 4 mm.

4. There was no correlation between the following and the subjective clinical result (relief of pain):

Age
Degree of preoperative slip
Degree of preoperative hourglass constriction
Degree of further slip occurring after surgery

5. There was no correlation between the degree of hourglass constriction and elevation of the CSF protein. However, elevated CSF protein portended a poorer result.

6. Slip progresses for at least 2 years post-surgery in some patients.

7. The level of the intercrestal line (line drawn between the tops of the iliac crests) fell either at the level of the L4 disc or below in 76% of the patients.[17]

There was a high correlation between relief of pain and whether a total posterior element removal or a midline decompression was done. If the entire posterior element (*i.e.*, spinous process, laminae, and articular processes of L4) was removed, the good or excellent long-range result was poor, in the neighborhood of 33%. If a midline decompression was done, saving the pars and articular processes, the result was good or excellent 78% of the time.

To summarize, it may be said that degenerative spondylolisthesis has never been seen in patients under age 40 and is symptomatic principally in women. The results of surgical decompression are good. We prefer a midline decompression, saving the pars and articular processes. As of this writing, if fusion is done, the author's group limits it to one level, the symptomatic one, and generally to patients under age 65. It is the L5 spinal nerve which is compressed in an L4–L5 olisthesis. This nerve is compressed between the inferior articular processes of L4 and the upper margin of the body of L5.

Bibliography

1. Amuso SJ, Mankin HJ: Hereditary spondylolisthesis and spina bifida. J Bone Jt Surg 49A:507–513, 1967
2. Anderson CE: Spondyloschisis following spine fusion. J Bone Jt Surg 38A:1142, 1956
3. Ascani E: Personal communication
4. Baker DR: Personal communication
5. Baker DR, McHolick W: Spondyloschisis and spondylolisthesis in children. J Bone Jt Surg 38A:933, 1956
6. Borkow SE, Kleiger B: Spondylolisthesis in the newborn, a case report. Clin Orthop 81:73–6, 1971
7. Boxall DW, Bradford DS, Moe JH, Winter RB: Management of severe spondylolisthesis (Grade III and Grade IV) in children and adolescents. J Bone Jt Surg 61A:479, 1979
8. Bradford D: Personal communication
9. Bradford DS: Treatment of severe spondylolisthesis: A combined approach for reduction and stabilization. Spine 4 (5):423, 1979
10. Clark K: Significance of small lumbar canal: Cauda equina compression syndromes due to spondylosis. Part 2. Clinical and surgical significance. J Neurosurg 31:495, 1969
11. Davis IS, Baily RW: Spondylolisthesis: Long-term followup study of treatment with total laminectomy. Paper presented at the annual meeting of Am Acad Orthop Surg, San Francisco, March, 1971

12. Daymond K, Sydney, Australia: Personal communication
13. DeWald R: Combined posterior and anterior correction and fusion for spondylolisthesis. Presented at the Scoliosis Research Society meeting, Ottawa, Canada, 1976
14. Duncan D: Alterations in the structure of the nerves caused by restricting their growth with ligature. J Neuropath Exp Neurol 7:261–273, 1948
15. Farfan HF: Mechanical Disorders of the Low Back. Philadelphia, Lea & Febiger, 1973
16. Fisk J, Moe J, Winter R: Scoliosis, spondylolysis and spondylolisthesis: Their relationship as reviewed in 539 patients. Spine (3): 234–245, 1978
17. Fitzgerald J, Newman P: Degenerative spondylolisthesis. J Bone Jt Surg 58B(2):184, 1976
18. Gill, Gerald: Avulsion of the first sacral nerve due to high grade olisthesis. Manuscript awaiting publication.
19. Gill GG, Manning JG, White HL: Surgical treatment of spondylolisthesis without spinal fusion. J Bone Jt Surg 33A:493–520, 1955
20. Harrington PR, Dickson JH: Spinal instrumentation in the treatment of severe progressive spondylolisthesis. Clin Orthop 117:157–163, 1976
21. Harrington PR, Tullos HS: Spondylolisthesis in children. Clin Orthop 79:75, 1971
22. Harris RI: Spondylolisthesis. Ann R Coll Surg (Engl) 8:259, 1951
23. Harris RI, Wiley JJ: Acquired spondylolisthesis as a sequel to spinal fusion. J Bone Jt Surg 45A:1159, 1963
24. Haukipuro K, Keranen N, Koivisto E, Lindholm R, Norio R, Punto L: Familial occurrence of lumbar spondylolysis and spondylolisthesis. Clinical Genetics 13:471–476, 1978
25. Henry A: Extensile Exposure applied to lumbar surgery, p. 161. Baltimore, Williams & Wilkins Co, 1945
26. Herbinaux G: Traite sur Divers Accouchement Laborieux et sur les Polypes de la Matrice. De Boubers, Bruxelles, 1782
27. Hoffman HJ, Hendrick EB, Humphrys RP: The tethered spinal cord: Its protean manifestations, diagnosis and surgical correction. Child's Brain 2:145–155, 1976
28. Hutton WC, Cyron BM: Spondylolysis: The role of the posterior elements in resisting the intervertebral compressive force. Acta Orthop Scand 49:604–609, 1978
29. Jenkins JA: Spondylolisthesis. Br J Surg 24:80, 1936
30. Junghanns H: Spondylolisthesis, 30 pathologischanatomisch untersuchte. Klin Chir 158:554, 1929
31. Karaharjii E, Hunnuksela M: Possible syphilitic spondylitis. Acta Orthop Scand 44:289, 1973
32. Kilian HF: Schilderungen neuer Beckenformen und ihres Verhalten im leben Bassermann und Mathy. Mannheim, 1854 (cit da Brocher)
33. Lambi, DA: Zehn Thesen über Spondylolisthesis. Zentralbl Gynaekol 9:250, 1955
34. Laurent LE, Einola S: Spondylolisthesis in children and adolescents. Acta Orthop Scand 31:45–64, 1961
35. Louis, R: Treatment of severe spondylolisthesis and spondyloptosis with reduction, internal fixation and arthrodesis. Paper read at the meeting of the International Society for the Study of the Lumbar Spine, Goteborg, Sweden, May, 1979
36. Macnab I: Paper read at the meeting of the International Society for the study of the lumbar spine, London, 1975
37. Macnab I: Spondylolisthesis with an intact neural arch. The so-called pseudospondylolisthesis. J Bone Jt Surg 32:325, 1950
38. Macnab I, Dall C: The blood supply of the lumbar spine and its application to the technic of intertransverse lumbar fusion. J Bone Jt Surg 53B:628, 1971
39. Matthias H: Reduction of spondylolisthesis. Paper read at the meeting of the International Society for the Study of the Lumbar Spine, Goteborg, Sweden, May, 1979
40. McPhee IP, O'Brien JP: Reduction of severe spondylolisthesis: A preliminary report. Spine 4(5):430, 1979
41. Neugebauer, F: Die Entschung der Spondylolisthesis. Zentrable Gynaekol 5:260–261, 1881
42. Neugebauer, FI: Zentrabl Gynaekol 5:260, 1881
43. Newman, PG: A clinical syndrome associated with severe lumbosacral subluxation. J Bone Jt Surg 47B:472, 1965
44. Newman PH: Paper read at the meeting of the International Society for the Study of the Lumbar Spine, London, 1975
45. Nisbet NW, Oswestry, England. Personal communication
46. O'Hata H: The familial incidence of spondylolisthesis. J Jap Orthop Assn, 1967
47. Ohki I, Mikanagi K, Shibuya K: Reduction and fusion of severe spondylolisthesis. Paper read at the meeting of SICOT, Oct, 1978, Kyoto, Japan
48. Peck H: Personal communication
49. Petajan J, Momberger G, Aase J, *et al*: Arthrogryposis syndrome (Kuskokwim disease) in the Eskimo. JAMA 209:1481, 1969
50. Prietto P: Personal communication
51. Reynolds, JR, Wiltse, L: Degenerative spon-

dylolisthesis. Paper presented at the meeting of the International Society for the Study of the Lumbar Spine, San Francisco, June, 1978

52. Risser J, Norquist D: Sciatic scoliosis in the growing child. Clin Orthop 21:156, 1961
53. Robert (zu Koblenz): Eine eigentumliche angeborene Lordose, wahrseheinlich bedingt eine Verschiebung des Korpers des letzten Lindenwirbels auf die vordere Flache des ersten Kreuzheinwirbels (Spondylolisthesis Kilian), nebst Bermerlsungen über die Mechanik dieser Beckenformation. Monatsschr Geburtskunde Frauenkrank 5:81–94, 1855
54. Rosenberg N: Degenerative spondylolisthesis, predisposing factors. J Bone Jt Surg 57A:467, 1975
55. Rosenberg, NJ: Degenerative spondylolisthesis, surgical treatment, Clin Ortho 117:112, 1976
56. Rowe GG, Roche MB: The etiology of separate neural arch. J Bone Jt Surg 35A:102, 1953
57. Ruge D, Wiltse LL: Spinal disorders, diagnosis and treatment. Philadelphia, Lea & Febiger, p 142, 1977
58. Schultz, AJ: Personal communication
59. Semon R, Spengler D: Significance of lumbar spondylolysis in college football players. Paper read at the meeting of the Western Orthopedic Assn, Las Vegas, Nevada, October, 1979
60. Sherman FC, Rosenthal RK, Hall JE: Spine fusion for spondylolysis and spondylolisthesis in children. Spine 4 (1):59, 1979
61. Snijder JGN, Seroo JM, Snijder CJ, Schijvens AWM: Therapy of spondylolisthesis by repositioning and fixation of the olisthetic vertebra. Clin Ortho 117:149, 1976
62. Stewart TD: The age incidence of neural arch defects in Alaskan natives, considered from the standpoint of etiology, J Bone Jt Surg 35A:937, 1953
63. Troup D: Paper read at the meeting of the International Society for the Study of the Lumbar Spine, London, 1975
64. Unander-Scharin L: A case of spondylolisthesis lumbalis adquisita. Acta Orthop Scand 19:536, 1950
65. West, F: Personal Communication
66. Wiltse LL: Etiology of spondylolisthesis. Clin Orthop 10:45, 1957
67. Wiltse LL: Paper read at the meeting of the International Society for the Study of the Lumbar Spine, London, 1975
68. Wiltse LL: Spondylolisthesis: Classification and etiology. Symposium of the Spine, Am Acad Ortho Surg, 143. St. Louis, CV Mosby, 1969
69. Wiltse, LL: Spondylolisthesis, etiology and classification. Sound slide program presented at the meeting of the American Acad Ortho Surgeons, New Orleans, Feb. 3, 1976
70. Wiltse LL, Bateman JG, Hutchinson RH: The paraspinal sacrospinalis-splitting approach to the lumbar spine. J Bone Jt Surg 50A:919, 1968
71. Wiltse LL, Hutchison RH: The surgical treatment of spondylolisthesis. Clin Orthop 34:116, 1964
72. Wynne-Davies R, Scott JHS: Inheritance and spondylolisthesis; A radiographic family survey. J Bone Jt Surg, (Br) 61B:301–305, 1979
73. Yano T, Meyagi S, Ikari T: Studies of familial incidence of spondylolisthesis. Singapore Med J, 8(3):203, 1967

Osteoporosis 16

Lawrence Wallach

Osteoporosis is the most common metabolic bone disease in adults. Seventy percent of all fractures occurring in the elderly population are secondary to osteoporosis. It has been estimated that six million spontaneous fractures occur annually, of which five million are in women. Minor trauma to the spine, even a cough or sneeze, may result in severe low back pain from collapse of weakened vertebrae. Fractures of the femoral heads or wrists are also common. Therefore, an understanding of osteoporosis is important in attempting to prevent and treat the significant morbidity that results from it.

Osteoporosis means "porous bone," but not all osteoporotic bone is roentgenologically, or histologically, identifiable as such. Therefore, the term osteopenia may be preferred, but this terminology has not replaced the usual term of osteoporosis in the medical literature. **Osteopenia** is the presence of a deceased bone mass in relationship to unit volume of bone. A simple visualization of this concept would be to imagine swiss cheese, with gradually increasing size of the holes (Fig. 16-1). The bone is histologically and chemically normal in composition. It is only that there is less bone than would be expected when compared to normal people.

There is no disagreement that all bone will become osteoporotic with age (Fig. 16-2). Bone mass reaches its maximum during the third decade, and then gradually declines as aging continues. Women attain less bone mass than men, and blacks attain more bone mass than other races. However, there are several groups that are not in the usual pattern, and they are classed by age at which the premature bone loss occurs: juvenile, idiopathic, post-menopausal, and senile type osteoporosis (Fig. 16-2). In addition, there are several diseases in which osteoporosis occurs as a secondary phenomenon (Table 16-1). The physician must exclude these illnesses before grouping his patients into any of these categories.

Theories of Pathogenesis

Although osteoporosis is a natural aging process, two principle theories exist to determine why some patients reach symptomatic levels of bone loss. Some believe that there may be subgroups of patients who lose bone mass more rapidly than the population at large.[21] Others believe that the rate of bone loss is approximately the same for all people, and only those with an inadequate or decreased bone mass at maturity will lose enough bone to ever become symptomatic from osteoporosis.[24]

If the latter theory is correct, those factors that lead to attainment of bone mass during growth are the only ones that are important in the development of osteoporosis in later years. Nutrition (especially adequate pro-

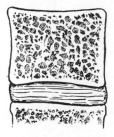

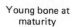

Young bone at maturity

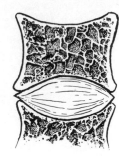

Osteoporotic Bone

Fig. 16-1. Osteoporosis, the loss of bone mass per unit volume, leads to porosity as shown. Pressure from intervertebral discs will deform the weakened vertebrae ("cod-fish" vertebrae).

tein, vitamin D, and calcium intake), exercise, and the racial and genetic factors mentioned above, would be important. In some animal experiments, it is possible to produce osteoporosis simply by decreasing calcium intake, but in most cases the predominant lesion produced is that of **osteomalacia,** or insufficient mineralization of bone.[10] In pure osteomalacia, the bone mass is usually normal. In human experiments, however, even prolonged intravenous calcium infusions will not lead to increased bone formation in osteoporosis.[36]

However, if the theory of variability in rates of bone loss is correct, factors that might increase this rate become most important in the etiology of osteoporosis. Early studies did show increased resorptive surfaces in comparison to active bony accretion, lending credence to theories of increased bone resorption as being important.[12] However, newer data show that resorptive surfaces are inactive,[22,26,33] and that the rates of resorption are not increased in osteoporosis. Apparently resorption continues at its usual rate.

It is now clear that a decrease in the rate of new bone formation is probably the key pathogenic factor in osteoporosis.[22,26] A decrease in the rate of new bone formation may simply be an aging process of bone which in some patients becomes more marked. If there is less bone formed during growth, the natural aging process may lead to premature bony mass depletion. An adequate skeleton at maturity may, on the other hand, become osteoporotic if rates of bone formation decrease.

Hormonal Factors

It is generally believed that new bone formation must occur in areas where bone resorption has just taken place.[26] Theoretically, there are stem cells, called **osteoprogenitor cells,** which first convert to osteoclasts, which induce resorption of bone. Other factors then convert the osteoclasts to osteoblasts, and bone accretion follows. The osteoblasts are active for several months; then they convert to a mature osteocyte. That area of the bone will then be quiescent until new bone remodeling occurs in the future. The factors that modulate the conversion from stem cell to osteocyte are schematically indicated in Figure 16-3.

For example, parathyroid hormone (PTH) will increase the conversion of osteoprogenitor cells to osteoclasts, but will decrease the conversion from that cell to osteoblasts. The net effect of these changes is increased bone resorption by increasing osteoclastic activity. Calcitonin, a hormone whose presence is universal but whose functional importance is still unclear, behaves in an opposite manner. Calcitonin will increase the conversion from osteoclasts to osteoblasts and decrease the flow of stem cells into the cycle. Therefore, the initial effect of calcitonin would be decreased bone resorption and increased bone formation. However, as the flow of stem cells decreases, the process of new bone formation will necessarily decrease as well.

Roles for other hormones and the factors that are mentioned in Figure 16-3 have been proposed in the pathogenesis of osteoporosis. Hormones do play an important role in the formation of new bone. Pathological states of hormone excess (of parathyroid hormone, thyroxine) and deficiencies (of estrogen, testosterone) may present with osteoporosis.

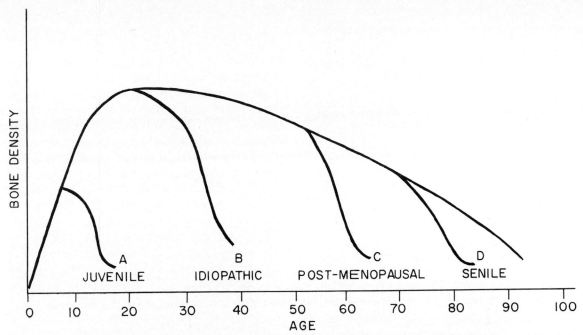

Fig. 16-2. Bone density reaches its peak and plateaus during the 2nd and 3rd decades, and then progressively falls with aging. Idiopathic forms of primary osteoporosis are classified by the age at which they occur.

However, the role of hormones in the development of primary osteoporosis remains unclear. At present, the factors that lead to decreased bone formation in primary osteoporosis are not so well understood as those in secondary forms of this disease. In addition, there may also be unknown humoral or local factors at the bone level that lead to decreased bone formation.

Differential Diagnosis of Secondary Osteoporosis

Known causes of bone loss must be excluded before one can diagnose primary osteoporosis (Table 16-1). Primary hyperparathyroidism may present as back pain, with or without vertebral crush fractures, as the initial manifestation.[4] Multiple myeloma may show diffuse osteoporosis and vertebral collapse, even in the absence of the other classical roentgenographic findings such as a "salt and pepper" skull. Hyperthyroidism, acromegaly, and hypercortisolemia (Cushings syndrome), especially the rare form micronodular adrenal hyperplasia, may present with osteoporosis as one of their manifestations.[30] Osteomalacia may coexist with osteoporosis and must always be considered. Juvenile diabetics have less bone mass than age-matched controls, but because of shortened longevity, they rarely present with symptomatic fractures.[32] Long-standing primary or secondary gonadal hypofunction is another entity that presents with osteoporosis. Malignancies, either by the secretion of humoral substances or infiltration of bone or bone marrow, may be roentgenographically interpreted as osteoporosis as well.

Laboratory Investigation

Laboratory investigation is required to exclude secondary causes of osteoporosis. Decreased serum calcium, decreased phosphate, and increased alkaline phosphatase

Table 16-1.   Differential Diagnosis of Osteoporosis

Primary	III. **Bone marrow replacement**
Juvenile	Malignant
Idiopathic	Nonmalignant (Gaucher's)
Postmenopausal	IV. **Malignancy**
Senile	Multiple myeloma
Secondary	Metastases
I. **Genetic**	Hormone-like secretion
Osteogenesis imperfecta	V. **Nutritional**
	Protein malnutrition
Homocytinuria	Calcium deficiency
II. **Endocrine**	Vitamin D deficiency
Cushing's syndrome	VI. **Localized**
Thyrotoxicosis	Disuse
Acromegaly	Post-traumatic
Primary hyperparathyroidism	VIII. **Drug Related**
	Heparin (long-term)
Hypogonadism	
Hypopituitarism	
Diabetes mellitus	

levels will demonstrate chemical evidence of osteomalacia. These studies should be normal in osteoporosis, but slight increases in alkaline phosphatase will occur if recent fractures are present. Parathyroid hormone levels may be needed if the patient is hypercalcemic. Serum thyroxine (T-4) may be helpful, but hopefully one would diagnose hyperthyroidism prior to its presentation as osteoporotic-induced fractures. Erythrocyte sedimentation rate, serum protein electrophoresis, CBC, and SMA-12 will aide in the diagnosis of multiple myeloma and other malignancies. In unusual cases, other studies may be needed, such as a bone marrow examination or even bone biopsy of undecalcified bone. In the biopsy, one would look for evidence of osteomalacia, which would be indicated by increased numbers of osteoid seams with inadequate mineralization. Biopsy of osteoporotic bone would show no such pathological changes.

Roentgenographic Diagnosis

Unfortunately, plain film roentgenography is an insensitive technique for the diagnosis of osteoporosis, because 30% or more of bone must be lost before changes are seen. Vertebral "codfishing," loss of height, collapse, and rarefaction of bone are noted. The horizontal trabeculae, or striations, are lost,

but the vertical ones remain. The end-plates remain well defined, and appear finely penciled. The skull is usually spared.

Because of the insensitivity of plain film roentgenograms, other methods of study have been developed for both the clinical and experimental purpose of studying osteoporosis. The loss of trabeculation of the femoral heads has been shown to occur not haphazardly, but in an orderly fashion. This loss of trabeculation correlates with the degree of bone loss and is termed the Singh index.[35] However, reproducibility of this index by various groups has been difficult. Bone mineral content can be studied by photodensitometry, absorptiometry, and neutron activation, but these procedures are not generally available except in research centers. Similarly, bone remodeling techniques, such as tetracycline labeling and calcium balance studies, are hardly routine procedures. These sophisticated methods aid the researcher; but clinicians must, of necessity, deal with plain films and routine laboratory tests to make a diagnosis and to exclude other illnesses such as osteomalacia or infiltration of bone. Technetium bone scanning may be of some help in differentiating an old from a more recent (and acute) compression deformity.

Signs and Symptoms

Is the simple loss of bone mass ever clinically apparent before roentgenographic fractures occur? Patients with low back pain may show rarefaction of the bone. Microfractures are known to occur and may be the cause of discomfort in cases where actual fractures are not seen on x-ray film. The symptoms of back pain are not fixed; they may be intermittent and difficult to correlate with the slow, progressive loss of bone mass. Pain certainly will occur with compressed vertebral fractures, because of pressure from fractured bone on spinal nerve roots and sensory fibers of the periosteum.

As previously mentioned, even minor trauma may cause the collapse of one or

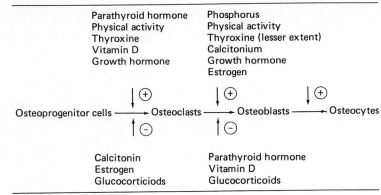

Fig. 16-3. Bone remodeling cycle. The various factors that stimulate this cycle are shown above the arrow; those that inhibit the cycle are below. (From Rasmussen H, Bordier P: Cellular basis of metabolic bone disease. NEJM 289:25–32, 1973)

more vertebral bodies. Occasionally, however, there is no history of trauma. Aching pain, with localized tenderness over the collapsed vertebra, may be seen. Kyphosis will occur if more than one vertebra collapses, and there will be loss of height as well. A quick guide to loss of height would be to look for decrease in the ratio of height to arm span. Paraspinal muscle spasms and decreased mobility may be present. It is a rare occurrence to see spinal cord compression from simple osteoporosis. Generalized bone pain may indicate osteomalacia but is usually not seen in osteoporosis. Therefore, one should look for the presence of pseudofractures on roentgenograms of the hip, clavicle, and scapula when osteomalacia is suspected.

Treatment

Once vertebrae have been weakened to the point of collapse, or the femur fractured because of osteoporosis, it must be conceded that restoration of bone to normal levels is impossible. However, it has been shown that various treatment modalities may prevent further bone loss, and perhaps, even increase bone density in some cases. The therapeutic modalities that are available are listed in Table 16-2. These agents have been used alone, or in combination, for the treatment of osteoporosis.

Estrogen Therapy

It has been repeatedly demonstrated that the administration of estrogen will prevent bone loss in postmenopausal women. Proponents of estrogen therapy for the treatment of osteoporosis have claimed clinical improvement in pain and restoration of bone after just 3 weeks of therapy.[6] In 1959, Henneman and Wallach suggested this, by showing that females who are replaced with estrogen lost less height and suffered fewer fractures than expected.[9] Many additional studies have supported this contention.[7,17,21,27] One recent large prospective study of a 10-year follow-up of similarly treated women supported the early data. It showed that estrogen therapy prevented bone loss and perhaps even increased bone formation, whereas placebo-treated controls increased their degree of osteoporosis (Fig. 16-4).[23]

The mode of action of estrogen in preventing bone loss remains uncertain. In the earlier model (Fig. 16-3), estrogen increased the conversion from osteoclasts to osteoblasts but slowed the stem cell entrance into the scheme of remodeling. Beyond this, estrogen may modulate the parathyroid hor-

Table 16-2. Therapeutic Modalities for Osteoporosis

Estrogens	Calcium
Anabolic steroids	Calcitonin
Fluoride	Growth hormone
Vitamin D	Diphosphonates

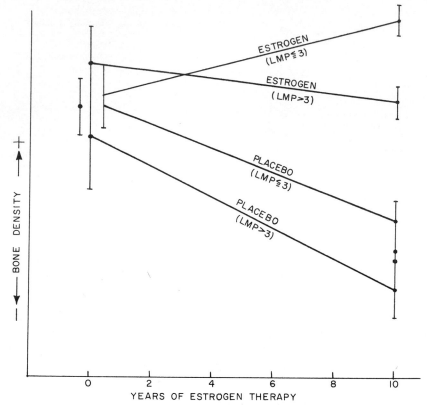

Fig. 16-4. The changes in bone density that followed 10 years' study of postmenopausal estrogen therapy. (LMP = last menstrual period) (From Nachtigall et al: Estrogen replacement therapy I: A 10-year prospective-study in the relationship to osteoporosis. Obstet Gynecol 53:277–281, 1979)

mone action on the bone to lessen osteoclastic activity. In addition, the relatively estrogen-deficient state of menopause may allow relative glucocorticoid excess to increase bone resorption.

Estrogen therapy has been enthusiastically promoted for postmenopausal females, but recent studies of a possible increase in endometrial carcinoma has certainly decreased its use, especially as a routine supplement for the menopausal state.[29] The federal government has labelled estrogen drugs as possibly carcinogenic. The risks and benefits of estrogen therapy for postmenopausal women have been debated in the literature.[31,34] The data proving increased risk of uterine carcinoma from estrogen is more convincing only for stage I or II (nonfatal) disease, and so some physicians are more concerned with the morbidity and possible mortality that may result from estrogen deficiency at the bone level than from endometrial cancer.

I believe the data, when taken in toto, indicate a role for estrogen therapy in postmenopausal females. The risk of osteoporosis-induced fractures seems to be greater for women who are castrated surgically at an early age, or who undergo a spontaneous premature menopause. Therapy with Premarin (1.25 mg daily for 21 days), followed by Provera (10 mg q.d. for 7) days will prevent the accumulation of continuously stimulated endometrial tissue that is believed to be the precancerous lesion. In patients who have had hysterectomies, there seems to be no reason not to employ estrogen therapy. In patients with symptomatic osteoporosis, doses of 2.5 mg of Premarin may be used.

Severely affected females should be treated with estrogen and anabolic steroids.

Anabolic Steroids

Modification of the steroid androgen nucleus has led to the development of steroids with less androgenicity but continued anabolic effectiveness. These anabolic steroids have a role in the treatment of osteoporosis. Although early studies were disappointing, with increased numbers of fractures noted in patients so treated, more recent studies using methandrostenolone (Dianabol) show decreased bone mineral loss in postmenopausal women.[3,28] Studies combining the use of anabolic steroids with estrogen and calcium carbonate have also decreased age-related bone loss.[27] I use Dianabol 5 mg daily for 3 of every 4 weeks. These drugs do impart other potentially beneficial clinical effects, such as increased sense of well-being, but they also may cause hirsutism in females. Anabolic steroids may induce hepatitis, so screening periodically for liver damage is necessary.

Fluoride

Fluoride treatment increases osteoblastic activity in bone, so it would seem that its use in osteoporosis would be assured. However, bone biopsy specimens in patients so treated indicate that the new bone that was formed was not normal but appeared similar to osteomalacic bone. Therefore, the use of fluoride has been combined with vitamin D and calcium in the hope that these drugs will decrease the formation of poorly mineralized bone.[14] The doses of fluoride employed are large, a hundred times the dose that is needed to prevent simple tooth decay. Giant cells have been noted in bone marrow specimens of patients on fluoride, and a recent editorial has cautioned against its use in the treatment of osteoporosis.[5,20] However, a new European study does report efficacy with fluoride treatment in osteo-

porosis.[15] In the United States, the use of fluoride for the treatment of osteoporosis is still experimental. At this time, it is of unproven benefit and therefore not recommended.

Vitamin D and Calcium, and Other Therapies

Marked benefits are occasionally ascribed to treatment of osteoporosis with vitamin D, or one of its more potent metabolites.[11] However, it is generally accepted that this improvement occurs in cases where osteomalacia (*i.e.*, vitamin D deficiency) is commonly present and possibly not previously diagnosed. Therapy with calcium infusions, growth hormone, and calcitonin are either of theoretical benefit or clinically helpful in short-term studies, but they have not proven effective over the long term in osteoporosis.[2,4,13,18,36] Such a case is that of calcitonin therapy. In the early months, definite improvement in bone density will occur, probably owing to decreased osteoclastic activity induced by the hormones' administration. However, calcitonin also decreases the flow of new stem cells into active bone remodeling units, so that the improvement in bone mass is evanescent at best. However, long-term calcitonin therapy is still under study.[8] One brief report suggests that calcitonin may be useful in the treatment of steroid-induced osteoporosis.[25]

Virtually all of the above-mentioned therapies have been used alone or in combination with vitamin D and calcium supplementation. These latter drugs are not benign, and severe hypercalcemia has resulted from their routine prescription to elderly patients.[16] If osteomalacia is suspected, laboratory and roentgenographic evaluation should be performed before prescribing pharmacologic doses of vitamin D or calcium.

Exercise has been shown to possibly increase bone formation, although the changes are of a mild degree.[7] Immobilation should be avoided, as decreasing bony stress leads to increased bone resorption. This is a prob-

Infections of the Lumbar Spine 17

Because infections of the lumbar spine are not common, they are often overlooked as a cause of back pain. Yet they are common enough to deserve consideration in the differential diagnosis of low back dysfunction of uncertain etiology. The infectious process can be bacterial, tuberculous, or mycotic, but in some instances no organism can be demonstrated on smear or culture. Spinal infections occur more commonly in adults than in children and in equal frequency between men and women. The infectious source may be postspinal surgery, a distant focus of infection, or an idiopathic one.

Infections Subsequent to Lumbar Disc Surgery

Soft Tissue Infections

In a personal series of 1000 cases of lumbar disc disease treated surgically, 241 patients developed wound infections (2.41%). The majority of these infections remained localized in the superficial soft tissues and did not involve, in a clinically identifiable way, the intervertebral disc space. When the infection does involve the disc space, these questions arise: did the interspace infection develop secondarily to the soft tissue infection; did the disc space infection develop first and subsequently spread outward to the soft tissues; or were both sites simultaneously infected? The sequence of events is of more than academic consideration, since it relates directly to the proper management of the complication. If disc infection is secondary to soft tissue infection, it follows that an incompletely drained soft tissue infection may spread into the intervertebral disc space, which otherwise would be spared.

SIGNS AND SYMPTOMS

An elevated temperature on the 4th to 8th postoperative day, in association with more than the anticipated postoperative incisional discomfort, should direct the physician's attention to the possibility of wound infection. Increased incisional tenderness and swelling may make it impossible for the patient to remain in a supine position which causes direct pressure upon the wound. Careful inspection usually reveals evidence of purulence at the edges of the incision, and sometimes drainage of pus is seen.[10]

MANAGEMENT

Purulent drainage is identified as soon as possible by culture and sensitivity tests and by microscopic examination. The generally accepted method of treatment is to open the wound to allow adequate drainage of purulent material, and to place the patient on appropriate antibiotics in accordance with the culture and sensitivity tests.

If the infection is confined to the superficial soft tissues, the incisional pain abates once the purulent collection is allowed to escape and wound abscess pressure is relieved. Persisting fever, signs of general septicemia, and increasing back and sciatic pain signal serious extension of the infectious process and require immobilization, massive doses of antibiotic, and major medical supportive efforts.

The vast majority of wound infections are confined to the superficial soft tissues, and some difference of opinion exists regarding the extent of wound reopening in such cases. Some physicians believe that in the presence of signs of wound suppuration, limited aspiration, probing, or bedside measures of wound evacuation should give way to a much more radical reopening of the wound in the operating room. Utilizing such wide exposure, all recesses of the wound which evidence infection or necrotic tissue or hematoma may then be saucerized and the wound lightly packed open. The wound will heal from the depths outward. With healing, gradual removal of the packing is carried out from the deepest portion of the wound outward. Soft rubber catheters are usually placed within the packing for daily instillations of topical antibiotics (equal parts of 0.1% polymyxin, 1.0% neomycin, and 500 units per cc bacitracin). Systematic antibacterial medication is administered in accordance with the organism culture and sensitivity tests.

The treatment of personal preference involves drainage of the wound through a limited and superficial opening of the incision, with no attempt to probe the depths of the wound. Frequent warm, wet soaks are utilized, and the patient is permitted to ambulate. In the absence of fever, signs of general septicemia, or increasing back and sciatic pain, the patient may be discharged and can continue warm, wet soaks at home without the use of antibiotics. Close outpatient follow-up on a twice weekly basis is continued until complete wound healing occurs.

Intervertebral Disc Space Infections

Two intervertebral disc space infections occurred in 241 superficial wound infections (0.8% of 241 superficial wound infections and 0.2% of 1000 cases). Most intervertebral disc space infections subsequent to lumbar disc surgery are associated with a superficial wound infection, which may develop before or after the interspace infection. Some cases have been reported with no external evidence of purulence.

SIGNS AND SYMPTOMS

Every intervertebral disc space infection is characterized by excruciating, diffuse back pain which often spreads into the hips and flanks in association with severe lumbar paraspinal muscle spasm. Any movement tends to aggravate the pain; weight bearing is intolerable; and even the most minor trauma, such as the inadvertent jarring of the bed by attendants, aggravates the pain. This clinical picture may occur within a week of surgery or may be delayed as long as 6 weeks after surgery. Ileus and abdominal distention may be associated with the clinical picture.

A low-grade temperature elevation may be present but is often normal. Leukocytosis may be present.

The sedimentation rate is invariably increased, but this may be a source of confusion, since the tissue trauma of surgery will generally result in an elevated of sedimentation level for 1 or 2 months. An increase in the sedimentation rate persisting 3 months after surgery in association with severe low back pain is strongly suggestive of a disc space infection. Blood cultures are usually negative, unless the infection extends into the adjacent soft tissues and creates a paraspinal abscess. Bone scans are not useful, because the increased uptake resulting from the tissue disruption of surgery may persist for as long as half a year.

Roentgenographic findings are unrevealing until at least 4 to 8 weeks, when the first changes are seen. At that time, in addition to slight narrowing of the involved interspace, some erosion of the adjacent articular surfaces can be visualized. Laminography in the lateral views is often helpful in defining these early changes. Progressive rarefaction of the anterior subchondral area, with irregular destruction of the end-plate, is seen. This is followed by further diminution of the disc space and destruction of the adjacent portion of the neighboring vertebral body. The end stages progress to bony ankylosis laterally and anteriorly over a variable period of time, from several weeks to several months. A significant number of cases do not demonstrate roentgenographic evidence of complete bony fusion.

MANAGEMENT

Maximal immobilization of the lumbar spine is essential to proper treatment of lumbar intervertebral disc space infection. Although absolute bed rest can be considered, persistence of pain may be an indication of inadequate immobilization, which may be augmented by maintaining the patient for 3 to 6 months in a plaster body spica extending from the midthorax to below the knees. Large doses of an appropriate, broad-spectrum antibiotic are given for 12 weeks.

When the spica is removed after 3 months, if the interspace infection is arrested, the patient should be reasonably comfortable at bed rest. Low back and mobilization exercises are initiated in bed, but the spine is supported by a low back support during weight bearing for approximately 3 or 4 additional months.

UNRECOGNIZED DISC SPACE INFECTION

Occasionally, a patient who has undergone lumbar disc surgery may develop a disc space infection which will neither be identified nor treated. Recovery will eventually occur and, under ordinary circumstances, no one will be the wiser. The following case history is illustrative.

F.S. A 36-year-old man underwent surgery for a herniated lumbar disc at the L4–5 level on the right, June 6, 1962. At surgery, a very large fragment of disc was found to be completely extruded into the spinal canal causing severe compression of the L5 nerve root. The operation went easily and I anticipated an excellent result.

Immediately after surgery, the patient was gratified by the dramatic disappearance of his right sciatica, and his 7-day hospital stay was uneventful. On the day of discharge, he appreciated moderate low back pain which was attributed to his incision and increased activities. After discharge, low back pain worsened; it was eased with bed rest and aggravated with weight-bearing activities. Because of these symptoms, lumbar spine films were obtained 3 weeks after surgery and these were nonrevealing. He required codeine and aspirin several times daily for 6 months after discharge. The codeine caused annoying chronic constipation, so he stopped this drug and relied solely on aspirin for the low back pain which was not very much improved. His original job as crew chief of a rigging group required him to pitch in with his men and participate in a variety of physically strenuous tasks. He requested and obtained a light duty job 8 months after surgery and was able to carry out this sedentary work, but he continued to experience intermittent low back discomfort. One year after surgery, he no longer required aspirin several times daily. One-and-a-half years after surgery, he was completely comfortable and was able to carry out all physical activities without pain. He was discharged from my care.

Three years after surgery, I saw him by chance, when he greeted me in the hospital roentgenography department. He was in the process of applying for a rigging job with a new company; the industrial physician, on being informed of his lumbar spine surgery, ordered lumbar spine films. These revealed obliteration and fusion of the L4–5 intervertebral space, certainly the result of a disc space infection.

This type of situation may occasionally explain a persistent and incapacitating back-

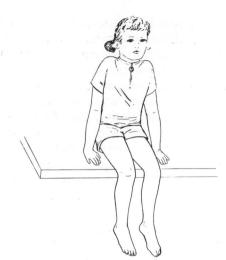

Fig. 17-1. Characteristic sitting position of children with intervertebral disc space infection, placing hands on either side of bed in an attempt to reduce weight-bearing of the spine.

intervertebral disc infection. A few of these infections arise from known foci, such as superficial wound infections or an appendectomy; but in most instances the disease develops spontaneously, without any recognizable antecedent infection elsewhere. Staphylococcus aureus is the organism usually responsible. In children under 5 years of age, the first symptom may be refusal to walk followed by back pain, stiffness, irritability, and fever, most often of less than 3 weeks' duration. Anorexia and weight loss often accompany these symptoms.

On examination the child has a rigid back with extremely restricted mobility. If the examiner attempts to sit the child, the child places his hands on either side of the bed behind his back in an attempt to stabilize the spine, because of increased pain on weight bearing (Fig. 17-1). Local tenderness of severe degree over the affected part of the spine may be noted. If the child can walk at all, ambulation is stiff, guarded, and performed in a gingerly fashion, since any motion or jarring causes an extreme exacerbation of pain. The child will often limp, favoring one or the other hip.[4,6,7]

When the lesion is within the lumbar spine, hamstring tightness is common and a positive iliopsoas sign is present, which may cause the examiner to consider hip disease. The iliopsoas sign is the production of pain when the hip joint is flexed beyond 30 degrees, causing the insertion of the iliopsoas into the lesser trochanter to move forward to the extent that its action becomes that of flexion. The Patrick's test involving external rotation of the hip is usually negative.

A low-grade temperature elevation is usually present early in the course of the disease. Laboratory studies usually reveal and elevated white cell count, and an elevated sedimentation rate is almost invariably present and may be the only laboratory abnormality. Bone scans are generally reliable and are helpful in identifying and localizing the septic process.

MODE OF INFECTION IN CHILDREN

The exact mode of infection of the intervertebral disc in children is not completely clear. It is thought that the infecting organism is carried through the intervertebral disc space by the blood stream or lymphatics. This can probably best be explained on a developmental basis. The intervertebral disc of the embryo and the young child receives its blood supply from the surfaces of the adjacent vertebral bodies. Blood vessels pass through the disc proper to permit perfusion of nutrients. These vessels gradually disappear with maturation of the vertebral body and the intervertebral disc, and the blood supply to the disc is completely obliterated by the end of the second decade. The vertebral plate of a preadolescent child, which is essentially a growth plate, demonstrates hyaline cartilage with vascular capillary buds penetrating through the cartilage. Organisms lodging in these capillaries may easily involve the disc space.

The vertebral plate of a 16-year-old demonstrates a transverse bony trabecular structure, with blood vessels approaching but not penetrating the vertebral disc cartilage. This closely resembles the adult anatomy with a

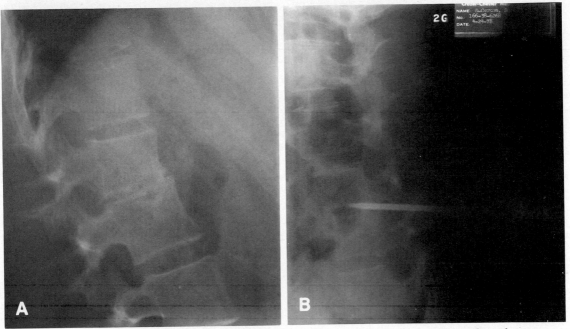

Fig. 17-2. **(A)** *Resolved (inactive) disc space infection L1–2 in 31-year-old female with chronic recurrant renal infection.* **(B)** *Percutaneous needle biopsy of A. No growth on culture.*

bony plate and closure or near closure of the growth plate. Intervertebral disc infection in the older child, therefore, closely resembles the process in the adult and may result in destruction along the margins of the vertebral body.

Review the section on Embryology for details of intervertebral disc vascularization, Chapter 1.

ROENTGENOGRAPHIC FINDINGS

Roentgenographic findings are meager in the early stages of the disease (Fig. 17-2). At least 2 or 4 weeks elapse after the onset of clinical symptoms before the disc space narrowing appears. There may be, however, a widening of the paravertebral shadows at the site of the involvement and occasional areas of marginal bony destruction in the older child. It is imperative, therefore, that any child with this symptom complex be closely followed at 1- or 2-week intervals for clinical examination and repeated roentgenograms

until the intervertebral disc narrowing at the site of maximum tenderness confirms the diagnosis. Tomograms are helpful in carefully defining the suspected interspace.

The symptomatic course of the disease varies from 2 to 6 weeks after treatment is initiated. However, the roentgenographic changes continue for a considerable period of time. In younger children, the initial reduction of the disc space may be followed in 6 to 12 weeks by a restoration of the original height of the intervertebral disc. In others, it may remain narrow indefinitely. Occasionally, in the older child, a gradual diminution of the disc space with eventual spontaneous fusion is the end result.

MANAGEMENT

Tuberculosis is not, currently, a very common disease, but pyogenic infections have not diminished and are much more likely to occur in children than in adults. If there is any doubt regarding the nature of the disease,

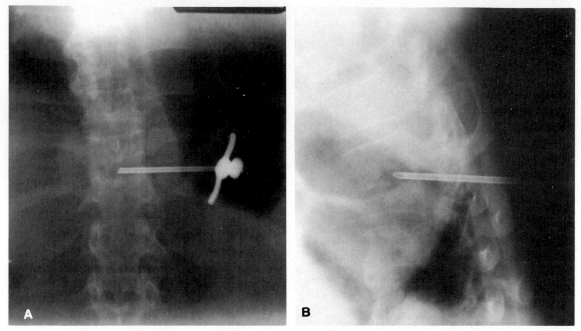

Fig. 17-3. Percutaneous needle biopsy of T10–11 of 58-year-old renal dialysis patient with spontaneous vertebral-disc space. Staphylococcus aureus infection (positive culture). **(A)** AP view. **(B)** Lateral view.

tuberculin skin tests are most helpful, since they are usually negative in children who ordinarily have minimal exposure to tuberculosis.

In addition to tuberculosis, the differential diagnosis must include spinal cord tumors, brucellosis, and salmonella infections. Aspirations and biopsy of the involved interspace with a Turkel needle, or surgical exposure for culture and biopsy purposes, are frequently indicated in adults but are not usually necessary in children.

Staphylococcus aureus is the organism usually responsible, and treatment with appropriate antibiotics and bed rest usually leads to a satisfactory outcome (Figs. 17-3 and 17-4). The antibiotics are continued empirically for 6 weeks, and the child is immobilized in a body spica extending from the midthorax to below the knees for 6 to 8 weeks. If the elevated sedimentation rate falls to a normal range and pain subsides, the spica can be removed within 6 to 8 weeks and replaced with a low back support, which can be worn during ambulation for an additional 4 months.

Nontuberculous Infections in Adults

CLINICAL PICTURE

Pyogenic spondylitis in adults may occur spontaneously without any recognizable antecedent infection elsewhere; it may follow skin infections; it may extend from an adjacent infection or urinary tract infection, either through catheterization or through genitourinary surgical procedures. When the urinary tract is the primary focus, the infection probably spreads to the vertebral bodies through the paravertebral veins described by Batson. A significant number of adults who develop this condition have preexisting diabetes mellitus.[11] Other associated medical conditions are illnesses that tend to debilitate patients and lower their resistance to infections. These include chronic alcoholism, metastatic carcinoma, drug addiction, and any illness that requires long-term steroid therapy such as rheumatoid arthritis.

Spinal infection in the adult is generally in the form of vertebral osteomyelitis as differentiated from the interspace infection of children. This difference in site predilection undoubtedly results from the presence of vascular channels perforating the vertebral end-plates in children, providing blood-borne organisms access to the intervertebral disc. The progressive obliteration of these channels after the age of 16 to 20 eliminates a direct vascular pathway to the disc.

In adults it is believed that the infectious organism spreads from a focus within that portion of the vertebral body adjacent to the cartilaginous end-plate. The exact etiology of the infection remains in some question.

Since the widespread use of antibiotics, a slowly developing bone infection has been encountered which is characterized by extensive destruction of bone. Following hip joint surgery, for example, the entire head and neck of the femur may erode and disappear over a period of weeks or months. This condition is invariably associated with an elevated white cell count and erythrocyte sedimentation rate. Although positive cultures are not always obtained from the abscess sites, in the final analysis *Staphylococcus aureus* is frequently found to be the causative organism. When these infections occur in the spine, their relative inaccessibility makes accurate establishment of the affecting organism even more difficult than in other areas.

The patient complains of severe pain in the lumbar region, which is aggravated by almost any movement or exertion but is not relieved by rest. The onset is usually abrupt but occasionally may be insidious.

Examination reveals local tenderness over the affected vertebrae, marked muscle spasm, and limitation of all spinal movements. An elevated white cell count and sedimentation rate and a low-grade fever are usually present.[5] The patient is often anemic.

ROENTGENOGRAPHIC FINDINGS

Early in septic spondylitis, roentgenograms are likely to be essentially normal. The bone scan, while not specific as to the nature of the condition, is most useful in localizing the disease process before x-ray film changes are evident. X-ray film changes do not develop until 3 or 4 weeks after the onset of pain. After that period of time, roentgenograms reveal rarefaction of the anterior subchondral area, with irregular destruction and erosion of the subchondral bone plate, rapid loss of the disc space, and destruction of the adjacent portion of the neighboring vertebral body. The process may advance to bony ankylosis laterally and anteriorly over the course of a few weeks or months.

Some cases do not go on to fusion but undergo progressive destruction of vertebrae, with possible extension of the infection anteriorly into the retroperitoneal space or through the natural barrier of the dura into the subarachnoid pathway, causing meningitis.

NEEDLE BIOPSY OF THE LUMBAR SPINE

Because of the potentially progressive nature of this disease in the adult, documentation of the infecting organism is advisable.

Aspiration and biopsy of the involved interspace with a Turkel or Craig needle may be necessary to establish a bacteriologic diagnosis and to exclude neoplasm or granulomatous disease, such as brucellosis and tuberculosis. The main difficulty with needle biopsy of the intervertebral disc is in not obtaining sufficient material for either culture or pathologic diagnosis. Complications such as bleeding or irreversible damage to neurological structures are not particularly common.[2]

Needle biopsy of the lumbar spine is especially useful in the management of pyogenic spondylitis (Figs. 17-2 and 17-3). Many of the patients suffering from this problem are seriously debilitated, presenting increased risk to general anesthesia and open biopsy. A needle biopsy performed under local anesthesia may provide information regarding the infecting organism and can be carried out with relative safety. The wide-

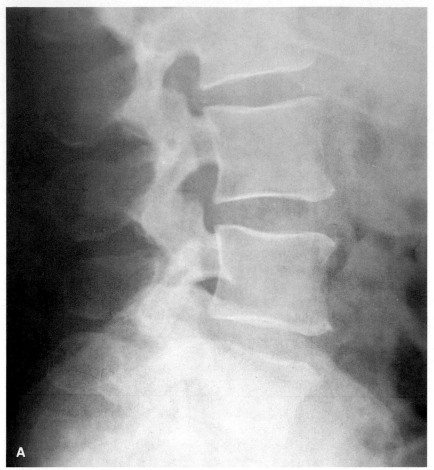

Fig. 17-4. *The insidious course of tuberculosis of the spine is demonstrated by these films. This 56-yr-old man with pulmonary tuberculosis first developed a dull aching low back pain in Oct 1954 and spine films obtained Nov 17, 1954, were nonrevealing. (A) Early vertebral body destruction of the L5 vertebra was visualized 4 months later. The film taken Dec 14, 1956, reveals extensive destruction of L5 with significant destructive changes involving L4. (B) The interspace is spared, indicating that the infection is primarily in the bone. (Continues on facing page.)*

spread availability of C-arm biplane fluoroscopic guidance allows careful and expeditious monitoring of the needle position. The Craig bone biopsy needle probably has the most widespread use, but there are a number of other bone biopsy needles on the market which have their advocates. The procedure can be carried out either in an operating room equipped with a C-arm fluoroscopic unit or in the x-ray film department. It is best performed with a standby anesthesiologist and a nurse or scrub technician from the operating room. The O.R. nurse or technician is helpful in preventing a lapse in sterile technique during the performance of this procedure. It is most important to avoid contaminating the specimen, which would yield a false positive culture and lead to an error in diagnosis and treatment.

The position of the patient can be either prone or lateral. Although my preference is the prone position, the final determinant is the patient's comfort; it is necessary for the patient to remain relatively immobile during the 45 minutes or 1 hour required to carry out this procedure. Prior to the biopsy, we

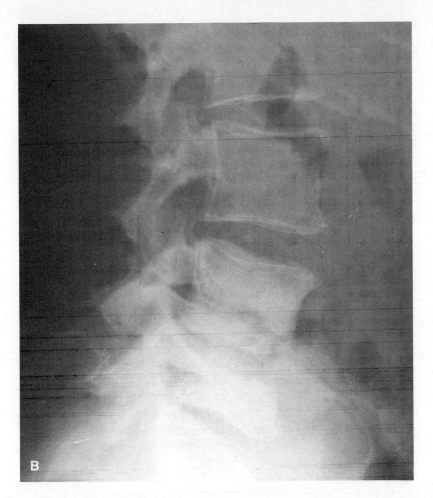

B

routinely cross and type for two bottles of blood and have an IV in place and running.

The suspected lesion is identified fluoroscopically, and a sterile metal marker is placed on the skin immediately over the involved vertebra. A Xylocaine skin wheal is made 6 cm lateral to the spinous process, and a 20-gauge LP needle is inserted through this wheal and directed toward the vertebral body at an angulation of approximately 45 to 50 degrees. If the body of L5 is biopsied, it may be necessary to overcome the obstruction presented by the ilium by angling the needle 30 degrees caudad as well. When satisfactory LP needle placement has been achieved, and the tip of the needle rests on the vertebral body, several cc's of Xylocaine injected via the LP needle will infiltrate the periosteum and reduce pain associated with the subsequent biopsy needle placement. The biopsy trocar is immediately introduced adjacent to the LP needle and closely following its direction. When fluoroscopic guidance reveals that the direction of the biopsy trocar is satisfactory, the LP needle is withdrawn.

The bone biopsy cannula, which has small serrated teeth, slides over the trocar so that it is positioned against the vertebral body, and the trocar is then removed. The cannula can be either rotated in one direction or twisted back and forth to cut a core of bone. During this maneuver, avoid exerting excessive downward pressure on the cannula, which may bend the small and relatively delicate teeth, and render the instrument inoperative. The bone core can often be retrieved without removing the cannula by inserting a "fish-tail" of two heavy, twisted wire sutures with the ends flared apart. After a suitable core of bone has been obtained from the desired site and if free pus is not present, a small amount of normal saline can be injected through the cannula and then reaspirated for purposes of culture.

When efforts to obtain such materials are unsuccessful, it might be necessary to consider open surgery. If tissue diagnosis and culture are needed in the thoracic region, a costotransversectomy is usually done.

MANAGEMENT

Some authorities defer invasive diagnostic measures to determine the organism and treat with bed rest, antibiotics, and a body spica. They rely on the clinical course as manifested by relief of pain, improvement in leukocytosis, sedimentation rate, and temperature, plus serial roentgenograms of the spine to determine success or failure of therapy. Almost all authorities on spinal infections presently favor documentation of the organism, so that appropriate antibiotic therapy can be utilized.[8,12] Occasionally myelography is necessary from a diagnostic point of view.

Most patients can be treated with antibiotic therapy, rest, and immobilization with a body spica. Occasionally this type of management is difficult to carry out because of the severe and intractable pain plus the prolonged duration of treatment extending over 3 or 4 months. Control of pain with medication becomes increasingly more difficult, and the associated emotional depression related to prolonged immobilization may create a progressively deteriorating environment. Open surgical debridement may be helpful in reducing both the duration of the illness and the intractable pain. A surgical approach is particularly appropriate if a soft tissue abscess is identified adjacent to the site of the vertebral infection. A variety of surgical approaches can be utilized, but a decompressive laminectomy is almost always contraindicated and best avoided. Such a procedure, which removes the posterior supporting bony elements in the face of a partially eroded and weakened vertebral body, has obvious disadvantages: once the patient resumed weight bearing, a serious spinal deformity creating neurological and mechanical problems would inevitably result.

If a computerized axial tomographic (CAT) scan of the spine reveals a soft tissue abscess extending anteriorly, an abdominal approach may be advisable. In the absence of a soft tissue abscess, a lateral approach similar to the costotransversectomy technique is preferable to the standard decompressive laminectomy. This enables open surgical debridement and subsequent irrigation of the infected site without total eradication of the posterior bony elements.

Efforts are presently in progress to place bone grafts in the infected areas to establish a segmental fusion of the involved interspace. This, of course, is counter to all traditional views holding that no foreign material, including new bone, should be placed adjacent to pyogenic osteomyelitis. However, preliminary reports indicate that some modification of this unbending rule may be forthcoming.

DISC SPACE ABSCESS

Very rarely, a disc space abscess is encountered which will simulate a disc herniation. My personal experience is limited to one case of this nature. The patient (T.D.), a 58-year-old man, was admitted to the hospital on March 8, 1957, with low back pain and radiation into the left lower extremity. Examination revealed a diminished but present left Achilles reflex and an inconstant zone of hypesthesia extending into the lateral aspect of the foot. The temperature was normal, blood count and laboratory studies unremarkable. The back pain was excruciating and aggravated by any movement; the sciatica was less painful. Pelvic traction was instituted but was discontinued because of increased discomfort. A myelogram revealed a filling defect at the L5-S1 interspace on the left which was thought to be compatible with a disc herniation. Because of the severity of his pain, surgery was performed March 12, 1957, the day following myelography. An interlaminar exploration of the L5-S1 interspace on the left was performed. Upon retracting the nerve root, 5 cc of creamy white purulent material escaped from the interspace; this, upon being cultured, grew *Staphylococcus aureus* coagulase-positive organisms. Inspection of the area revealed no free fragments of disc material; after aspiration of the pus, no attempt was made to enter the intervertebral space. The wound was irrigated with bacitracin solution and closed with stainless steel wire technique. Three drains were allowed to exit through the skin incision. The patient's postoperative course was remarkably benign and uneventful. He was maintained on antibiotics for 6 weeks. The patient was followed for 6 months after surgery, had a good clinical course, and returned to work in 3 months. Preoperative roentgenograms of the lumbar spine had revealed a somewhat narrowed L5–S1 interspace, but no evidence of bone destruction was noted. Postoperative x-ray films of the lumbar spine were not obtained. The patient left the geographical area and has not since been seen.

Tuberculosis of the Lumbar Spine

Tuberculous disc space infections are usually secondary to tuberculous infection of the adjacent vertebral body. The negative tuberculin skin test will usually, but not always, preclude the diagnosis of tuberculosis spondylitis. In occasional cases, the disc space will be the primary site of the infection. If this is the case, vascularity must be present in the disc, and thus it will occur in the younger age group.

SIGNS AND SYMPTOMS

A tuberculous infection of the lumbar spine is more insidious in its onset and course than a pyogenic infection. The patient complains of dull, aching pain in the low back that is aggravated by exertion but not relieved by rest. On examination there is localized tenderness over the affected vertebra, marked rigidity of the lumbar muscles, and an almost complete loss of all lumbar movements. There are usually some general signs of infection even in the early stages, the most reliable being a slight evening rise of temperature and a raised sedimentation rate.

ROENTGENOGRAPHIC FINDINGS

Roentgenographically, narrowing of the disc space will occur before bony destruction, when the disc is primarily involved. The characteristic osseous changes of osteolysis and sclerosis will be present before disc thinning, if the infection is primarily in the bone. The presence of a paraspinal mass is strongly suggestive of tuberculosis. Usually the loss of disc space occurs much later in tuberculosis than in pyogenic infections.

MANAGEMENT

Management of tuberculosis of the spine, as any other form of tuberculosis, requires the general treatment of the patient. The treatment directed toward the spine initially consists of immobilization with a body spica for a period of at least 3 months and the use of antitubercular drugs for 4 to 6 months.

Operative procedures, which are rarely necessary, involve excision of diseased tissue and placement of drains for instillation of specific chemotherapeutic agents directly into the focus. The approach for the exposure of the spinal focus may be posterolateral with partial removal of the transverse process, or abdominal, either lateroretroperitoneally or transperitoneally.

References

1. Anderson LD, Horn LG: Irrigation-suction technic in the treatment of acute hematogenous osteomyelitis, chronic osteomyelitis, and acute and chronic joint infections. South Med J 63:745–754, 1970
2. Craig FS: Vertebral-body biopsy. J Bone Joint Surg 38A:93, 1956
3. Garrido E: Closed irrigation-suction technique in the treatment of lumbar laminectomy infection: Case report. J Neurosurg 5 (3):354–355, 1979
4. Keiser RP, Grimes HA: Intervertebral disk space infections in children. Clin Orthop 30:163, 1963
5. Mella B: Inflammatory spondylitis. J Neurosurg 22:393, 1965
6. Smith RF, Taylor TKF: Inflammatory lesions of intervertebral discs in children. J Bone Joint Surg 49A:1508, 1967
7. Spiegal PG, Kengla KW, Isaacson AS, Wilson JC: Intervertebral disc-space inflammation in children. J Bone Joint Surg 54A:284, 1972
8. Stern WE: Preoperative evaluation; Complications, their prevention and treatment. In Youmans JR (ed): Neurological Surgery, Vol. 3, 1946–2009. Philadelphia, WB Saunders, 1973
9. Stern EW, Balch RE: Surgical aspects of nonspecific inflammatory and suppurative disease of the vertebral column. Am J Surg 112:314, 1966
10. Stern WE, Crandell PH: Inflammatory intervertebral disc disease as a complication of the operative treatment of lumbar herniations. J Neurosurg 16:261, 1959
11. Sullivan CR: Diagnosis and treatment of pyogenic infections of intervertebral disk. Surg Clin N Am 41:1077, 1961
12. Sullivan CF, Symmonds RE: Disk infections and abdominal pain. JAMA, 188:655, 1964
13. Taylor AR, Maudsley RH: Instillation-suction technique in chronic osteomyelitis. J Bone J Surg (Br) 52B:88–92, 1970
14. Wright RL: Septic Complications of Neurological Spinal Procedures. Springfield, Ill., Charles C Thomas, 1970

Tumors of the spine are rare compared to the great variety of non-neoplastic diseases that produce spinal symptoms. Because of its relative infrequency, the diagnostic possibility of neoplasm may be overlooked when assessing a patient with low back pain. The immediate proximity of these lesions to the spinal cord, nerve roots, and major blood vessels makes management of even the most benign spinal tumor potentially dangerous and crippling. Sometimes a problem of this nature is, at first glance, unpromising, and yet, with a planned approach, the results of proper treatment may be quite gratifying. Such management often requires close interdisciplinary cooperation between surgeon, radiologist, oncologist, and rehabilitation specialist.

Both primary and metastatic tumors involve the bony spine, with the ligaments and discs rarely effected. Intraspinal tumors originating from neural or meningeal cells may produce pressure erosion of the adjacent bony spine.

GENERAL OBSERVATIONS

Back pain is the most common complaint and, unlike most musculoskeletal backaches, it is not usually relieved by rest or recumbency. A unique and sometimes revealing symptom, which may indicate epidural extension, is aggravation of the pain when lying in a supine position (which exerts direct pressure on the lesion), and relief of pain when standing or walking. A spontaneous, gradually progressive onset is common, but occasionally the patient will attribute the onset of symptoms to a fall, a strenuous physical action, or other direct and indirect trauma. Such a history may be responsible for delay in diagnosis, since it tends to direct the physician's thoughts toward various musculoskeletal syndromes and reduces the suspicion of neoplasm. Neurological symptoms and signs may vary in accordance with the exact nature and location of the neoplasm, but the two entities most frequently confused with the early stages of tumor are herniated lumbar discs and stenotic lumbar spinal canal syndromes. Judicious use of the resources of the roentgenography department are most important in establishing the nature of the lesion. In addition to standard spine films, tomography, bone scan, computerized axial tomographic scan, and myelography all have their use in diagnosis and assessment of spinal neoplasm. Biplane C-arm fluoroscopic units facilitate the performance of percutaneous needle biopsy technique and provide valuable histological information on which to base subsequent management.

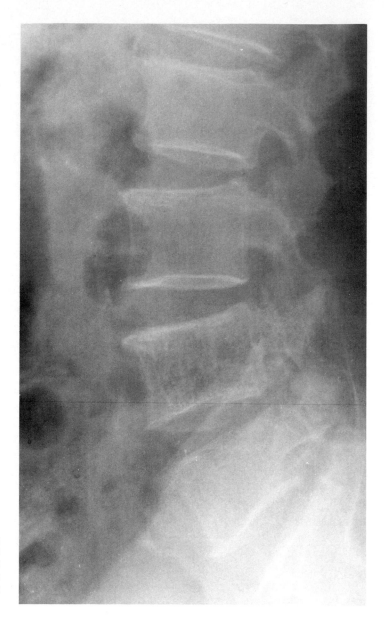

Fig. 18-1. Hemangioma of the fourth vertebral body. This lesion was noted as an incidental (symptom free) finding in a 71-yr-old man who was involved in a vehicular accident. (Continues on facing page.)

Benign Tumors

Hemangiomas

Hemangiomas are the most commonly occurring tumors of the vertebrae, found in approximately 10% of all spines when subjected to careful anatomical serial examination. They occur with greatest frequency between T12 and L4, and with least fre-

quency at the upper cervical spine and the lowermost part of the sacrum (Fig. 18-1). Women are more often affected than men by two-thirds. The incidence of hemangiomas increases with age, indicating that if these lesions are all truly congenital, they become progressively larger and more apparent with the passage of years. Most hemangiomas are revealed as incidental autopsy findings without clinically apparent symptoms.[14]

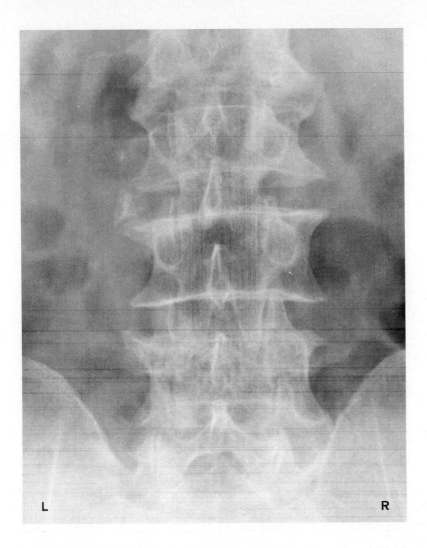

L   R

PATHOLOGY

Vertebral hemangiomas cause diminution in the number of bony trabeculae, coarsening of the remaining trabeculae, and transformation of some trabeculae into vertically extending stands which lend support to the diseased vertebral body. In addition to these characteristic vertical reticular stripes, one occasionally sees a coarse, honeycombed bony configuration. Large hemangiomas involving an entire vertebral body cause a "ballooning" of the body; the normally concave or indented sides of the vertebrae assume a straight or even convex configuration. Large hemangiomas occupying the entire vertebral body occasionally extend into the laminae and spinous processes. With involvement of a thoracic vertebra, hemangiomas sometimes involve an adjoining rib, causing these structures to become thickened and honeycombed.[4,3,10]

ROENTGENOGRAPHIC FINDINGS

The characteristic radiographic signs are the coarse vertical supportive strands, honeycombing and the ballooned configuration of the vertebral body.[13]

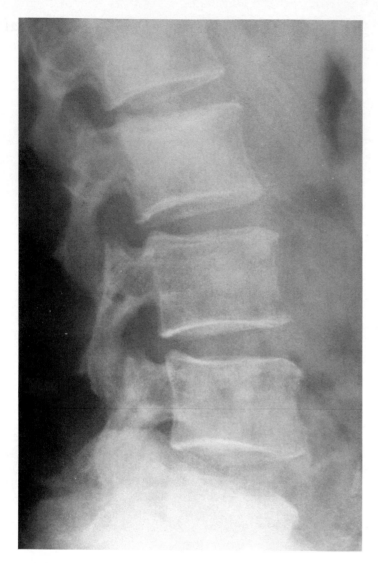

Fig. 18-2. Osteoblastic and osteoclastic metastasis simultaneously involving the vertebral bodies. Patient is a 59-yr-old man with carcinoma of the prostate.

Fig. 18-3. Destruction of pedicle T11 on right from metastatic bronchogenic carcinoma. (Opposite page.)

SIGNS AND SYMPTOMS

Most vertebral hemangiomas are noted as incidental findings, with clinical symptoms not commonly associated with the condition. The occasional symptoms that develop usually arise from nerve root pressure due to thickening of the vertebral body and arches or perforation of hemangiomatous tissue into the neural canal.[1,6]

Despite extensive vertebral involvement, compression fractures or wedging are rather uncommon because of the support provided by the vertical reinforcing lamellae. Interestingly enough, even in the face of trauma sufficient to fracture neighboring vertebral bodies, the diseased vertebra often remains intact.

TREATMENT

No treatment is required if the lesion is symptom free. When the condition is associated with nerve root pressure, radiation therapy may be effective.

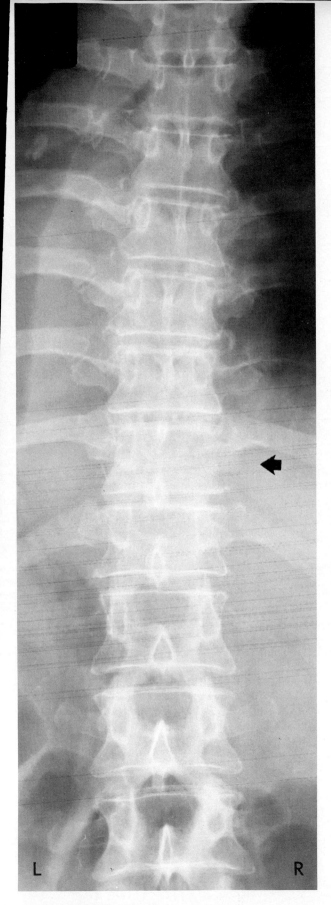

Osteomas

Osteomas may occur within any portion of the vertebra but are more apt to produce clinical symptoms when located within the laminae or spinous processes (Fig. 18-2). These exostosis-like lesions in the laminae will produce direct impingement upon the cauda equina or individual roots, and in the spinous processes may produce spinal malalignment and deformity.

Osteoid osteomas, also called benign osteoblastomas, destroy the bony parenchyma. Although they do not metastisize, they do extend locally and may be associated with compression of the nerve structures within the neural canal.[9,12]

These lesions, which often occur in children from 9 to 14 and which may be associated with scoliosis, can sometimes be confused with idiopathic scoliosis. Young patients with scoliosis, who complain of back pain which is worse at night and with recumbency, are osteoid osteoma suspects. These lesions may occasionally be difficult to demonstrate roentgenographically. If the x-ray films are equivocal, but clinical suspicions are present, a bone scan is in order. Increased uptake at the site of concern should be followed by tomography, which will usually demonstrate the existence of a lesion. Treatment is directed at a radical excision of the lesion and spinal fusion, followed by radiation therapy, if a complete removal of the neoplasm is not possible.

Malignant Tumors

Sarcomas

Sarcomas of the spine are extremely rare, with less than 1% of all bone sarcomas originating in the spine. These lesions cause extensive bony destruction within the vertebrae, which is associated with vertebral body collapse (Fig. 18-3). Occasionally, sarcomas produce osteosclerosis, the so-called "ivory vertebra," a roentgenographic term used to imply a pathologic bony condensing process of the vertebra. As a result of the proliferation of tumor tissue and malformation and malalignment of the spine, compression of the neural elements is almost invariably associated with this lesion. An increased paravertebral shadow is seen on x-ray film. This differs from the rather elongated spindle shape of the paravertebral shadow seen in tuberculosis, having a more ovoid mass which surrounds only the vertebra or vertebrae which are involved with tumor.

Roentgenologic evaluation of this lesion is generally nonspecific, so that a needle biopsy or possibly a surgical biopsy is necessary to obtain a satisfactory diagnosis. Because of the rapidly growing nature of this neoplasm, surgery is best confined to biopsy; minimal benefits are achieved by palliative decompression. The treatment of choice both to alleviate pain and to arrest the rapid progression of the disease is x-ray therapy.

Multiple Myeloma

A large percentage of patients with multiple myeloma present with low back pain, resulting from involvement of this disease within the lower lumbar vertebrae. As the vertebral bodies are penetrated and destroyed by the myeloma, all possible forms of vertebral body collapse with associated spinal deformities can be seen: wedging, marked flattening, and compression of the vertebral bodies (sometimes so flat that they are less than the height of the adjacent intervertebral discs). Osteosclerosis and periosteal proliferation, or reactive bony proliferation surrounding the site of metastasis are not seen in multiple myeloma. This differentiates it from other osseous metastatic lesions where they are common. This condition occurs most commonly between the ages of 35 and 65 and is rarely found in children.

The characteristic symptoms of multiple myeloma begin with somewhat vague and poorly localized low back pain, which is often worse when lying in bed at night. This diagnosis is not often made in its early stages because the x-ray films may be unrevealing or, if they are abnormal, may resemble diffuse osteoporosis. With the passage of time, sufficient destruction of the vertebra occurs to produce vertebral collapse, often associated with nerve root compression symptoms. At this stage of the disease, the character of the pain undergoes a change, both with regard to radiation from radicular compression and to its becoming more related to activity. Any movement, particularly jarring or percussion over the lumbar region, produces an acute aggravation of the pain. If the patient is followed by serial roentgenograms of the spine, the fairly rapid development of multiple lytic lesions can be identified, in addition to diffuse osteoporosis.[4]

In differentiating this condition from metastatic carcinoma, the roentgenologists, as a general rule of thumb, use the criterion that when a pedicle is destroyed, in association with a collapsed vertebral body, the cause is metastatic carcinoma rather than multiple myeloma. The latter usually causes vertebral body colapse without destroying the cortex of the pedicle; therefore, the pedicles appear intact on the x-ray film.

The diagnosis can be aided through the use of laboratory studies which demonstrate a markedly elevated sedimentation rate, a normocytic anemia, and a strikingly elevated gamma globulin concentration, with a characteristic configuration on the paper electrophoretic pattern. The urine may reveal Bence Jones protein. Bone marrow aspiration yields characteristic myeloma cells and is necessary to confirm the diagnosis. Occasionally, some cases of multiple myeloma present themselves as localized lesions, and the diagnosis may require a needle biopsy or even an open biopsy of the involved area.[7] Operative intervention is generally contraindicated; but treatment with cytostatic drugs and x-ray therapy may produce long-lasting improvement.

Metastatic Tumors

Metastatic disease of the spine is one of the most common abnormalities involving the bony elements of the spine. Almost 70% of all spinal tumors are metastatic. The remaining 30% are divided between primary spinal tumors and direct tumor invasion from adjacent structures or from neoplasm arising from dural tissues within the spinal canal. The magnitude of metastatic carcinoma to the bone becomes evident when one reviews the literature and finds that metastatic disease to the skeleton ranges from about 20% in one series to about 70% in autopsy cases reviewed by Jaffe.[11] The vertebrae are the most common site for metastatic disease, followed by the pelvis, proximal long bones, and ribs. It is quite rare to find metastatic disease distal to the elbow or knee joints. Certain cancers have distinct predilections for metastasis to bone, with breast and prostate being the most frequent, followed by lung, kidney, and thyroid. In the Institute for Spinal Column Research in Frankfurt, Germany, established by Dr. Georg Schmorl, it is the routine practice to remove the entire spinal column in every autopsy. Each spinal specimen is then subjected to a planned and most meticulous examination. Using this method, 1000 patients with cancer were investigated (500 women and 500 men) in order to establish the incidence of spinal involvement. This method revealed that 17.6% of patients with cancer had metastasis to the spine, representing a 19.6% incidence in men, and 15.6% in women. Most other series are considerably lower, but no other clinic follows the painstaking method utilized by the Schmorl Institute.

At one time, considerable confusion and speculation existed regarding the route by which carcinomas metastasized to the vertebrae. The hematogenous route was thought to be the principal pathway for metastatic disease, but no adequate explanation was offered for the frequent absence of lung lesions in the face of widespread bony metastasis. It was considered by some that lymphatics were the root of most metastatic diseases. However, advocates of this mechanism had difficulty explaining the frequency of bony metastasis, in view of the fact that bone is largely alymphatic. Batson, an anatomist, was responsible for rediscovering the vertebral vein complex. Through his specialized latex injection studies, he demonstrated that this venous system is quite complex, involving extensive anastomoses with the portal system, with the upper thorax by way of the intercostals, and with the superior vena cava system.[5] This is known to be a nonvalvular system. With any increase in intra-abdominal pressure, such as through coughing or straining, the flow of blood can be reversed through this system carrying tumor emboli with it. When tumor cells are experimentally injected into the femoral veins of rabbits, and the intra-abdominal pressure is increased, there is a marked increase in the number of vertebral bodies involved by tumor. We still are unable to fully explain why certain tumors, such as bladder carcinomas or carcinomas of the cervix, do not frequently metastasize to the spine as do prostatic tumors.

SYMPTOMS

A patient with a history of previous surgery for malignant disease who has the insidious onset of low back pain must be suspected of having metastatic disease to the spine. A prolonged lapse of time from the primary surgical procedure would not allay one's suspicions concerning metastatic disease, since it is well known that carcinomas of the breast frequently metastasize quite late following a radical mastectomy. It is not rare to see patients 5, 7, 10, and even more years following breast surgery who develop low back pain which turns out to be a metastatic tumor from the original breast lesion.

The pain produced by metastatic and primary tumors is characteristically of insidious onset, more frequently worse at night, and gradually increasing in severity with the passage of time. However, sudden onset of pain, or an acute exacerbation of pain in the back following little or no trauma, may represent a pathologic fracture. It occasionally may be the presenting complaint with metastatic disease to the spine.

PHYSICAL FINDINGS

Physical examination is of considerable importance, although it may not initially be rewarding, aside from noting some local tenderness over the area of pain and some paraspinal muscle spasm with limited spinal mobility. Occasionally, with advanced metastatic disease associated with wedging and collapse of a vertebra, one can detect the presence of a gibbous formation resulting from the malalignment of the spine. When a gibbous formation can be palpated and visualized, there is usually considerable point tenderness over the site. When malignant disease is suspected, a most comprehensive inspection and examination of the entire body is important to determine either the primary site or an accessible area of biopsy. This examination should, of course, include examination of the breasts, and if any suspicious areas of resistance or possible nodules are present, special techniques such as mammography may be helpful. The vaginal and rectal examination is important; the examiner must always keep in mind that many unnecessary biopsies of the spine have been done because the physician failed to slip on a rectal glove and missed a very obvious hard prostatic nodule or some other rectal mass.

ROENTGENOGRAPHIC DIAGNOSIS

Tumor metastasis to the spine may occur in two different forms: osteoclastic (bone-destructive) metastases, and osteoblastic, (bone-forming), metastases. Both of these forms may occur simultaneously and, in fact, sometimes the same vertebral body will display both forms of metastasis in apposition. The osteoblastic metastases are characteristically seen when the primary tumor is in the prostate or breast. They are seen on x-ray film as areas of increased density and are often described by the roentgenologist as "ivory-like" tumor foci. The osteoclastic tumor metastases are more frequently associated with vertebral body collapse. Metastatic lesions may involve any portion of the vertebrae and sometimes extend beyond the boundaries of the vertebrae and proliferate externally.

The x-ray film appearance of tumor metastasis to the spine is quite variable, owing to the frequent simultaneous existence of osteoclastic and osteoblastic metastases, which may present difficulties in differential diagnosis. It must be recognized that at least 30% of the vertebrae must be involved by neoplasm before these changes are readily appreciated by roentgenogram. Often, the axis of the defect in relationship to the axis of the x-ray beam is a factor in how readily the lesion can be seen roentgenographically. The bone scan will demonstrate increased uptake well before lesions can be identified on routine spine films. If there is an equivocal lesion, tomography will be most helpful in specifically determining the nature and extent of a metastatic lesion. Because of the difficulties in making a roentgenographic diagnosis and, since symptoms often precede roentgenographic changes, we must not stop in our diagnostic efforts with a presumably normal spine x-ray film if there is a suspicious history indicative of possible metastatic disease. When neoplasm is suspected, spine films must be carefully examined (each pedicle, each transverse process, each spinous process, the laminae) to eliminate the presence of lesions arising in these sites. There must also be a careful inspection of the vertebral bodies in which tumor pathology is more readily recognized, when a metastatic lytic lesion produces some vertebral wedging or collapse.[2]

Every patient suspected of having a spinal neoplasm should undergo a bone scan. This study will demonstrate increased uptake in vertebrae with relatively small lesions long before they can be visualized by routine spine films. Often an abnormal bone scan will direct our attention to a specific vertebra, and special views, including tomographic studies, will be helpful in demonstrating a lesion. If information is desired regarding the possible extension of a vertebral neoplasm into the surrounding soft tissues, computerized axial tomography of the spine is of great help.

MANAGEMENT

Histologic verification of these lesions is a necessity for proper management. If no other more accessible lesions are apparent, a biopsy of the affected vertebral body should be carried out. In some cases, a closed biopsy of the spine can be performed using several types of needles specifically designed for this purpose, such as the Craig needle with a 2-mm diameter bore. The advantage of this technique, which can usually be carried out under local anesthesia with biplane roentgenographic control, is its relative simplicity. It does not interfere with the patient's activities or with any treatment which is being carried out simultaneously. The greatest disadvantage of all needle biopsies is the relatively small fragment of tissue obtained, resulting in an indecisive diagnosis. When using a needle biopsy technique, the pathologist should have some understanding of the problem, be aware of the inherent difficulties, and be prepared to give extra attention to this small fragment of tissue. In addition, there are some potential dangers involving damage to surrounding structures and nerves. Occasionally, the lesion itself may be vascular, so a biopsy may result in considerable bleeding at that site. When needle biopsy is either not feasible or not successful, an open biopsy may be in order; this is usually accompanied by an attempt at operative decompression. When gross neurological deficit is caused by tumor compression from an absolute block, such de-

compression is often helpful. However, in many cases, relief obtained by decompression of the nerves from the enveloping tumor is temporary. Then cytostatic drugs and x-ray therapy, which remain the mainstay of treatment in most lesions, should be employed. Even when tumors are considered to be somewhat x-ray resistant, there is often significant alleviation of some pain, and the rapidity of growth tends to slow down. The fact that breast and prostatic tumors are hormonally dependent should be kept in mind; occasionally relief is achieved by pituitary ablation or hormonal therapy. In some cases, steroids are effective in relieving pain for limited durations; their action is primarily a reduction of edema resulting from tumor compression.

Intradural Tumors

Neurilemmomas (Schwannoma Neurofibroma)

Neurilemmomas are usually intradural and arise from the sheaths of the spinal nerve roots as oval or rounded tumors causing intradural compression of the neurological elements at the level of the tumor. These circumscribed, encapsulated growths, into which a portion of the nerve root can usually be traced, tend to be single and may grow to enormous size, particularly in the cauda equina, before they produce easily recognizable symptoms. By contrast, in von Recklinghausen's disease, there may be multiple tumors involving the cauda equina and conus medullaris, which are associated with cutaneous evidence of neurofibromatosis. It is felt by most authorities that the solitary neurilemmoma or schwannoma is indistinguishable from the multiple neurofibroma of von Recklinghausen's disease. Often neurilemmomas grow along the spinal nerve root through the dura mater and the vertebral foramen into the surrounding tissues, extending either into the abdomen in the lumbar region or into the thoracic cavity if involving the thoracic spine. As the tumor passes through the intervertebral foramen, it becomes constricted, taking an hourglass or dumbbell shape. Microscopically, the spinal cord neurilemmoma shows palisading of nuclei in association with degenerative changes, such as interstitial masses of lipoid deposits, hyaline substances, and cellular debris.

These tumors are usually separated from either the cord or the nerve roots and can be totally removed, along with any root fibers incorporated within the body of the tumor. In carrying out the surgery, magnification technique using an operating microscope, or sometimes high-powered operating telescopes, may be helpful. When a dumbbell tumor is found to extend into the abdomen or the higher spinal regions (the thorax), it should be pursued extradurally and removed during the same procedure, if possible. In extremely large tumors, where the extradural extension is so great that total excision through a laminectomy incision might be hazardous, it is helpful to use silver clip markers on the portion of the tumor that is visible through the laminectomy incision. The markers will help the general surgeon when he plans subsequent removal of this lesion as a secondary procedure. I have used this technique on several occasions, and have been surprised, on taking postoperative roentgenograms, to realize how far anterior or lateral to the spine my dissection had carried me. Following removal of a neurofibroma, a watertight dural closure is always performed.

Meningiomas

Meningiomas are occasionally seen in the cauda equina, arising in most instances from the inner surface of the dura mater or from the arachnoid membrane. These are usually a bit softer and occasionally more vascular than neurofibromas and are more likely to fit over the surface of the cauda equina and conform to its irregularities. They may vary from a round or oval shape to a large irregular mass, resembling the contour of that portion of the canal in which they are located. Histologically, spinal meningiomas closely resemble intracranial meningiomas and are composed of masses of cells which do not form an intercellular substance. Though this tumor is benign, if it is adherent to the dura, it may be necessary to excise the dura completely around the site of tumor origin to prevent recurrence. It will then be necessary to patch the dural defect in watertight fashion; a sheet of fascia, which can be obtained from the paraspinal muscles, is usually suitable. After the patch has been sutured in place, the original dural incision should, of course, be closed. As in excision of neurofibromas, magnification is most helpful in excising such lesions completely.

Surgery of Spinal Cord Tumors

The surgery of intraspinal tumors requires careful attention to certain details of technique. For instance, prior to surgery, one must consider the character and extent of the lesion and plan the location of the incision in relation to the lesion. The time-honored method of establishing the desired vertebral level in the lumbar region is to start from the sacrum and to count the interspaces from the solid sacral bone. For the upper lumbar level, the twelfth rib may serve as a useful guide; the spinous process of L1 is broader and larger than the thoracic spine. Further accuracy can be obtained in planning a laminectomy incision by placing a metal marker on the skin at the exact location of the tumor during myelography. An x-ray film is taken with the marker in place, that site is marked with indelible ink or in some cases, it is injected subcutaneously with a dot of methylene blue. It is most important to take the marking film while the patient is flexed in the prone position, which is the position planned for laminectomy, to avoid shift of the cutaneous mark when he is flexed on the operating

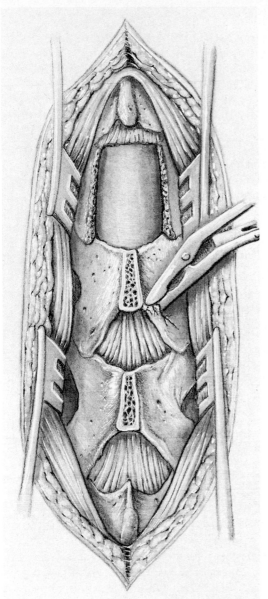

Fig. 18-4. Excision of spinous processes.

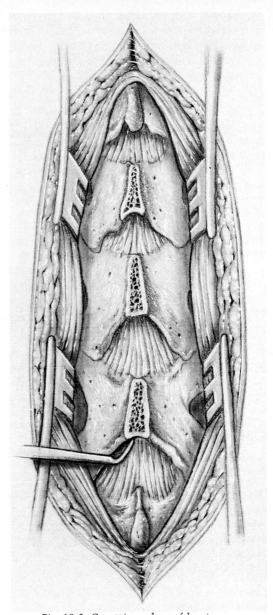

Fig. 18-5. Curetting edges of lamina.

table. The position of the patient for surgery is usually prone with moderate flexion of the spine at the level of the lesion.

During the performance of the laminectomy, a few factors should be considered. Blood loss is kept at a minimum by performing a strictly midline incision of the fascial attachments. Over the spinous processes and laminae great efforts should be made to peel the fascia cleanly without penetrating muscle, which is often the principal source of

bleeding. While carrying out a subperiosteal muscle dissection, care should be used with the periosteal elevators to avoid direct downward pressure. Such care is necessary because with both benign and malignant tumors, erosion and thinning of the laminal arches can occur, allowing a carelessly used instrument to plunge through this abnormal bone and produce damage to the underlying

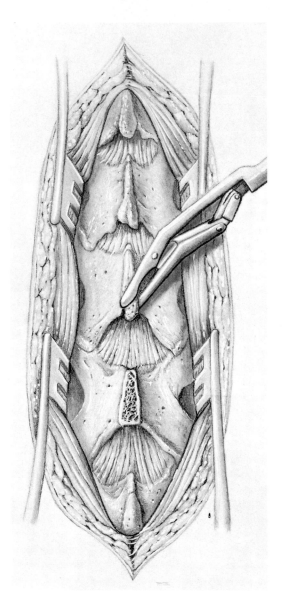

Fig. 18-6. Removing lamina "en face" to avoid excessive pressure upon dural contents.

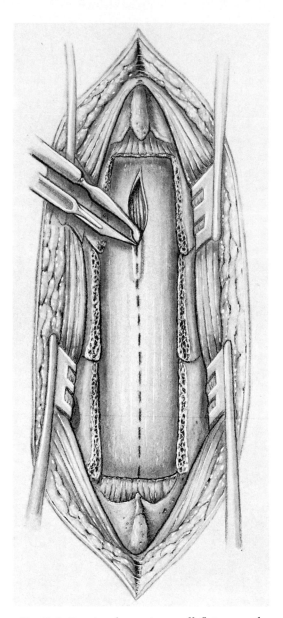

Fig. 18-7. Opening dura using small, flat, grooved director.

neural structures. Not long ago I carried out surgery on a neurofibroma in which the overlying lamina on the side of the tumor was paper thin.

Following complete exposure of the spinous processes and laminae, the spinous processes are removed with rongeurs; any bleeding from their base can be controlled with the use of bone wax (Fig. 18-4). Con-

trolling bleeding as it occurs allows a far more orderly procedure and, of course, avoids excessive loss of blood throughout the procedure. As an aid in identifying the upper and lower edges of each lamina, the edges may be curetted clear of ligamentum flavum (Fig. 18-5). The laminal removal is done "en face" to avoid introducing a rongeur blade beneath the lamina. This is done by holding the rongeur vertically so that the bone is actually rongeured away from above downwards (Fig. 18-6). When the surgeon cannot avoid introducing a rongeur blade beneath the lamina, he should use a thin underblade, such as a thin-bladed laminectomy punch with an angled tip. Adherence to this technique will prevent added cauda equina compression that may result in permanent neurological dysfunction. After carrying out the medial portion of the laminectomy, it is then helpful to go to either side and carry out a more lateral decompression. Again the angled, thin-bladed laminectomy punch is most helpful in performing this procedure without producing dural compression. Following this portion of the procedure, complete hemostasis of all bleeding structures should be achieved. Bleeding from muscles may be controlled with cautery; venous oozing from the rongeured bony edges with bone wax; epidural venous bleeding, in most cases, with a small pledget of Gelfoam. If epidural bleeding persists, cauterization with the use of a Mallis bipolar cautery may be necessary.

At this point a search for an extradural tumor, disc, or bony spur can be carried out. Most extradural spinal tumors are malignant, with metastatic tumors being the most frequent. Usually both meningiomas and neurofibromas are intradural. However, an occasional neurofibroma or meningioma may be extradural and is frequently referred to as a "dumbbell tumor," with extension through the intervertebral foramen into tissues adjacent to the spine. This type of lesion extends along either side of the dura, and the extradural extension can project through the intervertebral foramen into the peritoneal space. Or, if it is in the thoracic or cervical region, the lesion may extend into the lung and sometimes into the soft tissue of the neck. Lipomas, congenital cysts, and osteomas are rarely found as benign extradural tumors.

The dura should almost always be opened in the midline, beginning the incision at the safest point above the area of obstruction, and extending it past the lesion, so that the tumor can be completely exposed. The dura

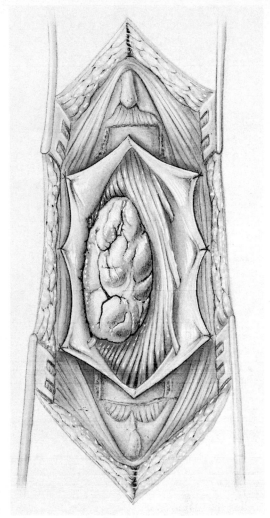

Fig. 18-8. *Retraction of incised dural margins using stay sutures. The neurilemmoma is exposed.*

is opened with a No. 11 blade, attempting to keep the arachnoid intact. A small flat grooved director can be introduced between the dura and the arachnoid and may be used to guide the No. 11 blade over the lesion (Figs. 18-7 through 18-9). After opening the dura, if it is found that the tumor had not been completely exposed, the laminectomy should, of course, be extended further until an adequate exposure can be obtained.

Surgery of an extradural malignancy should be done without undue delay. A decompressive laminectomy is carried out as widely and as thoroughly as possible using

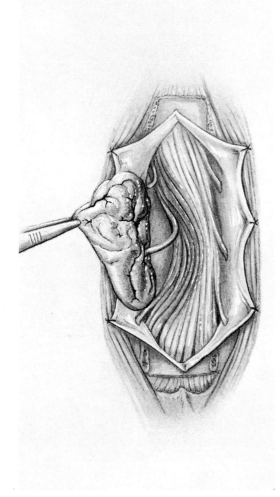

Fig. 18-9. Tumor excision. The L4 nerve root is incorporated within the body of the tumor and will be sectioned.

is to fill the bony defect with a plastic substance, methyl methacrylate. In his technique, he partially inserts a metal screw into the center of each healthy vertebral body, above and below the defect; these screws provide an anchor for the methyl methacrylate that is poured in to fill the defect. To prevent the heat of polymerization of this plastic from damaging the cord, he uses a protective layer of Gelfoam over the dura and continues to irrigate the wound during polymerization with cool saline solution. Following surgery, x-ray therapy or chemotherapy may be considered if indicated by the nature of the pathology.

References

1. Askenasy H, Behmoaram A: Neurological manifestations in hemangioma of the vertebrae. J Neurol 20:276, 1957
2. Austin GM: The Spinal Cord. Springfield (Ill), Charles C Thomas, 1961
3. Baily P, Bucy P: Cavernous hemangioma of the vertebrae. JAMA 92:27, 1929
4. Barnard N: Primary hemangioma of the spine. Am Surg 97:19, 1933
5. Batson OV: The vertebral vein system. Am J Roentgenol 78:195, 1957
6. Bell R: Hemangioma of a dorsal vertebra with collapse and compression myelopathy. J Neurosurg 12:570, 1955
7. Cohen DM, Dahlin DC, MacCarty CS: Apparently solitary tumors of the vertebral column. Mayo Clin Proc 39:509, 1964
8. Davison B: Myeloma and its neurological complications. Arch Surg 35:913, 1937
9. Freiberger RE: Osteoid osteoma of the spine. A cause of backache and scoliosis in children and young adults. Radiology, 75:232, 1960
10. Ireland J: Hemangioma of the vertebrae. Am J Roentgenol 28:372, 1932
11. Jaffe HL: Tumors and Tumorous Conditions of the Bones and Joints. Philadelphia, Lea & Febiger, 1958
12. Lichtenstein L, Sawyer WR: Benign osteoblastoma. J Bone J Surg, 46A:755, 1964
13. Lindqvist I: Vertebral hemangioma with compression of the spinal cord. Acta Radiol (Stockh) 35:400, 1951
14. Schmorl G, Junghanns H, Besemann EE: The human spine in health and disease. New York, Grune and Stratton, 1971

all means, including rongeurs and curettage, to achieve as extensive a tumor removal as can be done. On completing the laminectomy and tumor removal, particularly when the vertebral bodies are grossly involved, the spinal column may be so weakened that a spinal fusion should be considered at the time of operation. A method which has been utilized by Dr. William Scoville, with patients who had advanced malignant involvement of one or more contiguous vertebrae,

Uncommon Causes of Low Back Pain and Sciatica

19

The diseases included in this section are either rarely encountered or not commonly considered in connection with low back pain and sciatica. However, an awareness of their existence may be helpful in considering the occasional clinical problem that does not lend itself to ready classification.

Pelvic Disease

Low back pain of variable severity is manifested during menstrual periods by approximately 10% to 20% of females. These pains often described as "bearing down," a sensation of heaviness, a tired feeling, are not particularly severe and are usually adequately managed with mild analgesics, so that the patient is able to carry on with routine activities of daily living. In rare cases, the pain, often referred to by gynecologists as "pelvic backache," is of such severity that the patient may be confined to bed for 1 or 2 days each month. Examination usually reveals nothing, even during the painful intervals.

Pelvic tumors, particularly those within the retroperitoneal space, may cause irritation and compression of the lumbosacral plexus and be productive of low back pain and sciatica. Occasionally, endometriosis may invade the lumbar or sciatic plexus or the sciatic nerve itself, producing severe hip

and sciatic pain. In such cases, reflex, motor, and sensory changes may be elicited on physical examination.

Low Back Pain and Pregnancy

At the end of pregnancy a moderate degree of low back pain is common, in part because of the increased mechanical demands on the low back imposed by carrying the fetus. During the latter half of pregnancy also, there is a generalized softening of the fibrous structures in the lumbosacral spine and pelvis, attributed to hormonal effect. This produces some tissue laxity and allows increased stretching of the involved ligaments. Several months may elapse before these fibrous structures regain their original tensile strength.

The vast majority of pregnant women who complain of low back pain are easily managed with a program of reduced physical activities, mild analgesics, and a supporting corset. In some instances, the low back symptoms are so severe that prolonged periods of bed rest are necessary. Occasionally, joint diastasis is seen on roentgenograms, with some separation of the symphysis pubis and a slight widening of the sacroiliac joints.[2]

The most severe problems are usually in multiparas who have had a diastasis during a previous pregnancy. The pain is often quite

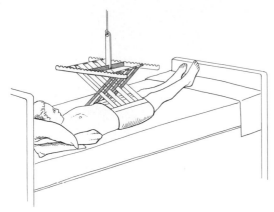

Fig. 19-1. Pelvic sling.

severe in the low back and both hips and may also be present in the lower abdomen and over the symphysis pubis. Sometimes, the pain is not adequately relieved by resting in a nonweight-bearing position and will require the use of a canvas pelvic sling suspended from an overhead bar (Fig. 19-1). The sling is attached to traction weights and is most effective if it crosses in front of the body, reducing the sacroiliac and symphysis pubis separations.

Postpartum improvement in low back dysfunction is generally seen and is attributed to passage of the mechanical burden imposed by the fetus and recovery of the fibrous structures to normal tensile strength. Infrequently, the sacroiliac and pubic pain persist and, with increased physical activity, even worsen. The typical sacroiliac waddling gait is associated with increased lumbar lordosis and protrusion of the abdomen resulting from relaxation of the lower abdominal muscles, which are painful at the site of pubic attachment. The "reverse" Patrick's test, using internal rotation rather than external rotation, is painful, since it tends to distract the sacroiliac joint. Treatment of this condition requires approximately 2 weeks in a pelvic sling, after which a pelvic support is worn for 3 or 4 months.

In addition to softening of the ligaments at the symphysis pubis and sacroiliac joint, similar changes occur in the ligamentous supporting structures of the lower lumbar spine, including the annulus fibrosis of the lower intervertebral discs. Preexisting annular weakness may be aggravated during pregnancy, leading to severe protrusion of the nucleus pulposus, and all of the signs and symptoms of lumbar disc disease will follow. Some low back and sciatic pains, attributed by the obstetrician to pressure of the fetal head, are caused by lumbar disc disease.

This type of problem is best managed prophylactically, when dealing with a patient who has a history compatible with lumbar disc disease. Restriction of all activities likely to cause undue stress on the low back structures is helpful.

Severe pain is best treated with prolonged bed rest and mild analgesics. The only indication for disc surgery during pregnancy is severe neurologic dysfunction, such as a cauda equina syndrome.

Intra-abdominal Vascular Disease

Thrombosis of the terminal aorta may be the cause of lumbar pain, while occlusion of the common iliac or internal iliac may produce low back and hip pain. Occasionally, this pain is quite severe and may be the predominant symptom. It is described as a constant, deep, severe, aching pain and is poorly localized. Other symptoms of arterial obstruction, including intermittent claudication with numbness and tingling of the legs and temperature changes in the feet, are seen on examination. The femoral and dorsalis pedis pulses are diminished or absent.[1]

Compression of the lumbosacral plexus by an aneurysm of the common iliac artery is a rare cause of sciatica. A dissection aneurysm of the aorta may produce, as its initial symptom, excruciating low back pain which spreads into the buttocks and legs. The pain is usually associated with pallor, sweating, and the patient's being close to shock. The femoral pulses may be absent, and bruits may be heard along the course of the aorta or its branches. Occasionally, paraplegia may develop suddenly as a result of ischemia to the spinal cord. All of these vascular lesions are delineated by aortography.

Sacroiliac Sprain

During the first third of this century, a large proportion of low back pains were identified as sacroiliac disorders. Low back syndromes in the second third of the century have been equally misidentified as herniated lumbar discs, now that the sacroiliac diagnosis has fallen out of fashion. Although sacroiliac sprain can not be resurrected as a wastebasket diagnosis used to explain the majority of backaches, this condition does exist and can be identified.

History

The typical history describes severe direct or indirect trauma to the pelvis, such as a fall from a height or a heavy-impact, vehicular accident. The patient is almost invariably younger than 50 years of age, since after that time the sacroiliac joint is completely fused and not subject to either sliding or rotary movements, no matter how severe the trauma. The pain is unilateral, involving the hip, buttock, and upper posterior thigh, with minimal discomfort extending to the mid-low back area. Occasional pain radiation below the upper thigh is somewhat diffuse, not in accordance with a specific dermatomal pattern, and decreasing in severity as it extends distally. In addition to pain in the general area of the sacroiliac joint, discomfort in the area of the symphysis pubis is not unusual and may be mistaken for iliohypogastric or ilioinguinal neuritis.

Walking, standing, and sitting are more uncomfortable than bed rest in a supine position. When in the sitting position, cross-ing the painful leg over the uninvolved leg is pain provoking, as is lying in a lateral position with the painful side down.

Examination

Sacroiliac strain is easily confused with hip dysfunction since several tests are painful to both conditions. These include a variety of hip maneuvers such as hip flexion, extension, rotation, and abduction against resistance. Squatting and local sacroiliac joint tenderness are likewise painful in both conditions. The two tests that are specific for this condition are related to the anatomical construction of the pelvic ring, the bony integrity of which is interrupted at three sites: the two sacroiliac joints posteriorly and the pubic symphysis anteriorly.

1. With the painful side uppermost, downward pressure upon the iliac crest will provoke sacroiliac joint pain.
2. Pressure over the symphysis pubis is painful both locally at the symphysis and over the sacroiliac region (Fig. 19-2).
3. Roentgenograms are not usually helpful aside from ruling out other conditions, such as rheumatoid arthritis or either a pyogenic or tubercular sacroiliac joint infection.

Management

The acute phase of this condition requires bed rest, analgesic drugs, and anti-inflammatory medications. When pain has eased, progressive mobilization with a trochanter belt is in order. This condition is one of the few indications for a trochanter belt, although I see many patients who have had this appliance prescribed for them when a much wider garment would have been preferable. Rarely, in the face of persistent pain, injection of steroids into the sacroiliac joint is necessary.

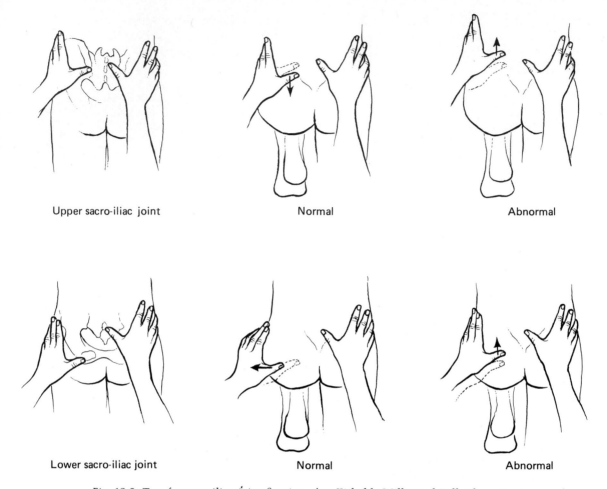

Upper sacro-iliac joint   Normal   Abnormal

Lower sacro-iliac joint   Normal   Abnormal

Fig. 19-2. Test for sacroiliac joint fixation after Kirkaldy-Willis and Hill. The patient is examined in a standing position and is asked to flex both hip and knee, lifting the leg as high as possible.

Sciatic Neuritis

Piriformis Syndrome

This syndrome is characterized by pain behind the greater trochanter extending down the course of the sciatic nerve. Differentiating this condition from lumbar disc disease is difficult, since many of the tests and physical findings that are positive for the piriformis syndrome are also seen with lumbar disc disease. In addition, the nerve root irritation from lumbar disc disease can produce spasm of the piriformis muscle as well as of the lumbar paraspinal muscle groupings. A valid piriformis syndrome can occur as a secondary condition from a disc protrusion or be a primary condition unrelated to lumbar disc dysfunction. Pain on straight leg raising and numbness along the lateral surface of the foot are common to both lumbar disc disease and the piriformis syndrome. The most specific diagnostic sign is pain on internal rotation of the hip with the hips and knees in flexion. A rectal examination is often helpful in identifying this condition. The examiner should apply digital pressure initially on the nonpainful side which ordinarily elicits no unusual pain response. Pressure on the painful side produces direct pressure upon the piriformis muscle and will elicit a painful sciatic radiation.

Some authorities advocate injection of a local anesthetic into the piriformis muscle both as a diagnostic procedure and for therapeutic value. I am not satisfied with the validity of this injection technique as a diagnostic tool. The close proximity of the sciatic nerve to the piriformis muscle allows some "spill" of the local anesthetic onto the sciatic nerve, so that pain relief following this injection may be due to a partial sciatic block. Bed rest, analgesic medications, and anti-inflammatory drugs are usually adequate to ease the pain. Surgery involving a sciatic neurolysis and section of the piriformis muscle is rarely necessary.

Trauma

Probably the most frequent cause of sciatic trauma is an inadvertently placed intramuscular injection in the buttock, with the needle situated too low and medial (Fig. 19-3). At the time of the injection, the patient may experience a painful radiation down the leg. Depending on the severity of damage to the nerve from the injection, the symptoms can vary from mild discomfort and "tingling" paresthesia along the course of the sciatic nerve, to severe motor changes, with a complete foot drop and anesthesia along the lateral aspect of the calf and the dorsum of the foot.

Sciatic trauma may occur from a posterior dislocation of the femur. Occasionally, a fall in the sitting position on a hard projecting object will traumatize the nerve where it is quite superficial, just below the edge of the gluteus maximus. This sudden trauma not only may cause direct injury to the nerve but also may impinge the nerve against the sharp edge of the sciatic notch. This may be a significant factor in the prolongation of persisting symptoms. Contusions of the sciatic nerve, in addition to causing pain, may produce motor and sensory dysfunction. Given a history of injury either from blunt trauma or injection, the diagnosis is generally obvious.

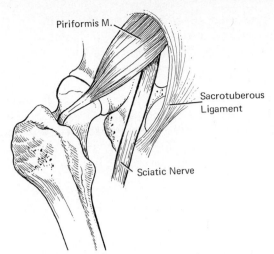

Fig. 19-3. Relationship of the piriformis muscle and the sciatic nerve.

Primary Sciatica

This is an extremely rare condition involving pain along the distribution of the sciatic nerve, which varies in intensity from a dull ache to severe, episodic, lancinating pain. The exact nature of this condition remains unknown. I have treated two patients who complained of extreme lancinating pains, similar in intensity and character to the pain of tic douloureux. Improvement occurred with bed rest, sedation, and Dilantin (often helpful in controlling the pain of tic douloureux, 100 ml every 6 hr) within several days. This condition seems to be self-limiting in nature, and symptomatic measures seem to suffice.

Tumors Involving the Sciatic Nerve

Tumors involving the sciatic nerve are quite painful and often difficult to diagnose, particularly if the lesion is hidden by the mass of the buttock. Tumors of the nerve sheath, such as a neurofibroma, may occur, and they should be suspected if the patient has von Recklinghausen's disease. Occasionally, the sciatic nerve is invaded by metastatic tumor. I have seen one such patient who complained of hip and sciatic pain as the only manifestation of this condition. He continued to complain of this pain for 6 months and was considered by his physician to be a neurotic. Unfortunately, I did not diagnose the cause of his pain, and he was later seen by a medical neurologist, who palpated along the course of the sciatic nerve and located a tender area of swelling. The patient was subsequently explored, and biopsy revealed evidence of a neoplasm which was eventually determined to be a renal carcinoma.

Coccydynia

Most cases of coccydynia follow some traumatic injury to the coccyx. Because the coccyx is usually protected from direct trauma by the buttocks, a fall onto a projecting object (such as a tent stake), or an unusually prominent coccyx in a thin individual are likely precursors to this condition. In general, syndromes related to trauma are predominantly seen in males because of their increased exposure both in industry and sport. Post-traumatic coccydynia is somewhat unique, since it is predominantly seen in females. I can offer no satisfactory explanation for this, since males probably sustain trauma to the coccyx more frequently than females. In addition to direct trauma to the coccyx, this condition will infrequently occur following obstetrical delivery and, even more rarely, in association with lumbar disc syndromes and lumbosacral strains.

The predominant symptom is pain in the coccygeal area, aggravated by coccygeal pressure which is produced by sitting and eased when standing or walking. Patients with prominent buttocks often prefer to sit on firm, non-yielding surfaces and avoid soft upholstered chairs which may produce coccygeal pressure. Thin individuals with flat buttocks often carry about cushions or foam rubber rings to provide extra padding when sitting.

The diagnosis of coccydynia is associated with an element of chronicity. The acute pain following trauma to the coccyx which progressively lessens with the passage of time and is gone within a month or two may theoretically be labelled coccydynia but is not really consistent with what is generally implied by this diagnosis. Most physicians identify this condition as one in which the coccygeal pain persists long beyond the anticipated duration of such a traumatic injury.

In addition to the pain at the end of the coccyx, associated symptoms are not uncommon. Persistent rectal pain and fullness, plus a variety of rectal sphincter complaints including pain on defecation, reduced sphincter control, and constipation, may be elicited.

Examination of the coccyx is best performed bimanually, with the examining finger of one hand in the patient's rectum and the other on the perineum. The coccyx is gently palpated and manipulated, with any pain response to this maneuver carefully assessed and compared to the patient's symptoms. During rectal examination, prior to coccygeal manipulation, palpation of the surrounding viscera and piriformis muscles on either side is performed.

If manipulation and movement of the coccyx reproduces the patient's pain syndrome, injection of the sacrococcygeal joint with lidocaine and 40 mg of methyl prednisolone acetate is often helpful. If pressure over the tip of the coccyx and the coccygeal muscle reduplicates the pain without movement of the coccyx, then a lidocaine-methyl prednisolone injection to either side of the coccyx into the coccygeus muscle may be helpful. When performing an injection in the vicinity of the coccyx, it is advisable to keep an index finger within the rectum and to advance the needle slowly and carefully to prevent inadvertent needle perforation of the rectal mucosa which may lead to subsequent infection.

Many patients with longstanding coccydynia demonstrate a significant emotional component to their symptoms, so that psychological support and reassurance are necessary. Gluteal muscle exercises are often helpful. These are performed in a standing position. The gluteal muscles are maintained in a state of contracture for a count of five and then relaxed for the same duration, for a total of ten contractures. These are repeated three times daily.

Dry or moist heat alternated with ice packs to the area of discomfort may be beneficial, as is intermittent use of anti-inflammatory medications. The stronger and potentially addictive analgesic medications are best avoided.

Logically, one would expect this condition to be cured by a coccygectomy, since the pain is so specifically localized to the coccyx and no loss of function results from removal of this vestigial remnant of a tail. However, as in many other medical conditions, logic does not always prevail, and a coccygectomy often results merely in adding a painful scar to the preexisting symptoms.

Entrapment Neuropathies

Obturator Neuropathy

Obturator neuritis may occur either from an obturator hernia or from osteitis pubis (Fig. 19-4). The pain characteristically radiates from the groin along the inner aspect of the thigh. In the case of an obturator hernia, coughing or sneezing increase the abdominal pressure and are productive of pain.[3]

Why obturator neuritis is so often seen in association with osteitis pubis is not completely clear, but it is attributed to the surrounding tissue edema associated with this condition. Osteitis pubis, like intervertebral disc space infection, must be diagnosed on the basis of history and physical findings, since in both conditions the characteristic x-ray film changes are not apparent for 3 to 6 weeks after onset of pain. By the time roentgenographic evidence is discernible, the clinical syndrome is usually improving and is another example of an after-the-fact roentgenographic diagnosis.

In addition to pain, obturator neuritis is associated with weakness of thigh adduction. However, even in patients with long-standing obturator neuritis, thigh adductor atrophy is not seen, because the adductor magnus is supplied by the sciatic nerve, and the adductor longus frequently has supplementary innervation by the femoral nerve.

In association with the pain radiating along the inner aspect of the thigh, a dysesthesia or paresthesia may be appreciated. Sensory examination may reveal some loss of sensation, but more frequently there is none, despite painstaking examination.

A characteristic obturator neuritis gait abnormality, with an increased outward swing of the involved leg owing to the partially unopposed action of the thigh abductors, is helpful in diagnosing this condition (Fig. 19-5).

If rest and medication do not relieve the symptoms, an obturator nerve block may be helpful on two counts. Relief of pain, following the block, provides further verification of the diagnosis. Also, the block can be utilized as a therapeutic trial for intrapelvic section of the obturator nerve, if intractable pain makes this procedure necessary.

TECHNIQUE OF OBTURATOR NERVE BLOCK

With the patient lying in the supine position, both thighs are abducted (Fig. 19-6 and 19-7). The pubic tubercle on the side to be blocked is palpated, and a local anesthetic wheal is made ½ inch lateral and inferior to it. A 22-gauge, 3½-inch, spinal needle is introduced through this wheal perpendicular to the skin, until the upper portion of the inferior ramus of the pubis is contacted. The depth gauge is placed 1 inch above the skin. The needle is withdrawn to permit an altered lateral and slightly superior needle direction, allowing the needle bevel to glide along the inferior border of the superior ramus of the pubis. When the depth gauge is flush with the skin, the stylet is removed and aspiration attempted, in order to rule out blood vessel penetration. If aspiration is negative, 10 cc of 1% Xylocaine is injected; the obturator nerve is blocked by diffusion of the anes-

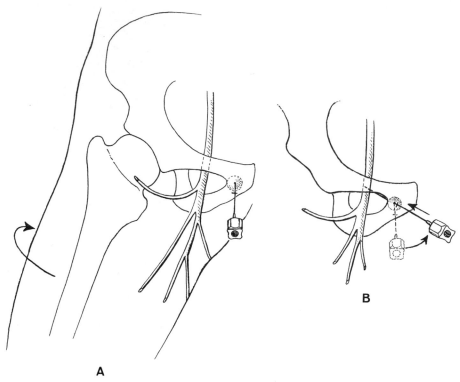

Fig. 19-7. Technique of obturator nerve block.

the nerves from one abdominal muscle interface to another makes them vulnerable to abdominal muscle spasm. I have difficulty completely accepting this theory but have nothing better to offer by way of explanation. Whatever the cause, the spontaneous onset of this condition occasionally occurs and can be mistaken for various forms of renal disease, because of its pain distribution; or, the patient is sometimes labeled a psychoneurotic. If inguinal neuritis is a diagnostic possibility, a nerve block at the anterior iliac spine may be helpful.

TECHNIQUE OF BLOCK

A line drawn from the umbilicus to the anterior superior iliac spine is divided into thirds. An anesthetic wheal is formed at the lateral third of this line. Through this 3 cc of local anesthetic is deposited in five closely approximated sites as the needle is progressively moved perpendicular to the original line.

MANAGEMENT

If relief is obtained with a local block, a series of blocks may be utilized with hydrocortisone. Rest and oral anti-inflammatory medication may also be helpful. If conservative measures are ineffective, a neurolysis may be in order.

Meralgia Paresthetica

Neuralgia of the lateral femoral cutaneous nerve causes burning pain and numbness in the anterolateral aspect of the thigh, and may be confused with sciatica (Fig. 19-9).

Pathophysiology

Pressure on the lateral femoral cutaneous nerve at any point along its long course may produce the meralgia paresthetica syndrome.

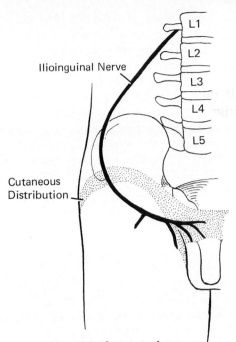

Fig. 19-8. Ilioinguinal nerve.

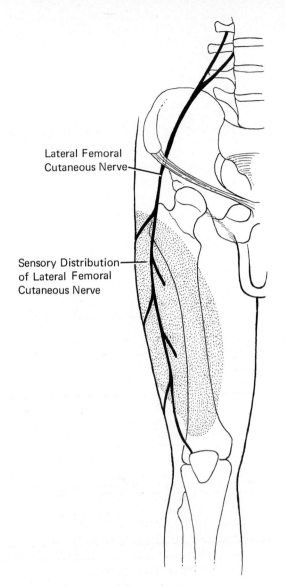

Fig. 19-9. Lateral femoral cutaneous nerve.

The nerve arises from the L2 and L3 nerve roots, and hypertrophic arthritis of the upper lumbar spine may cause nerve root compression. The nerve emerges at the lateral border of the psoas major muscle, and can be involved at this site by a psoas abscess. The nerve then runs across the iliac muscle in the pelvis just beneath the iliac fascia. Because of the superficial position in its long course within the pelvis, it is quite vulnerable to pressure produced by intrapelvic lesions, including pregnancy, tumors, and infections. A traction neuritis of the nerve may occur as it passes over the brim of the iliac crest and emerges from the fascia under Poupart's ligaments, just medial to its attachment to the anterior superior spine of the ilium. At this site, the nerve may be angulated and stretched as the patient stands or walks. Patients who have gained weight and have developed pendulous abdomens are particularly susceptible to involvement at this site. Braces, corsets, and trusses may cause compression in this region. We once treated a dentist for this problem who was accustomed to standing for long periods with his right anterior iliac spine pressed against the arm of the dental chair, producing compression neuritis of the lateral femoral cutaneous nerve.

Signs and Symptoms

The pain of meralgia paresthetica, frequently described as burning, glowing, tingling, and "pins and needles," involves the anterolateral thigh. The onset is usually

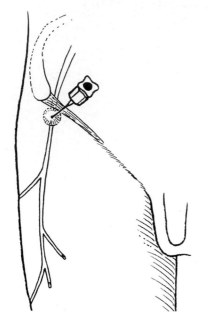

Fig. 19-10. Lateral femoral cutaneous nerve block.

spontaneous, but occasionally the patient may relate the development of pain to an unusually long walk or a prolonged period of standing. Symptoms are usually unilateral, although both thighs may be involved. The pain is usually decreased by lying down or sitting and is aggravated by walking about or prolonged standing. Although firm pressure upon the affected area may not be uncomfortable, light stroking of the skin may provoke an unpleasant tingling sensation. Men often complain that the fabric of their trousers brushes their thighs when they walk and causes this unpleasant dysesthesia.

Diagnosis

Although little difficulty is encountered in diagnosing this rather distinct clinical entity, determining the nature and site of the causative factor may be a problem. If the nerve is involved as it passes over the brim of the iliac crest, an analgesic block of the lateral femoral cutaneous nerve will relieve the pain; this block will be ineffective if the

lesion is located proximally. In such instances, a complete neurologic survey, including roentgenograms of the lumbar spine, should be carried out. When the lesion is within the spine and is due to compression of the nerve roots by osteoarthritis or a herniated disc in the upper lumbar region, diminution of the patellar reflex, weakness, and atrophy of the quadriceps muscle may be evident. Rectal and vaginal examination should be done, and in some cases, myelography may be necessary.

Treatment

If the lesion is located at the antero-superior iliac spine and is confirmed by subsidence of pain after analgesic block, repeated injections may create progressively longer pain-free intervals. If after three blocks no significant improvement beyond the pharmacologic action of the local anesthetic is noted, they are not likely to be of therapeutic value.

LATERAL FEMORAL CUTANEOUS NERVE BLOCK

The technique of blocking the lateral femoral cutaneous nerve in the thigh is simple (Fig. 19-10). A 25-gauge, 1-inch hypodermic needle is inserted at a site ½ inch medial and 1 inch below the anterior superior iliac spine. The needle is carefully advanced through the skin until paresthesia occurs from contact with the nerve; at this point 10 ml of Xylocaine is infiltrated. There is a tendency to insert the needle too deeply, thus causing the anesthetic to be injected into the sartorius muscle and resulting in an ineffective block.

The patient should be placed on a reducing diet directed at elimination of the pendulous abdomen. Constricting straps around the abdomen must be eliminated: women must discard tight corsets or girdles; men must substitute suspenders for belts.

At one time, section of the lateral femoral cutaneous nerve, or neurolysis and transposition into a slot in the ilium, was the treatment of choice. These procedures have not withstood the tests of time particularly well. When the nerve is sectioned, the pain may return because of the formation of a painful neuroma, which may also occur with transposition of the nerve. Spontaneous subsidence of the pain is likely to occur if a conservative regimen as previously outlined is carried out. When the syndrome is caused by a proximal lesion of the nerve or its spinal roots, proper therapy is directed appropriately.

Adhesive Arachnoiditis

A number of patients with low back and sciatic pain have had their symptoms attributed to adhesive arachnoiditis which was demonstrated by myelography. In many instances, the etiology of this condition was attributed to spinal anesthesia, which had been carried out years previously; in some cases, no history of spinal anesthesia was obtained.[4,5]

A number of physicians have advocated performing a laminectomy, opening the dura, and separating the roots from their adhesive constrictions. This is no longer a widely accepted or commonly performed procedure. It is now believed that some of those patients who improved following this procedure did so as a result of the decompressive laminectomy. Some of them may have had an unrecognized stenotic lumbar spinal canal, with a misinterpreted myelogram.

Arthritis of the Hips

Pain of arthritis of the hips is usually quite characteristic and readily identified. It is usually confined to the hip and is aggravated by all hip movements.

Occasionally, this pain radiates not only down the posterior thigh to the knee but

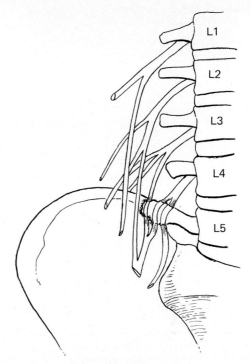

Fig. 19-11. The relationship of the ilium-transverse process pseudoarthrosis and lower lumbar roots.

also up into the buttock and lumbar region. In such infrequent instances, the physician may confuse hip pain with sciatica. Sometimes, the associated muscle spasm of hip disease may cause diminution of deep tendon reflexes.

Hip pain is almost invariably aggravated by external hip rotation, and the Patrick's test is probably the single most reliable sign to aid in the diagnosis. X-ray film evidence of hip disease is sometimes equivocal in the early stages of the condition.

Ilium-Transverse Process Pseudoarthrosis

A rare cause of low back pain occurs when an elongated transverse process of the L5 vertebra comes into contact with, but is not fused to, the ilium. As a result of normal L5 movement, the site of such bony impaction

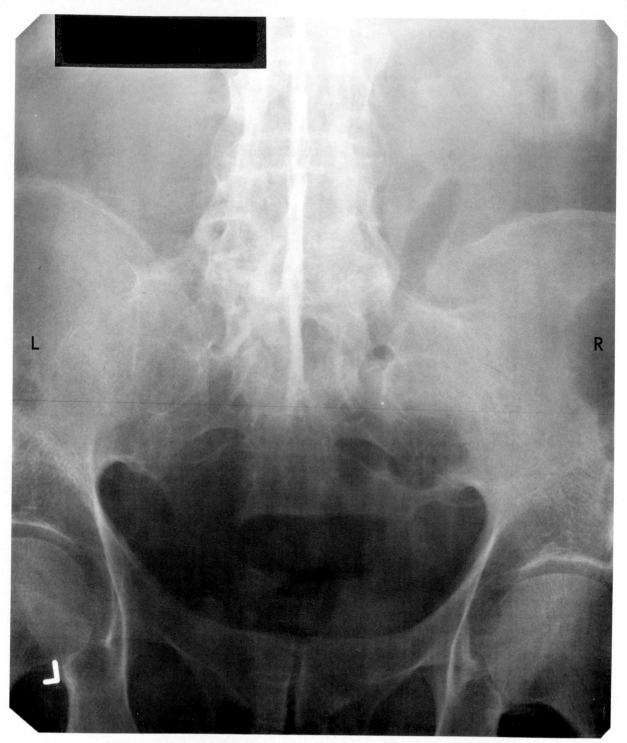

Fig. 19-12. Ankylosing spondylitis. Note the almost obliterated sacroiliac joint margins, fusion of the apophyseal joints, and interspinous ligamentous ossification. This 62-yr-old patient was hospitalized subsequent to relatively moderate trauma which produced a compression fracture of L1. The rigidity of the spine makes this structure vulnerable to mechanical stresses which are easily tolerated by a normally mobile skeleton. (Continued opposite page).

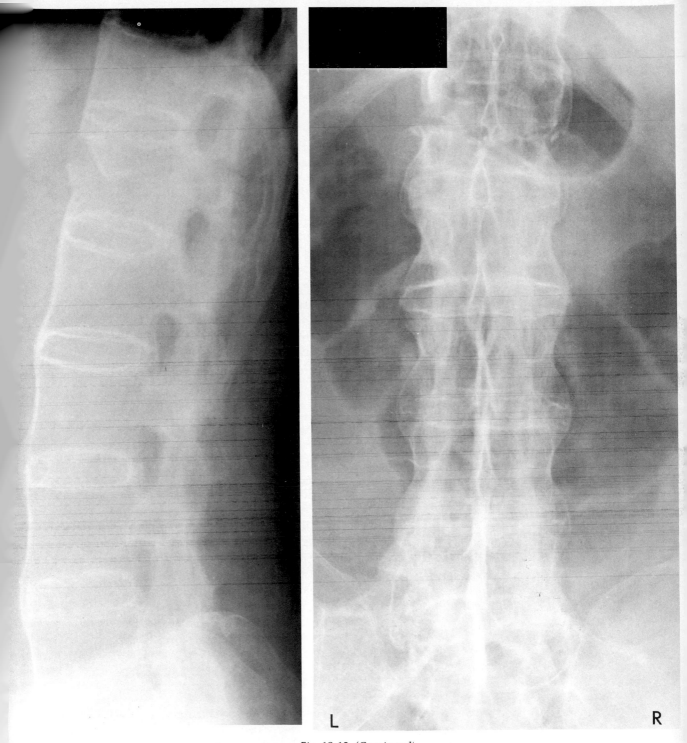

L   R

Fig. 19-12. (Continued)

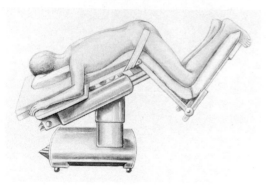

Fig. 19-13. Positioning of the patient for unroofing of the sacrum. If the patient is obese, it may be necessary to use adhesive strapping to retract the gluteii laterally.

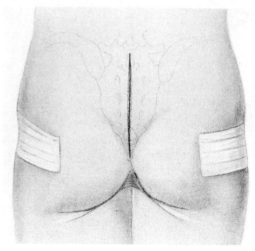

Fig. 19-14. Incision.

is subject to trauma; hypertrophic osteoarthritic changes at the site of contact occur.

The primary symptom resulting from such a pseudoarthrosis is low back pain with rather specific referral to the site of pseudoarthrosis (Fig. 19-11). Examination reveals tenderness to pressure over the site, with paraspinal muscle spasm particularly on the involved side. The pain is aggravated by specific movements of the lumbar spine, especially lateral flexion and rotation, which in most other causes of low back dysfunction are not hampered or productive of increased discomfort.

Occasionally, either the L4 or L5, nerve root in its extrathecal course may become involved with the mass of degenerated fibrocartilaginous tissue formed in reaction to the pseudoarthrosis. This may produce a radiculitis of the affected nerve root, with lower extremity pain and a positive straight leg raising test on the affected side. The root affected depends upon the relative position of the sacrum with regard to the pelvis.

Treatment

Pseudoarthritis is improved with bed rest, anti-inflammatory and analgesic medication, and the wearing of a low back support. If pain persists, injection of hydrocortisone into the site of the pseudoarthrosis may be in order.

If pain continues despite adequate conservative management, surgery may be necessary. At surgery, the site of the pseudoarthrosis is exposed and the elongated transverse process rongeured away.

Ankylosing Spondylitis

Ankylosing spondylitis, also called Marie-Strumpell disease, is a form of rheumatoid arthritis with certain features identifying it as a specific entity. The disease is often familial, is predominant in males at a five to one ratio, and presents with an absence of rheumatoid factor or rheumatoid nodules. In common with rheumatoid arthritis, typical rheumatoid peripheral joint disease occurs sporadically in more than half of these patients, and a significant proportion suffer from chronic peripheral joint disease.

Symptoms

The onset usually occurs between 25 and 35 years of age and is manifested by low back discomfort involving one or both buttocks. It is usually described as an aching or stiffness which is often more apparent after remaining in the same position for prolonged

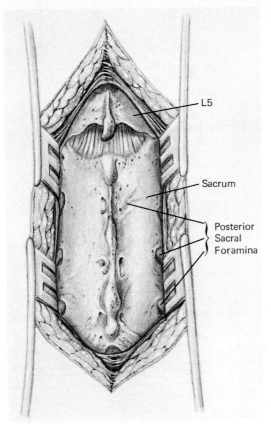

Fig. 19-15. In retracting and carrying out a sub-periosteal muscle dissection, avoid dissecting beyond the posterior sacral foramina to prevent damage to the dorsal division of the sacral nerves emerging through the foramina under cover of the multifidus.

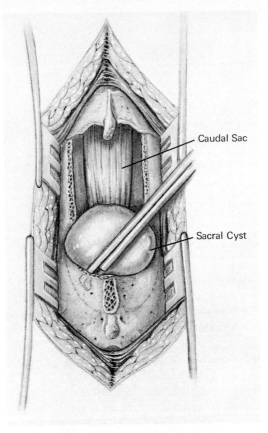

Fig. 19-16. Unroofing of sacrum.

periods and particularly so upon awakening in the morning (Fig. 19-12). This onset is rather insidious, tends to be episodic, is not likely to require medical attention initially. It is usually vaguely recalled by the patient during the history. With the passage of time, the episodes of discomfort become progressively more severe and may awaken the patient from a sound sleep during the night. Unlike most pains associated with low back dysfunction, it is not particularly aggravated by physical activity.

Approximately 75% of the patients with this condition have some form of sciatica (unilateral, alternating, or bilateral), usually occurring during the early phases of the disease. Eventually, these radicular pains are

superceded by increased aching and stiffness, and aggravated by inactivity.

The increasingly severe episodes of pain over a period of years will be associated with increasing rigidity of the spine. Occasionally, an episode of iritis occurs as one of the early symptoms.

Examination

In the early stages of this disease, physical examination may reveal nothing, but later findings include paraspinal muscle spasm, with flattening of the lumbar lordosis. Tenderness over the sacroiliac joints may be quite striking and can be elicited not only by pressure or percussion posteriorly but also by digital pressure applied through the rectum. Eventually, a flattening of the lower thoracic curvature and restriction of cervical

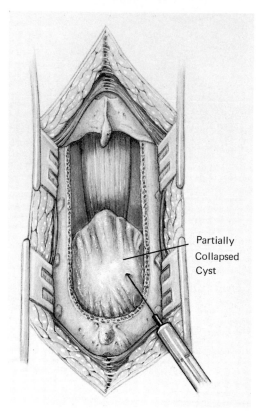

Fig. 19-17. *Tapping the cyst to reduce the pressure, permitting cyst wall mobilization in all directions for visualization of the exiting sacral nerves.*

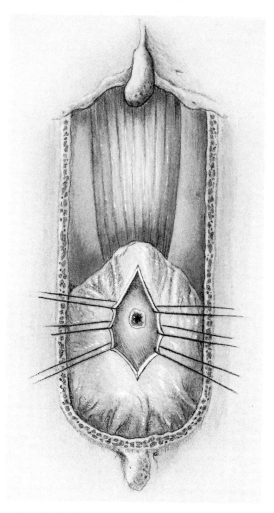

Fig. 19-18. *Incision into cyst and visualization of connection between neck of cyst and the terminal position of the caudal sac.*

mobility are noted, with restriction of chest expansion being a relatively late sign. Despite a history of radicular signs, sensory, motor, or reflex changes are rare. Eventually, the entire vertebral column becomes fixed. Intermittent low-grade fevers may occur.

Laboratory Tests

An elevated sedimentation rate may be most helpful, but this may remain normal even during active exacerbations in 10% to 20% of patients. Serologic tests for the rheumatoid factor are helpful when positive, but false negatives may occur in more than 90% of the cases of ankylosing spondylitis.

Roentgenograms

Convincing roentgen diagnosis of ankylosing spondylitis is usually apparent only after several years. The earliest x-ray film abnormalities are usually seen in the sacroiliac joints. The joint space at first is somewhat wider than usual, with irregular margins due to bony erosion and a slight increase in density at the margins of the joints. In almost every case this condition ultimately progresses to destructive sacro-ilitis. The spine eventually progresses to ligamentous ossification with narrowing and fusion of the apophyseal joints.

Treatment

In the early stages of the disease, symptomatic relief is obtained with local heat, salicylates, and mild exercise. Long-term management requires a supervised exercise program to retard the onset of osteoporosis and ankylosis, plus the use of anti-inflammatory drugs to reduce pain and muscle spasm.

Confusion with Lumbar Disc Disease

Each year I encounter a patient or two with ankylosing spondylitis who has been subjected to lumbar disc surgery in the early stages of disease. A positive familial history for spondylitis, a history of peripheral joint disease or iritis, the typical morning stiffness and absence of positive neurological signs should warn off the surgeon. In the late stages of this disease, the diagnosis is apparent.

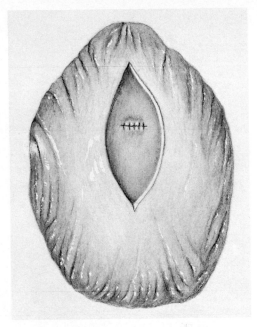

Fig. 19-20. Cyst wall is allowed to remain open so that it will not reform.

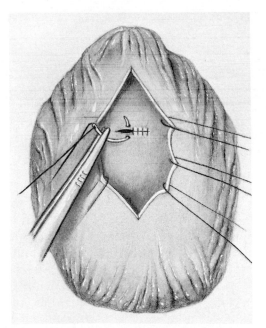

Fig. 19-19. Closure of terminal portion of caudal sac.

Charcot's Disease of the Spine (Vertebral Osteoarthropathy)

One of the rare causes of low back pain is tertiary syphilis which produces bony changes in the vertebral bodies. The bone and joint changes involving the lumbar spine resemble those of osteoarthritis in the earlier stages of this disease. However, with progression in the tabetic arthropathy, the eburnation of bone and the proliferative changes at the margins of the vertebral bodies are more extensive than those seen in ordinary osteoarthritis.

The appreciation of pain, which normally protects the joints from injury or from excessive use after injury, lessens as a result of tabes dorsalis. It is thought to be responsible for fragmentation of the hypertrophied margins of the vertebrae and extensive degeneration of the intervertebral discs at multiple levels. There are those who feel that this neurotrophic disease affects the vertebrae directly through disturbance of bone

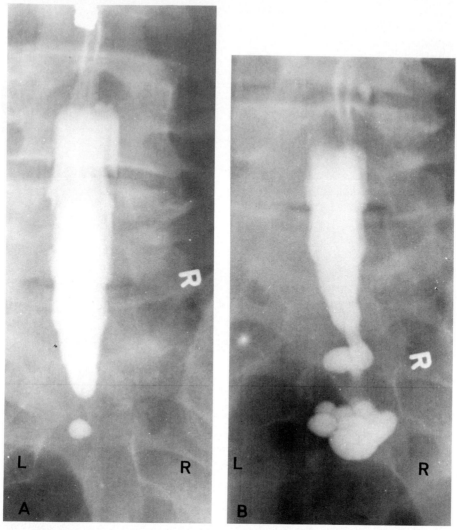

Fig. 19-21. Myelography of sacral cyst. **(A)** Normal lumbar myelogram with droplet of Pantopaque indicative of possible sacral cyst. **(B)** Sacral cyst gradually filling by placing patient in upright (standing) position and having him strain ("bear down"). (Continued opposite page)

metabolism and who point to the fact that the bones of patients with tabes are not exposed to extraordinarily excessive trauma.

As a result of considerable new bone formation with posterior and posterolateral bony ridges, cauda equina compression may occur, thus further complicating the neurological dysfunction caused by tabes dorsalis. Myelography in these instances reveals marked generalized narrowing of the subarachnoid space as a result of bony proliferation and thickening of the ligaments of the vertebral canal. Bilateral constriction resulting from this narrowing is seen at multiple layers in both the AP and the lateral views. Frequently, the bony encroachment is severe enough to cause a partial or complete myelographic block. When this occurs, surgical decompression for relief of cauda equina compression is indicated.

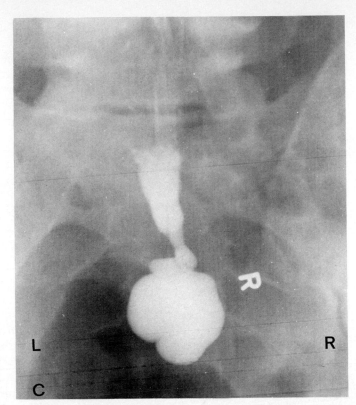

Fig. 19-21. (Continued) *(C) Sacral cyst filled with Pantopaque. (D) After withdrawal some Pantopaque remained trapped within the sacral cyst. (E) Lateral view of the "trapped" Pantopaque within the sacral cyst. Note the bony erosion of the sacrum at the site of the cyst.*

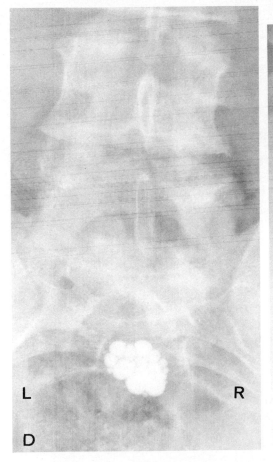

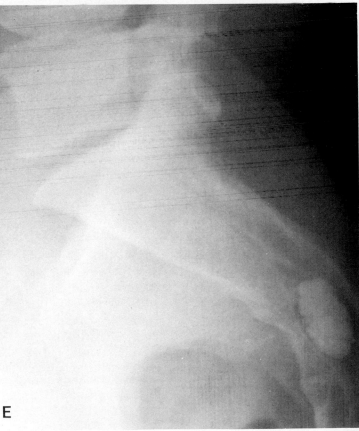

Sacral Cysts

Uncommonly, patients with low back and sciatic pain will be found to have sacral cysts on myelography. The etiology and pathogenesis of these lesions are obscure, as is the mechanism of symptom production. These cysts usually occur at the junction of the posterior root and the dorsal ganglion and can be found on the dorsal ganglia of any of the spinal nerve roots. They are most commonly seen on the S2 and S3 roots. They may be either asymptomatic or associated with low back and sciatic pain, and may be single or multiple.

Since 1938, Dr. I. M. Tarlov has written extensively on cysts of the posterior sacral roots. He believes that these lesions are caused by hydrostatic pressure dissecting the nerve root sheath at a site where the arachnoid which invests the nerve roots is relatively weak. This results in a splitting of the nerve root sheath and formation of a space between the pia-derived endoneurium and the arachnoid-derived perineurium. Others attribute the formation of these cysts to trauma, and some consider them purely congenital in etiology.

Plain roentgenograms are usually negative; but occasionally, with extremely large cysts, localized thinning and erosion of the sacrum occurs and is seen in the lateral view.

Myelography is essential to establishing the diagnosis. It may demonstrate a free and readily patent communication between the subarachnoid space and the cyst; there may be a partial communication; and, in some instances, no communication between the subarachnoid space and the cyst can be demonstrated. When the communication is partial, the Pantopaque may be forced into the cyst by either bilateral jugular compression or a Valsalva-type maneuver with the patient straining. If the partial communication between the subarachnoid space and the cyst is minimal, Pantopaque will not enter the cyst until 24 or 48 hours after the initial subarachnoid injection of the radiocontrast material. Some authorities advocate intentionally leaving 1 cc of dye within the subarachnoid space and obtaining a follow-up film 48 hours later, in order to determine the possible existence of such lesions. A number of these cysts were discovered when a complete withdrawal of Pantopaque was technically unsuccessful and follow-up x-ray films unexpectedly revealed their presence. When no communication exists between the subarachnoid space and the cyst, the presence of such a lesion can only be inferred by displacement of the caudal sac in association with bony erosion.

One should be relatively cautious in the surgical removal of these lesions for two reasons (Figs. 19-13 through 19-21). First, in many instances they are asymptomatic; after obliteration of the cyst, the patient notes no abatement of the pain. Second, excision of a sacral nerve root cyst may result in some sensory dysfunction within the sacral distribution. If this numbness extends over the shaft of the penis in males, it may be associated with alteration and impairment of sexual functions. Before considering surgery on a sacral cyst, particularly in a male, this potential complication should be discussed at some length with the patient. Failure to alert the patient to this potential problem has led to a number of lawsuits.

The following case history will indicate my caution with regard to this lesion. G.L. (49542), a 34-year-old policeman, was hospitalized on July 19, 1970, because of long-standing low back pain and right sciatica which did not respond to conservative management. A myelogram revealed a large sacral cyst measuring approximately 1½ inches in diameter. After Pantopaque removal (some remained within the cyst and could not be removed), 80 ml of methyl prednisolone acetate was injected through the LP needle used for myelography, prior to needle withdrawal.

The patient noted some improvement with this medication and was discharged from the hospital on July 24, 1970. He was followed at intervals on an outpatient basis for 2 years. During this interval he continued to complain of severe, intense low back pain and right sciatica. Because of the persistence of his symptoms, he was rehospitalized and the sacral cyst was excised June 7, 1972. The postoperative course was benign and uneventful, and the patient has had no recurrence of pain. During the 2-year interval between discovery of the sacral cyst and its excision, the patient was followed regularly and was fully aware of the potential sexual complications of surgery. After patient and surgeon were satisfied that he would not appreciate any significant improvement, we mutually agreed that surgery was in order.

References

1. Filtzer DL, Bhanson HH: Low back pain due to arterial obstruction. J Bone Joint Surg 41B:244, 1959
2. Finneson BE: Diagnosis and Management of Pain Syndromes, ed. 2. Philadelphia, WB Saunders, 1969
3. Kopell HP, Thompson WAL: Peripheral Entrapment Neuropathies. Baltimore, William & Wilkins, 1963
4. Schwarz GA, Bevilacqua JE: Paraplegia following spinal anesthesia. Clinicopathologic report and review of literature. Arch Neurol 10:308, 1964
5. Thorsen G: Neurological complications after spinal anesthesia and results from 2493 follow-up cases. Acta Chir Scand (Suppl 121) 95:1–272, 1947

Experimental and Unorthodox Treatments for Low Back and Sciatic Pain

20

Evaluating Treatment

The ever-present problem of low back pain illustrates how very thin and unsubstantial are theories, as compared with tangible experience. The physician must be constantly mindful that no one disease or condition is responsible for low back dysfunction, nor can one single form of treatment be considered universally effective for the variety of causal entities. The goal of proper management is individualization of the treatment of the patient's specific needs. When deciding upon treatment for such a relatively benign condition, the potential hazards of the contemplated treatment, the residual dysfunction produced by the treatment, and the convalescent interval following the treatment must be considered.

In 1949, as an assistant neurology resident, I was exposed to my first clinical research experience. This effort involved the use of a drug which some investigators claimed would arrest the progress of multiple sclerosis. The natural history of this disease, characterized by occasionally prolonged periods of remission, is well known to create short-term, overoptimistic results. However, after 2 years my enthusiasm for what turned out to be a valueless treatment was cooled.

Some years ago, in an effort to document the "natural history" of lumbar disc disease, a number of my patients with verified lumbar disc protrusions, who were not treated surgically but who received conservative management, were contacted by mail. Slightly more than 50% of these patients indicated that they were physically active and reasonably pain free. Three years later a second mailed questionnarie was sent to a somewhat larger group including most of the previously polled patients. The second mailing again indicated that approximately 50% of the patients were satisfied with their status, but that these were different patients. Careful scrutiny revealed that a sizable shift had occurred, with formerly pain-free patients now being incapacitated, and many of the previously incapacitated patients now being comfortable.

At any given time approximately half of all untreated patients with low back dysfunction will be in remission. For a method of treatment to be considered effective, it must improve on the natural history of the disease; that is, achieve a "cure rate" significantly better than 50%.

Intervertebral Discolysis

The concept of nonsurgically diminishing the overall bulk of protruding intervertebral disc, with the presumption that such a contraction of tissue mass would reduce nerve root pressure, has been considered for more than 20 years. A variety of methods to convert the intervertebral disc to scar tissue

557

were considered, including damaging the disc with heavy needles or trocars, injecting bacteria into the disc space, and injecting sclerosing solutions into the disc.

Chymopapain

In 1959, Dr. Carl Hirsch discussed the feasibility of injecting a discolytic enzyme into the intervertebral space; this was further discussed by Dr. Mitchell, Dr. Hendry, and Dr. Billewicz. In 1961, Dr. Lyman Smith injected chymopapain, the major proteolytic component of *Carica papaya* latex, into the intervertebral discs of rabbits and dogs. On the basis of this animal experimentation, the first humans were so treated by him in July of 1963. Since that time, a number of investigators have conducted similar clinical investigative experiments in man. This substance attacks chondromucoprotein-producing keratosulfate, chondroitin sulfate, and protein.

Over the next 14 years approximately 17,000 patients received injections of chymopapain. These injections were carried out by approximately 40 physician investigators who adhered to gudielines established by the Food & Drug Administration. Assistance was provided by Travenol Laboratories, the manufacturer of the substance. The reported results of this large investigative effort were as follows: 68% of these patients achieved marked improvement; 15% achieved slight improvement; 3.2% experienced adverse reactions; 0.5% sustained sensitivity reactions. Two deaths followed anaphylactic reactions. The results were questioned by some because this study was nonblind and uncontrolled. As a result of this criticism, a double-blind study of 105 patients was carried out. It compared chymopapain injections with similar volumes of the presumably inert diluent or carrier solution (cysteine and EDTA) without the chymopapain. When the code was broken and the reports assessed, it was determined that no statistically significant difference existed between the two groups. Shortly after completion of this double-blind study, all human investigation of chymopapain was halted in the United States.

Use of this material has continued in areas outside the United States. Between 1973 and 1978, approximately 6000 patients have received Chymopapain injections in Canada. This group of patients is reported as having 61% good or excellent results, 17% fair results; the balance were unimproved. The injections were performed by 60 Canadian physicians, either orthopedic surgeons or neurosurgeons, working in 40 different hospitals throughout Canada. A number of adverse reactions were reported. There were 18 immediate sensitivity reactions, six of which were severe, requiring administration of IV fluids, adrenalin, Benadryl, and hydrocortisone to counteract the hypotensive state successfully. Another 16 patients developed a delayed sensitivity reaction in the form of hives, rash, edema, and itching. Six patients had an intervertebral disc space infection. There were no fatalities.

Chymopapain has recently been approved for use by the United Kingdom Ministry of Health, and clinical investigations are presently underway in Belgium, Germany, and France. Clinical trials are in the planning stage in several other countries. A triple-blind study is presently going on at 11 different medical centers in the United States.

The ups and downs encountered by this investigative drug demonstrates the difficulty of assessing the true efficacy of treatment for any low back problem. Hopefully, the new triple-blind study will be of some benefit in determining the relative effectivenss of chymopapain.

Collagenase Injection

Collagenase, extracted from culture of *Clostridium histolyticum* and *C. welchii*, is an enzyme which attacks the collagen molecule. It has been utilized in the debridement of dermal ulcers, necrotic tissues, and burns.

It has been implicated as a possible etiological factor in the early stages of degenerative joint disease. This material has been used to date in studies in vitro and in the operative intradiscal injection of dogs.

Dr. Bernard Sussman, who advocates the use of collagenase as opposed to chymopapain, states that the chemical changes undergone by degenerating discs, both from aging or herniation, increase the collagen content in the nucleus pulposus and the annulus fibrosus. He further states that since chymopapain has no solubilizing effect upon collagen, collagenase would seem the logical discolytic agent of choice. He states too that chymopapain exerts its principal enzymatic action upon the nucleus pulposus, but many symptom-producing discs are actually a protrusion of the annulus fibrosus over the underlying nucleus pulposus. This strengthens his thesis that collagenase is more suitable as a discolytic agent in the degenerated disc. Clinical investigation of this drug in humans is anticipated in the near future.

Intradiscal Hydrocortisone Injection

Dr. Henry L. Feffer first injected hydrocortisone into an intervertebral disc in 1954. He stated that degeneration of this structure inevitably leads to radial tears and fissures, which cause an inflammatory reaction in the surrounding longitudinal ligaments of the spine and produce a syndrome of low back pain. Progression of this lesion will cause increased widening of the angular fissures and, eventually, sufficient weaken the annulus fibrosus, so that herniation of nuclear material will occur through this tear. Dr. Feffer assumed that the polymerizing effect of hydrocortisone would reverse or block the degenerative changes within the intervertebral disc and would help recreate the normal physiological role of the nucleus pulposus in supporting the vertical load. He further assumed that the fissures and tears of the annulus fibrosus associated with the clinical syndrome of low back pain

would have an opportunity to heal and that this treatment, in association with routine low back rehabilitative measures, would be of value in preventing recurrence of low back pain.

His technique involved discograms which were performed by means of a posterior lateral approach using a 23-gauge spinal needle. The injected mixture consists of 25 mg of hydrocortisone with 1.5 cc of radiopaque, water-soluble contrast material (Diodrast, and more recently Hypaque). The selection of patients was primarily from those who did not improve with conservative management and in whom the question of low back surgery was considered.

He reported a series of 244 patients who were followed for a minimum of 4 years and a maximum of 10 years. A fraction less than half of these patients (46.7%) obtained permanent remission, or at most a minor backache on occasion, from this injection. A fraction more than half (53.3%) either showed no initial response or suffered recurrence of symptoms from 1 week to 6 years later. The patients whose pain was primarily in the back rather than radicular, those mainly within the older age groups, seemed to do better. One intervertebral disc space infection was reported as a complication.

On the basis of these reports it seems that the patients with primarily low back pain without sciatic radiation do better with the intradiscal injection of hydrocortisone, while those with radicular symptoms are best served by intervertebral discolysis.

Some authorities object to the use of hydrocortisone in degenerative disc disease, since hydrocortisone, which is widely used in the treatment of soft tissue injuries of all kinds, inhibits fibrous tisssue formation and as a result, in certain circumstances, may help to prevent the formation of painful scarring. If one assumes that the eventual desired result in a degenerative disc lesion is to establish formation of a stable fibrous tissue reaction, injecting hydrocortisone locally into the disc would appear to run counter to this end result.

Prolotherapy

In 1956, a monograph was published indicating that the cause of low back pain in many patients was relaxation of the ligaments about the joints of the spine and pelvis.[1] Dr. George S. Hackett, the author of this text, proposed that as a result of "strain, sprain, tearing, or degeneration," a weakening of the fibrous tissue at the fibro-osseous junction occurs. This causes relaxation of the affected ligaments, impairs the stability of the joints supported by these "incompetent" ligaments, and results in a painful disability. He defined ligament relaxation as a "condition in which the strength of the ligament fibers has become impaired so that a stretching of the fibrous strands occurs when the ligament is submitted to normal or less than normal tension." The treatment advocated by Dr. Hackett was the intraligamentous injection of a sclerosing solution to develop a maximum amount of fibrous tissue and bone, thereby affording joint stabilization. He called his method "prolotherapy" based on the Latin *proli* meaning offspring, from which the word proliferate derives. He implied by this term "the rehabilitation of an incompetent structure by the generation of new cellular tissue."

Proliferating Solutions

Several proliferating solutions can be used. Sylnasol (G. D. Searle & Co.) is a solution of the sodium salt of a psyllium oil fatty acid. For office treatment, this is combined with an equal amount of local anesthetic solution, usually 1% Xylocaine. For hospitalized patients, the Sylnasol is combined with normal saline, which apparently is productive of a greater amount of reactive fibrous tissue and bone. The increased pain appreciated in the absence of a local anesthetic is controlled by the administration of analgesics in the hospital.

Zinc sulfate may be used in combination with either phenol or Pontocaine, or a combination of all three (zinc sulfate, phenol, and Pontocaine).

A dextrose proliferating solution, which is said to give adequate fibro-osseous proliferation with a minimum of discomfort, can be made up by a pharmacist as follows:

Dextrose BP	25.0%
Phenol BP	2.5%
Glycerine BP	25.0%
Distilled water to	100.0%

This solution, which is "self-sterilizing," may be placed on 100-cc, rubber-stoppered bottles. Prior to injection one part of this solution is mixed with three parts of 1% Xylocaine.

Injection Technique

The injection technique utilizes a 22-gauge Luerlock needle of sufficient length to contact bone at the site of the fibro-osseous attachment. The needle is attached to a 10-cc syringe containing the sclerosing solution combined with a local anesthetic solution. After inserting the needle to contact bone within the fibro-osseous attachment, 0.25 cc to 1.0 cc of solution is injected, and the needle is withdrawn sufficiently to redirect without bending and to recontact bone at approximately ½ inch distance from the original injection. Usually three to eight injections are made through one cutaneous needle insertion, depending on the size of the area and the amount of solution injected at each needle placement. Forced aspiration prior to injection is stressed, as is the dictum "always touch bone" during the injection.[4] These precautions are taken to avoid inadvertent injection into a blood vessel, nerve root, or the subarachnoid space.

Site of Injection

Selection of injection site is based on rather unique guidelines and diagnostic criteria formulated by Dr. Hackett. Confirmation of this diagnosis is obtained during the intraligamentous needling by the precipitation of intense trigger point pain, which disappears within 2 minutes from the effect of the local anesthetic solution.

Posterior sacroiliac "relaxation" is identified by local tenderness over the sacroiliac joint in association with referred pain to the "outer anterior thigh and the outer side of the leg."[2] The treatment for posterior sacroiliac "relaxation" is injection of sclerosing solution into the fibro-osseous attachment of the posterior sacroiliac, sacrospinous, and sacrotuberous ligaments. Other ligaments which are presumably prone to "relaxation" and require treatment with injection are the interspinous ligaments, the lumbosacral ligaments, and the lumbar articular capsular ligaments.

Some advocates of this method are less selective in their approach and, rather than injecting one specific ligament, will treat "the entire low back area." This involves injecting the intraspinous ligaments from L3 to S1, the lumbar articular capsular ligaments, the sacroiliac, sacrosciatic, and sacrotuberous ligaments. Injections are made at weekly intervals until all of the ligaments are injected, doing as "many as the patient permits or the operator feels the patient can tolerate." After a series of from three to six weekly injections is completed, a "rest period" of 6 to 8 weeks is suggested, after which the patient may return for monthly "follow-up" injections for recurrent pain. Postinjection pain is treated with substantial doses of Demerol.

The advocates of this method consider all patients with low back pain suitable candidates, including those who have previously undergone surgery.

Complications

After publication of Dr. Hackett's monograph in 1956, a number of physicians involved in the management of low back problems explored his method of treatment. Generally, the results were disappointing, much below the 82% improvement rate reported by Dr. Hackett. On the heels of indifferent results, two reports of serious complications arising from this method were published in the *Journal of the American Medical Association;* the first in August, 1959, and the second a year later.[3,4]

The first case involved a 50-year-old woman with a long history of lumbar and sciatic pain who improved on two occasions on a regimen of pelvic traction, bed boards, bed rest, a back brace, and sedation. Following each remission of pain, she developed intermittent recurrence of her symptoms. In June of 1957, she underwent interligamentous injection of sclerosing agent. The patient was placed in a prone position and the sclerosing agent (zinc sulfate in 2.5% phenol solution) was injected in the midline into the ligaments about the lumbosacral joint. She developed immediate severe pain in the legs, became paralyzed from the waist downward and had loss of bladder control. On attempting to arise from the table she fell to the floor. She gradually regained almost complete use of her legs over the next few days but required an indwelling catheter for bladder function and cleansing enemas for bowel care. On October 27 of 1957, she was readmitted to the hospital complaining of nausea, vomiting, paresthesia over the buttocks and legs, perioral numbness, blurred vision, headaches, and generalized malaise. She had developed diplopia due to a right sixth nerve palsy. On examining the fundi, two diopters of papilledema were found, with retinal hemorrhages and engorged retinal veins bilaterally. She had a mild peripheral facial paresis on the right, progressive weakness of the right leg, nuchal rigidity, and slurred speech. A diagnosis of basilar adhesive arachnoiditis was made. On November 1, 1957, ventriculograms demonstrated a widely dilated ventricular system, and a ventriculostomy was performed to gradually reduce the markedly increased intracranial pressure. On November 4, 1957, exploration of the posterior fossa was performed, which revealed a markedly adhesive arachnoiditis about the rim of the cisterna magna. Technical difficulties were encountered during surgery, and the patient died several hours after surgery. The immediate cause of death was an extradural hematoma in the occipital area, which was a complication of the suboccipital craniectomy. In addition to the changes secondary to surgery, chronic changes involving the spine and brain were attributed to the introduction of sclerosing solution into the subarachnoid space. Adhesive arachnoiditis and chronic scarification were found in the cauda equina, spinal cord, medulla, cerebellopontine angle, and the base of the brain.

The second case report of a serious complication from this method involved a 53-year-old woman suffering from low back pain. In March, 1957, she received an injection of "vegetable oil and anesthetic" into each sacroiliac region. After the injection, she developed severe pain which radiated from the site of injection around to the anterior and medial aspect of both thighs and down the medial aspect of the lower extremities to the ankles. The pain in the sacroiliac region persisted for 3, but the radiating pain into the lower extremities subsided by the next morning. In May, 1957, she received two more injections into each sacroiliac area and a third injection into "one side of the spine." She immediately experienced severe pain in the low back, which radiated down both legs, and a numbness over her body below the umbilicus. When she tried to walk, her legs would not support her, and she was unable to urinate for several hours. These symptoms subsided by the next morning. One week later she awakened with a severe headache which recurred daily for 2 weeks. During this period she had a stiff neck and pain in the right shoulder. In July, 1957, she began to drag both feet as she walked, and within 3 to 4 weeks she required a can and had to hold onto furniture or walls. Numbness returned to her lower extremities and grew more severe. In August, 1957, a lumbar myelogram was normal except for an elevated spinal fluid protein of 68 mg%. In September, 1957, she was unable to walk. Urinary frequency and occasional incontinence developed; fi-

nally, she could not urinate and became severely constipated. By October, 1957, the patient had complete spastic paraplegia with the usual reflex changes. There was analgesia below the fifth rib on the left side and the sixth on the right, complete anesthesia from the eighth thoracic through the third lumbar dermatomes on the left side, and hypesthesia in the remainder of the analgesic area. Vibratory sensibility, sense of position, and the perception of numbers written on the skin were all absent bilaterally below the costal margins. Roentgenographic examination revealed a small residue of radiopaque material in the spinal canal at the level of T6. This did not move as the patient was tipped on the fluoroscopic table.

On October 7, 1957, a laminectomy of T5, T6, and T7 was performed. The dura was closely adherent to the underlying structures throughout the area exposed by the laminectomy. A subarachnoid cyst was evacuated at the level of T6 and considerable thickened arachnoidal tissue was cut away, including the walls of the cyst.

Following surgery the patient's condition improved slightly, but soon the spastic paraplegia returned to its original intensity and ultimately grew more severe. The microscopic examination of the surgical specimens revealed adhesive arachnoiditis.

Present Status of Prolotherapy

The authors of the two case reports were critical of this method in regard both to the authenticity of its value and to the potential dangers. It was emphasized that "there are areas in the lower part of the back where a needle can accidentally and easily enter the subarachnoid space. This can occur directly at the lumbosacral joint or laterally at the dural sleeve of the spinal nerve root."

After the second case report was published in 1960, the number of physicians utilizing this method declined sharply, but in the past few years it has enjoyed a mild revival. Most of the patients referred to me who had previously received this treatment did not seem to demonstrate any beneficial deviation from the expected natural course of their dysfunction. Such unevenly weighted material may lead to a biased conclusion, but my overall personal opinion of the technique is not favorable.

Facet Rhizotomy

In 1971 Dr. W. E. Shyrme Rees, an Australian physician, reported on a large series of cases with low back and sciatic pain which he treated with an original and unique technique of cutting the nerve rootlets to the spinal facets.[5,7] Dr. C. Norman Shealy of LaCrosse, Wisconsin, was impressed by the excellent results and he invited Dr. Rees to the United States to demonstrate his procedure. Encouraged by the results of the technique, he performed the Rees procedure on 29 patients. Dr. Shealy subsequently modified this procedure, using a radio frequency lesion rather than a scalpel to perform the rhizotomy.

Principles of Facet Rhizotomy

Many patients with low back pain, who have extension of this pain into a lower extremity, present with more diffuse and vague sciatic symptoms than the characteristic "single root syndrome" associated with nerve root compression. Such nonspecific leg pain does not remain within the distribution of a single root and is usually not associated with reflex changes or valid motor weakness. It is speculated that "facet dysfunction" may be a factor in these problems. A clinical finding associated with facet dysfunction is acute tenderness to pressure over the affected facet. Sometimes this pressure will not only reproduce pain within the back but also aggravate extension of the pain into a lower extremity. It is further speculated that the facet dysfunction may occur from derangement and instability of the facet joint, resulting from overriding secondary to

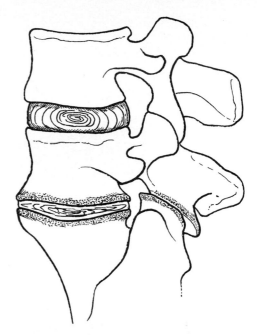

Fig. 20-1. Facet joint overriding, secondary to the collapsed degenerated intervertebral disc.

a collapsed degenerated intervertebral disc (Fig. 20-1).

The clinical success of this procedure in selected cases causes one to speculate upon the entire symptom complex of many patients with low back and leg pain. It reemphasizes the importance of strict correlation of myelographic findings with the clinical findings before determining that the patient's symptoms are primarily due to a protruding lumbar disc causing the root pressure. Further speculation is invited regarding the clinical improvement occasionally derived from prolotherapy (injection of sclerosing solution). It is possible that sclerosing solution injected in the vicinity of the articular facet is associated with clinical improvement, not because of a beneficial effect on the stability of the facet joint, but because of destruction of the nerve rootlet innervating the facet (Fig. 20-2).

Technique of Facet Rhizotomy

The technique advocated by Dr. Rees involves making a deep stab incision 2 cc lateral to the spinous process. This incision

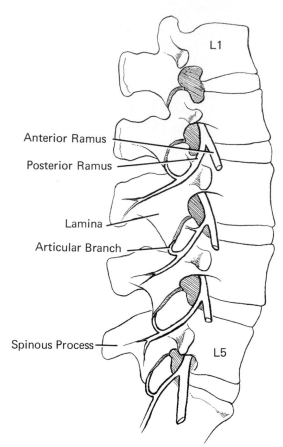

Fig. 20-2. Diagrammatic representation of the articular rootlets entering the capsule of the intervertebral joints. (After Pedersen, Blunck, Gardener: The anatomy of lumbosacral posterior rami and meningeal branches of the spinal nerves. J Bone Joint Surg 38A:377, 1956)

is extended just lateral to the articular facet to the level of the transverse process. At this level, a sweep of the tip of the knife blade is made to assure sectioning of the facet innervation. A determination as to the site of the stab incision is made primarily by finding the sites of tenderness to deep pressure over the facets. Following this type of stab incision, a considerable hematoma often developed in the paraspinal muscles of the lumbar region, particularly if this procedure was carried out at multiple levels.

Because of the excessive subcutaneous bleeding that occurred in two patients, Dr. Shealy modified the procedure. Using fluoroscopic and roentgenographic control, a ra-

dio frequency electrode is inserted down to the intertransverse ligament slightly lateral to the facets (Fig. 20-3). Local anesthesia is used only to make a skin wheal with no anesthetic injected into the deeper tissues. Avoidance of deep local anesthetic will allow a further clinical correlation of the facet syndrome, since, when the electrode reaches the intertransverse ligament, it invariably elicits pain similar to that which the patient originally complained of.

Electrical stimulation with a pulse of 1 millisecond duration, 25 to 50 cycles, evokes tingling at 1 to 2 volts, pain at 2 to 4 volts. If the electrode is inserted too deeply and is impinging upon the nerve root, pain will occur with less than 1 volt and muscle contractions will occur at 1 or 2 volts. This test is done to avoid damaging the root with a radio frequency lesion. A further safety check is a lateral Polaroid x-ray film to confirm that the depth of electrode penetration is short of the intervertebral foramen and the exiting nerve root.

After the electrode is positioned to satisfaction, a radio frequency generator is activated with the power raised slowly to produce a temperature of 75°C at the electrode tip for 90 seconds. If the elevation of the temperature to 75° is excessively painful, the temperature is reduced to 50°. After a minute at this temperature, it can then usually be raised to 75° with little or no discomfort. The lesion created with this technique varies from 8 × 10 to 10 × 12 mm.

Diagnostic blocks involving one or more facets at the L3–4, L4–5, and L5–S1 levels are usually advised as an aid in patient selection for this procedure. The specific facet that is blocked is dependent on the location of pain. If pain is limited to one side, a unilateral block is employed. Twenty-gauge spinal needles are positioned upon the facet joint under fluoroscopic guidance. Exactly 1 cc of 1% Xylocaine is injected at each facet. Satisfactory relief of pain for an hour following the injection is considered an effective block.

In the 8 years since this technique was

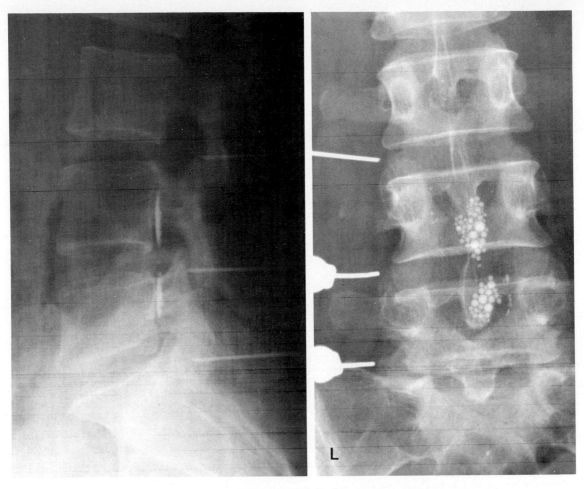

Fig. 20-3. AP and lateral films of a radio frequency electrode placement.

introduced, considerable discussion has occurred regarding both the value of the treatment and exactly what is being denervated. The rather large lesion created by the Shealy radio frequency technique can certainly involve any or all of the articular branches of the posterior ramus plus some injury to the posterior ramus itself.

My personal experience with this technique began shortly after Doctor Shealy introduced it in 1972 and by 1975 involved a total of 73 patients. I was initially enthusiastic, but after several years my enthusiasm cooled and I regretfully gave it up as valueless. The primary reason I was sorry to eliminate this technique from my armamentarium is that I encountered no significant complications with it and it seemed to be singularly safe when performed in the lumbar region.

Neurostimulator Implantation

The technique of neurostimulator implantation was originally based on a theory of pain mechanism advanced in 1966 by Dr. Ronald Melzack, Professor of Psychology, McGill University, Montreal, Canada, and Dr. Patrick D. Wall, Professor of Psychology, M.I.T., Cambridge, Massachusetts. This theory has been popularly referred to as the "gate theory of pain transmission," and it introduced a number of new concepts regarding pathways of pain. The traditional

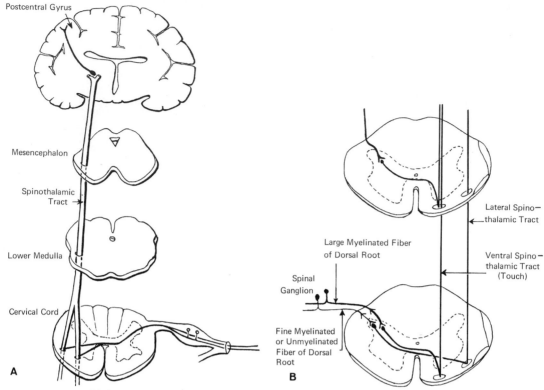

Fig. 20-4. Diagrammatic illustration of the traditional concept of pain conduction. (Courtesy of WB Saunders)

concept of pain conduction implied that the pain impulses were transmitted into the spinal cord through the dorsal roots; once reaching the cord they crossed within several spinal segments to the opposite anterolateral quadrant of the cord (Fig. 20-4). Fibers within the anterolateral quadrant of the cord gathered into a specific bundle identified as the spinothalamic tract, which conducted pain sensation upward to the thalamus. The anatomical basis of this concept of pain transmission was developed by tracing neural pathways, using the traditional method of following the course of myelin sheath and nerve degeneration with a variety of silver tissue stains and other histologic techniques. These traditional anatomical degenerative studies presented a rather simplistic pain pathway schema and did not allow for consideration of the multiple synaptic connections within the cord and the fact that most of the pain input fibers were of the smaller, unmyelinated type.

It has been demonstrated that pain impulses are transmitted to the spinal cord by way of the smaller gamma-delta or C-fibers, and that stimulation of the larger A-beta fibers is never painful (Fig. 20-5). Physiologically, the painful response consists of prolonged firing of many units activating the C-fibers throughout the entire spinal axis, through the medulla, into the medial reticular formation of the midbrain, and into the cerebellum. It is theorized that activity in the larger beta fibers inhibits, at the first spinal synapse, immediate subsequent activity from the smaller C-fibers which is considered essential to pain production. Melzack and Wall suggested that this mechanism normally acts as a gate to balance the input of pain and nonpain sensations (Fig. 20-6). Wall and Sweet tested this theory by employing low-voltage electrical stimulation to the large fibers within a peripheral nerve and reported inhibition of the response to C-fiber input. Painful stimuli to

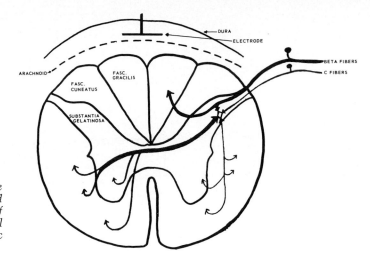

Fig. 20-5. Diagrammatic illustration of the synapse between the large beta fibers and the small C-fibers. Note the position of the stimulating electrode over the dorsal columns. (Shealy, Long, Kahn Pan-Pacific Surgical Association, 1972)

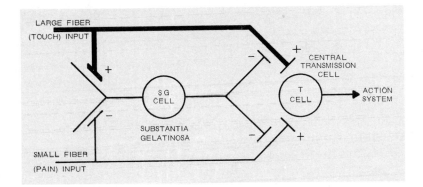

Fig. 20-6. Simplified Melzack-Wall model. (Medtronic, Inc)

a site within the sensory distribution of the nerve were not appreciated as pain so long as electrical stimulation to the large fibers continued. Conversely, it can be demonstrated that if one blocks the large and intermediate beta-gamma and delta peripheral nerve fibers, there is an increase in the amount of the prolonged after-discharge with stimulation of the isolated C-fiber in a peripheral nerve.

Because most pain arises from anatomically widespread tissues, and it is impractical to use peripheral nerve stimulation for control of such pain, it was logical to extend experimental work to a more central transmission site of pain: the spinal cord. Since the dorsal columns within the spinal cord contain an almost pure and concentrated grouping of beta fibers, Dr. Shealy hypothesized that the dorsal columns offered the best site for selective stimulation of pain fibers. Experimentally, he applied a stimulating current to the dorsal column of cats. During such dorsal column stimulation, noxious stimuli did not provoke any apparent pain response in conscious animals. However, if the noxious stimulus was continued and the dorsal column stimulation removed, the experimental animals would react with the normal violent reaction within 5 seconds of cessation of dorsal stimulation. This technique was subsequently applied to human patients with chronic intractable pain.

Prior to the technical implementation of the Melzack-Wall theory, the treatment of chronic intractable pain relied mainly on procedures involving destruction of some portion of the pain-transmitting pathway (thalamotomy, cordotomy, rhizotomy, neu-

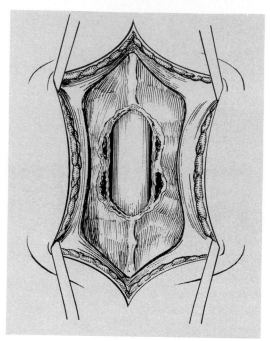

Fig. 20-7. Thoracic laminectomy. (Medtronic, Inc)

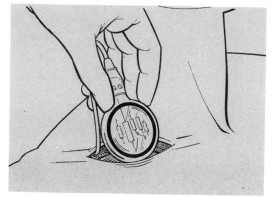

Fig. 20-8. Subcutaneous implantation of the receiver below the right clavicle. (Medtronic, Inc)

rectomy) or the use of narcotics in progressively increasing doses. The goal of dorsal column stimulation was to interfere with pain impulses without destroying any portion of the pain conduction system.

Indications

The prime indication for the application of a dorsal column stimulator is the long-standing and intractable nature of the pain. The pain should not be amenable to the more traditional methods of management. For example, in the management of a patient with low back pain secondary to malignancy, if the neoplasm is x-ray sensitive, a trial of radiation is in order prior to consideration of this method. When this device is considered for patients with low back and sciatic pain who have been failures following disc surgery, a most exhaustive study is required. It must be well established that further low back surgery, or other treatment locally to the involved root or nerve roots, would be fruitless.

Psychoneurosis of severe degree is a sig-

nificant contraindication to use of a dorsal column stimulator. Narcotic addiction of long-standing duration is a contraindication; however, the severity of the pain should be such that it is refractory to non-narcotic drug therapy. The physician should be particularly hesitant to use this device in those patients whose pain is unusual, suspected of being nonorganic, and without any definite explainable etiology.

Routine preoperative screening of the patient involves both psychological and psychiatric evaluation, including the Minnesota Multiphasic Personality Inventory (MMPI). Patients with MMPI's showing elevations or depressions of two or more standard deviations in four or more personality scales are generally considered poor candidates for dorsal column stimulation. It must be realized, however, that some patients often have changes in the MMPI related to their long-standing suffering, so that absolute values and rigid standards relating to emotional factors are difficult to establish.

An essential preoperative screening factor is the patient's response to some form of trial electrical stimulation. In most instances, this is easily done by applying skin electrodes at sites which will induce a tingling sensation in some portion of the painfully involved area. Often, a patient who will derive significant improvement from dorsal column stimulation will also appreciate some degree of improvement within

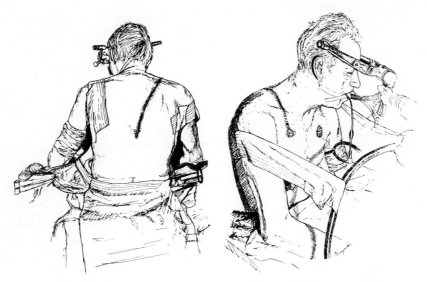

Fig. 20-9. Subcutaneous tunnel extending from thoracic spine to subclavicular region.

the limited anatomical area affected by transcutaneous stimulation. Of even greater importance to identify are those patients who will find the transcutaneous stimulation unpleasant, since they will almost invariably have a poor result from the dorsal column stimulator.

Surgical Technique

Clinical evaluation results indicate that the stimulating electrode is best placed four to six spinal segments above the highest pain input, and the site of preference for low back and sciatic pain is the T3 to T4 level.

With the patient in the sitting position, a laminectomy of T3, T4, and T5 is performed (Fig. 20-7). The bony removal is carried out to the facets to assure adequate exposure of the dura mater to position the electrode. After this portion of the procedure has been completed and all bleeding controlled, a sponge is lightly packed within the laminectomy wound and the subclavicular receiver site is prepared.

A 3-in transverse incision is made over the right clavical, and a small, subcutaneous pocket, just large enough to accommodate the receiver, is developed beneath the lower

flap of the clavicular incision (Fig. 20-8). With blunt dissection, using a long double-curved uterine packing forceps, a subcutaneous tunnel is extended from the clavicular incision over the right shoulder to the laminectomy site (Fig. 20-9). Through this tunnel, a ¼-in Penrose drain is passed. Using the drain as a guide, the electrode is pulled back through the tunnel into the laminectomy incision.

The dura is then opened in the midline, and the electrode is positioned over the dorsal columns between the dura and the arachnoid (Figs. 20-10 and 20-11). The electrode is secured in place using four sutures at each corner, and closure of the wound is carried out in the usual fashion.

Postoperatively, the transmitting antenna is placed on the skin overlying the receiver, and dorsal column stimulation is instituted with a radio frequency transmitter (Figs. 20-12 through 20-14). When the transmitter is activated, the patient appreciates a tingling sensation below the level of electrode implantation and simultaneous reduction of pain. Patients have individually varying needs regarding duration and frequency of stimulation, from several times daily to almost constant stimulation.

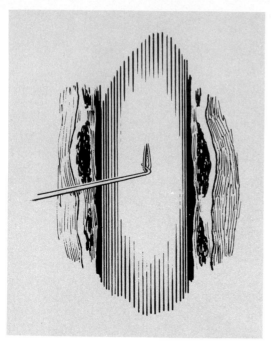

Fig. 20-10. Opening dura in midline. (Medtronic, Inc)

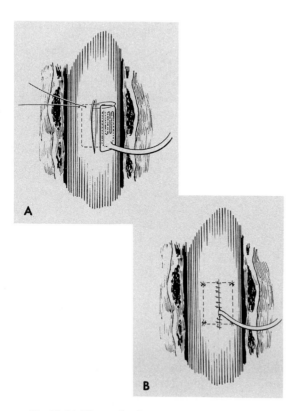

Fig. 20-11. Electrode placement. (Medtronic, Inc)

In addition to the use of this mechanical appliance, the patient requires considerable support to be helped to withdraw from narcotics as rapidly as possible. In addition, a total program of physical and emotional rehabilitation is generally necessary.

The original Melzack-Wall concept has undergone a number of modifications in the past 15 years. Experience with implantation of electrical stimulating devices for 12 years has also resulted in significant technical and conceptual changes. Specifity of effect of the electrical stimulation upon the dorsal columns has been questioned, so that the stimulating electrode is identified by some as a neurostimulator rather than a dorsal column stimulator.

Neurostimulating devices have undergone several modifications including miniaturization, so it is now possible to introduce them through a modified Touhy needle into the spinal epidural space without performing a laminectomy. Under fluoroscopic control the electrode can be guided to the appropriate spinal level. The disadvantage of this technique is the undesirable mobility of the electrode; a shift in its position might cause it to become ineffective.

The initial promise that seemed to have been offered by this technique has not been fully realized. The appeal of achieving pain relief without destruction of important sensory pathways once encouraged many neurosurgeons to implant intraspinal neurostimulating devices. The frequently disappointing long-term results of this method have caused a substantial decrease in its use. Yet several pain treatment centers and neurosurgeons who have a special interest in pain control surgery continue utilizing this technique.

Posterior Lumbar Rhizotomy

Patient Selection

Posterior lumbar rhizotomy has been employed for many years in patients who have continued to complain of radicular pain after

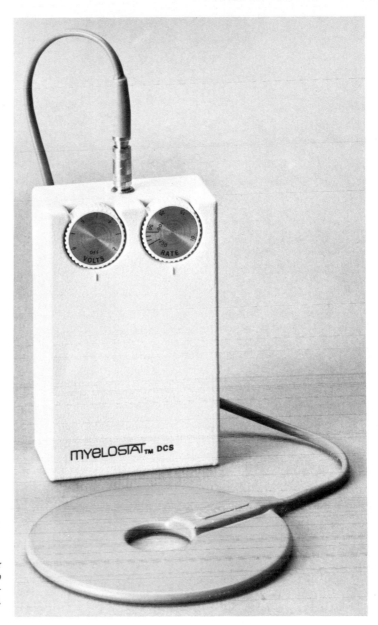

Fig. 20-12. *Radiofrequency transmitter and antenna. The antenna is taped onto the skin directly over the subcutaneously implanted receiver. (Medtronic, Inc)*

low back surgery. One or another surgeon who would utilize this technique might derive an occasional good result with the procedure and then, because of several less than satisfactory results, would give it up. Although this operation may have a use, its application is best limited to a specific type of problem. This is the patient who, subsequent to multiple surgical procedures designed to alleviate nerve root pressure, continues to manifest nerve root pain. The results are not likely to be satisfactory unless the pain is confined to a single root. If the pain syndrome includes low back discomfort in addition to radicular symptoms, the likelihood of success for this procedure is poor.

Prior to consideration of a dorsal rhizotomy, a diagnostic paravertebral block, using roentgenographic guidance for needle place-

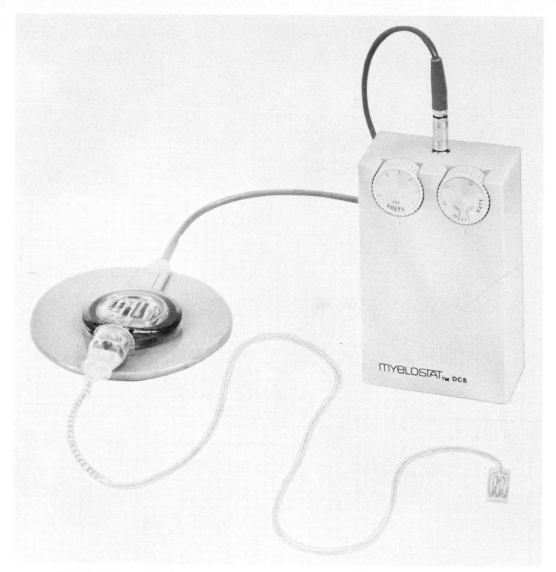

Fig. 20-13. The radio frequency transmitter-antenna, together with the receiver and electrode. (Medtronic, Inc)

ment, should be performed. Only after obtaining pain relief with anesthetic blockade of the suspected nerve root should posterior lumbar rhizotomy be considered. Before making a surgical decision, a second injection, using saline to rule out a placebo effect, should be done, followed by a third confirmatory Xylocaine injection. (See section on analgesic blocks, Chapter 13.)

Procedure

Under general anesthesia with the patient in prone position, a bilateral subperiosteal muscle dissection is performed exposing the spines and laminae above and below the nerve root to be sectioned (Figs. 20-15 through 20-17). If the S1 dorsal root is to be sectioned, a laminectomy of L5 and the

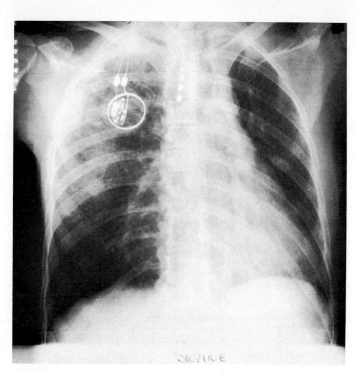

Fig. 20-14. X-ray film of implanted spinal cord electrode and subcutaneous receiver.

superior margin of S1 must be accomplished; for the L5 dorsal root, a laminectomy of L4 and the superior portion of L5. The dura is opened in the midline and the edge on the side of the proposed root section is retracted by sewing to the paraspinal muscles. Identification of the specific root is vital to the procedure and is best done by tracing the combined motor and sensory root to its dural exit. Only after this has been clearly demonstrated should separation of the motor and sensory rootlets be carried out (Fig. 20-18). The operating microscope or high-power magnifying loops are necessary in identifying and separating the motor from the sensory rootlets. Oftentimes, there are two sensory rootlets and one motor root. Identification is best done with a nerve stimulator. A small silver clip can be placed on either side of the sensory roots to be sectioned, and they are then cut with fine scissors (Fig. 20-19).

Dr. R. K. Jones has devised what he describes as a "provisional" posterior rhizotomy. If obvious pathology such as a recur-

rent disc protrusion is encountered and excised when surgery is undertaken to relieve persistent lower extremity pain, particularly in recurrent disc disease, one hesitates to section the involved posterior root and hopes that the removal of the offending pathology will result in the relief of pain. To obviate the necessity for cutting a posterior root when it is not necessary, Dr. Jones places an absorbable No. 3–0 catgut suture around the posterior root and brings both ends of this suture out through the skin incision including it in the wound dressings (Fig. 20-20). If the radicular pain in the first 4 or 5 postoperative days is noted to be persistent and unrelieved, the suture is withdrawn and the rhizotomy accomplished. If after that period of time the patient is satisfied with the relief of the radicular pain, the suture is cut flush with the skin and left to dissolve. In carrying out this procedure, Dr. Jones exposes the root by carrying out a generous hemilaminectomy and foraminotomy exposing the dural root sleeve. An incision is made in the dural

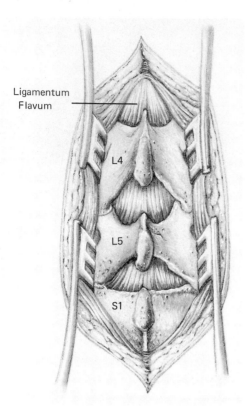

Fig. 20-15. Exposure of spines and laminae for lumbar rhizotomy.

sleeve and the dorsal roots identified and separated by means of this minute dural exposure.

Results of Posterior Lumbar Rhizotomy

The sensory deficit following section of one root is often quite minimal and in some cases equivocal. Following the section of the L5 and S1 roots, there is greater sensory dysfunction, particularly with regard to position sense. This proprioceptive impairment is serious and is associated with a very disabling gait disturbance and a high incidence of foot and ankle sprains and strains. Therefore, for the first 4 to 6 months the patient must wear an ankle and foot brace to facilitate ambulation and weight-bearing in the presence of such significant sensory loss around the ankle and foot. After 6 months, this loss may be to some degree

(Text continues on p. 576.)

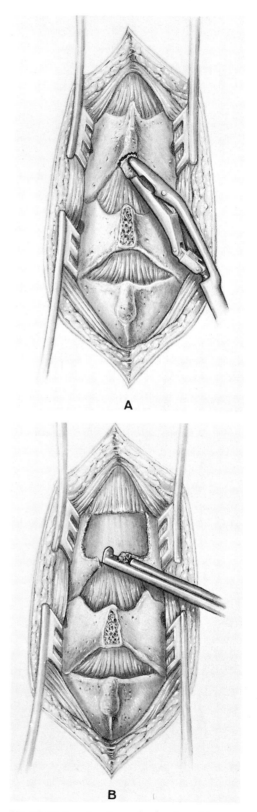

Fig. 20-16. Laminectomy for lumbar rhizotomy.

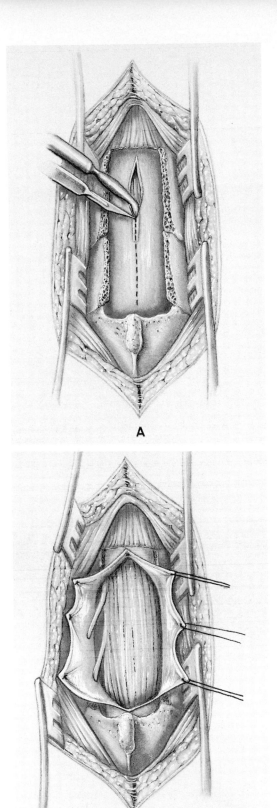

A

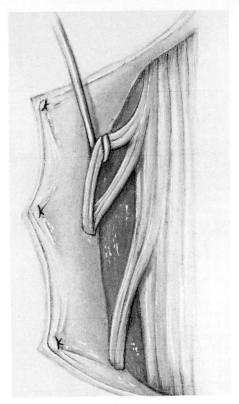

Fig. 20-18. *Separation of motor and sensory rootlets.*

B

Fig. 20-17. **(A)** *Midline dural incision.* **(B)** *Dural retraction.*

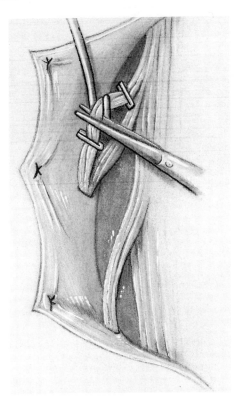

Fig. 20-19. *Sensory root section.*

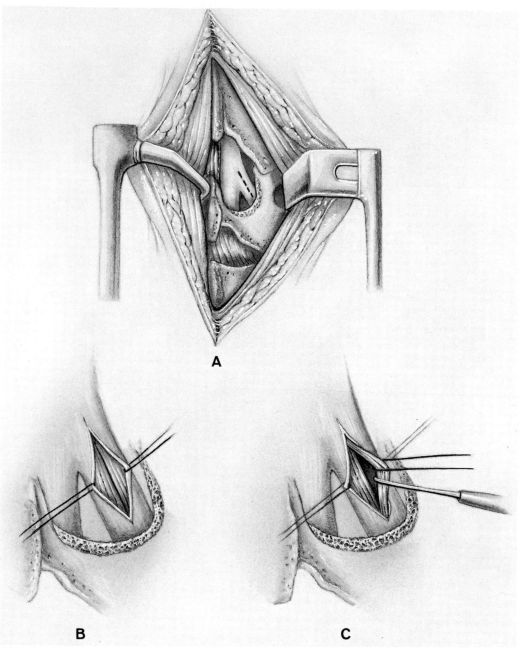

*Fig. 20-20. **(A)** Incision into dural root sleeve. **(B)** Identification of dorsal rootlets. **(C)** Suture around sensory rootlets.*

compensated and this appliance can sometimes be discarded.

This procedure should not be recommended lightly. If there is any suspicion that the patient's symptoms are nonorganic, if there is a question regarding secondary gain,

or if the physician is uncertain in his mind regarding the anatomical limitations of the dysfunction, it should be deferred.

In common with all procedures that fall into the category of "salvage spine surgery" the long-term results of posterior lumbar rhizotomy are never totally gratifying. When the predominant pain can be demonstrated to arise from a specific nerve root, severing the sensory fibers of that root should theoretically create a tolerable situation that will set the patient at ease. For a limited interval of time, usually not exceeding a half year, the patient may be reconciled to the exchange of the original pain for the unwelcome and undesired hypesthesia. All too often, however, this new numbness becomes progressively more disagreeable and after a year has passed may be described by the patient as unendurable.

Low Back School

In 1977, the results of a controlled prospective study on 217 back pain patients who were employees of the Volvo Corporation in Goteborg, Sweden, were published as a supplement (Number 170) to the ACTA Orthopaedica Scandenavica. The study was carried out by Marianne Bergquist-Ullman from Doctor Alf Nachemson's Department of Orthopedic Surgery at Sahlgren Hospital in Goteborg. One of the principal aims of the investigation was to evaluate and compare the therapeutic effect of: (1) **physiotherapy** consisting primarily of manual therapy, (2) **placebo** using low-intensity, shortwave diathermy, and (3) the **Back School.**

All of the 217 patients included in the study had consulted the Volvo medical department because of low back symptoms and were given an intensive history and physical examination plus psychological tests. After admission to the investigative program, they were then randomly allocated to one of the three test groups. The following four criteria were preselected to demonstrate relative therapeutic effectiveness of each of the three treatment groups:

1. Duration of symptoms following the first treatment

Physiotherapy:	15.8 days
Placebo:	28.7 days
Back School:	14.8 days

2. Duration of absence from work during the initial episode

Physiotherapy:	26.5 days
Placebo:	26.5 days
Back School:	20.5 days

3. Change of pain during the initial episode

All groups equal

4. Sick leave time resulting from recurrences of pain during the first year

All groups equal

Several factors are related to the effectiveness of the low back school. An understanding of "low back hygiene" involves several easily followed alterations in routine activities of daily living. The informed patient can utilize these to reduce low back pain and increase the range of physical activities without detriment to his or her clinical state. Implicit in the group environment is the positive reinforcement, understanding, and sympathy that one receives from a group of fellow low back sufferers. Such group dynamics have achieved considerable popularity and acceptance in the management of psychological problems; similar principles can be adopted for organic problems. The three goals for the Back School program in Sweden are: to create self-confidence so that the patient may most effectively adjust to and manage the back condition; to avoid potentially harmful treatment and particularly to avoid consideration of unnecessary surgery; to reduce the continuously increasing cost of medical care.

The Swedish program consists of four separate 1-hour sessions within a 2-week interval. The student-patients usually lie on the floor on mats during the teaching demonstrations. The course outline is as follows:

I. Anatomy and function of spine back pain. Cause, incidence, treatment effects

II. Biomechanics of spine. Effects of various activities on intradiscal pressure; importance of decreasing loads on back

III. Ergonomics and practical application. Individual advice about working, resting, and other activities; teaching isometric abdominal and back exercises

IV. Repetition, synopsis, and test. Instilling self-confidence; encouraging sports and other activities

Similar back schools have been instituted in the United States. Some follow the Swedish course outline quite rigidly. Others place considerably more emphasis on the group dynamics and certain peripheral issues. These include programs for weight loss, encouragement of social activities, and increased emphasis on psychological factors. The Back School concept may be helpful when dealing with the chronic low back pain patient. This individual falls into a pattern of progressively increasing dependence on the medical establishment. In the case of a workmen's compensation situation, the patient relies on the medical establishment not only for treatment and advice regarding his medical condition, but also for signatures on medical forms to maintain his compensation income. This creates a situation in which the patient is both medically and financially dependent on the medical establishment. Such total dependence often tends to ensnare both the doctor and the patient, with the passive patient waiting for the doctor to "make me feel better." The Back School environment may alter this relationship. After being provided with a number of practical reliable guidelines, the now-knowledgeable patient may take more active control of his own destiny and assume increased responsibility for his medical program. In view of the progressively increasing number of patients who are afflicted with chronic and incapacitating low back pain, the Back School approach will receive increased attention.

References

1. Feffer HL: Therapeutic intradiscal hydrocortisone, symposium chemonuclolysis. Clin Orthop 67, 1969
2. Ford LT: Clinical use of chymopapain in lumbar and dorsal disk lesions, symposium chemonuclolysis. Clin Orthop 67, 1969
3. Garvin PJ, Jennings RB, Smith L, Gesler RM: Chymopapain: A pharmacologic and toxicologic evaluation in experimental animals. Clin Orthop 41:204, 1965
4. Hackett GS: Joint Ligament Relaxation Treated by Fibro-osseous Proliferation with Special Reference to Low Back Disability—Trigger Point Pain and Referred Pain. Springfield, Ill, Charles C Thomas, 1956
5. Hackett GS, Huang TC: Prolotherapy of sciatica from weak pelvic ligaments and bone dystrophy. Clinical Medicine 8 (12), 1961
6. Hoppenstein R: Percutaneous implantation of chronic spinal cord electrodes for control of intractable pain: Preliminary Report. Surg Neurol 4:195–198, 1975
7. Jansen EF, Balls AK: Chymopapain: A new crystalline protease from papaya-latex. J Biol Chem 137:459, 1941
8. Keplinger JE, Bucy PC: Paraplegia from treatment with sclerosing agents. JAMA 173:1333, 1960
9. Long DM, Hagfors N: Electrical stimulation in the nervous system: The current status of electrical stimulation of the nervous system for relief of pain. Pain 1:109–123, 1975
10. Melzack R, Wall PD: Pain mechanism: A new theory. A gate control system modulates sensory input from the skin before it evokes pain perception and response. Science 150:971–979, 1965
11. Myers A: Prolotherapy treatment of low back pain and sciatica. Bulletin of the Hospital for Joint Disease 22:48, 1961
12. Nashold BS Jr: Dorsal column stimulation for control of pain: A 3-year follow-up. Surg Neurol 4:146–147, 1975
13. Pedersen HE, Blunck SFJ, Gardner E: The anatomy of lumbosacral posterior rami and meningeal branches of the spinal nerves (sinu-vertebral nerves). J Bone Joint Surg 38A:377, 1956
14. Rees WES: Multiple bilateral subcutaneous rhizolysis of segmental nerves in the treatment of the intervertebral disc syndrome. Ann Gen Tract 16:126, 1971
15. Richardson RR, Sigueira E, Cerullo L: Spinal epidural neurostimulation for treatment of acute and chronic intractable pain: Initial and long-term results. Neurosurgery 5 (3):344–348, 1979
16. Schneider RC, Williams JJ, Liss L: Fatality after injection of sclerosing agent to precipitate fibro-osseous proliferation. JAMA 170, 1768, 1959
17. Shealy CN: Tissue reaction to chymopapain in cats. J Neurosurg 26:327, 1967

18. Smith L: Enzyme dissolution of the nucleus pulposus in humans. JAMA 187:137, 1964
19. Smith L, Brown JE: Treatment of lumbar intervertebral disc lesions by direct injection of chymopapain. J Bone Joint Surg 49B:502, 1967
20. Smith L, Garvin PJ, Jennings RB, Gesler RM: Enzyme dissolution of the nucleus pulposus. Nature 198:1311, 1963
21. Stern IJ, Smith L: Dissolution by chymopapain *in vitro* of tissue from normal or prolapsed intervertebral disks. Clin Orthop 40:269, 1966
22. Sweet WH, Wespic JG: Stimulation of the posterior columns of the spinal cord for pain control. Surg Neurol 4:133, 1975
23. Urban BJ, Nashold BS: Percutaneous epidural stimulation of the spinal cord for relief of pain: Long-term results. J Neurosurg 48:323–328, 1978